Rheumatic Diseases: Clinical Perspectives

Rheumatic Diseases: Clinical Perspectives

Editor: Nicholas Greyson

AMERICAN
MEDICAL PUBLISHERS
www.americanmedicalpublishers.com

AMERICAN
MEDICAL PUBLISHERS
www.americanmedicalpublishers.com

Cataloging-in-Publication Data

Rheumatic diseases : clinical perspectives / edited by Nicholas Greyson.
p. cm.
Includes bibliographical references and index.
ISBN 979-8-88740-438-7
1. Rheumatism. 2. Rheumatism--Diagnosis. 3. Rheumatism--Treatment.
4. Musculoskeletal system--Diseases. I. Greyson, Nicholas.
RC927 .R44 2023
616.723--dc23

American Medical Publishers,
41 Flatbush Avenue,
1st Floor, New York,
NY 11217, USA

ISBN 979-8-88740-438-7 (Hardback)

Contents

Preface

Rheumatic diseases or rheumatism are disorders that cause inflammation of the joints or connective tissue. The main cause of rheumatic disease is the malfunctioning of the immune system that attacks body's own tissues, affecting the joints, tendons, ligaments, muscles, bones and organs. Osteoarthritis, rheumatoid arthritis, capsulitis, palindromic rheumatism, etc. are among the most common types of rheumatic disorders. Osteoarthritis is a type of degenerative joint disease that results from the breakdown of joint cartilage and underlying bone. The major factors that lead to it are previous joint injury and abnormal joint or limb development. The diagnosis of rheumatic disorders is done through physical examination and specialized laboratory and imaging tests. These include blood test, urine test, creatinine level test, uric acid test, and the ESR and CRP tests. This book provides significant information to help the readers develop a good understanding of the clinical perspectives of rheumatic diseases. It is a collective contribution of a renowned group of international experts. Those with an interest in the treatment and study of rheumatic diseases would find this book helpful.

The information shared in this book is based on empirical researches made by veterans in this field of study. The elaborative information provided in this book will help the readers further their scope of knowledge leading to advancements in this field.

Finally, I would like to thank my fellow researchers who gave constructive feedback and my family members who supported me at every step of my research.

Editor

1

Validation of GWAS-Identified Variants for Anti-TNF Drug Response in Rheumatoid Arthritis: A Meta-Analysis of Two Large Cohorts

*Jose Manuel Sánchez-Maldonado[1,2,3], Rafael Cáliz[1,3,4], Miguel Ángel López-Nevot[3,5], Antonio José Cabrera-Serrano[1,2,3], Ana Moñiz-Díez[1,2,3], Helena Canhão[6,7], Rob Ter Horst[8], Luca Quartuccio[9], Signe B. Sorensen[10,11], Bente Glintborg[12,13], Merete L. Hetland[12,13], Ileana Filipescu[14], Eva Pérez-Pampin[15], Pablo Conesa-Zamora[16], Jerzy Swierkot[17], Alfons A. den Broeder[18], Salvatore De Vita[9], Eva Rabing Brix Petersen[19], Yang Li[8,20], Miguel A. Ferrer[3], Alejandro Escudero[21], Mihai G. Netea[8,22], Marieke J. H. Coenen[23], Vibeke Andersen[9,10,24], João E. Fonseca[25,26], Manuel Jurado[1,2,3], Katarzyna Bogunia-Kubik[27], Eduardo Collantes[21] and Juan Sainz[1,2,3,28]**

[1] Genomic Oncology Area, Centre for Genomics and Oncological Research (GENYO), Parque tecnológico de la Salud (PTS) Granada, Granada, Spain, [2] Hematology Department, Virgen de las Nieves University Hospital, Granada, Spain, [3] Instituto de Investigación Biosanitaria (IBs) Granada, Granada, Spain, [4] Department of Rheumatology, Virgen de las Nieves University Hospital, Granada, Spain, [5] Immunology Department, Virgen de las Nieves University Hospital, Granada, Spain, [6] EpiDoC Unit, CEDOC, NOVA Medical School and National School of Public Health, Universidade Nova de Lisboa, Lisbon, Portugal, [7] Comprehensive Health Research Center (CHRC), NOVA Medical School, Lisbon, Portugal, [8] Department of Internal Medicine and Radboud Center for Infectious Diseases, Radboud University Nijmegen Medical Center, Nijmegen, Netherlands, [9] Department of Medical Area, Clinic of Rheumatology, University of Udine, Udine, Italy, [10] Molecular Diagnostic and Clinical Research Unit, IRS-Center Sonderjylland, University Hospital of Southern Jutland, Aabenraa, Denmark, [11] Institute of Molecular Medicine, Faculty of Health Sciences, University of Southern Denmark, Odense, Denmark, [12] The Danish Rheumatologic Biobank and Copenhagen Center for Arthritis Research (DANBIO) Registry, The Danish Rheumatologic Biobank and Copenhagen Center for Arthritis Research (COPECARE), Center for Rheumatology and Spine Diseases, Centre of Head and Orthopaedics, Rigshospitalet, Glostrup, Denmark, [13] Department of Clinical Medicine, Faculty of Health and Medical Sciences, University of Copenhagen, Copenhagen, Denmark, [14] Rheumatology Department, University of Medicine and Pharmacy "Iuliu Hatieganu", Cluj-Napoca, Romania, [15] Rheumatology Unit, University Hospital of Santiago de Compostela, Santiago de Compostela, Spain, [16] Clinical Analysis Department, Santa Lucía University Hospital, Cartagena, Spain, [17] Department of Rheumatology and Internal Medicine, Wroclaw Medical University, Wroclaw, Poland, [18] Radboud Institute for Health Sciences, Department of Rheumatology, Radboud University Medical Center, Nijmegen, Netherlands, [19] Department of Biochemistry and Immunology, University Hospital of Southern Jutland, Aabenraa, Denmark, [20] Centre for Individualised Infection Medicine (CiiM) & Centre for Experimental and Clinical Infection Research (TWINCORE), Helmholtz-Centre for Infection Research (HZI) and The Hannover Medical School (MHH), Hannover, Germany, [21] Rheumatology Department, Reina Sofía Hospital/Instituto Maimónides de Investigación Biomédica de Córdoba (IMIBIC)/University of Córdoba, Córdoba, Spain, [22] Department for Immunology & Metabolism, Life and Medical Sciences Institute (LIMES), University of Bonn, Bonn, Germany, [23] Radboud Institute for Health Sciences, Department of Human Genetics, Radboud University Medical Center, Nijmegen, Netherlands, [24] Institute of Regional Research, Faculty of Health Sciences, University of Southern Denmark, Odense, Denmark, [25] Rheumatology and Metabolic Bone Diseases Department, Hospital de Santa Maria, Centro Hospitalar Universitário Lisboa Norte (CHLN), Lisbon, Portugal, [26] Rheumatology Research Unit, Instituto de Medicina Molecular, Faculty of Medicine, University of Lisbon, Lisbon Academic Medical Center, Lisbon, Portugal, [27] Hirszfeld Institute of Immunology and Experimental Therapy, Polish Academy of Sciences, Wrocław, Poland, [28] Department of Biochemistry and Molecular Biology I, University of Granada, Granada, Spain

Correspondence:
Juan Sainz
juan.sainz@genyo.es

We aimed to validate the association of 28 GWAS-identified genetic variants for response to TNF inhibitors (TNFi) in a discovery cohort of 1361 rheumatoid arthritis (RA) patients monitored in routine care and ascertained through the REPAIR consortium and DANBIO registry. We genotyped selected markers and evaluated their association with response to

TNFi after 6 months of treatment according to the change in disease activity score 28 (ΔDAS28). Next, we confirmed the most interesting results through meta-analysis of our data with those from the DREAM cohort that included 706 RA patients treated with TNFi. The meta-analysis of the discovery cohort and DREAM registry including 2067 RA patients revealed an overall association of the *LINC02549*$_{rs7767069}$ SNP with a lower improvement in DAS28 that remained significant after correction for multiple testing (per-allele OR_{Meta}=0.83, P_{Meta}=0.000077; P_{Het}=0.61). In addition, we found that each copy of the *LRRC55*$_{rs717117G}$ allele was significantly associated with lower improvement in DAS28 in rheumatoid factor (RF)-positive patients (per-allele OR_{Meta}=0.67, *P*=0.00058; P_{Het}=0.06) whereas an opposite but not significant effect was detected in RF-negative subjects (per-allele OR_{Meta}=1.38, *P*=0.10; P_{Het}=0.45; $P_{Interaction}$=0.00028). Interestingly, although the identified associations did not survive multiple testing correction, the meta-analysis also showed overall and RF-specific associations for the *MAFB*$_{rs6071980}$ and *CNTN5*$_{rs1813443}$ SNPs with decreased changes in DAS28 (per-allele $OR_{Meta\_rs6071980}$ = 0.85, *P*=0.0059; P_{Het}=0.63 and $OR_{Meta\_rs1813443\_RF+}$=0.81, *P*=0.0059; P_{Het}=0.69 and $OR_{Meta\_rs1813443\_RF-}$=1.00, *P*=0.99; P_{Het}=0.12; $P_{Interaction}$=0.032). Mechanistically, we found that subjects carrying the *LINC02549*$_{rs7767069T}$ allele had significantly increased numbers of CD45RO+CD45RA+ T cells (*P*=0.000025) whereas carriers of the *LINC02549*$_{rs7767069T/T}$ genotype showed significantly increased levels of soluble scavengers CD5 and CD6 in serum (*P*=0.00037 and *P*=0.00041). In addition, carriers of the *LRRC55*$_{rs717117G}$ allele showed decreased production of IL6 after stimulation of PBMCs with *B burgdorferi* and *E coli* bacteria (*P*=0.00046 and *P*=0.00044), which suggested a reduced IL6-mediated anti-inflammatory effect of this marker to worsen the response to TNFi. In conclusion, this study confirmed the influence of the *LINC02549* and *LRRC55* loci to determine the response to TNFi in RA patients and suggested a weak effect of the *MAFB and CNTN5* loci that need to be further investigated.

Keywords: GWAS, genetic variant, rheumatoid arthritis, drug response, TNF inhibitors

INTRODUCTION

Rheumatoid Arthritis (RA) is a complex and chronic disease marked by symptoms of inflammation and pain in the joints that eventually lead to joint destruction, loss of function and disability. These symptoms of inflammation are mostly driven by certain central cytokines that modulate both cellular and humoral immune responses in the synovial fluid and synovium of patients (1). Although RA remains as a chronic and incurable autoimmune disease that occurs in as much as 0.5-1% of the general population (2), the introduction of biological agents to target deregulated cytokines has substantially improved the signs and symptoms of the disease (3). Among these cytokines, tumor necrosis factor alpha (TNFα) has attracted most attention as it has been found to be deregulated in patients with autoimmune diseases including RA (4). It has been reported, for instance, that TNFα activates macrophages, synoviocytes, chondrocytes, and osteoclasts in a dose-dependent manner (5) and that high levels of circulating TNFα correlate with disease activity and disease progression (6).

The increasing number of biological agents approved by the FDA and the increased prevalence of the disease all around the world (7) have placed a substantial economic burden for health care systems. Although the introduction of biosimilars in clinical practice reduced the cost of these treatments in many countries (8), there is still an unmet need to optimize biologic therapies, avoiding unnecessary adverse effects risks and reducing costs (9).

The interplay between genetics and drug response has been the subject of intense investigations during last decades. Response to biologics has been shown to vary between individuals and that a large proportion of patients show no clinical improvement (10). Given the high cost of these drugs and the potential impairment of non-responding patients, the identification of genetic biomarkers associated with drug response to specific biological agents would help to know which patients might benefit from a particular treatment. However, to date, only a few genome-wide association studies (GWAS) (11–17) or well powered candidate gene association studies have been conducted (18–26). We are far from being able to optimize drug dosing or prioritize drug combinations based on genetic findings. In fact, attempts to validate the association of most of the genetic markers identified in these association studies have failed (27), which confirms the limited application of genetic findings in a clinical setting. Considering that the validation of previous GWAS findings is an essential step to tailor treatments for RA and to approach personalized medicine, we aimed to validate the association of GWAS-identified variants for response to TNF inhibitors (TNFi) in a two-stage nested case-control association study including a cohort of 1361 anti-TNF naïve RA patients ascertained through the REPAIR consortium and DANBIO registry and an independent replication cohort of 706 RA patients treated with TNFi from the DREAM registry. We also investigated whether the effect of selected markers on the response to TNFi could be modified by rheumatoid factor (RF) status, and whether genetic variants could influence immune responses and affect the serological concentration of 108 plasmatic inflammatory proteins, 7 serum steroid hormones or counts of 91 blood-derived immune cell populations.

MATERIAL AND METHODS

Study Populations and Response to TNFi

The discovery population consisted of 1361 RA patients ascertained through the REPAIR consortium and the DANBIO registry (**Table 1**) (28, 29). RA patients fulfilled the 1987 revised American College of Rheumatology (ACR) (30) and/or the ACR/EULAR 2010 classification criteria (31). In order to further replicate the most interesting results, we validated the association with response to anti-TNF drugs of those SNPs showing a *P*<0.05 in the discovery cohort in 706 Dutch RA patients treated with TNFi from the DREAM (Dutch RhEumatoid Arthritis Monitoring) registry (**Supplementary Table 1**). The study followed the Declaration of Helsinki. Study participants were of European origin and gave their written informed consent to participate in the study, which was approved by the ethical review committee of participant institutions: Virgen de las Nieves University Hospital (2012/89); Santa Maria Hospital-CHLN (CE 877/121.2012); University Clinical Hospital of Santiago de Compostela (2013/156); Wroclaw Medical University (KB-625/2016); Radboud university medical center (2011/299) and by the Regional Ethics Committee of Central Denmark Region (S-20120113). A detailed description of the discovery population has been reported elsewhere (19, 20, 22, 24). All RA patients were naïve for TNFi and response to TNFi for each patient in all study populations was calculated using the change in disease activity score (DAS28CRP) between baseline and 6 months after treatment. Overall and RF-stratified linear regression analyses adjusted for age, sex and country of origin were used to determine the association between GWAS-identified SNPs and changes in DAS28. RA patients with missing values either for DAS28 (in at the time points of interest) or RF were not included in the analysis.

TABLE 1 | Demographic and clinical characteristics of anti-TNF patients.

Anti-TNF patients (n=1361)	
Demographic characteristics	***REPAIR consortium + DANBIO registry***
Age (years)	52 ± 14
Sex ratio (female/male)	3.4 (1050/310)
Clinical assessment	
Percentage of patients with RF positivity †	721 (67.45)
Percentage of ACPA-positive patients ◊	728 (64.03)
DAS28 at baseline	5.91 ± 1.23
Disease duration (years)	12.92 ± 12.90
Treatments	
First biologic agent	
Infliximab (%)	386 (28.36)
Etanercept (%)	466 (34.24)
Adalimumab (%)	413 (30.35)
Golimumab (%)	48 (03.53)
Certolizumab (%)	67 (04.04)
Biosimilars (%)	16 (01.76)

Number of patients (%).
†RF status was available for 1069 patients.
◊ACPA status was available for 1137 patients.

DNA Extraction, SNP Selection, Genotyping, and Quality Control

Genomic DNA from RA patients was extracted from blood samples using the QIAamp DNA Blood Mini kit (Valencia, CA, EEUU) according to manufacturer's instructions. The single-nucleotide polymorphisms (SNPs) were selected through an extensive literature search of relevant GWAS and meta-analyses published by February 2019 using publicly available online databases. Additional criteria were potential functionality and linkage disequilibrium between the reported SNPs. Biological function was predicted according to the data publicly available in the integrated Regulome database (www.regulomedb.org), and eQTL data browsers (www.gtexportal.org/home/ and https://genenetwork.nl/bloodeqtlbrowser/). A total of 28 SNPs in 25 genes were selected for genotyping in the discovery cohort (**Table 2**). Genotyping of selected SNPs was performed using KASP® probes according to manufacturer's instructions (LGC Genomics, Hoddesdon, UK). For quality control, ~5% of DNA samples were randomly included as duplicates and concordance between duplicate samples was ≥99.0%. Replication of the most interesting association was conducted in the DREAM registry (n=706) following a similar quality control genotyping strategy.

Hardy-Weinberg Equilibrium, Genetic Association Analysis, and Meta-Analysis

Deviation from Hardy-Weinberg Equilibrium (HWE) was tested in the control group (responders and moderate responders according to the EULAR response criteria) by chi-square ($\chi 2$), and linear regression analysis adjusted for age, sex and country of origin was used to assess the associations of the GWAS-identified polymorphisms with absolute changes in DAS28 assuming log-additive, dominant and recessive models of inheritance. Those SNPs with the lowest P-value in the discovery population according to each genetic model were advanced for replication in the DREAM cohort and meta-analysis of the discovery and replication populations using a fixed effect model was performed

TABLE 2 | Selection of GWAS-identified SNPs for response to anti-TNF drugs.

dbSNP rs#	Chr.	Position (GRCh38.p7)	Nearest gene	Nucleotide substitution	Effect allele	SNP location	Reference
rs885813	1	21550581	ALPL	C/T	T	Intronic	(14)
rs885814	1	21549423	ALPL	C/T	T	Intronic	(14)
rs1813443	11	100140279	CNTN5	G/C	C	Intronic	(16)
rs8046065	16	3788297	CREBBP	C/T	T	Intronic	(14)
rs6138150	20	23866372	CST2||CST5	C/T	C	Intergenic	(15)
rs6028945	20	40192165	HSPEP1||MAFB	G/T	T	Intergenic	(15)
rs6071980	20	40239936	HSPEP1||MAFB	C/T	C	Intergenic	(15)
rs3849942	9	27543283	IFNK||C9orf72	T/C	T	ncRNA	(15)
rs13393173	2	168532581	LASS6	A/G	A	Intronic	(15)
rs4411591	18	6550118	LINC01387	C/T	A	Intronic	(16)
rs983332	1	87666697	LMO4||PKN2	A/C	A	Intergenic	(15)
rs1875620	9	88925144	C9orf47||LOC100128660||LOC100128911	A/G	A	Intergenic	(14)
rs1539909	18	71581359	CBLN2||LOC100132647	A/G	A	Intronic	(14)
rs7767069	6	68060671	LOC102723883||LINCO2549	A/T	T	Downstream	(16)
rs1568885	7	13597906	LOC107986770||ETV1	A/T	T	Intronic	(16)
rs10520789	15	95598638	LINC00924	A/G	A	Downstream	(14)
rs11870477	17	69806211	MAP2K6||KCNJ16	A/C	C	Intronic	(14)
rs2378945	14	31831584	NUBPL	G/A	A	Intronic	(16)
rs717117	11	57127131	OR5BP1P||LRRC55	A/G	G	Intronic	(14)
rs1532269	5	32018735	PDZD2	C/G	G	Intronic	(17)
rs4651370	1	187269960	PLA2G4A||FDPSL1	A/T	A	Intronic	(16)
rs854547	7	95294544	PPP1R9A	A/G	G	3'UTR	(15)
rs854548	7	95296508	PPP1R9A||PON1	A/G	A	Downstream	(15)
rs10945919	6	163765645	QKI||LOC728275	A/G	G	Intronic	(15)
rs437943	4	35370476	CENTD1	A/G	G	Upstream	(15)
rs3794271	12	20707159	SLCO1C1	C/T	C	Intronic	(14)
rs4694890	4	48224250	TEC	A/C	C	Intronic	(17)
rs1447722	3	139835611	TRMT112P5	C/G	C	Intergenic	(16)

SNP, single nucleotide polymorphism; MAF, minor allele frequency; UTR, untranslated region.
References: (14–17).

to validate the association observed. I2 statistic was used to assess heterogeneity between studies. Correction for multiple testing was performed using the Bonferroni method but also considering the two inheritance models tested. Given that log-additive and dominant models showed a high degree of collinearity, the significant threshold for the meta-analysis was set to 0.00089 considering log-additive/dominant and recessive inheritance models (0.05/28SNPs/2models). Overall statistical power was calculated using Quanto (v.12.4) assuming a log-additive model and a baseline risk of 30% for response to TNFi (32, 33).

Cell Isolation, Differentiation and Cytokine Quantitative Trait Loci, and Hormone Analysis in Relation to the GWAS-Identified Variants for Response To TNFi

With the aim of determining whether those SNPs associated with response to TNFi had a role in modulating immune responses, we performed *in vitro* stimulation experiments and measured cytokine production (IFNγ, IL1Ra, IL1β, IL6, IL8, IL10, TNFα, IL17, and IL22) after stimulation of peripheral blood mononuclear cells (PBMCs), whole blood or monocyte-derived macrophages (MDMs) from 408 healthy subjects of the 500FG cohort from the Human Functional Genomics Project (HFGP) with LPS (1 or 100 ng/ml), PHA (10μg/ml), Pam3Cys (10μg/ml), CpG (ODN M362; 10μg/ml) and *B. burgdorferi* and *E. coli*, as experimental model for cytokine production capacity. Given the sex disparities in the prevalence and course of RA and the impact of steroid hormones in modulating immune responses, we also evaluated the correlation of SNPs with serum levels of 7 steroid hormones (androstenedione, cortisol, 11-deoxy-cortisol, 17-hydroxy progesterone, progesterone, testosterone and 25 hydroxy vitamin D3) in a subset of the 500FG cohort without hormonal replacement therapy or oral contraceptives (n=280). After log transformation, cytokine or serum steroid hormone levels were correlated with the SNPs of interest using a linear regression model with age and sex as co-factors in R (http://www.r-project.org/). This analysis led to cytokine quantitative trait loci (cQTL) and hormone quantitative trait loci (hQTL). Significance thresholds were set to be 0.000463 and 0.00357 (0.05/6stimulants/9cytokines or 0.05/7hormones and 2 inheritance models) for cQTL and hQTL, respectively.

Correlation Between GWAS-Identified Polymorphisms and Cell Counts of 91 Blood-Derived Immune Cell Populations and Serum/Plasmatic Proteomic Profile

We also investigated whether selected polymorphisms had an impact on blood cell counts by analyzing a set of 91 manually annotated immune cell populations and genotype data from the 500FG cohort that consisted of 408 healthy subjects (**Supplementary Table 2**). Cell populations were measured by 10-color flow cytometry (Navios flow cytometer, Beckman

Coulter) after blood sampling (2-3 hours) and cell count analysis was performed using the Kaluza software (Beckman Coulter, v.1.3). In order to reduce inter-experimental noise and increase statistical power, cell count analysis was performed by calculating parental and grandparental percentages, which were defined as the percentage of a certain cell type within the cell-populations one or two levels higher in the hierarchical definitions of cell sub-populations (34). Detailed laboratory protocols for cell isolation, reagents, gating and flow cytometry analysis have been reported elsewhere (35) and the accession number for the raw flow cytometry data and analyzed data files are available upon request to the authors (http://hfgp.bbmri.nl). A proteomic analysis was also performed in serum and plasma samples from the 500FG cohort. Circulating proteins were measured using the commercially Olink® Inflammation panel (Olink, Sweden) that resulted in the measurement of 103 different biomarkers (**Supplementary Table 3**). Proteins levels were expressed on a log2-scale as normalized protein expression values, and normalized using bridging samples to correct for batch variation. Considering the number of proteins (n=103) and cell populations (n=91) tested, *P*-values of 0.00049 and 0.00055 were set as significant thresholds for the proteomic and cell-level variation analysis, respectively.

RESULTS

A total of 1361 anti-TNF patients were included in the discovery population. The mean age of the RA patients was 52±14 and they showed a female/male ratio of 3.4 (1050/310). Sixty-seven percent of the RA patients were positive for RF and 64% had anti-citrullinated protein antibodies (ACPA). The median disease duration was of 12.92 years and the disease activity score 28 (DAS28CRP) calculated at patient recruitment was of 5.91 (**Table 1**).

Association of GWAS-Identified SNPs With Response to Anti-TNF Drugs

All SNPs were in Hardy-Weinberg equilibrium in the control group (responders according to EULAR response criteria; $P>0.001$) and showed a high genotyping call rate (>90%) with the exception of the $LINC01387_{rs4411591}$ SNP that was excluded from the statistical analysis. The overall linear regression analysis of the discovery cohort including 1361 RA patients treated with TNFi showed that the $MAFB_{rs6028945}$, $MAFB_{rs6071980}$, $LINC02549_{rs7767069}$, and $LRRC55_{rs717117}$ SNPs had an overall significant effect on the response to TNFi at P<0.05 level ($OR_{Dominant}$=0.81, 95%CI 0.68-0.97, P=0.020; per-allele OR=0.83, 95%CI 0.72-0.97, P=0.020; per-allele OR=0.85, 95% CI 0.76-0.96, P=0.008; per-allele OR=0.76, 95%CI 0.60-0.97, P=0.026; **Table 3**). Importantly, the meta-analysis of the discovery and replication cohorts confirmed the overall association of the $LINC02549_{rs7767069}$ SNP with lower DAS28 improvement that remained significant after multiple testing correction (per-allele OR_{Meta}=0.83, 95%CI 0.76-0.91, P_{Meta}=0.000077; P_{Het}=0.61; **Table 4**). Although it did not survive multiple testing correction, the meta-analysis also showed a potentially interesting overall associations for the $MAFB_{rs6071980}$ SNP with less DAS28 improvement (per-allele $OR_{Meta\_rs6071980}$ = 0.85, 95%CI 0.76-0.95, P=0.0059; P_{Het}=0.63; **Table 4**).

A RF-stratified analysis showed a RF-specific association for the $LRRC55_{rs717117}$ SNP with response to TNFi that remained statistically significant after correction for multiple testing in the discovery population. Thus, RF-positive RA patients carrying the $LRRC55_{rs717117G}$ allele additively decreased the drop in DAS28 (per-allele OR=0.54, 95%CI 0.39–0.74, P=0.00012) whereas RF-negative RA patients showed an opposite but not statistically significant effect (per-allele OR=1.52, 95%CI 0.96–2.42, P=0.07; $P_{Interaction}$=0.00028; **Table 3**). Interestingly, the meta-analysis of our data with those from the DREAM registry including 2067 RA patients confirmed the RF-specific effect of this SNP to modulate the response to anti-TNF drugs (per-allele OR_{Meta_RF+}=0.67, 95% CI 0.54-0.84, P_{Meta}=0.00058; P_{Het}=0.06 and per-allele OR_{Meta_RF-}=1.38, 95%CI 0.94-2.02, P=0.10; P_{Het}=0.45; $P_{Interaction}$=0.00028; **Table 4**). Although it did not survive multiple testing, the meta-analysis also showed potentially interesting RF-specific association for the $CNTN5_{rs1813443}$ SNP with a decreased drop in DAS28 ($OR_{Meta\_rs1813443\_RF+}$=0.81, 95% CI 0.70-0.94, P=0.0059; P_{Het}=0.69 and $OR_{Meta\_rs1813443\_RF-}$=1.00, 95%CI 0.79-1.27, P=0.99; P_{Het}=0.12; $P_{Interaction}$=0.032; **Table 4**).

Functional Characterization of the Most Interesting Findings

Considering these results, we attempted to shed some light into the functional consequences of the overall or RF-specific effects of the $LINC02549_{rs7767069}$, $LRRC55_{rs717117}$, $MAFB_{rs6071980}$ and $CNTN5_{rs1813443}$ SNPs to modulate the response to TNFi. Interestingly, our functional experiments showed that, when considering the total number of leukocytes as reference, the $LINC02549_{rs7767069}$ polymorphism significantly correlated with increased numbers of CD45RO+CD45RA+ T cells in blood (P=0.00047; **Figure 1A**). Subjects carrying the $LINC02549_{rs7767069T}$ allele (associated with poor response to TNFi in RA patients) had significantly increased numbers of CD45RO+CD45RA+ T cells (P=0.000025), which suggested that this genetic marker might influence the response to TNFi by mediating the number of this specific T cell subset in blood and, thereby contribute to inflammation. In addition, we observed that those subjects carrying two copies of the $LINC02549_{rs7767069T}$ allele showed significantly increased serum levels of soluble scavenger receptors CD5 and CD6 when compared with those carrying the A/T or A/A genotypes (P=0.00037 and P=0.00041; **Figures 1B, C**). These results also suggested a functional role of the $LINC02549_{rs7767069}$ SNP in RA likely through the CD5/CD6-mediated modulation of T cells and certain subsets of B cells that control multiple processes including cellular adhesion and migration across endothelial and epithelial cells, antigen presentation by B cells and the subsequent proliferation of T cells.

Furthermore, although we could not stratify our functional analyses by RF status because of the healthy nature of the blood donors, we found that carriers of the $LRRC55_{rs717117G}$ allele

TABLE 3 | Overall and RF-specific associations of selected polymorphisms and response to anti-TNF drugs (ΔDAS28) in the REPAIR consortium.

Gene	SNP ID	Effect allele	Overall		RF-positive patients		RF-negative patients		$P_{Interaction}$
			REPAIR+DANBIO (n=1361)		REPAIR+DANBIO (n=721)		REPAIR+DANBIO (n=347)		
			OR (95% CI)[δ]	P	OR (95% CI)[δ]	P	OR (95% CI)[δ]	P	
ALPL	rs885813	T	0.96 (0.86-1.07)	0.48	1.06 (0.91-1.22)	0.47	**0.80 (0.65-0.99)**	**0.040**	0.13
ALPL	rs885814	T	0.96 (0.85-1.07)	0.45	0.91 (0.78-1.06)	0.24	1.18 (0.95-1.47)	0.14	0.08
CNTN5	rs1813443	C	0.97 (0.84-1.13)[†]	0.72	**0.79 (0.65-0.97)[†]**	**0.023**	1.14 (0.86-1.53)[†]	0.34	**0.032**
CREBBP	rs8046065	T	1.01 (0.87-1.19)	0.85	1.18 (0.96-1.45)	0.11	0.82 (0.60-1.10)	0.19	0.07
CST2||CST5	rs6138150	C	1.06 (0.92-1.22)	0.40	1.04 (0.87-1.26)	0.66	1.01 (0.77-1.32)	0.96	0.72
HSPEP1||MAFB	rs6028945	T	**0.81 (0.68-0.97)[†]**	**0.020**	0.89 (0.70-1.21)[†]	0.31	0.78 (0.53-1.09)[†]	0.14	0.57
HSPEP1||MAFB	rs6071980	C	**0.83 (0.72-0.97)**	**0.020**	0.85 (0.70-1.03)	0.10	0.81 (0.58-1.14)	0.23	0.73
IFNK||C9orf72	rs3849942	T	1.02 (0.90-1.15)	0.74	0.93 (0.79-1.10)	0.39	1.21 (0.95-1.55)	0.13	0.27
LASS6	rs13393173	A	1.10 (0.96-1.25)	0.19	1.08 (0.91-1.28)	0.41	1.18 (0.89-1.55)	0.25	0.48
LMO4||PKN2	rs983332	A	1.12 (0.97-1.29)	0.11	1.14 (0.95-1.38)	0.16	1.07 (0.84-1.38)	0.58	0.68
C9orf47	rs1875620	A	0.94 (0.84-104)	0.24	0.93 (0.81-1.08)	0.34	**0.80 (0.65-0.99)**	**0.037**	0.29
CBLN2|| LOC100132647	rs1539909	A	0.96 (0.81-1.13)	0.62	0.88 (0.70-1.10)	0.27	0.84 (0.61-1.16)	0.29	1.00
LOC102723883||LINC02549	rs7767069	T	**0.85 (0.76-0.96)**	**0.008**	0.91 (0.78-1.08)	0.28	0.81 (0.65-1.01)	0.058	0.11
LOC107986770||ETV1	rs1568885	T	0.67 (0.40-1.10)[§]	0.11	0.84 (0.42-1.66)[§]	0.61	**0.44 (0.20-0.98)[§]**	**0.046**	0.23
LOC400456||LOC100132798	rs10520789	A	1.03 (0.86-1.22)	0.76	1.14 (0.90-1.44)	0.29	1.01 (0.72-1.41)	0.97	0.48
MAP2K6||KCNJ16	rs11870477	C	1.07 (0.91-1.25)	0.42	0.92 (0.74-1.14)	0.46	1.18 (0.85-1.65)	0.33	0.13
NUBPL	rs2378945	A	1.02 (0.91-1.13)	0.79	1.06 (0.91-1.24)	0.44	0.97 (0.79-1.20)	0.81	0.41
OR5BP1P||LRRC55	rs717117	G	**0.76 (0.60-0.97)**	**0.026**	**0.54 (0.39-0.74)**	**0.00012**	1.52 (0.96-2.42)	0.07	**0.00028**
PDZD2	rs1532269	G	1.01 (0.88-1.16)	0.86	1.03 (0.89-1.20)	0.68	1.02 (0.82-1.26)	0.87	0.95
PLA2G4A||FDPSL1	rs4651370	A	1.05 (0.90-1.23)	0.53	1.09 (0.88-1.35)	0.42	0.92 (0.69-1.24)	0.60	0.15
PPP1R9A	rs854547	G	1.00 (0.89-1.11)	0.95	1.03 (0.89-1.19)	0.71	0.92 (0.74-1.14)	0.43	0.46
PPP1R9A||PON1	rs854548	A	1.01 (0.89-1.15)	0.89	1.04 (0.87-1.24)	0.67	0.85 (0.66-1.10)	0.22	0.39
QKI||LOC728275	rs10945919	G	0.88 (0.76-1.03)[†]	0.11	**0.79 (0.64-0.97)[†]**	**0.027**	1.03 (0.77-1.38)[†]	0.85	0.14
SEC63P3	rs437943	G	1.10 (0.95-1.28)[†]	0.21	0.98 (0.80-1.20)[†]	0.82	**1.37 (1.02-1.85)[†]**	**0.037**	0.25
SLCO1C1	rs3794271	C	0.95 (0.85-1.07)	0.39	0.96 (0.82-1.11)	0.57	1.02 (0.82-1.27)	0.87	0.34
TEC	rs4694890	C	0.96 (0.86-1.07)	0.42	1.01 (0.87-1.17)	0.86	0.84 (0.67-1.05)	0.12	0.37
TRMT112P5	rs1447722	C	1.03 (0.92-1.15)	0.61	1.01 (0.87-1.18)	0.85	1.08 (0.87-1.35)	0.48	0.81

SNP, single nucleotide polymorphism; OR, odds ratio; CI, confidence interval.
Data on RF was available in 1069 RA patients. Estimates were adjusted for age, sex and country of origin. $P < 0.05$ in bold.
[δ]Estimates calculated according to a log-additive model of inheritance.
[†]Estimates calculated according to a dominant model of inheritance.
[§]Estimates calculated according to a recessive model of inheritance.

showed significantly decreased levels of IL6 production after stimulation of PBMCs with either *B. burgdorferi* (P=0.00046; **Figure 2A**) or *E. coli* (P=0.00044; **Figure 2B**), which suggested an implication of the *LRRC55* locus in the modulation of the response to TNFi by regulating IL6 production and likely IL6-mediated T cell differentiation into effector Th2 cells. Functional data from Haploreg also showed that the $LRRC55_{rs717117}$ variant correlates with mRNA *P2RX3* expression levels, a well-known gene involved in controlling T cell proliferation. Finally, our functional experiments revealed that carriers of the $MAFB_{rs6071980}{}^{C}$ allele showed decreased levels of Chemokine (C-C motif) ligand 23 (CCL23; P=0.0060; **Figure 3A**) and increased levels of serum Fibroblast growth factor 19 (FGF-19; P=0.0034; **Figure 3B**). Whereas FGF-19 protein modulates inflammation by mediating IL6 production, CCL23 has been implicated in monocyte recruitment during inflammation and it has been previously shown to positively correlate with drop in DAS28 after treatment with TNFi. Although the effect of the *MAFB* SNP to modulate either serum FGF-19 or CCL23 levels did not remain significant after correction for multiple testing, these results might indicate a weak, but still functional, effect of the *MAFB* locus in modulating response to anti-TNF drugs.

DISCUSSION

Although treatment of RA patients using monoclonal anti-TNF drugs has been a particularly successful approach to control inflammation and to prevent joint destruction and the appearance of bone erosions, non-responsiveness is prevalent and no effective biomarkers for drug response prediction have been consistently identified (36). This comprehensive validation study aimed at confirming the association of GWAS-identified variants with response to TNFi and to shed some light into the biological mechanisms underlying the most interesting associations. For that purpose, we conducted a two-stage case control study including 2067 RA patients treated with anti-TNF drugs ascertained through the REPAIR consortium but also DANBIO and DREAM registries. The most significant result was the overall association of the $LINC02549_{rs7767069}$ SNP with a poor response to anti-TNF drugs. The meta-analysis of the discovery and replication cohorts showed that each copy of the $LINC02549_{rs7767069T}$ allele significantly decreased the improvement in DAS28 by 17% after the treatment with a TNFi. Importantly, the association of the $LINC02549_{rs7767069}$ variant with poor response to TNFi was significant in the two

TABLE 4 | Overall and RF-specific meta-analysis of the *CNTN5*$_{rs1813443}$, *MAFB*$_{rs607198}$, *LINCO2549*$_{rs7767069}$ and *LRRC55*$_{rs717117}$ polymorphisms and response to anti-TNF drugs.

Gene	SNP ID	Effect allele	Overall REPAIR+DANBIO (n=1361)		Overall DREAM (n=706)		Meta-analysis (n=2067)		$P_{Heterogeneity}$
			OR (95% CI)$^{\delta}$	*P*	OR (95% CI)$^{\delta}$	*P*	OR (95% CI)$^{\delta}$	*P*	
CNTN5	rs1813443	C	0.97 (0.84-1.13)†	0.72	**0.82 (0.68-1.00)†**	**0.046**	0.91 (0.81-1.03)†	0.12	0.18
HSPEP1‖MAFB	rs6071980	C	**0.83 (0.72-0.97)**	**0.020**	0.88 (0.73-1.06)	0.18	**0.85 (0.76-0.95)**	**0.0059**	0.63
LOC102723883‖LINC02549	rs7767069	T	**0.85 (0.76-0.96)**	**0.008**	**0.80 (0.70-0.93)**	**0.004**	**0.83 (0.76-0.91)**	**0.00007**	0.61
OR5BP1P‖LRRC55	rs717117	G	**0.76 (0.60-0.97)**	**0.026**	0.89 (0.67-1.20)	0.46	**0.81 (0.67-0.98)**	**0.026**	0.41
		Effect allele	**RF-positive patients REPAIR+DANBIO (n=721)**		**RF-positive patients DREAM (n=532)**		**RF-positive patients Meta-analysis (n=1253)**		
Gene	**SNP ID**		**OR (95% CI)$^{\delta}$**	***P***	**OR (95% CI)$^{\delta}$**	***P***	**OR (95% CI)$^{\delta}$**	***P***	$P_{Heterogeneity}$
CNTN5	rs1813443	C	**0.79 (0.65-0.97)†**	**0.023**	0.84 (0.67-1.04)†	0.12	**0.81 (0.70-0.94)†**	**0.0059**	0.69
HSPEP1‖MAFB	rs6071980	C	0.85 (0.70-1.03)	0.10	0.85 (0.69-1.04)	0.11	**0.85 (0.73-0.98)**	**0.023**	1.00
LOC102723883‖LINC02549	rs7767069	T	0.91 (0.78-1.08)	0.28	**0.82 (0.69-0.97)**	**0.022**	**0.87 (0.77-0.97)**	**0.016**	0.39
OR5BP1P‖LRRC55	rs717117	G	**0.54 (0.39-0.74)**	**0.00012**	0.83 (0.60-1.15)	0.28	**0.67 (0.54-0.84)**	**0.00058**	0.06
		Effect allele	**RF-negative patients REPAIR+DANBIO (n=347)**		**RF-negative patients DREAM (n=154)**		**RF-positive patients Meta-analysis (n=501)**		
Gene	**SNP ID**		**OR (95% CI)$^{\delta}$**	***P***	**OR (95% CI)$^{\delta}$**	***P***	**OR (95% CI)$^{\delta}$**	***P***	$P_{Heterogeneity}$
CNTN5	rs1813443	C	1.14 (0.86-1.53)†	0.34	0.76 (0.50-1.16)†	0.20	1.00 (0.79-1.27)†	0.99	0.12
HSPEP1‖MAFB	rs6071980	C	0.81 (0.58-1.14)	0.23	1.10 (0.71-1.71)	0.67	0.91 (0.69-1.19)	0.48	0.28
LOC102723883‖LINC02549	rs7767069	T	0.81 (0.65-1.01)	0.058	0.76 (0.55-1.04)	0.08	**0.79 (0.66-0.95)**	**0.012**	0.75
OR5BP1P‖LRRC55	rs717117	G	1.52 (0.96-2.42)	0.07	1.10 (0.55-2.19)	0.80	1.38 (0.94-2.02)	0.10	0.45

SNP, single nucleotide polymorphism; OR, odds ratio; CI, confidence interval.
Response to anti-TNF defined as ΔDAS28. Data on RF was available in 1068 and RA patients in the discovery (REPAIR+DANBIO) and replication cohorts (DREAM).
Association estimates were adjusted for age, sex and country of origin in the discovery cohort and age and sex in the replication cohort (all Dutch patients). $P < 0.05$ in bold.
$^{\delta}$*Estimates calculated according to a log-additive model of inheritance.*
†*Estimates calculated according to a dominant model of inheritance.*

populations analyzed and remained significant after correction for multiple testing, which confirmed a role of the *LINC02549* locus in the modulation of response to anti-TNF drugs.

LINC02549 (Long Intergenic Protein Coding RNA 2549) is an RNA gene that is affiliated with the lncRNA class, which represents a large proportion of the human transcriptome. *LINC02549* maps to chromosome 6 and it is expressed in resting T cells and CD4 activated T cells. Although its function is still largely unknown, our data suggest that it might exert a role in determining the number of circulating CD45RO+CD45RA+ T cells, which are a subset of cells frequently found in the synovial fluid of both chronic arthritis (37) and RA patients (38). According to the results of Koch et al. (1990), CD45RA+ CD45RO+ T lymphocytes are mostly detected in perivascular regions, which suggest that these lymphocytes might access the RA synovial tissue *via* the synovial vasculature (38) and that, once there, they could play a role in promoting synovial tissue inflammation mainly by the induction of memory immune responses. Therefore, it seems to be plausible to suggest that the negative impact of the *LINC02549*$_{rs7767069}$ SNP on the response to TNFi might be mediated by its role in modulating numbers of CD45RA+CD45RO+ T lymphocytes that could migrate to the synovial tissue and promote inflammatory responses and, thereby hamper the control of inflammation during treatment with anti-TNF drugs. In support of this hypothesis, we found that carriers of two copies of the *LINC02549*$_{rs7767069T}$ allele also showed significantly increased levels of soluble scavenger receptors CD5 and CD6 (sCD5 and sCD6) in serum that are proteins highly expressed in regulatory T cells and a specific subset of B cells (CD5+ or B1a) (39). Although the origin of these soluble scavenger receptors in RA is poorly understood, it has been suggested that they are shed in the serum by proteases from the surface of activated lymphocytes that subsequently infiltrate synovium structures (40). In fact, increased serum levels of sCD5 and sCD6 has been found in subjects diagnosed with RA (41–44) but also other autoimmune diseases such as primary Sjögren's syndrome (42, 45, 46), systemic inflammatory response syndrome (47), multiple sclerosis (44) or dermatitis (48). Although the functional role of both soluble scavengers in autoimmune diseases is still under investigation, it is well established that sCD5 and sCD6 are regulators of T cell functions and induce autoreactivity. It is known that they are required for the initiation, differentiation and maintenance of T cell immune responses (49, 50) but also T cell migration and extravasation to the synovial tissue (51). Furthermore, it has been reported that both sCD5 and sCD6 are involved in the modulation of TCR and BCR signaling and determinate T- and B-cell survival (52) and Th17 differentiation (53, 54). Furthermore, clinical trials using humanized anti-CD6 mAbs have provided valuable information regarding the potential targeting of CD6 for the treatment of RA but also psoriasis and potentially other T cell–driven autoimmune diseases (55–57). Recent investigations have also suggested that genetic alterations within the CD6 gene associated with clinical outcome of several autoimmune diseases (44, 58) and correlated with the response to TNFi (59), which pointed to a role of these soluble scavenger receptors in modulating response to anti-TNF drugs. Considering these findings, we hypothesize that, besides

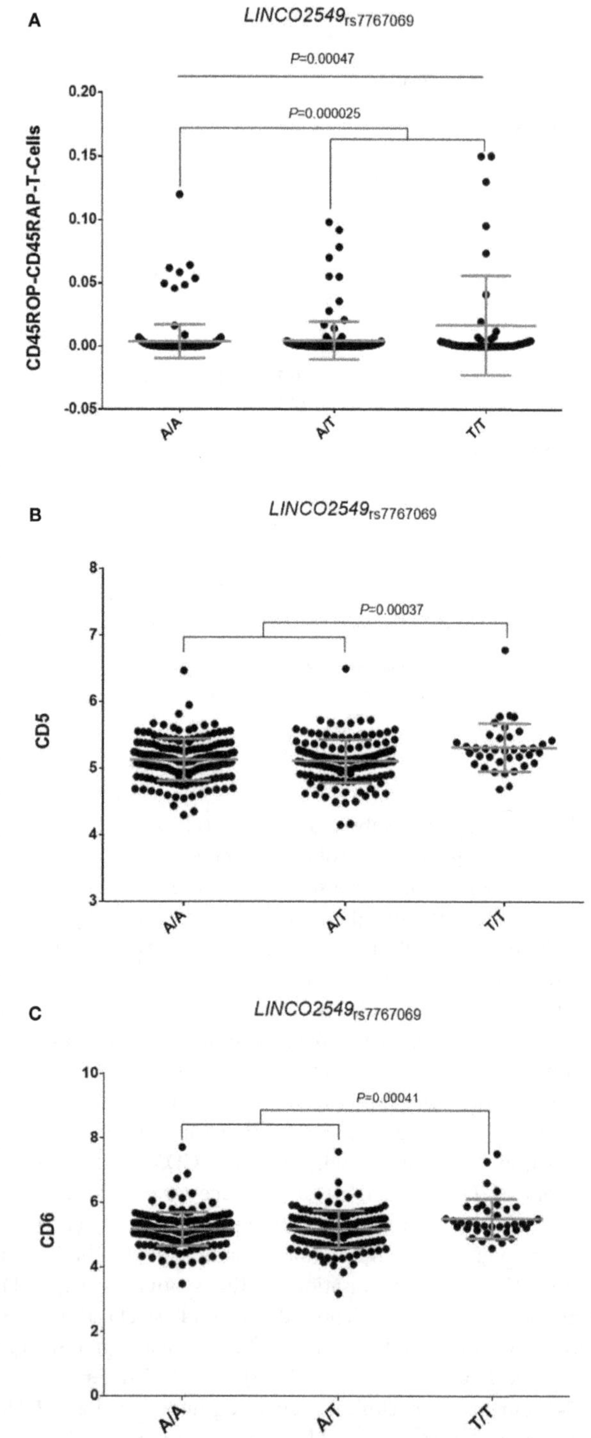

FIGURE 1 | Correlation of the LINC02549$_{rs7767069}$ polymorphism with absolute numbers of CD45RO+CD45RA+ T cells in blood **(A)** and serum levels of soluble scavenger receptors CD5 **(B)** and CD6 **(C)**.

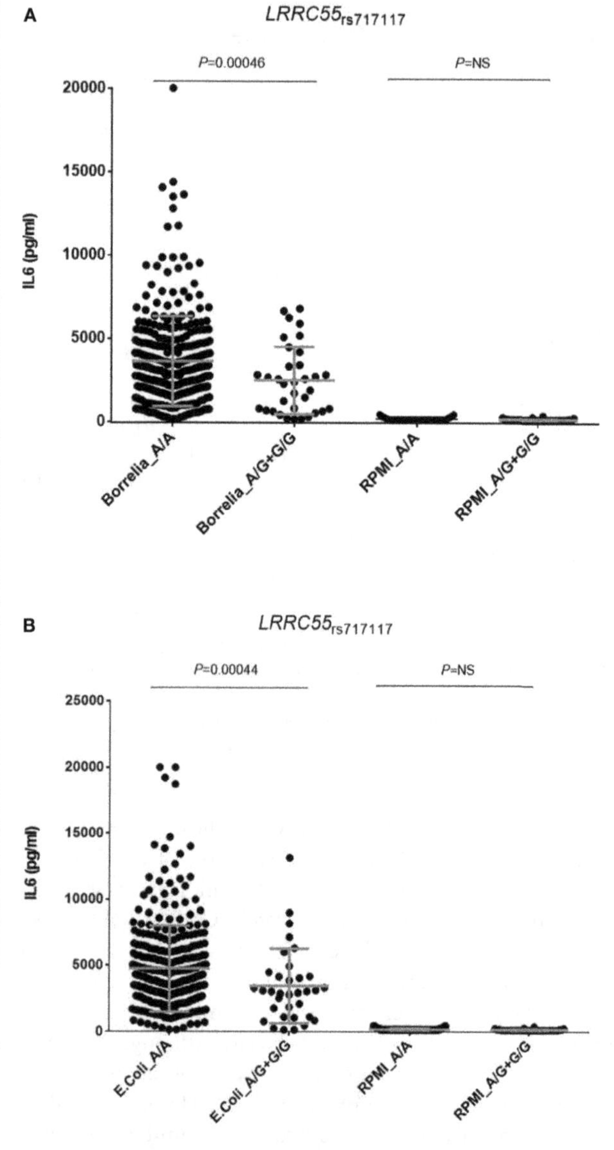

FIGURE 2 | Correlation of the LRRC55$_{rs717117G}$ allele and levels of IL6 after stimulation of PBMCs either with *B. burgdorferi* **(A)** or *E. coli* **(B)**.

its effect on modulating number of the CD45RA+CD45RO+ T lymphocytes, the *LINC02549*$_{rs7767069}$ SNP might negatively influence the response to anti-TNF drugs by stimulating directly or indirectly the production of sCD5 and sCD6 and thereby inducing long-term T cell-mediated immune responses.

Another interesting result that remained significant after correction for multiple testing was the RF-specific association of the *LRRC55*$_{rs717117}$ SNP with lower changes in DAS28 after the treatment with TNFi. The meta-analysis of the discovery and replication cohorts showed that RF-positive patients carrying the *LRRC55*$_{rs717117G}$ allele have a significantly decreased drop in DAS28 after treatment with a TNFi, whereas an opposite but not statistically significant effect was observed in RF-negative RA patients. Noticeably, functional experiments showed that, after stimulation of PBMCs from healthy subjects with *B. burgdorferi* and *E. coli* bacteria, carriers of the *LRRC55*$_{rs717117G}$ allele showed significantly decreased production of IL6 when compared to

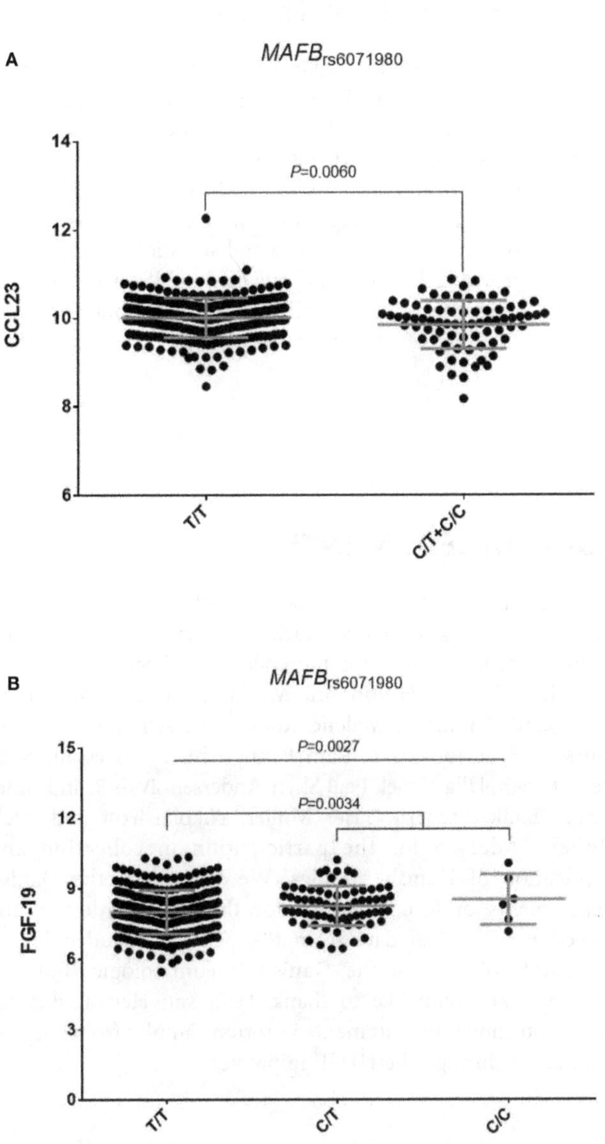

FIGURE 3 | orrelation of the $MAFB_{rs6071980C}$ allele with serum levels of CCL23 **(A)** and FGF-19 proteins **(B)**.

those carrying the most common genotype. Although functional experiments could not be stratified by RF because of the healthy nature of blood donors, these results suggested a role of the *LRRC55* locus in modulating IL6-mediated immune responses. On the other hand, functional data from Haploreg also suggested an implication of the $LRRC55_{rs717117}$ variant in controlling *P2RX3*-mediated T cell proliferation.

LRRC55 gene maps on chromosome 11 and it encodes for the leucine-rich repeat-containing protein 55, a protein that belongs to the LRRC superfamily that include hundreds of proteins mainly expressed in brain. Several LRRC proteins have been linked to the regulation of ion channels (60) but it has been also demonstrated that LRRC proteins are also implicated in modulating immune responses against bacterial pathogens (61) and modulate cell trafficking of membrane receptors such as toll-like receptors (62). Although the interplay between LRRC55 and IL6 has not been demonstrated, our experimental data suggest that the $LRRC55_{rs717117}$ SNP modulates IL6 production in response to bacteria and, therefore, might be involved in other IL6-dependent immune processes that could worsen the response to TNFi.

It is widely known that IL6 can induce both anti-inflammatory and pro-inflammatory immune responses, which depend entirely on the signalling pathway triggered. Whereas anti-inflammatory responses are mostly mediated by the classic signalling cascade (through binding to the transmembrane IL6 receptor), pro-inflammatory responses and chronic inflammation are mediated by trans-signalling (through binding to the soluble IL6 receptor) or by the interaction of IL6R with gp130 (63, 64). Considering our functional data, it is conceivable to suggest that the $LRRC55_{rs717117}$ SNP might affect the response to TNFi by decreasing IL6 production and thus inhibiting the classical IL6-dependent anti-inflammatory pathway and dysregulating pro-inflammatory responses. In support of this hypothesis, several mouse models have shown that the activation of the IL6 classic signaling pathway is essential for the activation of STAT3-mediated signaling pathways which reduce inflammation and induce the regeneration of the affected tissues (65). In addition, it has been reported that IL6 is one of the earliest factors that trigger the differentiation of naive T cells into effector Th2 cells *in vitro* and that, when absent, aggravates the development of the inflammatory processes (64).

Finally, although the genetic association of the $MAFB_{rs6071980}$ SNP with lower response to TNFi did not remain significant after correction for multiple testing, we found that the $MAFB_{rs6071980}$ SNP correlated with higher levels of serum FGF-19 and decreased levels of CCL23. Given that FGF-19 is a master protein involved in the inhibition of intestinal inflammation (66, 67) and CCL23 has been positively correlated with the DAS28 score in RA patients (68), we think that it would worth to investigate more in detail the impact of this SNP on drug response in future studies. In addition, it might be interesting to further analyze the weak association of the $CNTN5_{rs1813443}$ SNP with poor response to TNFi. However, given that we could not find any significant impact of this marker on immune responses, blood cell counts or serum inflammatory proteins or steroid hormones, we are prone to think that this SNP might not have a relevant role in modulating response to TNFi.

This study has both strengths and weaknesses. Among the strengths we can highlight the use of large and well-characterized RA patient populations that allowed the development of a well-powered overall association analysis but also to investigate the effect modification by RF status. Overall, we had 80% of power to detect an OR of 1.18 (α=0.00089) for a SNP with a frequency of 0.25. On the other hand, it is worth mentioning the comprehensive analysis of the functional effect of the most interesting genetic variants on modulating immune responses, which was performed using a large sample size for this kind of studies. We analysed cQTL and hQTL data but also counts of 91 blood-derived cell populations and serum levels of 103 immunological proteins. An important limitation of this study was the impossibility to adjust linear regression analyses for potential confounding factors including concomitant treatments that might influence the response to TNFi. In addition, given the healthy nature of the subjects included in the HFGP cohort, we could not control our functional experiments by RF status.

In conclusion, this study validates the overall or RF-specific association of *LINC02549* and *LRRC55* loci with the response to TNFi and provides new insights into the functional role of these polymorphisms in modulating immune responses and response to anti-TNF drugs.

DATA AVAILABILITY STATEMENT

All data used in this project have been meticulously catalogued and archived in the BBMRI-NL data infrastructure (https://hfgp.bbmri.nl/) using the MOLGENIS open-source platform for scientific data (69). This allows flexible data querying and download, including sufficiently rich metadata and interfaces for machine processing (R statistics, REST API) and using FAIR principles to optimize Findability, Accessibility, Interoperability and Reusability (70, 71).

ETHICS STATEMENT

The study was approved by the ethical review committee of participant institutions: Virgen de las Nieves University Hospital (2012/89); Santa Maria Hospital-CHLN (CE 877/121.2012); University Clinical Hospital of Santiago de Compostela (2013/156); Wroclaw Medical University (KB-625/2016); Radboud university medical center (2011/299) and by the Regional Ethics Committee of Central Denmark Region (S-20120113). The patients/participants provided their written informed consent to participate in this study.

AUTHOR CONTRIBUTIONS

RC and JSa designed the study and drafted the manuscript. JMSM, AM-D, and AJCS were responsible for genotyping. MALN, HC, LQ, SS, BG, MH, IF, EP-P, PC-Z, JSw, AB, SV, EP, MF, AE, MC, VA, JF, MJ, KBK, EC, and JSa coordinated the sample collection and HC, IF, and MF were involved in the records review and data acquisition. JMSM and JSa performed data quality control of genetic data and statistical analysis. MN, RTH, YL provided the functional raw data and JSa performed the analysis of functional data. All authors contributed to and approved the final version of the manuscript.

ACKNOWLEDGMENTS

We thank all participants who have agreed to participate in this study. Authors also thank María Dolores Casares, Ángeles Molina, Carmen Oloriz for the collection of Spanish samples and Hans Jurgen Hoffmann, Marianne Thomsen, Vibeke Østergaard Thomsen, Malene Rohr Andersen, Lise Lotte B. Laursen, Helle Jørgensen, Ram Benny Christian Dessau, Niels Steen Krogh, Ulla Vogel, Paal Skytt Andersen, Ivan Brandslund, Steffen Bank, Frederik Trier Møller, Nikolai Toft and Niels Møller Andersen for the participation in collection and purification of Danish samples. We also thank the Danish Departments of Rheumatology for their implication in the collection of clinical data from RA patients included in the DANBIO cohort and the Danish Rheumatologic Biobank. Likewise, we would like to thank Teun van Herwaarden for steroid hormone measurements in serum samples from subjects ascertained through the HFGP initiative.

REFERENCES

1. Bluml S, Scheinecker C, Smolen JS, Redlich K. Targeting TNF Receptors in Rheumatoid Arthritis. *Int Immunol* (2012) 24(5):275–81. doi: 10.1093/intimm/dxs047
2. Scott DL, Wolfe F, Huizinga TW. Rheumatoid Arthritis. *Lancet* (2010) 376 (9746):1094–108. doi: 10.1016/S0140-6736(10)60826-4
3. Pisetsky DS, Ward MM. Advances in the Treatment of Inflammatory Arthritis. *Best Pract Res Clin Rheumatol* (2012) 26(2):251–61. doi: 10.1016/j.berh.2012.03.001
4. Di Giovine FS, Nuki G, Duff GW. Tumour Necrosis Factor in Synovial Exudates. *Ann Rheum Dis* (1988) 47(9):768–72. doi: 10.1136/ard.47.9.768
5. Tracey D, Klareskog L, Sasso EH, Salfeld JG, Tak PP. Tumor Necrosis Factor Antagonist Mechanisms of Action: A Comprehensive Review. *Pharmacol Ther* (2008) 117(2):244–79. doi: 10.1016/j.pharmthera.2007.10.001
6. Azuma Y, Kaji K, Katogi R, Takeshita S, Kudo A. Tumor Necrosis Factor-Alpha Induces Differentiation of and Bone Resorption by Osteoclasts. *J Biol Chem* (2000) 275(7):4858–64. doi: 10.1074/jbc.275.7.4858
7. Safiri S, Kolahi AA, Hoy D, Smith E, Bettampadi D, Mansournia MA, et al. Global, Regional and National Burden of Rheumatoid Arthritis 1990-2017: A Systematic Analysis of the Global Burden of Disease Study 2017. *Ann Rheum Dis* (2019) 78(11):1463–71. doi: 10.1136/annrheumdis-2019-215920
8. Tesar T, Golias P, Kobliskova Z, Wawruch M, Kawalec P, Inotai A. Potential Cost-Savings From the Use of the Biosimilars in Slovakia. *Front Public Health* (2020) 8:431. doi: 10.3389/fpubh.2020.00431
9. Atzeni F, Benucci M, Salli S, Bongiovanni S, Boccassini L, Sarzi-Puttini P. Different Effects of Biological Drugs in Rheumatoid Arthritis. *Autoimmun Rev* (2013) 12(5):575–9. doi: 10.1016/j.autrev.2012.10.020
10. Plenge RM, Bridges SL Jr. Personalized Medicine in Rheumatoid Arthritis: Miles to Go Before We Sleep. *Arthritis Rheum* (2011) 63(3):590–3. doi: 10.1002/art.30126

11. Honne K, Hallgrimsdottir I, Wu C, Sebro R, Jewell NP, Sakurai T, et al. A Longitudinal Genome-Wide Association Study of Anti-Tumor Necrosis Factor Response Among Japanese Patients With Rheumatoid Arthritis. *Arthritis Res Ther* (2016) 18:12. doi: 10.1186/s13075-016-0920-6
12. Cui J, Stahl EA, Saevarsdottir S, Miceli C, Diogo D, Trynka G, et al. Genome-Wide Association Study and Gene Expression Analysis Identifies CD84 as a Predictor of Response to Etanercept Therapy in Rheumatoid Arthritis. *PloS Genet* (2013) 9(3):e1003394. doi: 10.1371/journal.pgen.1003394
13. Julia A, Fernandez-Nebro A, Blanco F, Ortiz A, Canete JD, Maymo J, et al. A Genome-Wide Association Study Identifies a New Locus Associated With the Response to Anti-TNF Therapy in Rheumatoid Arthritis. *Pharmacogenom J* (2016) 16(2):147–50. doi: 10.1038/tpj.2015.31
14. Krintel SB, Palermo G, Johansen JS, Germer S, Essioux L, Benayed R, et al. Investigation of Single Nucleotide Polymorphisms and Biological Pathways Associated With Response to TNFalpha Inhibitors in Patients With Rheumatoid Arthritis. *Pharmacogenet Genomics* (2012) 22(8):577–89. doi: 10.1097/FPC.0b013e3283544043
15. Liu C, Batliwalla F, Li W, Lee A, Roubenoff R, Beckman E, et al. Genome-Wide Association Scan Identifies Candidate Polymorphisms Associated With Differential Response to Anti-TNF Treatment in Rheumatoid Arthritis. *Mol Med* (2008) 14(9-10):575–81. doi: 10.2119/2008-00056.Liu
16. Umicevic Mirkov M, Cui J, Vermeulen SH, Stahl EA, Toonen EJ, Makkinje RR, et al. Genome-Wide Association Analysis of Anti-TNF Drug Response in Patients With Rheumatoid Arthritis. *Ann Rheum Dis* (2013) 72(8):1375–81. doi: 10.1136/annrheumdis-2012-202405
17. Plant D, Bowes J, Potter C, Hyrich KL, Morgan AW, Wilson AG, et al. Genome-Wide Association Study of Genetic Predictors of Anti-Tumor Necrosis Factor Treatment Efficacy in Rheumatoid Arthritis Identifies Associations With Polymorphisms at Seven Loci. *Arthritis Rheum* (2011) 63 (3):645–53. doi: 10.1002/art.30130
18. Canet LM, Caliz R, Lupianez CB, Canhao H, Martinez M, Escudero A, et al. Genetic Variants Within Immune-Modulating Genes Influence the Risk of Developing Rheumatoid Arthritis and Anti-TNF Drug Response: A Two-Stage Case-Control Study. *Pharmacogenet Genomics* (2015) 25(9):432–43. doi: 10.1097/FPC.0000000000000155
19. Canet LM, Filipescu I, Caliz R, Lupianez CB, Canhao H, Escudero A, et al. Genetic Variants Within the TNFRSF1B Gene and Susceptibility to Rheumatoid Arthritis and Response to Anti-TNF Drugs: A Multicenter Study. *Pharmacogenet Genomics* (2015) 25(7):323–33. doi: 10.1097/FPC.0000000000000140
20. Canet LM, Sanchez-Maldonado JM, Caliz R, Rodriguez-Ramos A, Lupianez CB, Canhao H, et al. Polymorphisms at Phase I-Metabolizing Enzyme and Hormone Receptor Loci Influence the Response to Anti-TNF Therapy in Rheumatoid Arthritis Patients. *Pharmacogenom J* (2019) 19(1):83–96. doi: 10.1038/s41397-018-0057-x
21. Canhao H, Rodrigues AM, Santos MJ, Carmona-Fernandes D, Bettencourt BF, Cui J, et al. TRAF1/C5 But Not PTPRC Variants Are Potential Predictors of Rheumatoid Arthritis Response to Anti-Tumor Necrosis Factor Therapy. *BioMed Res Int* (2015) 2015:490295. doi: 10.1155/2015/490295
22. Manuel Sanchez-Maldonado J, Martinez-Bueno M, Canhao H, Ter Horst R, Munoz-Pena S, Moniz-Diez A, et al. NFKB2 Polymorphisms Associate With the Risk of Developing Rheumatoid Arthritis and Response to TNF Inhibitors: Results From the REPAIR Consortium. *Sci Rep* (2020) 10(1):4316. doi: 10.1038/s41598-020-61331-5
23. Potter C, Cordell HJ, Barton A, Daly AK, Hyrich KL, Mann DA, et al. Association Between Anti-Tumour Necrosis Factor Treatment Response and Genetic Variants Within the TLR and NF{kappa}B Signalling Pathways. *Ann Rheum Dis* (2010) 69(7):1315–20. doi: 10.1136/ard.2009.117309
24. Sanchez-Maldonado JM, Caliz R, Canet L, Horst RT, Bakker O, den Broeder AA, et al. Steroid Hormone-Related Polymorphisms Associate With the Development of Bone Erosions in Rheumatoid Arthritis and Help to Predict Disease Progression: Results From the REPAIR Consortium. *Sci Rep* (2019) 9(1):14812. doi: 10.1038/s41598-019-51255-0
25. Sode J, Vogel U, Bank S, Andersen PS, Hetland ML, Locht H, et al. Genetic Variations in Pattern Recognition Receptor Loci Are Associated With Anti-TNF Response in Patients With Rheumatoid Arthritis. *PloS One* (2015) 10 (10):e0139781. doi: 10.1371/journal.pone.0139781
26. Sode J, Vogel U, Bank S, Andersen PS, Hetland ML, Locht H, et al. Confirmation of an IRAK3 Polymorphism as a Genetic Marker Predicting Response to Anti-TNF Treatment in Rheumatoid Arthritis. *Pharmacogenom J* (2018) 18(1):81–6. doi: 10.1038/tpj.2016.66
27. Suarez-Gestal M, Perez-Pampin E, Calaza M, Gomez-Reino JJ, Gonzalez A. Lack of Replication of Genetic Predictors for the Rheumatoid Arthritis Response to Anti-TNF Treatments: A Prospective Case-Only Study. *Arthritis Res Ther* (2010) 12(2):R72. doi: 10.1186/ar2990
28. Ibfelt EH, Jensen DV, Hetland ML. The Danish Nationwide Clinical Register for Patients With Rheumatoid Arthritis: DANBIO. *Clin Epidemiol* (2016) 8:737–42. doi: 10.2147/CLEP.S99490
29. Ibfelt EH, Sorensen J, Jensen DV, Dreyer L, Schiottz-Christensen B, Thygesen PH, et al. Validity and Completeness of Rheumatoid Arthritis Diagnoses in the Nationwide DANBIO Clinical Register and the Danish National Patient Registry. *Clin Epidemiol* (2017) 9:627–32. doi: 10.2147/CLEP.S141438
30. Arnett FC, Edworthy SM, Bloch DA, Mcshane DJ, Fries JF, Cooper NS, et al. The American Rheumatism Association 1987 Revised Criteria for the Classification of Rheumatoid Arthritis. *Arthritis Rheum* (1988) 31:315–24. doi: 10.1002/art.1780310302
31. Aletaha D, Neogi T, Silman AJ, Funovits J, Felson DT, Bingham CO3rd, et al. Rheumatoid Arthritis Classification Criteria: An American College of Rheumatology/European League Against Rheumatism Collaborative Initiative. *Arthritis Rheum* (2010) 62:2569–81. doi: 10.1002/art.27584
32. Keystone EC, Kavanaugh AF, Sharp JT, Tannenbaum H, Hua Y, Teoh LS, et al. Radiographic, Clinical, and Functional Outcomes of Treatment With Adalimumab (A Human Anti-Tumor Necrosis Factor Monoclonal Antibody) in Patients With Active Rheumatoid Arthritis Receiving Concomitant Methotrexate Therapy: A Randomized, Placebo-Controlled, 52-Week Trial. *Arthritis Rheum* (2004) 50(5):1400–11. doi: 10.1002/art.20217
33. Weinblatt ME, Kremer JM, Bankhurst AD, Bulpitt KJ, Fleischmann RM, Fox RI, et al. A Trial of Etanercept, a Recombinant Tumor Necrosis Factor Receptor:Fc Fusion Protein, in Patients With Rheumatoid Arthritis Receiving Methotrexate. *N Engl J Med* (1999) 340(4):253–9. doi: 10.1056/NEJM199901283400401
34. Orru V, Steri M, Sole G, Sidore C, Virdis F, Dei M, et al. Genetic Variants Regulating Immune Cell Levels in Health and Disease. *Cell* (2013) 155(1):242–56. doi: 10.1016/j.cell.2013.08.041
35. Aguirre-Gamboa R, Joosten I, Urbano PCM, van der Molen RG, van Rijssen E, van Cranenbroek B, et al. Differential Effects of Environmental and Genetic Factors on T and B Cell Immune Traits. *Cell Rep* (2016) 17(9):2474–87. doi: 10.1016/j.celrep.2016.10.053
36. Cuppen BV, Welsing PM, Sprengers JJ, Bijlsma JW, Marijnissen AC, van Laar JM, et al. Personalized Biological Treatment for Rheumatoid Arthritis: A Systematic Review With a Focus on Clinical Applicability. *Rheumatol (Oxford)* (2016) 55(5):826–39. doi: 10.1093/rheumatology/kev421
37. Summers KL, O'Donnell JL, Hart DN. Co-Expression of the CD45RA and CD45RO Antigens on T Lymphocytes in Chronic Arthritis. *Clin Exp Immunol* (1994) 97(1):39–44. doi: 10.1111/j.1365-2249.1994.tb06576.x
38. Koch AE, Robinson PG, Radosevich JA, Pope RM. Distribution of CD45RA and CD45RO T-Lymphocyte Subsets in Rheumatoid Arthritis Synovial Tissue. *J Clin Immunol* (1990) 10(4):192–9. doi: 10.1007/BF00918651
39. Aruffo A, Melnick MB, Linsley PS, Seed B. The Lymphocyte Glycoprotein CD6 Contains a Repeated Domain Structure Characteristic of a New Family of Cell Surface and Secreted Proteins. *J Exp Med* (1991) 174(4):949–52. doi: 10.1084/jem.174.4.949
40. Calvo J, Places L, Espinosa G, Padilla O, Vila JM, Villamor N, et al. Identification of a Natural Soluble Form of Human CD5. *Tissue Antigens* (1999) 54(2):128–37. doi: 10.1034/j.1399-0039.1999.540203.x
41. Lydyard PM, Youinou PY, Cooke A. CD5-Positive B Cells in Rheumatoid Arthritis and Chronic Lymphocytic Leukemia. *Immunol Today* (1987) 8 (2):37–9. doi: 10.1016/0167-5699(87)90235-0
42. Youinou P, Mackenzie L, Broker BM, Isenberg DI, Drogou-Lelong A, Gentric A, et al. The Importance of CD5-Positive B Cells in Nonorgan-Specific Autoimmune Diseases. *Scand J Rheumatol Suppl* (1988) 76:243–9. doi: 10.3109/03009748809102975

43. Jamin C, Magadur G, Lamour A, Mackenzie L, Lydyard P, Katsikis P, et al. Cell-Free CD5 in Patients With Rheumatic Diseases. *Immunol Lett* (1992) 31 (1):79–83. doi: 10.1016/0165-2478(92)90014-F
44. Consuegra-Fernandez M, Lin F, Fox DA, Lozano F. Clinical and Experimental Evidence for Targeting CD6 in Immune-Based Disorders. *Autoimmun Rev* (2018) 17(5):493–503. doi: 10.1016/j.autrev.2017.12.004
45. Ramos-Casals M, Font J, Garcia-Carrasco M, Calvo J, Places L, Padilla O, et al. High Circulating Levels of Soluble Scavenger Receptors (Scd5 and Scd6) in Patients With Primary Sjogren's Syndrome. *Rheumatol (Oxford)* (2001) 40 (9):1056–9. doi: 10.1093/rheumatology/40.9.1056
46. Dauphinee MJ, Tovar Z, Ballester A, Talal N. The Expression and Function of CD3 and CD5 in Patients With Primary Sjogren's Syndrome. *Arthritis Rheum* (1989) 32(4):420–9. doi: 10.1002/anr.1780320411
47. Aibar J, Martinez-Florensa M, Castro P, Carrasco E, Escoda-Ferran C, Fernandez S, et al. Pattern of Soluble CD5 and CD6 Lymphocyte Receptors in Critically Ill Patients With Septic Syndromes. *J Crit Care* (2015) 30(5):914–9. doi: 10.1016/j.jcrc.2015.04.120
48. Noh GW, Lee KY. Circulating Soluble CD5 in Atopic Dermatitis. *Mol Cells* (1998) 8(5):618–22.
49. Zimmerman AW, Joosten B, Torensma R, Parnes JR, van Leeuwen FN, Figdor CG. Long-Term Engagement of CD6 and ALCAM Is Essential for T-Cell Proliferation Induced by Dendritic Cells. *Blood* (2006) 107(8):3212–20. doi: 10.1182/blood-2005-09-3881
50. Nair P, Melarkode R, Rajkumar D, Montero E. CD6 Synergistic Co-Stimulation Promoting Proinflammatory Response Is Modulated Without Interfering With the Activated Leucocyte Cell Adhesion Molecule Interaction. *Clin Exp Immunol* (2010) 162(1):116–30. doi: 10.1111/j.1365-2249.2010.04235.x
51. Alonso-Ramirez R, Loisel S, Buors C, Pers JO, Montero E, Youinou P, et al. Rationale for Targeting CD6 as a Treatment for Autoimmune Diseases. *Arthritis* (2010) 2010:130646. doi: 10.1155/2010/130646
52. Burgueno-Bucio E, Mier-Aguilar CA, Soldevila G. The Multiple Faces of CD5. *J Leukoc Biol* (2019) 105(5):891–904. doi: 10.1002/JLB.MR0618-226R
53. Li Y, Singer NG, Whitbred J, Bowen MA, Fox DA, Lin F. CD6 as a Potential Target for Treating Multiple Sclerosis. *Proc Natl Acad Sci USA* (2017) 114(10): 2687–92. doi: 10.1073/pnas.1615253114
54. Consuegra-Fernandez M, Julia M, Martinez-Florensa M, Aranda F, Catala C, Armiger-Borras N, et al. Genetic and Experimental Evidence for the Involvement of the CD6 Lymphocyte Receptor in Psoriasis. *Cell Mol Immunol* (2018) 15(10):898–906. doi: 10.1038/cmi.2017.119
55. Rodriguez PC, Prada DM, Moreno E, Aira LE, Molinero C, Lopez AM, et al. The Anti-CD6 Antibody Itolizumab Provides Clinical Benefit Without Lymphopenia in Rheumatoid Arthritis Patients: Results From a 6-Month, Open-Label Phase I Clinical Trial. *Clin Exp Immunol* (2018) 191(2):229–39. doi: 10.1111/cei.13061
56. Rodriguez PC, Torres-Moya R, Reyes G, Molinero C, Prada D, Lopez AM, et al. A Clinical Exploratory Study With Itolizumab, an Anti-CD6 Monoclonal Antibody, in Patients With Rheumatoid Arthritis. *Results Immunol* (2012) 2:204–11. doi: 10.1016/j.rinim.2012.11.001
57. Krupashankar DS, Dogra S, Kura M, Saraswat A, Budamakuntla L, Sumathy TK, et al. Efficacy and Safety of Itolizumab, a Novel Anti-CD6 Monoclonal Antibody, in Patients With Moderate to Severe Chronic Plaque Psoriasis: Results of a Double-Blind, Randomized, Placebo-Controlled, Phase-III Study. *J Am Acad Dermatol* (2014) 71(3):484–92. doi: 10.1016/j.jaad.2014.01.897
58. Kofler DM, Farkas A, von Bergwelt-Baildon M, Hafler DA. The Link Between CD6 and Autoimmunity: Genetic and Cellular Associations. *Curr Drug Targets* (2016) 17(6):651–65. doi: 10.2174/1389450117666160201105934
59. Krintel SB, Essioux L, Wool A, Johansen JS, Schreiber E, Zekharya T, et al. CD6 and Syntaxin Binding Protein 6 Variants and Response to Tumor Necrosis Factor Alpha Inhibitors in Danish Patients With Rheumatoid Arthritis. *PloS One* (2012) 7(6):e38539. doi: 10.1371/journal.pone.0038539
60. Yan J, Aldrich RW. BK Potassium Channel Modulation by Leucine-Rich Repeat-Containing Proteins. *Proc Natl Acad Sci USA* (2012) 109(20):7917–22. doi: 10.1073/pnas.1205435109
61. Shi XZ, Feng XW, Sun JJ, Zhao XF, Wang JX. Leucine-Rich Repeats Containing Protein Functions in the Antibacterial Immune Reaction in Stomach of Kuruma Shrimp Marsupenaeus Japonicus. *Fish Shellfish Immunol* (2017) 61:130–7. doi: 10.1016/j.fsi.2016.12.029
62. Tatematsu M, Funami K, Ishii N, Seya T, Obuse C, Matsumoto M. LRRC59 Regulates Trafficking of Nucleic Acid-Sensing TLRs From the Endoplasmic Reticulum *via* Association With UNC93B1. *J Immunol* (2015) 195(10):4933–42. doi: 10.4049/jimmunol.1501305
63. Gabay C. Interleukin-6 and Chronic Inflammation. *Arthritis Res Ther* (2006) 8 Suppl 2:S3. doi: 10.1186/ar1917
64. Scheller J, Chalaris A, Schmidt-Arras D, Rose-John S. The Pro- and Anti-Inflammatory Properties of the Cytokine Interleukin-6. *Biochim Biophys Acta* (2011) 1813(5):878–88. doi: 10.1016/j.bbamcr.2011.01.034
65. Becker C, Fantini MC, Schramm C, Lehr HA, Wirtz S, Nikolaev A, et al. TGF-Beta Suppresses Tumor Progression in Colon Cancer by Inhibition of IL-6 Trans-Signaling. *Immunity* (2004) 21(4):491–501. doi: 10.1016/j.immuni.2004.07.020
66. Gadaleta RM, Garcia-Irigoyen O, Cariello M, Scialpi N, Peres C, Vetrano S, et al. Corrigendum to 'Fibroblast Growth Factor 19 Modulates Intestinal Microbiota and Inflammation in Presence of Farnesoid X Receptor': [EBioMedicine 54 (2020) 102719]. *EBioMedicine* (2020) 57:102873. doi: 10.1016/j.ebiom.2020.102719
67. Gadaleta RM, Garcia-Irigoyen O, Cariello M, Scialpi N, Peres C, Vetrano S, et al. Fibroblast Growth Factor 19 Modulates Intestinal Microbiota and Inflammation in Presence of Farnesoid X Receptor. *EBioMedicine* (2020) 54:102719. doi: 10.1016/j.ebiom.2020.102719
68. Rioja I, Hughes FJ, Sharp CH, Warnock LC, Montgomery DS, Akil M, et al. Potential Novel Biomarkers of Disease Activity in Rheumatoid Arthritis Patients: CXCL13, CCL23, Transforming Growth Factor Alpha, Tumor Necrosis Factor Receptor Superfamily Member 9, and Macrophage Colony-Stimulating Factor. *Arthritis Rheum* (2008) 58(8):2257–67. doi: 10.1002/art.23667
69. Swertz MA, Dijkstra M, Adamusiak T, van der Velde JK, Kanterakis A, Roos ET, et al. The MOLGENIS Toolkit: Rapid Prototyping of Biosoftware at the Push of a Button. *BMC Bioinf* (2010) 11 Suppl 12:S12. doi: 10.1186/1471-2105-11-S12-S12
70. Wilkinson MD, Dumontier M, Jan Aalbersberg I, Appleton G, Axton M, Baak A, et al. Addendum: The FAIR Guiding Principles for Scientific Data Management and Stewardship. *Sci Data* (2019) 6(1):6. doi: 10.1038/s41597-019-0009-6
71. Wilkinson MD, Dumontier M, Aalbersberg IJ, Appleton G, Axton M, Baak A, et al. The FAIR Guiding Principles for Scientific Data Management and Stewardship. *Sci Data* (2016) 3:160018. doi: 10.1038/sdata.2016.18

2

Circ_0088194 Promotes the Invasion and Migration of Rheumatoid Arthritis Fibroblast-Like Synoviocytes *via* the miR-766-3p/MMP2 Axis

Yujie Cai[1], Renge Liang[1], Shibai Xiao[1], Qin Huang[1], Dingji Zhu[1], Guo-Ping Shi[2], Qingqing Ouyang[1] and Min Yang[1*]*

[1] *Department of Rheumatology and Immunology, Nanfang Hospital, Southern Medical University, Guangzhou, China,*
[2] *Department of Medicine, Brigham and Women's Hospital and Harvard Medical School, Boston, MA, United States*

***Correspondence:**
Qingqing Ouyang
ouyangqing1988@163.com
Min Yang
minyanggz@163.com

Dysregulation of circular RNAs (circRNAs) is involved in various human diseases. Fibroblast-like synoviocytes (FLSs), which form the lining of the joint, are epigenetically imprinted with an aggressive phenotype and contribute to joint destruction in rheumatoid arthritis (RA). In the present study, we identified a novel circRNA, Circ_0088194, which was upregulated in RA fibroblast-like synoviocytes (RA-FLSs) and correlated with the disease activity score in 28 joints. Overexpression of Circ_0088194 promoted RA-FLS migration and invasion, while inhibition of Circ_0088194 had the opposite effect. Mechanistically, Circ_0088194 acted as a miR-766-3p sponge to relieve the repressive effect of miR-766-3p on its target, *MMP2* (encoding matrix metalloproteinase 2), thereby promoting migration and invasion. The expression level of Circ_0088194 was inversely correlated with that of miR-766-3p in RA-FLSs. Importantly, overexpression of miR-766-3p partially blocked the migration and invasion induced by Circ_0088194 overexpression. Collectively, this study identified a novel circRNA Circ_0088194 that promotes RA-FLS invasion and migration *via* the miR-766-3p/MMP2 axis. Circ_0088194 might represent a novel therapeutic target to prevent and treat RA.

Keywords: rheumatoid arthritis, fibroblast-like synoviocytes, CircRNA, Circ_0088194, miR-766-3p, matrix metalloproteinase 2

INTRODUCTION

Rheumatoid arthritis (RA) is one of the most prevalent chronic inflammatory diseases, and is characterized by progressive destruction of cartilage and bone, with concomitant disability (1). This disease carries a substantial burden for both the affected individuals and for society (2). Recently, the treatment of RA has improved, such as the use of combination anti-rheumatic drug strategies that modify the disease and the development of biological therapies; however, overall remission rates are still unsatisfactory (3). Therefore, it is imperative to determine the molecular mechanisms responsible for the development and progression of RA, and to identify new target molecules for early treatment.

In the formation of invasive synovial tissue, the key cells are RA fibroblast-like synoviocytes (RA-FLSs), which play a major role in the RA pathological processes (4). In RA pathogenesis, activated RA-FLSs exhibit similar characteristics to tumor cells, such as enhanced migration and invasion abilities, which promote RA progression, ultimately leading to joint destruction (5). Thus, investigating the mechanisms responsible for RA-FLs invasion and migration might identify potential therapeutic strategies to treat RA.

RNA transcripts forming covalently closed loops produced by direct non-canonical back-splicing are known as circular RNAs (circRNAs) (6, 7). CircRNAs are very stable and are highly abundant in various tissues because of their circular structure (8). CircRNA sequences are highly conserved and circRNAs are expressed in a tissue or cell-specific manner (9, 10). Recent studies indicated that circRNAs have diverse biological functions and are associated with the pathogenesis of various diseases, including cancer (11), cardiovascular disease (12), neurological disorders (13), and osteoarthritis (OA) (14). Importantly, the regulation of human cancer cell migration and invasion involves several circRNAs. For example, in non-small cell lung cancer, migration and invasion are promoted by the circRNA F-circEA-2a, which is expressed from the *EML4-ALK* fusion gene (15); and circRNA circNHSL1 promotes gastric cancer cell migration and invasion through the miR-1306-3p/SIX1/Vimentin axis (16). These reports suggested that circRNAs play an important role in the regulation of migration and invasion. However, the roles of circRNAs in RA-FLSs are largely unknown.

The most abundant internal modification of mRNAs and long non-coding RNAs is N6-methyladenosine (m^6A) (17, 18), which plays vital roles in stabilizing circRNAs and mRNAs (19, 20), in alternative splicing (21), and in miRNA (microRNA) biogenesis (22). Furthermore, m^6A methylation is found in various physiological and pathological processes, such as neurogenesis (23) and cancer (24). However, whether the N6-methyladenosine modification affects the stability of circRNAs in RA-FLSs remains unknown.

In the present study, a novel circRNA, Circ_0088194, was identified in human RA-FLSs that was associated positively with RA disease activity and was responsible for RA-FLS migration and invasion by binding to miR-766-3p, thus promoting matrix metalloproteinase 2 *(MMP2)* expression.

MATERIALS AND METHODS

Patients and Specimens

Osteoarthritis (OA), a degenerative disease with generally less severe clinical symptoms and pathology, has been utilized as a control in studies of RA pathology. From January 2017 to December 2017, nine RA synovial tissues and seven OA synovial tissues were acquired from patients with end-stage symptomatic hip RA or OA at the time of total hip replacement surgery, as performed at the Department of Orthopedic Surgery, Nanfang Hospital, Southern Medical University, Guangzhou, China. The Ethics Committee of the Southern Medical University approved the study and its associated protocols (Guangzhou, China, NFEC-20120201). All participants satisfied the criteria from the American College of Rheumatology to classify RA (25) or OA (26). Prior to enrollment, each participant provided written informed consent. The participants' clinical parameters are shown in **Table 1**.

Fibroblast-Like Synoviocytes (FLSs) Culture

FLSs were isolated from human synovial tissue specimens and cultured in Dulbecco's modified Eagle's medium (DMEM) (Thermo Fisher Scientific, Inc., Waltham, MA, USA) with 10% added fetal bovine serum (FBS) (Gibco BRL, Grand Island, NY, USA). FLSs were passaged three to five times before being used and the RA-FLSs were confirmed using vimentin immunofluorescent staining as a homogenous population with purity >98% (**Supplementary Figure 1**).

CircRNA Microarray Analysis

Three different samples of RA-FLSs and OA-FLSs were used for microarray analysis, which was performed by Kangcheng Biotech Inc. (Shanghai, China). Briefly, RNase R (Epicentre Inc., Madison, WI, USA) was used to digest the total RNA, which removed linear RNAs, thus enriching circRNAs. An Arraystar Super RNA Labeling Kit (Arraystar Inc., Rockville, MD, USA), together with the random-priming method, was used to amplify and transcribe the enriched circRNAs into fluorescent circRNAs. Complementary DNA (cDNA) was synthesized and labeled before array hybridization. Then, the fluorescent circRNAs were hybridized to the Arraystar Human circRNA Microarray V2.0 (8 × 15K, Arraystar Inc.). Thereafter, the slides were washed and an Agilent Scanner G2505C (Agilent Technologies, Santa Clara, CA, USA) was used to scan the arrays. Analysis of the acquired array images was carried out using Agilent Feature Extraction software (version 11.0.1.1). The R software package (R version 3.1.2) was used for quantile normalization and subsequent data processing.

Quantitative Real-Time Polymerase Chain Reaction (qRT-PCR)

Total RNA was obtained from cultured cells using the TRIzol reagent (Takara, Shiga, Japan), according to the manufacturer's instructions, and reverse transcribed into cDNA. The qPCR step was carried out using the cDNA as the template and SYBR Premix DimerEraser (Takara) with the ABI7500 system (Applied Biosystems, Foster City, CA, USA). Relative expression was calculated using the relative quantification ($2-\Delta\Delta Ct$)

TABLE 1 | Clinical characters and laboratory measures of the participants.

	RA (n = 9)	OA (n = 7)
Age (year, mean ± SD)	51.11 ± 2.72	51.71 ± 2.10
Gender (male/female)	2/7	2/5
Anti-CCP* (U/ml)	37.59 (7.80–1,121.50)	NA*
DAS28* (scores)	7.01 (3.08–7.71)	NA*

**DAS28, disease activity score in 28 joints; anti-CCP, anti-cyclic citrullinated peptide antibodies; NA, not available.*

method (27). *GAPDH* (encoding glyceraldehyde-3-phosphate dehydrogenase) was used as an internal control for circRNAs and mRNAs, and U6 was employed as an endogenous control for the miRNAs. **Supplementary Table S1** shows the details of the primers used for qRT-PCR.

Electrophoresis of Nucleic Acids

Agarose gel electrophoresis (4%) with Tris acetate-ethylenediaminetetraacetic acid running buffer (Thermo Fisher Scientific) was used to analyze genomic DNA (gDNA), PCR products, and cDNAs. Electrophoresis was performed at 110 V for 50 min to isolate DNA. A 20 bp DNA marker (Takara) was used and bands were examined by ultraviolet irradiation.

Fluorescence *In Situ* Hybridization (FISH)

FISH analysis of RA-FLSs used biotin-labeled probes specific to Circ_0088194 (GenePharma Co. Ltd., Shanghai, China). FISH (GenePharma) was used to detect the signals of these probes according to the manufacturer's instructions. 4, 6-diamidino-2-phenylindole (DAPI) was used to counterstain the nuclei. A Leica TCS SP2 AOBS confocal microscope (Leica Microsystems, Mannheim, Germany) was used to acquire images. The probe sequences are listed in **Supplementary Table S1**.

Western Blotting Analysis

Cultured RA-FLSs were lysed in ice-cold radioimmunoprecipitation assay buffer (BestBio, Shanghai, China) containing phosphatase inhibitors and a protease inhibitor cocktail (Sigma-Aldrich, St. Louis, MO, USA). The proteins in the cell lysates were separated using 10% SDS-PAGE, followed by electroblotting onto a polyvinylidene difluoride membrane (Millipore, Billerica, MA, USA). Incubation for 1 h at room temperature in Tris-buffered saline with Tween-20 and 5% skim milk was used to block the membrane. The membrane was then probed using primary antibodies recognizing rabbit matrix metalloproteinase 2 (MMP2) (1:5,000; Bioworld, Bloomington, MN, USA) and GAPDH (1:10,000; Bioworld) overnight at 4°C. Next day, the blot was incubated with horseradish peroxidase-conjugated secondary antibodies (1:10,000; Fdbio science, Hangzhou, China). The signals from the immunoreactive proteins were quantified using the Quantity One Software (Bio-Rad, Hercules, CA, USA).

Adenoviral Construction and Transduction

The adenoviral expression vectors for Circ_0088194 were constructed by Genepharma (Shanghai, China). To overexpress Circ_0088194, RA-FLSs were transduced with an adenoviral expression vector expressing Circ_0088194 or an empty adenoviral vector control following the manufacturer's protocol. QRT-PCR was used to determine the Circ_0088194 expression levels.

Oligonucleotides and siRNA Transfection

Small interfering RNAs (siRNAs), miRNA mimics, and miRNA inhibitors were obtained from the RiboBio (Guangzhou, China). Cells were transfected with 50 nM of Circ_0088194 siRNAs, *MMP2* siRNAs, miR-766-3p mimics, miR-766-3p inhibitors, or the corresponding controls using RNAiMAX (RiboBio) according to the manufacturer's instructions. All relevant sequences are listed in **Supplementary Table S1**.

Assays for Cell Migration and Invasion

For the migration assay, cells [1×10^4 in 200 µl of DMEM (serum free)] were seeded onto the top chamber of a Transwell insert, then DMEM with 10% FBS (600 µl) was added to the bottom chamber. The invasion assay started the same, except that in addition to the above, 50 µl of Matrigel (BD Biosciences, Franklin Lakes, NJ, USA) was layered onto the top chamber. The chambers were then incubated for 48 h. Thereafter, a cotton swab was used to remove the cells remaining on the on the surface of the upper membrane surface. Crystal violet was used to stain the cells that had crossed the membrane. Under a microscope, cells in six random fields were counted. These assays were carried out three times independently.

RNA Immunoprecipitation (RIP)

RIP experiments were conducted following the manufacturer's instructions of the Magna RIP RNA-Binding Protein Immunoprecipitation Kit (Millipore, Bedford, MA, USA). Briefly, MiR-766-3p mimics or the negative control were transfected into RA-FLSs. After 48 h, the RA-FLSs were lysed using RIPA buffer (Cell Signaling Technology, Danvers, MA, USA). Magnetic beads (Invitrogen, Waltham, MA, USA) were pre-incubated with anti-AGO2 antibodies or anti-rabbit IgG (Cell Signaling Technology) for 30 min, and then the lysates were immunoprecipitated using the beads, with rotation overnight at 4°C. Next day, the RNA was purified from the RNA–protein complexes bound to the beads, and then the levels of Circ_0088194 and miR-766-3p were determined using qRT-PCR followed by agarose gel electrophoresis.

Protein Array Analysis

RA-FLS cell lysate protein samples were assayed using a Human Cytokine Array GS440 (Cat#GSH-CAA-440, RayBiotech, Inc., Norcross, GA, USA) and processed according to the manufacturer's instructions. Briefly, the array slide was incubated with 65 µl of RA-FLS cell lysate overnight at 4°C. The glass array slide was equilibrated to room temperature on the following day, and washed extensively before incubating with an array-specific biotinylated antibody cocktail for 2 h. Unbound antibody was washed away, and the slide was developed for 1 h with Cy3-equivalent dye-conjugated streptavidin. Images were captured using an InnoScan 300 Microarray Scanner (Innopsys, Chicago, IL, USA), and positive clones were identified using the ScanArray Express analysis software (PerkinElmer, Boston, MA, USA). To minimize false positive hits, each sample was screened twice and only the hits that appeared in both screens were analyzed. In this manner, a unique antibody profile was generated for each sample. Experiments were carried out in duplicate.

Bioinformatic Analysis

Potential miRNA targets were predicted using three publicly available databases: TargetScan, miRanda (http://www.microrna.org/microrna/home.do), and circular RNA interactome (https://

circinteractome.nia.nih.gov). Targets were accepted only when they appeared in all three databases.

Dual-Luciferase Reporter Assay

The Circ_0088194 segment and a fragment of *MMP2* mRNA were synthesized from either mutant (MUT) or wild-type (WT) seed regions and cloned into the psiCHECK-2 vector (Promega, Madison, WI, USA). To generate mutant Circ_0088194 sequences, 11 nucleotides of the seed region were changed (WT seed sequence: 5′-CTGT ... GCTGGAG-3′, MUT seed sequence: 5′-GACA ... CGACCTC-3′). To generate the mutant *MMP2* mRNA sequence, we mutated five nucleotides of the seed region (WT seed sequence: 5′-CTGGA-3′; MUT seed sequences: 5′-GACCT-3′). RA-FLSs (1×10^5) were transfected with either WT or MUT Circ_0088194, miR-766-3p mimics or mimics control, and WT or MUT *MMP2* mRNA, using Lipofectamine 2000 (Thermo Fisher Scientific). After induction for 48 h, luciferase activity was assessed using a dual-luciferase reporter kit (Promega).

Measurement of m^{6}A-modified Circ_0088194

Quantification of m^{6}A-modified Circ_0088194 was achieved using methylated RNA immunoprecipitation. An aliquot (1.5 μg) of anti-m^{6}A antibody (Santa Cruz Biotechnology, Santa Cruz, CA, USA) or anti-IgG antibody (Santa Cruz Biotechnology) was incubated with protein A/G magnetic beads overnight at 4°C. An aliquot (100 ng) of total RNA and m^{6}A spike-in control mixture were added to 300 μl of an IP buffer (50 mM Tris-HCl, pH 7.4, 150 mM NaCl, 0.1% NP40, 40 U/μl RNase Inhibitor) containing 2 μg of anti-m^{6}A rabbit polyclonal antibody. RNA was eluted using elution buffer, purified using phenol-chloroform extraction, and subjected to qRT-PCR analysis.

Immunofluorescent Staining

RA-FLSs were fixed for 20 min using 4% paraformaldehyde, and then permeabilized for 5 min at room temperature using 0.2% Triton X-100. The cells were then washed and blocked for 1 h at room temperature using 10% normal goat serum (BioSS, Beijing, China), followed by incubation at 4°C overnight with antibodies recognizing vimentin (1:100). Next day, the cells were washed with phosphate buffered saline three times, followed by incubation for 1 h at room temperature with goat anti-rabbit IgG/Alexa Fluor 647 antibodies (1:200). Nuclei were counterstained with DAPI and images were acquired on a Leica TCS SP2 AOBS confocal microscope (Leica Microsystems).

Statistical Analysis

All experiments were carried out three times. Data are shown as the mean ± the standard deviation (SD). For comparisons between two groups or among multiple groups, we used Student's t-test and one-way analysis of variance (ANOVA), respectively. Spearman rank correlation was used to analyze the association of Circ_0088194 expression with disease activity. All statistical analyses were performed using the SPSS 20.0 software (IBM Corp. Armonk, NY, USA). $P < 0.05$ was considered statistically significant.

RESULTS

Expression Profile of Circular RNAs in OA-FLSs and RA-FLSs

FLSs samples from three patients with RA and samples from three age- and sex-matched patients with OA were subjected to microarray analysis of circRNAs to assess their expression (**Supplementary Figure S2**). Hierarchical clustering showed variations in circRNA expression between RA-FLSs and OA-FLSs (**Figure 1A**). Seven circRNAs were identified as being differentially expressed (fold change > 2.5 and $p < 0.05$) between RA-FLSs and OA-FLSs (**Table 2**). Next, we selected exonic circRNAs that exhibited >3-fold change ($p < 0.05$) and detected their expression levels in nine RA-FLSs and seven OA-FLSs to verify the microarray results. The results showed that the expression levels of Circ_0088194 and Circ_0088200 were elevated in RA-FLSs compared with those in OA-FLSs, while the expression levels of Circ_0012103 and Circ_0034953 did not differ between the two cell populations (**Figure 1B**). These differentially expressed circRNAs between RA-FLSs and OA-FLSs may have potential functions in RA progression.

Circ_0088194 Is Highly Expressed in the Cytoplasm of RA-FLSs and Correlated With the Disease Activity Score in 28 Joints

The expression levels of Circ_0088194 were the highest among the differentially expressed circRNAs in RA-FLSs compared with that in OA-FLSs (**Figure 1B**). Therefore, Circ_0088194 was chosen for further investigation. The gene encoding this circRNA is located at chr9:117798376–117808961 and this circRNA is formed by the reverse splicing of exons 17 to 21 of the tenascin C (*TNC*) gene (**Figure 1C**). We found that the expression levels of *TNC* were downregulated significantly in RA-FLSs compared with those in OA-FLSs (**Figure 1D**). The existence of Circ_0088194 was confirmed in numerous circRNA databases. According to the circBase database (http://circrna.org/cgi-bin/singlerecord.cgi?id=hsa_circ_0088194), Circ_0088194 exists in many tissue and cell types, such as normal human epidermal keratinocytes. We then used Sanger sequencing to confirm the head-to-tail splicing (formed from a 5′-end splice site and the corresponding 3′-end site of exons) using the Circ_0088194 qRT-PCR product, which was identified by its expected size (**Figure 1C**).

To rule out the possibility that genomic rearrangements or trans-splicing caused the head-to-tail splicing, two groups of primers were designed: Divergent primers were used to amplify Circ_0088194, and convergent primers were used to amplify the *TNC* mRNA. The cDNA and gDNA samples were used as templates for qRT-PCR. Using the divergent primers, we could amplify Circ_0088194 using the cDNA as a template, but not using the gDNA (**Figure 1E**). To assess the correlation between Circ_0088194 expression levels and RA disease activity in nine RA-FLS samples, Spearman's rank correlation was used. We found that the Circ_0088194 levels correlated positively with the disease activity score in 28 joints (DAS28) ($r = 0.683$, $p = 0.043$) (**Figure 1F**). Moreover, a FISH assay revealed that Circ_0088194 was localized mostly in the cytoplasm of RA-FLSs, but not in the nucleus (**Figure 1G**). Thus, Circ_0088194 is associated with RA disease severity and is highly expressed in the cytoplasm of RA-FLSs.

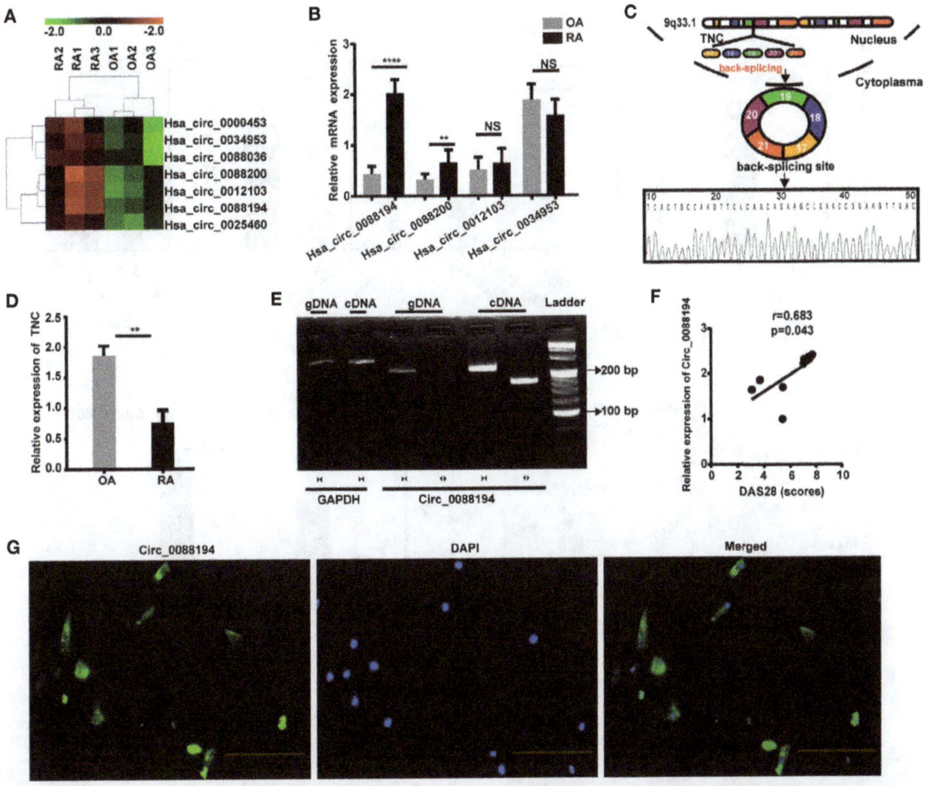

FIGURE 1 | Circ_0088194 is upregulated in RA-FLSs. **(A)** Hierarchical clustering analysis of differentially expressed CircRNAs between RA-FLSs and OA-FLSs. **(B)** QRT-PCR was used to detect the circRNA expression levels in nine RA-FLSs and seven OA-FLSs. (RA-FLSs = 9, OA-FLSs = 7). **(C)** Schematic illustration of how the Circ_0088194 is back-spliced from tenascin C (*TNC*) exons 17 to 21. The existence of Circ_0088194 was validated using qRT-PCR, followed by Sanger sequencing. **(D)** The *TNC* mRNA expression level, as detected using qRT-PCR in nine RA-FLSs and seven OA-FLSs. (RA-FLSs = 9, OA-FLSs = 7). **(E)** Divergent primers could amplify Circ_0088194 from cDNA but not from gDNA. **(F)** Circ_0088194 expression in RA-FLSs correlated positively with the RA disease activity score in 28 joints (DAS28 score). (n = 9; r = 0.683, $P = 0.043$). **(G)** Circ_0088194 showed a predominantly cytoplasmic localization upon RNA FISH. Scale bar, 500 μm. Data are shown as mean ± SD. NS, not significant. **indicates $p < 0.01$, and ****indicates $p < 0.0001$.

TABLE 2 | Microarray analysis of dysregulated circRNAs in three RA patients compared with three OA patients.

CircRNA	P-value	Fold change	Regulation	CircRNA type	Gene Symbol
Hsa_circ_0088200	0.027778	3.503261	up	exonic	*TNC*
Hsa_circ_0012103	0.018074	3.401054	up	exonic	*ST3GAL3*
Hsa_circ_0034953	0.023194	3.202578	up	exonic	*TUBGCP4*
Hsa_circ_0088194	0.015054	3.095609	up	exonic	*TNC*
Hsa_circ_0000453	0.03798	2.733945	up	antisense	*BCL7A*
Hsa_circ_0088036	0.048633	2.673338	up	exonic	*SUSD1*
Hsa_circ_0025460	0.004475	2.601944	up	exonic	*YBX3*

Circ_0088194 Promotes RA-FLS Migration and Invasion

To evaluate the functions of Circ_0088194 in human RA-FLSs, an adenoviral vector encoding Circ_0088194 was constructed and three siRNAs targeting the junction sites of Circ_0088194 were designed. Circ_0088194 expression in RA-FLSs increased significantly after transduction with adenoviral vector expressing Circ_008819 (**Figure 2A**). The expression levels of Circ_0088194 decreased significantly after transfection with siRNAs targeting Circ_0088194 (**Figure 2B**). Interestingly, overexpression or knockdown of Circ_0088194 did not affect *TNC* mRNA levels (**Figure 2C**). However, overexpression of Circ_0088194 significantly promoted the migration and invasion of RA-FLSs (**Figures 2D, E**). Conversely, knockdown of Circ_0088194 significantly inhibited RA-FLS migration and invasion (**Figures 2F, G**). Taken together, these results indicated that Circ_0088194 promotes the migration and invasion of RA-FLSs.

Circ_0088194 Regulates MMP2 Expression in RA-FLSs

To investigate how Circ_0088194 promotes RA-FLS invasion, we performed a protein array analysis in RA-FLSs that overexpressed

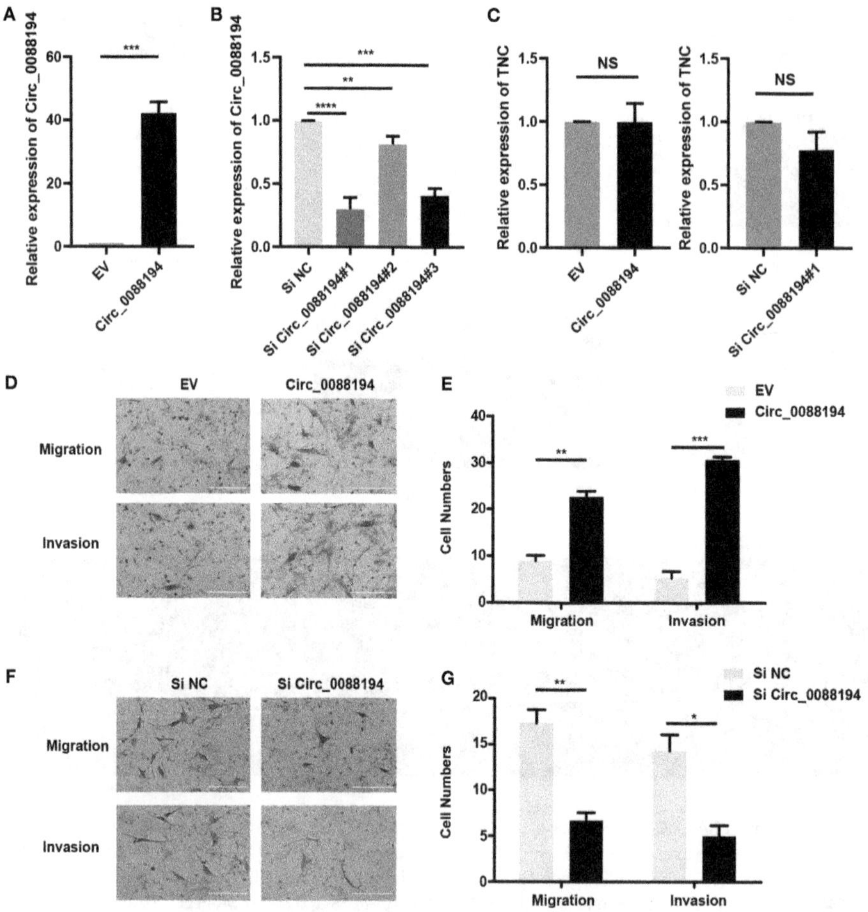

FIGURE 2 | Circ_0088194 promotes RA-FLS migration and invasion. **(A)** RA-FLSs were infected with adenovirus expressing Circ_0088194 or with the empty vector (EV). The expression levels of Circ_0088194 were detected using qRT-PCR. **(B)** RA-FLSs were transfected with three Circ_0088194 siRNAs or the negative control (NC). The Circ_0088194 expression level was measured using qRT-PCR **(C)** RA-FLSs were infected with adenovirus expressing Circ_0088194 or Circ_0088194#1 siRNA, respectively. The Tenascin C (*TNC*) expression level was measured using qRT-PCR. **(D, E)** Transwell migration and Matrigel invasion assays were used to evaluate the migratory and invasive activity of RA-FLSs. RA-FLSs were infected with adenovirus expressing Circ_0088194 or the EV. Scale bar, 500 μm. **(F, G)** RA-FLSs transfected with Circ_0088194#1 siRNA, or NC. Transwell migration and Matrigel invasion assays were used to evaluate the migratory and invasive activity of RA-FLSs. Scale bar, 500 μm. Data are shown as mean ± SD. NS, not significant. *indicates $p < 0.05$, **indicates $p < 0.01$, ***indicates $p < 0.001$, and ****indicates $p < 0.0001$.

Circ_0088194. The protein array analysis revealed that the levels of nine proteins were downregulated, while four proteins were upregulated in cells overexpressing Circ_0088194 (fold change > 3, $p < 0.05$) (**Table 3**). Furthermore, qRT-PCR was used to analyze the mRNA expression of three upregulated proteins (fold change > 4 and $p < 0.05$): Tumor necrosis factor-α (TNF-α) converting enzyme (TACE), matrix metalloproteinase 2 (MMP2), and platelet derived growth factor subunit AA (PDGF-AA), all of which might promote RA-FLS invasion. The results showed that only MMP2 levels, and not TACE or PDGF-AA, levels, increased in RA-FLSs after Circ_0088194 overexpression (**Figure 3A**). Moreover, western blotting analysis confirmed the elevated MMP2 levels in Circ_0088194-overexpressing RA-FLSs (**Figure 3B**). In addition, western blotting and qRT-PCR showed that knockdown of Circ_0088194 reduced the expression of MMP2 (**Figures 3C, D**).

TABLE 3 | Protein array analysis of dysregulated proteins in three overexpressing Circ_0088194 RA-FLSs compared with three control RA-FLSs.

Proteins	Fold change
Tumor necrosis factor α converting enzyme	5.53
Matrix metalloproteinase 2	5.05
Platelet derived growth factor subunit AA	4.96
A disintegrin and metalloproteinase 9	3.03
Fibroblast growth factor 6	0.29
Interleukin-1 receptor antagonist	0.28
Transferrin	0.28
Fibroblast growth factor 4	0.26
Bone morphogenetic protein 9	0.25
Interferon-γ-inducible protein 10	0.23
Ectodysplasin A2 receptor	0.20
Albumin	0.15
C-C motif chemokine ligand 16	0.14

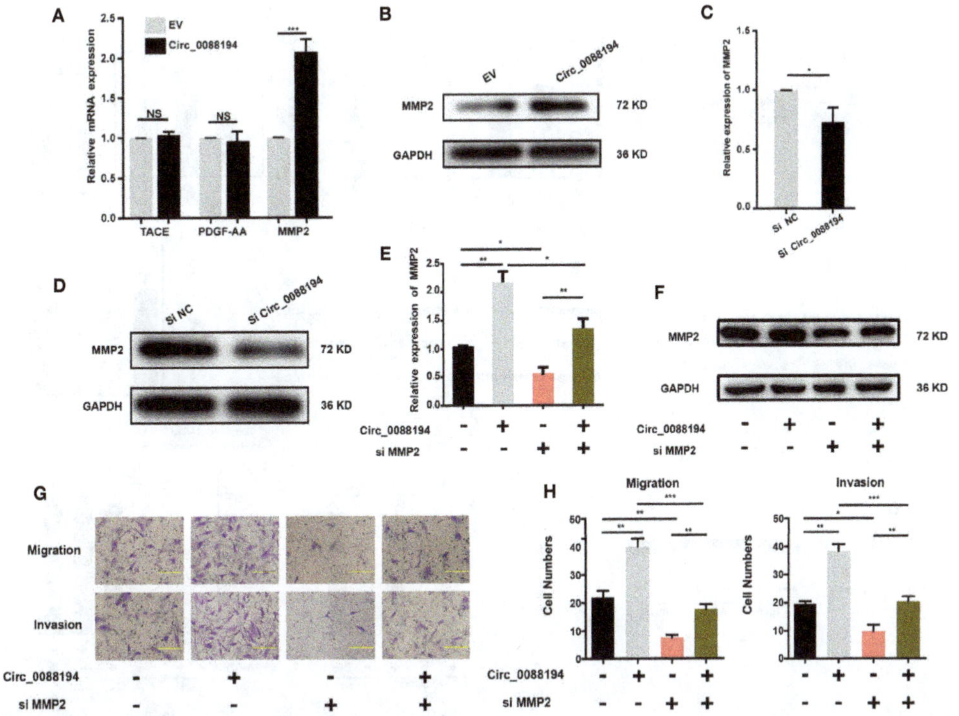

FIGURE 3 | MMP2 expression in RA-FLSs is regulated by Circ_0088194. **(A)** Adenovirus expressing Circ_0088194 or empty vector (EV) were transfected into RA-FLSs. QRT-PCR determined tumor necrosis factor-α converting enzyme (*TACE*), platelet derived growth factor subunit AA (*PDGF-AA*), and matrix metalloproteinase 2 (*MMP2*) mRNA levels. **(B)** Adenovirus expressing Circ_0088194 or EV were transfected into RA-FLSs. Western blotting was used to detect MMP2 expression. **(C, D)** The *MMP2* mRNA and protein expression levels were examined in RA-FLSs transfected with Circ_0088194#1 siRNAs or the negative control (NC). **(E, F)** Western blotting and qRT-PCR detection of *MMP2* expression. RA-FLSs were co-transfected with the adenovirus expressing Circ_0088194 or MMP2 siRNA. **(G, H)** Transwell migration and Matrigel invasion assays were used to evaluate the migratory and invasive activity of RA-FLSs. Adenovirus expressing Circ_0088194 or MMP2 siRNA were co-transfected into RA-FLSs. Scale bar, 500 μm. Data are shown as mean ± SD. NS, not significant. *indicates $p < 0.05$, **indicates $p < 0.01$, and ***indicates $p < 0.001$.

MMP2 is one of the most important proteases that mediate fibrillar collagen degradation. Several studies have indicated that MMP2 promotes the migration and invasion of glioma cells (28), lung cancer cells (29), and RA-FLSs (30, 31). Thus, we sought to determine whether Circ_0088194 promotes RA-FLSs migration and invasion by increasing MMP2 expression. Downregulation of MMP2 decreased the expression level of MMP2 induced by overexpression of Circ_0088194 (**Figures 3E, F**). Consistently, we found that inhibition of MMP2 in RA-FLSs blocked Circ_0088194 overexpression-induced migration and invasion (**Figures 3G, H**). Taken together, these results showed that Circ_0088194 promotes the migration and invasion of RA-FLSs at least partly dependent on MMP2.

Circ_0088194 Sponges miR-766-3p in RA-FLSs

It has been reported that CircRNAs can regulate gene expression *via* their miRNA responsive elements (MREs), which function as miRNA sponges in the cytoplasm (32). Circ_0088194 is localized mostly in the cytoplasm of RA-FLSs and bioinformatic analysis using three publicly available databases (TargetScan, miRanda, and circular RNA interactome) indicated that miR-766-3p and miR-635 might bind to Circ_0088194 and the 3′-untranslated region (UTR) of *MMP2* mRNA (**Figure 4A**). This led us to hypothesize that Circ_0088194 functions as a miRNA sponge to promote MMP2 expression in RA-FLSs. Firstly, we found that miR-766-3p expression increased in RA-FLSs after Circ_0088194 knockdown, while miR-766-3p expression decreased when Circ_0088194 was overexpressed (**Figure 4B**). However, the expression of miR-635 did not change after Circ_0088194 overexpression or knockdown (**Figure 4C**). Furthermore, we performed dual-luciferase assays to confirm the binding between Circ_0088194 and miR-766-3p (**Figures 4D, E**). The results showed that miR-766-3p mimics decreased the luciferase activity of the wild-type Circ_0088194 vector, but not that of the mutant Circ_0088194 vector (**Figure 4F**). A previous study indicated that miRNAs bind to MREs in an Argonaute 2 (AGO2)-dependent manner (33). Thus, we performed an RNA immunoprecipitation (RIP) experiment using anti-AGO2 antibodies to confirm the direct binding between miR-766-3p and Circ_0088194. Indeed, Circ_0088194 and miR-766-3p were enriched in the AGO2 immunoprecipitates relative to the IgG immunoprecipitates (**Figures 4G, I**). Importantly, we observed that overexpression of Circ_0088194 with mutated miR-766-3p binding sites had no significant effect on the migration and invasion

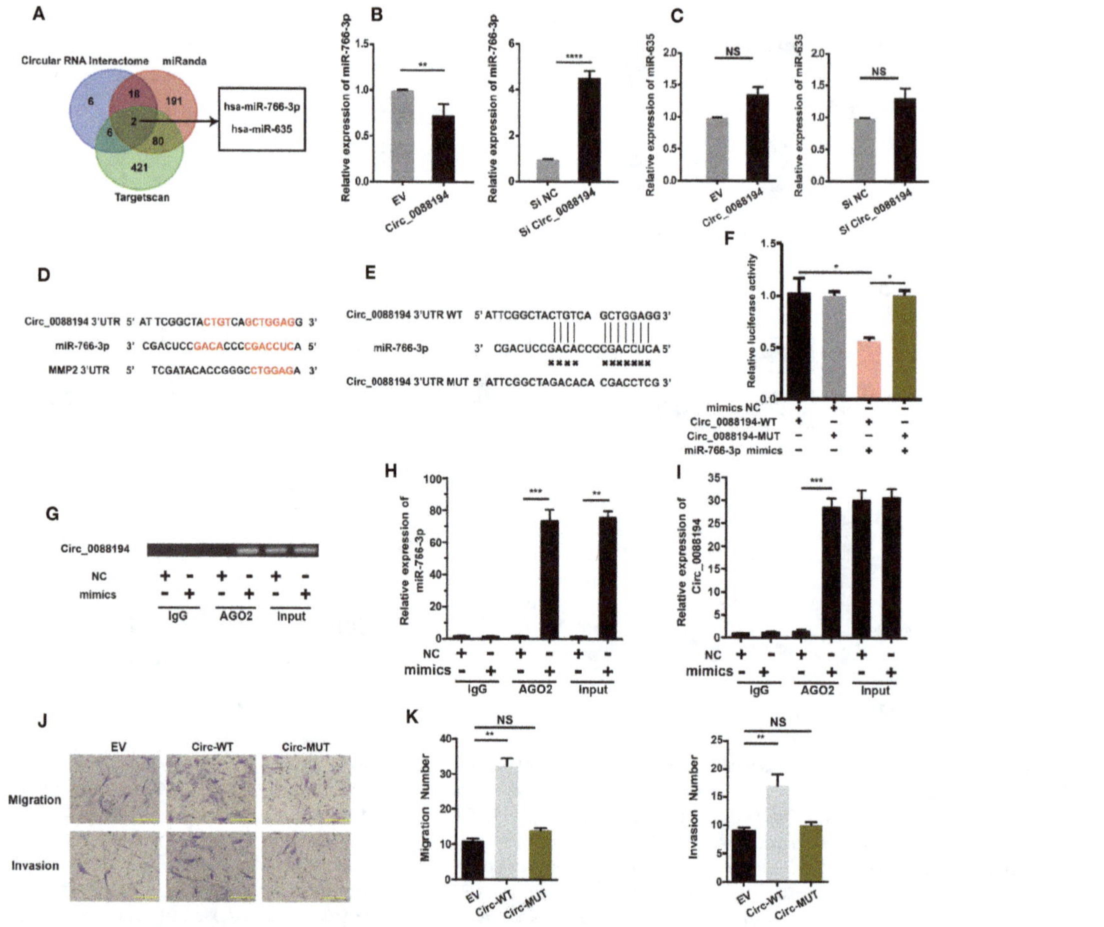

FIGURE 4 | Circ_0088194 act as sponge of miR-766-3p in RA-FLSs. **(A)** Schematic illustration showing the identification of two miRNAs, hsa-miR-766-3p and hsa-miR-635, predicted from three available databases (miRanda, circular RNA interactome, and Targetscan). **(B, C)** QRT-PCR determination of the expression of miR-766-3p **(B)** and miR-635 **(C)** in RA-FLSs. The cells were transfected with adenovirus expressing Circ_0088194 or Circ_0088194#1 siRNA. **(D)** The miR-766-3p MREs in the sequences of Circ_0088194 and *MMP2* as identified using bioinformatic analysis. **(E)** Wild-type (WT) or mutant (MUT) miR-766-3p target sequences of Circ_0088194. **(F)** The miR-766-3p mimics reduced the luciferase activities of WT not MUT Circ_0088194 reporter genes, as assessed using dual-luciferase reporter assays. **(G)** RA-FLSs were transfected with the miR-766-3p mimics or the negative control. Anti-AGO2 RIP was used to investigate AGO2 binding to Circ_0088194 and miR-766-3p; IgG was used as a negative control. **(H, I)** The expression levels of Circ_0088194 and miR-766-3p, as detected using qRT-PCR. **(J, K)** The migratory and invasive activities of RA-FLSs were evaluated by Transwell migration and Matrigel invasion assays. RA-FLSs were transfected with the adenovirus encoding Circ_0088194 or the adenovirus encoding Circ_0088194 with mutated miR-766-3p binding sites. Scale bar, 500 μm. Data are shown as mean ± SD. NS, not significant. *indicates $p < 0.05$, **indicates $p < 0.01$, ***indicates $p < 0.001$, and ****indicates $p < 0.0001$.

of RA-FLSs (**Figures 4J, K**). Collectively, our findings suggested that Circ_0088194 acts as a sponge for miR-766-3p.

MiR-766-3p Inhibits the Invasion and Migration of RA-FLSs

The impact of miR-766-3p mimics on *MMP2* expression and RA-FLS migration and invasion was studied by transfecting RA-FLSs cells with miR-766-3p mimics or inhibitors, respectively. Transfection of miR-766-3p mimics (**Figure 5A**) reduced the expression of *MMP2* mRNA and protein in RA-FLSs (**Figure 5B**). Conversely, transfection of miR-766-3p inhibitors increased the expression of *MMP2* mRNA and protein (**Figure 5C**). Next, we constructed luciferase reporter plasmids containing the WT 3′-UTR of the *MMP2* mRNA and a version of the 3′-UTR of the *MMP2* mRNA in which the miR-766-3p binding sites were mutated (**Figure 5D**). The results demonstrated that in the presence of the miR-766-3p mimics, the luciferase activity from the WT construct decreased. However, the mimics had any effect on the luciferase activity from the MUT construct (**Figure 5E**). These results indicated that *MMP2* is a target of miR-766-3p. Importantly, Transwell assays revealed that overexpression of miR-766-3p reduced RA-FLS migration and invasion (**Figure 5F**); while the miR-766-3p inhibitors increased RA-FLS migration and invasion (**Figure 5G**). Thus miR-766-3p was confirmed to reduce *MMP2* expression and inhibit the migration and invasion of RA-FLSs.

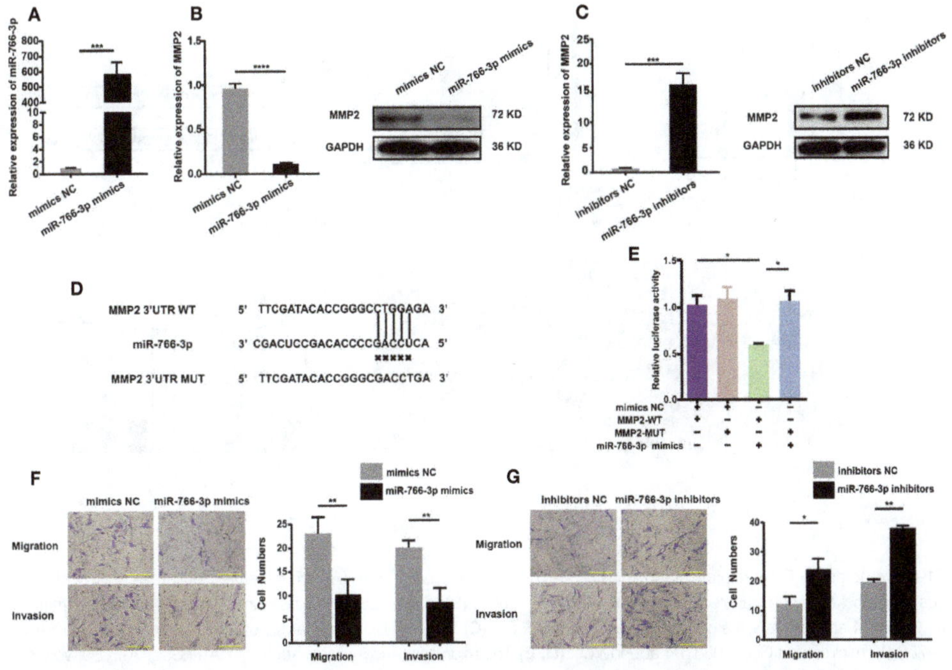

FIGURE 5 | MiR-766-3p inhibits RA-FLS migration and invasion. **(A)** RA-FLSs were transfected with the miR-766-3p mimics or the negative control (NC) at a final concentration of 50 nM. The expression level of miR-766-3p was determined using qRT-PCR. **(B)** QRT-PCR and Western blotting determination of *MMP2* expression in RA-FLSs. RA-FLSs were transfected with miR-766-3p mimics. **(C)** QRT-PCR and Western blotting detection of MMP2 expression in RA-FLSs. RA-FLSs were transfected with miR-766-3p inhibitors. **(D)** Wild-type (WT) or mutant (MUT) miR-766-3p target sequences in the *MMP2* 3′ UTR. **(E)** The miR-766-3p mimics reduced the luciferase activities of WT but not MUT *MMP2* reporter gene, as detected using dual-luciferase reporter assays. **(F)** Assays of RA-FLSs migration and invasion in cells transfected with miR-766-3p mimics. Scale bar, 500 μm. **(G)** Assays of RA-FLSs migration and invasion in cells transfected with miR-766-3p inhibitors. Scale bar, 500 μm. Data are shown as mean ± SD. *indicates $p < 0.05$, **indicates $p < 0.01$, ***indicates $p < 0.001$, and ****indicates $p < 0.0001$.

Circ_0088194 Promotes RA-FLSs Migration and Invasion *via* the miR-766-3p/MMP2 Axis

To test whether Circ_0088194 promotes *MMP2* expression by sponging miR-766-3p, we performed dual-luciferase reporter assays. The result showed that the miR-766-3p mimics reduced the luciferase activities from the reporter plasmid containing the potential binding sequence of Circ_0088194-WT or MMP2-WT (**Figure 4F**, **5E**). However, luciferase activities were not affected when mutant Circ_0088194-MUT and MMP2-MUT were used. Circ_0088194 overexpression increased the luciferase activity of MMP2-WT relative to the corresponding MMP2-MUT. Interestingly, when the miR-766-3p mimics were co-transfected, the increased luciferase activity from MMP2-WT in response to Circ_0088194 overexpression was abrogated (**Figure 6A**). MiR-766-3p mimic co-transfection blocked the upregulation of the *MMP2* mRNA and protein levels induced by Circ_0088194 overexpression in RA-FLSs (**Figures 6B, C**). Consistently, transfection of Circ_0088194 promoted RA-FLSs migration and invasion, which could be blocked by co-transfection with miR-766-3p mimics (**Figures 6D, E**). Taken together, these results indicated that Circ_0088194 regulates the expression of *MMP2* by sponging miR-766-3p, thereby promoting migration and invasion.

The m^{6}A Modification of Circ_0088194 Exists in RA-FLSs

The m^{6}A modification occurs in circRNAs as a mechanism to drive translation initiation (34, 35). Using the SRAMP website (http://www.cuilab.cn/sramp), we predicted the m^{6}A modification sites on Circ_0088194. Next, we verified the mRNA levels of four essential components of the m^{6}A methylase complex: alkB homolog 5 (ALKBH5), methyltransferase-like 14 (METTL14), fat mass and obesity associated protein (FTO), and methyltransferase-like 3 (METTL3), in RA-FLSs and OA-FLSs using qRT-PCR. The mRNA levels of *METTL3* and *ALKBH5* in RA-FLSs were markedly higher than those in OA-FLSs (**Figure 7A**). However, the *METTL14* and *FTO* expression levels did not differ between OA-FLSs and RA-FLSs. To test whether the m^{6}A modification of Circ_0088194 differed in RA-FLSs compared with that in OA-FLSs control cells, we performed methylated RNA immunoprecipitation using the rabbit anti-m^{6}A polyclonal antibody to enrich m^{6}A-modified total RNA, followed by qRT-PCR of Circ_0088194. We found that the relative contents of m^{6}A-modified Circ_0088194 did not differ between RA-FLSs and OA-FLSs (**Figure 7B**). These results suggested a negligible effect of this modification on Circ_0088194's activity in miR-766-3p binding and *MMP2* expression.

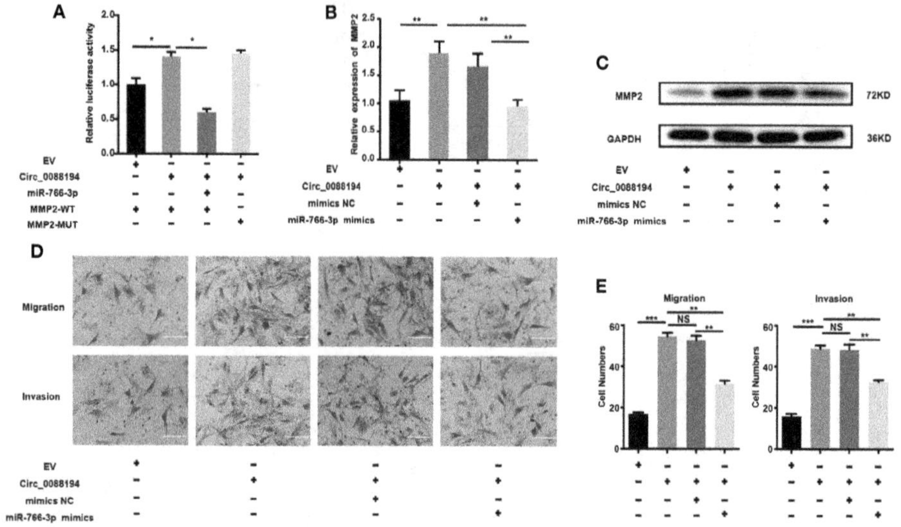

FIGURE 6 | Circ_0088194 promotes RA-FLSs migration and invasion *via* miR-766-3p/MMP2 axis. **(A)** The increased luciferase activity of WT-MMP2 treated with Circ_0088194 adenovirus was blocked by co-transfection with miR-766-3p mimics. **(B)** In RA-FLSs, the *MMP2* mRNA levels were determined using qRT-PCR. MiR-766-3p mimics and Circ_0088194 adenovirus were co-transfected into RA-FLSs. **(C)** Western blotting analysis of MMP2 protein levels in RA-FLSs. RA-FLSs were co-transfected with miR-766-3p mimics and Circ_0088194 adenovirus. **(D, E)** The migratory and invasive ability of RA-FLSs. RA-FLSs were co-transfected with miR-766-3p mimics and Circ_0088194 adenovirus. Scale bar, 500 μm. Data are shown as mean ± SD. NS, not significant. *indicates $p < 0.05$, **indicates $p < 0.01$, and ***indicates $p < 0.001$.

DISCUSSION

Recently, thousands of circRNAs have been identified from mammalian transcriptomes, and dysregulation of circRNAs is involved in the pathogenesis of various diseases, including RA (36–38). However, the roles of circRNAs in RA-FLSs are largely unknown. In this study, we identified a novel circRNA, Circ_0088194, which was upregulated in RA-FLSs and correlated positively with the RA disease activity score in 28 joints. Overexpression of Circ_0088194 promoted the migration and invasion of RA-FLSs. Mechanistically, Circ_0088194 acted as a miRNA sponge to reduce the level of miR-766-3p, thereby relieving miR-766-3p's repressive effect on its target, MMP2, ultimately promoting migration and invasion. These results indicated that the Circ_0088194/miR-766-3p/MMP2 axis has an important function in regulating RA-FLS migration and invasion (**Figure 7C**).

Invasion and migration of RA-FLSs leads to cartilage degradation and subsequent bone destruction, which cause a high level of disability in patients with RA. Therefore, it is imperative to identify invasion-related factors and determine the molecular mechanisms of RA-FLS invasion and migration. Herein, molecular experiments showed that overexpression of Circ_0088194 promoted migration and invasion of RA-FLSs, while downregulation of Circ_0088194 had the reverse effect. Importantly, in RA, Circ_0088194 levels correlated with the disease activity score in 28 joints. These data implied that in RA-FLSs, Circ_0088194 might contribute to increased rheumatoid synovial aggression and hyperplasia, ultimately leading to joint destruction.

CircRNAs may play specific roles in cellular physiology, and several possible functions have been proposed, including miRNA sponges (33), protein binding (39), and regulation of translation and translation into proteins (40). When acting as miRNA sponges, MREs in circRNAs reduce the levels of endogenous miRNAs capable of binding to their target mRNAs, thereby increasing mRNA translation, which is the most important and frequently reported function of circRNAs. For example, circRNA ciRS-7, which contains 74 binding sites for miR-7, was the first circRNA to be established as a miRNA sponge and has been reported to participate in the development of many cancers (41). In this study, we found that Circ_0088194 promoted RA-FLSs migration and invasion by increasing the expression of invasion-related gene, *MMP2*. Bioinformatic analyses demonstrated that *MMP2* and Circ_0088194 share an MRE for miR-766-3p. Therefore, we hypothesized that Circ_0088194 promotes RA-FLS migration and invasion *via* the miR-766-3p/MMP2 axis. To verify our hypothesis, luciferase reporter assays confirmed the direct interaction between Circ_0088194 and miR-766-3p, and between miR-766-3p and *MMP2*. Importantly, miR-766-3p reverses the ability of Circ_0088194 to upregulate *MMP2* expression and promote RA-FLS migration and invasion. Thus, we demonstrated that Circ_0088194 acts as a sponge toward miR-766-3p to promote RA-FLSs migration and invasion by upregulating *MMP2* expression at the post-transcription level. This consists with previous studies which showed knockdown of MMP2 reduced the invasion and migration of RA-FLSs (30, 42, 43).Moreover, MMP (including MMP-2) is considered as the primary therapy for RA (44, 45). However, the other study indicated that MMP-2 suppresses RA synovial fibroblast-mediated cartilage degradation; MMP-2 KO mice developed arthritis of greater clinical and histological severity than wild-type mice (46). Therefore, the role of MMP2 in

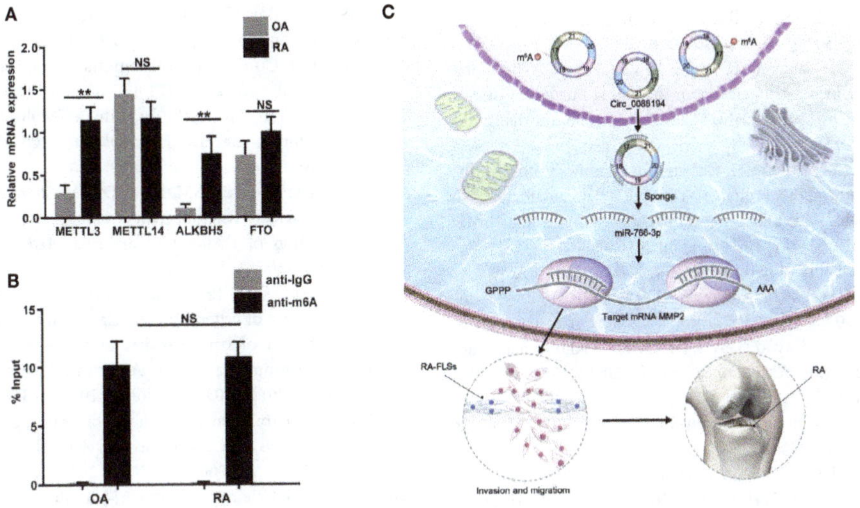

FIGURE 7 | Circ_0088194 m^{6}A modification in RA-FLSs. **(A)** QRT-PCR determined the mRNA level of four components of the m^{6}A methylase complex methyltransferase-like 3 (METTL3), alkB homolog 5 (ALKBH5), methyltransferase-like 14 (METTL14), and fat mass and obesity associated genes (FTO) in RA-FLSs and OA-FLSs. **(B)** Anti-m^{6}A antibody-enriched m^{6}A-modified total RNA immunoprecipitation followed by qRT-PCR determined the m^{6}A-modified Circ_0088194 levels in RA-FLSs and OA-FLSs. The negative control for immunoprecipitation comprised rabbit IgG. The percentages of input are shown. **(C)** A working model of the Circ_0088194/miR-766-3p/MMP2 signaling axis in the promotion of the migration and invasion of RA-FLSs and RA pathogenesis. Data are shown as mean ± SD. NS: not significant. **indicates $p < 0.01$.

the progression of RA-FLS is still controversial. We speculate that the varied roles of MMP2 in the progression of RA may be associated with the inconsistency of microenvironment and experimental conditions. Additionally, we cannot exclude the possibility that other pathways might also be involved Circ_0088194's effects in addition to the miR-766-3p/MMP2 axis, which might also play important roles in RA-FLSs progression. These the other potential functions of Circ_0088194 beyond acting as a miRNAs sponge in RA-FLSs merit further exploration.

A recent study showed that the m^{6}A modification on circRNAs mediate their stability by increasing circRNA association with YTH N6-methyladenosine RNA binding protein 2 (YTHDF2) in a heat-responsive protein 12 (HRSP12)-dependent manner (20). We found that upregulation of Circ_0088194 correlated with elevated RA-FLSs invasion and migration. Therefore, we suspected that the m^{6}A modification might affect the stability of Circ_0088194 and account for Cir_0088194 differences between RA-FLSs and OA-FLSs. The prediction website showed there are three methylation sites with high confidence on Circ_0088194. As expected, our study showed that the mRNA levels of two components from the m^{6}A methylase complex, METTL3 and ALKBH5, were significantly higher in RA-FLSs than in OA-FLSs. To our surprise, such differences did not affect the total amount of m^{6}A-modified Circ_0088194. These observations suggested that the elevated levels of Circ_0088194 in RA-FLSs compared with those in OA-FLSs might have resulted from different mechanisms to control Circ_0088194 production, such as Circ_0088194 alternative splicing, a hypothesis that requires further exploration.

To the best of our knowledge, this is the first report that Circ_0088194 acts as a pathogenic element in the progression of human RA by regulating the expression of collagenase MMP2 and promoting RA-FLS migration and invasion. However, we did not test this hypothesis in experimental RA models, and additional studies with large sample size and patients of different ethnicities and regions might be required. Our findings identified the Circ_0088194/miR-766-3p/MMP2 pathway as a novel therapeutic target to prevent and treat human RA. The significant positive correlation between the RA disease score and the RA-FLS Circ_0088194 contents supported our hypothesis.

ETHICS STATEMENT

The ethics committee of Southern Medical University approved the study and associated protocols (Guangzhou, China, NFEC-20120201). The patients/participants provided their written informed consent to participate in this study. Written informed consent was obtained from the individual(s) for the publication of any potentially identifiable images or data included in this article.

AUTHOR CONTRIBUTIONS

YC, QO, RL, SX, and DZ performed the molecular genetic analyses. MY, QO, and QH participated in experimental design and statistical analyses. YC drafted the manuscript, and G-PS edited the manuscript. All authors contributed to the article and approved the submitted version.

ACKNOWLEDGMENTS

The authors thank the donors who provided the specimens.

REFERENCES

1. Smolen JS, Aletaha D, McInnes IB. Rheumatoid arthritis. *Lancet* (2016) 388:2023–38. doi: 10.1016/S0140-6736(16)30173-8
2. Cross M, Smith E, Hoy D, Carmona L, Wolfe F, Vos T, et al. The global burden of rheumatoid arthritis: estimates from the global burden of disease 2010 study. *Ann Rheum Dis* (2014) 73:1316–22. doi: 10.1136/annrheumdis-2013-204627
3. Chen SY, Hsu WT, Chen YL, Chien CH, Chiang BL. Lymphocyte-activation gene 3(+) (LAG3(+)) forkhead box protein 3(-) (FOXP3(-)) regulatory T cells induced by B cells alleviates joint inflammation in collagen-induced arthritis. *J Autoimmun* (2016) 68:75–85. doi: 10.1016/j.jaut.2016.02.002
4. Bottini N, Firestein GS. Duality of fibroblast-like synoviocytes in RA: passive responders and imprinted aggressors. *Nat Rev Rheumatol* (2013) 9:24–33. doi: 10.1038/nrrheum.2012.190
5. Huber LC, Distler O, Tarner I, Gay RE, Gay S, Pap T. Synovial fibroblasts: key players in rheumatoid arthritis. *Rheumatol (Oxford)* (2006) 45:669–75. doi: 10.1093/rheumatology/kel065
6. Chen LL, Yang L. Regulation of circRNA biogenesis. *RNA Biol* (2015) 12:381–8. doi: 10.1080/15476286.2015.1020271
7. Qu S, Yang X, Li X, Wang J, Gao Y, Shang R, et al. Circular RNA: A new star of noncoding RNAs. *Cancer Lett* (2015) 365:141–8. doi: 10.1016/j.canlet.2015.06.003
8. Rybak-Wolf A, Stottmeister C, Glazar P, Jens M, Pino N, Giusti S, et al. Circular RNAs in the Mammalian Brain Are Highly Abundant, Conserved, and Dynamically Expressed. *Mol Cell* (2015) 58:870–85. doi: 10.1016/j.molcel.2015.03.027
9. Salzman J, Chen RE, Olsen MN, Wang PL, Brown PO. Cell-type specific features of circular RNA expression. *PLoS Genet* (2013) 9:e1003777. doi: 10.1371/journal.pgen.1003777
10. Jeck WR, Sorrentino JA, Wang K, Slevin MK, Burd CE, Liu J, et al. Circular RNAs are abundant, conserved, and associated with ALU repeats. *RNA* (2013) 19:141–57. doi: 10.1261/rna.035667.112
11. Lei M, Zheng G, Ning Q, Zheng J, Dong D. Translation and functional roles of circular RNAs in human cancer. *Mol Cancer* (2020) 19:30. doi: 10.1186/s12943-020-1135-7
12. Lim TB, Lavenniah A, Foo RS. Circles in the heart and cardiovascular system. *Cardiovasc Res* (2020) 116:269–78. doi: 10.1093/cvr/cvz227
13. Floris G, Zhang L, Follesa P, Sun T. Regulatory Role of Circular RNAs and Neurological Disorders. *Mol Neurobiol* (2017) 54:5156–65. doi: 10.1007/s12035-016-0055-4
14. Shen S, Wu Y, Chen J, Xie Z, Huang K, Wang G, et al. CircSERPINE2 protects against osteoarthritis by targeting miR-1271 and ETS-related gene. *Ann Rheum Dis* (2019) 78:826–36. doi: 10.1136/annrheumdis-2018-214786
15. Tan S, Sun D, Pu W, Gou Q, Guo C, Gong Y, et al. Circular RNA F-circEA-2a derived from EML4-ALK fusion gene promotes cell migration and invasion in non-small cell lung cancer. *Mol Cancer* (2018) 17:138. doi: 10.1186/s12943-018-0887-9
16. Zhu Z, Rong Z, Luo Z, Yu Z, Zhang J, Qiu Z, et al. Circular RNA circNHSL1 promotes gastric cancer progression through the miR-1306-3p/SIX1/vimentin axis. *Mol Cancer* (2019) 18:126. doi: 10.1186/s12943-019-1054-7
17. Jia G, Fu Y, He C. Reversible RNA adenosine methylation in biological regulation. *Trends Genet* (2013) 29:108–15. doi: 10.1016/j.tig.2012.11.003
18. Meyer KD, Jaffrey SR. The dynamic epitranscriptome: N6-methyladenosine and gene expression control. *Nat Rev Mol Cell Biol* (2014) 15:313–26. doi: 10.1038/nrm3785
19. Wang X, Lu Z, Gomez A, Hon GC, Yue Y, Han D, et al. N6-methyladenosine-dependent regulation of messenger RNA stability. *Nature* (2014) 505:117–20. doi: 10.1038/nature12730
20. Park OH, Ha H, Lee Y, Boo SH, Kwon DH, Song HK, et al. Endoribonucleolytic Cleavage of m(6)A-Containing RNAs by RNase P/MRP Complex. *Mol Cell* (2019) 74:494–507. doi: 10.1016/j.molcel.2019.02.034
21. Zhao X, Yang Y, Sun BF, Shi Y, Yang X, Xiao W, et al. FTO-dependent demethylation of N6-methyladenosine regulates mRNA splicing and is required for adipogenesis. *Cell Res* (2014) 24:1403–19. doi: 10.1038/cr.2014.151
22. Alarcon CR, Lee H, Goodarzi H, Halberg N, Tavazoie SF. N6-methyladenosine marks primary microRNAs for processing. *Nature* (2015) 519:482–5. doi: 10.1038/nature14281
23. Yoon KJ, Ringeling FR, Vissers C, Jacob F, Pokrass M, Jimenez-Cyrus D, et al. Temporal Control of Mammalian Cortical Neurogenesis by m(6)A Methylation. *Cell* (2017) 171:877–89. doi: 10.1016/j.cell.2017.09.003
24. Pan Y, Ma P, Liu Y, Li W, Shu Y. Multiple functions of m(6)A RNA methylation in cancer. *J Hematol Oncol* (2018) 11:48. doi: 10.1186/s13045-018-0590-8
25. Arnett FC, Edworthy SM, Bloch DA, McShane DJ, Fries JF, Cooper NS, et al. The American Rheumatism Association 1987 revised criteria for the classification of rheumatoid arthritis. *Arthritis Rheum* (1988) 31:315–24. doi: 10.1002/art.1780310302
26. Altman R, Asch E, Bloch D, Bole G, Borenstein D, Brandt K, et al. Development of criteria for the classification and reporting of osteoarthritis. Classification of osteoarthritis of the knee. Diagnostic and Therapeutic Criteria Committee of the American Rheumatism Association. *Arthritis Rheum* (1986) 29:1039–49. doi: 10.1002/art.1780290816
27. Livak KJ, Schmittgen TD. Analysis of relative gene expression data using real-time quantitative PCR and the 2(-Delta Delta C(T)) Method. *Methods* (2001) 25:402–8. doi: 10.1006/meth.2001.1262
28. Pereira MS, Celeiro SP, Costa AM, Pinto F, Popov S, de Almeida GC, et al. Loss of SPINT2 expression frequently occurs in glioma, leading to increased growth and invasion via MMP2. *Cell Oncol (Dordr)* (2020) 43:107–21. doi: 10.1007/s13402-019-00475-7
29. Wu DM, Deng SH, Liu T, Han R, Zhang T, Xu Y. TGF-beta-mediated exosomal lnc-MMP2-2 regulates migration and invasion of lung cancer cells to the vasculature by promoting MMP2 expression. *Cancer Med* (2018) 7:5118–29. doi: 10.1002/cam4.1758
30. Li G, Zhang Y, Qian Y, Zhang H, Guo S, Sunagawa M, et al. Interleukin-17A promotes rheumatoid arthritis synoviocytes migration and invasion under hypoxia by increasing MMP2 and MMP9 expression through NF-kappaB/HIF-1alpha pathway. *Mol Immunol* (2013) 53:227–36. doi: 10.1016/j.molimm.2012.08.018
31. Xue M, McKelvey K, Shen K, Minhas N, March L, Park SY, et al. Endogenous MMP-9 and not MMP-2 promotes rheumatoid synovial fibroblast survival, inflammation and cartilage degradation. *Rheumatol (Oxford)* (2014) 53:2270–9. doi: 10.1093/rheumatology/keu254
32. Chen LL. The biogenesis and emerging roles of circular RNAs. *Nat Rev Mol Cell Biol* (2016) 17:205–11. doi: 10.1038/nrm.2015.32
33. Hansen TB, Jensen TI, Clausen BH, Bramsen JB, Finsen B, Damgaard CK, et al. Natural RNA circles function as efficient microRNA sponges. *Nature* (2013) 495:384–8. doi: 10.1038/nature11993
34. Yang Y, Fan X, Mao M, Song X, Wu P, Zhang Y, et al. Extensive translation of circular RNAs driven by N(6)-methyladenosine. *Cell Res* (2017) 27:626–41. doi: 10.1038/cr.2017.31
35. Zhou C, Molinie B, Daneshvar K, Pondick JV, Wang J, Van Wittenberghe N, et al. Genome-Wide Maps of m6A circRNAs Identify Widespread and Cell-Type-Specific Methylation Patterns that Are Distinct from mRNAs. *Cell Rep* (2017) 20:2262–76. doi: 10.1016/j.celrep.2017.08.027
36. Ouyang Q, Wu J, Jiang Z, Zhao J, Wang R, Lou A, et al. Microarray Expression Profile of Circular RNAs in Peripheral Blood Mononuclear Cells from Rheumatoid Arthritis Patients. *Cell Physiol Biochem* (2017) 42:651–9. doi: 10.1159/000477883
37. Zheng F, Yu X, Huang J, Dai Y. Circular RNA expression profiles of peripheral blood mononuclear cells in rheumatoid arthritis patients, based on microarray chip technology. *Mol Med Rep* (2017) 16:8029–36. doi: 10.3892/mmr.2017.7638
38. Tang X, Wang J, Xia X, Tian J, Rui K, Xu H, et al. Elevated expression of ciRS-7 in peripheral blood mononuclear cells from rheumatoid arthritis patients. *Diagn Pathol* (2019) 14:11. doi: 10.1186/s13000-019-0783-7
39. Memczak S, Jens M, Elefsinioti A, Torti F, Krueger J, Rybak A, et al. Circular RNAs are a large class of animal RNAs with regulatory potency. *Nature* (2013) 495:333–8. doi: 10.1038/nature11928

40. Li Z, Huang C, Bao C, Chen L, Lin M, Wang X, et al. Exon-intron circular RNAs regulate transcription in the nucleus. *Nat Struct Mol Biol* (2015) 22:256–64. doi: 10.1038/nsmb.2959
41. Peng L, Yuan XQ, Li GC. The emerging landscape of circular RNA ciRS-7 in cancer (Review). *Oncol Rep* (2015) 33:2669–74. doi: 10.3892/or.2015.3904
42. Ma JD, Jing J, Wang JW, Yan T, Li QH, Mo YQ, et al. A novel function of artesunate on inhibiting migration and invasion of fibroblast-like synoviocytes from rheumatoid arthritis patients. *Arthritis Res Ther* (2019) 21:153. doi: 10.1186/s13075-019-1935-6
43. Shi DL, Shi GR, Xie J, Du XZ, Yang H. MicroRNA-27a Inhibits Cell Migration and Invasion of Fibroblast-Like Synoviocytes by Targeting Follistatin-Like Protein 1 in Rheumatoid Arthritis. *Mol Cells* (2016) 39:611–8. doi: 10.14348/molcells.2016.0103
44. Jackson C, Nguyen M, Arkell J, Sambrook P. Selective matrix metalloproteinase (MMP) inhibition in rheumatoid arthritis–targetting gelatinase A activation. *Inflamm Res* (2001) 50:183–6. doi: 10.1007/s000110050743
45. Martel-Pelletier J, McCollum R, Fujimoto N, Obata K, Cloutier JM, Pelletier JP. Excess of metalloproteases over tissue inhibitor of metalloprotease may contribute to cartilage degradation in osteoarthritis and rheumatoid arthritis. *Lab Invest* (1994) 70:807–15.
46. Itoh T, Matsuda H, Tanioka M, Kuwabara K, Itohara S, Suzuki R. The role of matrix metalloproteinase-2 and matrix metalloproteinase-9 in antibody-induced arthritis. *J Immunol* (2002) 169:2643–7. doi: 10.4049/jimmunol.169.5.2643

3

Current Understanding of Circular RNAs in Systemic Lupus Erythematosus

Hongjiang Liu [1,2], *Yundong Zou* [1], *Chen Chen* [1], *Yundi Tang* [1] *and Jianping Guo* [1*]

[1] Department of Rheumatology and Immunology, Peking University People's Hospital & Beijing Key Laboratory for Rheumatism Mechanism and Immune Diagnosis (BZ0135), Beijing, China, [2] Department of Rheumatology and Immunology, The People's Hospital of China Three Gorges University/The First People's Hospital of Yichang, Yichang, China

***Correspondence:**
Jianping Guo
jianping.guo@bjmu.edu.cn

Systemic lupus erythematosus (SLE) is a common and potentially fatal autoimmune disease that affects multiple organs. To date, its etiology and pathogenesis remains elusive. Circular RNAs (circRNAs) are a novel class of endogenous non-coding RNAs with covalently closed loop structure. Growing evidence has demonstrated that circRNAs may play an essential role in regulation of gene expression and transcription by acting as microRNA (miRNA) sponges, impacting cell survival and proliferation by interacting with RNA binding proteins (RBPs), and strengthening mRNA stability by forming RNA-protein complexes duplex structures. The expression patterns of circRNAs exhibit tissue-specific and pathogenesis-related manner. CircRNAs have implicated in the development of multiple autoimmune diseases, including SLE. In this review, we summarize the characteristics, biogenesis, and potential functions of circRNAs, its impact on immune responses and highlight current understanding of circRNAs in the pathogenesis of SLE.

Keywords: circRNAs, endogenous regulation, biological function, biomarker, systemic lupus erythematosus

INTRODUCTION

Systemic lupus erythematosus (SLE) is a chronic systemic autoimmune disease characterized by production of multiple autoantibodies and involvement of multi-systemic organ damage (1). Although genetic and environmental factors have been implicated in the development of SLE, its exact etiology and pathogenesis remain unclear (2). Furthermore, the early diagnosis and effective therapies for SLE have been a challenge, which maybe partly attributed to the poor understanding of the disease pathogenesis. Therefore, dissecting the molecular mechanisms underlying SLE pathogenesis will provide clues for identifying novel diagnostic markers and therapeutics for SLE patients. Recent evidence indicates that the non-coding RNAs (ncRNAs), such as the microRNAs (miRNAs), long non-coding RNAs (lncRNAs), and circular RNAs (circRNAs), can function as epigenetic factors and play important roles in the development and progression of SLE (3, 4). Among these non-coding RNAs, the circRNAs are the novel class of ncRNAs with covalently closed RNA circles by non-canonical backsplicing events (5). These circular RNAs are highly conserved, stable, and resistant to RNase (6, 7). Thus, the circRNAs could be considered as better biomarkers than the linear ncRNAs for diagnosis and management of diseases. In this review, we summarize circRNA biogenesis, classification, biological functions and its implication in immune responses and diseases, with a particular emphasis on the emerging roles of circRNAs in SLE.

CIRCRNA DISCOVERY

CircRNAs were first discovered in pathogens in 1976 (8). In the study, Sanger and colleagues characterized the structure for viroids, which are single-stranded and covalently closed circular RNA molecules. A few years later, a second study observed that circRNAs were existed in the cytoplasm of eukaryotic cell lines with an electron microscopy (9). Thereafter, a handful of circRNAs were reported in the early 1990 (10–12). However, these findings were not followed up, as at the time circRNAs were mainly considered to be byproducts generated by splicing error of pre-mRNA processing without significant biological effect (13). Until recent years, with the advance of high-throughput sequencing and bioinformatics algorithms, researchers have identified thousands of circRNAs in eukaryotes and found some circRNAs expressed in a tissue-specific manner with potential functions (14–16).

Since the landmark finding of CDR1as and circSry in 2013, which could function as microRNA sponge (17, 18), the circRNAs have become a novel hotspot in non-coding RNAs (19). Accumulating evidence has demonstrated that circRNAs are an abundant and conserved subclass of RNAs and are widely expressed in a cell-/tissue-specific, and development-dependent manner (15, 16, 20–22). As stated before, the circRNAs are distinguished from the linear RNAs by the structure of covalently closed loop lacking 5' cap and 3' poly-adenylated tails. This unique feature makes the circRNAs much more stable than their linear counterparts and resistant to degradation by exonuclease and RNases (6). Therefore, the circRNAs are proposed as novel and promising diagnostic biomarkers and potential therapeutic targets for diseases. So far, circRNAs have been reported to be involved in the pathogenesis of multiple diseases, such as neurological disorders, cardiovascular diseases, cancer, and chronic inflammatory and autoimmune diseases (23–26).

CIRCRNA BIOGENESIS AND CLASSIFICATION

Alternative splicing of RNA is a key event for gene expression in eukaryotes. Precursor mRNA (pre-mRNAs) is processed by the spliceosome to remove introns and thereby exons are rapidly linked to form a functional mature mRNA (**Figure 1A**). It was widely accepted that circRNAs are derived from canonical splice sites (15, 18, 27). When pre-mRNA catalyzing events are slowed down, the nascent RNAs may be directed to alternative paths that accelerate back-splicing (5, 28). CircRNAs are generated by back-splicing that joins a 5' splice donor to an upstream 3' splice acceptor site, thus forming a single-strand covalently closed loop (15, 18, 29, 30). However, the exact mechanisms by which the spliceosome selects certain exons to circularize are not completely elucidated. Jeck and colleagues proposed two models for exon-derived circRNA formation: "lariat-driven circularization" and "intron-pairing-driven circularization" (15, 29). In the lariat-driven circulating model (**Figure 1B**), exon-skipping is required and leads to an exon-containing lariat, which will then itself be internally processed to form exon-derived circRNAs (15, 29). In intro-pairing-driven circularization (**Figure 1C**), cyclization is prompted presumably by intronic motifs such ALU complementarity bordering the circularized exon(s), which may bring the two exons (or the ends of the same exon) into close proximity to form the loop (15, 29). Meanwhile, Zhang et al. reported a novel subclass of circRNAs

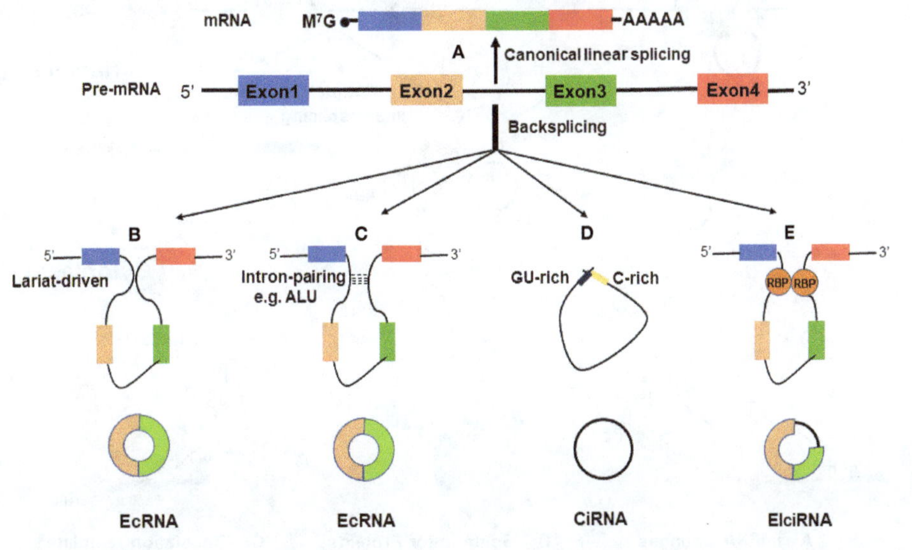

FIGURE 1 | Biogenesis of three major types of circRNAs. **(A)** A linear mRNA is formed by canonical splicing from pre-messenger RNA (pre-mRNA). **(B–E)** CircRNAs are generated by backsplicing from pre-mRNA. **(B)** Lariat-driven circularization, exon-skipping leads to an exon-containing lariat whose restricted structure facilitates circularization. **(C)** Intro-pairing-driven circularization is mediated by base-pairing between inverted repeat elements such as ALU complementarity. **(D)** CiRNA biogenesis is mainly dependent on GU-rich motif and C-rich sequence. **(E)** RNA-binding proteins (RBP) serving as trans-acting factors can bring two splicing sites close together to promote circularization.

originating from introns (31). Such intronic circRNA generated from the intronic lariat contains a 7-nucleotide GU-rich element at the 5' splice site and an 11-nucleotide C-rich element near the branchpoint site, which makes them resistant to the debranching enzyme and leads to the formation of an intro-derived circRNA (31) (**Figure 1D**). In some cases, if the intron between exons is retained, the cyclizing transcript tends to form exon-intron circRNAs (31, 32). In addition, some RNA binding proteins (RBPs) such as Quaking 1 (QKI) (33), muscleblind (MBL) (34), adenosine deaminase acting on RNA (ADAR) (35) and FUS (36) were reported to regulate the circRNA biogenesis (**Figure 1E**).

CircRNAs can be categorized into three major types based on their structural sequence: exonic circRNAs (EcRNAs), exon-intro circRNAs (ElciRNAs), and circular intronic RNAs (ciRNAs) (18, 31, 32). It has been observed that EcRNAs are predominantly localized in the cytoplasm, while ElciRNAs and ciRNAs are mainly restricted in the nucleus (18, 31, 32). EcRNAs are thought to be the most abundant circRNAs, which account for ~80% among currently discovered circRNAs (5, 37). In addition to the aforementioned types, it was reported that circRNAs can also be generated from intergenic genomic DNA (known as intergenic circRNAs) (18), the splicing of pre-tRNA [termed tRNA intronic circRNAs (tricRNAs)] (38), and from long ncRNAs (for example, circPINTexon2) (39).

CIRCRNA FUNCTIONS

In recent years, growing evidence indicates that circRNAs may play important roles in regulation of gene expression and participate in a series of pathophysiological processes (**Figure 2**).

CircRNAs Act as Competing Endogenous RNA or miRNA Sponges

MicroRNAs (miRNAs) are a class of endogenous, noncoding RNAs of approximately 22 nucleotides in length, and can play crucial regulatory roles in post-transcription by targeting mRNAs for cleavage or translational repression (40). It has been proposed that the competing endogenous RNAs (ceRNAs) including pseudogenes and long-chain non-coding RNA (lncRNA) can act as sponges for miRNAs through their binding sites of miRNA recognition elements (MREs) (41–43). Subsequently, Hansen et al. reported that several abundant circRNAs can function as ceRNAs (17) (**Figure 2A**). CiRS-7 (also termed CDR1as) was first demonstrated to harbor more than 70 conserved binding sites for miR-7 (17, 18). Overexpression of ciRS7 can efficiently recruit miR-7 to promote the specific AGO2 interaction, thus resulting in decreased miR-7 function and up-regulation of its target mRNAs. Moreover, ciRS7 was highly expressed in brains and its function was conserved, overexpression of ciRS7 or knockdown of miR-7 could impair the development of midbrain and nerve in mice and zebrafish (17, 18). In esophageal squamous cell carcinoma, ciRS-7 accelerated tumor growth and metastasis by regulation of miR-7/HOXB13 (44).

Besides ciRS-7, many other circRNAs in eukaryotes have been suggested as potential miRNA sponges. For instance, circSRY, the testis-specific circRNA derived from sex-determining region Y (SRY), contained 16 MREs of miR-138 and acted as miR-138 sponge in mouse testis (12, 17). Also, circHIPK2 could work as a sponge for miR124-2HG to regulate the activation of astrocytes *via* the synergistic effect of autophagy and endoplasmic

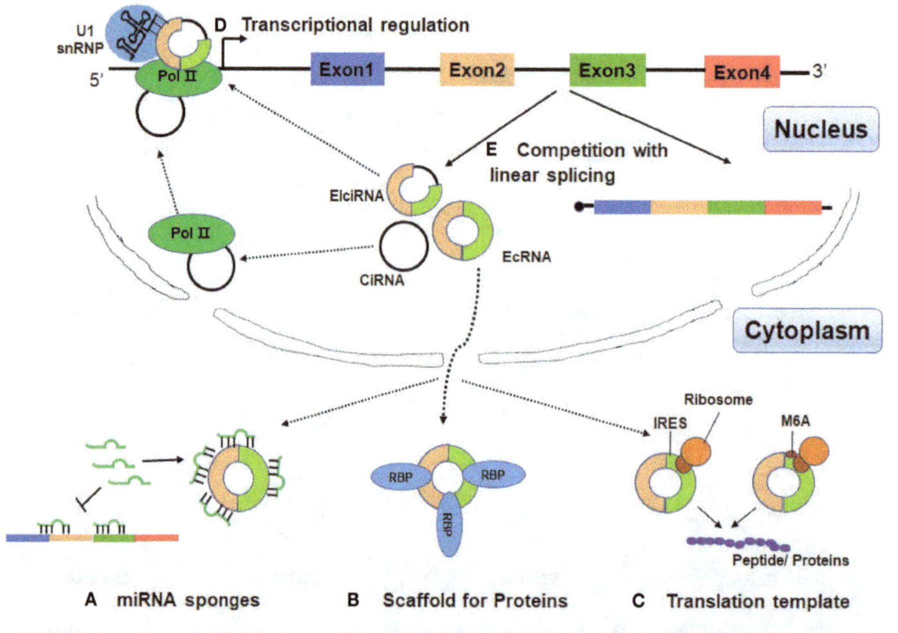

FIGURE 2 | Functions of circRNAs. **(A)** CircRNAs can act as miRNA sponges to diminish the effects of miRNAs on target mRNAs. **(B)** CircRNAs can serve as scaffolds or decoys for RBPs to modulate their functions, thus affecting the related biological processes. **(C)** CircRNAs may be translated if they contain an internal ribosome entry site (IRES) or extensive N6-methyladenosines (m6A) modification. **(D)** CircRNAs can promote transcription by interacting with U1 small nuclear ribonucleoprotein (U1 snRNP) and the RNA polymerase II (Pol II) in the nucleus. **(E)** The processing of circRNAs could affect host gene expression by competing with their linear mRNA splicing.

reticulum stress (45). In addition, circHIPK3, circCCDC66 and circPVT1 have been reported to have tumor-suppressive or oncogenic functions by serving as miRNA sponges (46–48). However, many circRNAs in mammals are expressed at relatively low levels and harbor few binding sites for miRNA (7, 49), suggesting them highly unlikely to act as ceRNAs or by working as miRNA sponges. Therefore, whether the miRNA sponge is a universal biological function of circRNAs needs to be further confirmed by more investigation.

CircRNAs Interact With Proteins

In addition to miRNAs, circRNAs can also interact with proteins to form specific circRNA–protein complexes which affect the activity of related proteins (**Figure 2B**). The first example of circRNA acting as a protein sponge was a RNA transcript encoding the splicing factor protein–muscleblind (MBL) (34). The circular Mbl (circMbl) derived from its own gene contains multiple binding sites for MBL. This circRNA was found to regulate the linear splicing of the gene by functioning as a decoy for MBL. When MBL protein levels are high, MBL binds to the pre-mRNA and causes it to splice into circMbl. Subsequently, circMbl could sponge out the excess MBL by binding to it (34). Other circRNAs, such as circANRIL and circPABPN1, have also been reported to function as protein sponge by interacting with target proteins (50, 51). CircANRIL can bind to Pescadillo homologue 1 (PES1), a vital 60S pre-ribosomal assembly factor, and then dampens ribosome biogenesis and exonuclease-mediated pre-rRNA processing in human macrophages and vascular smooth muscle cells (50). CircPABPN1 represses the translation of nuclear poly (A) binding protein 1 mRNA in human cervical cancer (HeLa) cells through binding to the RNA binding protein Hu-antigen R (HUR) (51).

In some cases, circRNAs may function as protein scaffolds or alter modes of action of the proteins. For instance, circ-Foxo3 and circAmotl1 can function as scaffolds of protein to potentiate the colocalization of enzymes and their substrates (52, 53). In mouse cancer cells, circ-Foxo3 suppresses cell cycle progression by interacting with cyclin-dependent kinase 2 (CDK2) and cyclin-dependent kinase inhibitor 1 (p21) to form a circFoxo3-p21-CDK2 ternary complex, thereby arresting the functions of p21 and CDK2 in cell cycle regulation (52). In addition, circ-Foxo3 also has high binding affinity to senescence-related proteins ID-1 and E2F1 as well as anti-stress proteins FAK and HIF1a, and accelerates the location of these proteins in the cytoplasm and accordingly leads to increased cellular senescence (54). In a mouse model, circAmotl1 simultaneously binds to phosphoinositide- dependent kinase 1 (PDK1) and protein kinase AKT1 *via* its spatial structure, leading to PDK1-dependent AKT1 phosphorylation and nuclear translocation, thus enhancing the cardio-protective role of pAKT1 (53).

Although a growing number of circRNAs have been shown to interact with proteins, the exact mechanisms underlying these interactions remain obscure (55). Additionally, one general question is to what extent lowly expressed circRNAs can confer measurable regulation on their binding proteins.

CircRNAs Can be Translatable

CircRNAs were initially believed to be non-coding RNA due to the absence of 5' cap and 3' ploy A tail that were normally required for linear mRNA translation. Given that most circRNAs were produced from protein-coding exons and mainly located in the cytoplasm. An intriguing question raises whether they are translatable. Recently, increasing evidence has shown that some circRNAs can be translatable molecules if they harbor an internal ribosome entry site (IRES) (56–58) (**Figure 2C**). In some cases, the presence of N6-methyladenosine (m6A) modification in the circRNAs can help to recruit the ribosome and promote the translation of circRNAs in cap-independent manner, but the underlying mechanisms remain largely unknown (59–61) (**Figure 2C**).

As early as the 1990s, Chen and Sarnow have proposed that synthetic engineered circRNAs may recruit ribosomal subunits and initiate peptide translation *in vitro* (62). However, this study did not support that circRNAs could also be translatable *in vivo*. In 2015, Abe and colleagues provided strong evidence that endogenous circRNAs can act as a template for translation in an IRES-dependent manner (56). Thereafter, several other groups have utilized mass spectrometry, ribosome profiling, and/or expression plasmids to demonstrate that a subset of circRNAs may indeed produce proteins (61, 63, 64). Nevertheless, to date only a few endogenous circRNAs, such as Mbl, circ-ZNF609, circFBXW7, cir-SHPRH, circPINTexon2, and circ-AKT3, have been reported to serve as protein templates (39, 63–67). Although thousands of circRNAs were predicted to have putative open reading frame (ORF) and IRES elements, not all of these circRNAs can perform translatingfunctions (68). The translational ability and mechanism of circRNAs are not fully understood and need to be further investigated. Furthermore, the functions of peptides/proteins encoded by circRNAs are still unknown. Since most circRNA-derived peptides are usually short peptides which lack important functional domains, they may function as decoys or dominant-negative protein variants (63). For example, several peptides, including FBXW-185aa, SHPRH-146aa, and PINT87aa, were reported to serve as tumor suppressors in glioblastoma (39, 65, 66). Although translation seems not to be a universal function for circRNAs, it is important to identify the physiological and pathological roles for the proteins translated by circRNAs.

CircRNAs Regulate Transcription and Alternative Splicing

The CiRNAs and EIciRNAs, which consist of either introns or both intron and exon, are dominantly restricted in the nucleus. These circRNAs can regulate transcription through interaction with U1 small nuclear ribonucleoprotein (U1 snRNA) and the RNA polymerase II (Pol II) (31, 32) (**Figure 2D**). For instance, ci-ankrd52 can accumulate to its transcription sites and positively regulate the transcriptional activity of parental coding gene through association with elongation Pol II machinery (31). In addition, two ElcircRNAs, circEIF3J, and circPAIP2, were identified to interact with host U1 snRNP to form circRNA-U1 snRNP complexes. The complexes further interact with the Pol II to increase gene expression in the promoter region of parental genes (32).

CircRNA biosynthesis naturally affects host gene expression. From this point of view, two studies have shown that the circRNAs processing strongly competes with linear mRNA splicing (28, 34) (**Figure 2E**). Ashwal-Fluss et al. observed that circMbl derived from the second exon of Mbl can compete with conventional pre-mRNA to keep the balance between linear alternative splicing and circRNAs production (34). Another study has demonstrated that depletion or inhibition of canonical pre-mRNA processing events resulted in increased levels of circRNAs, suggesting that the negative association between circRNA and their linear mRNAs (28). Additionally, a nuclear-retained circSEP3 derived from SEPALLATA3 (SEP3) gene was reported to regulate its cognate mRNA splicing by forming an R-loop or RNA : DNA hybrid (69). Taken together, some nuclear retained circRNAs can participate in gene regulation in both transcription and splicing mechanisms. However, how these circRNAs are accumulated or localized in the nucleus and how exactly they modulate gene expression remains elusive.

CIRCRNAS IN INNATE AND ADAPTIVE IMMUNE RESPONSE

The immune system is classically divided into two categories, i.e. innate and adaptive immunity. Innate immune response is the first line of host defense against pathogens, such as antibacterial and antiviral immune responses. Adaptive immune response is the second line of defense against specific antigens. It creates immunological memories to the encountered antigens and initiates a highly efficient response to specific antigens in the future. Notably, recent studies have suggested that circRNAs are involved in the regulation of both innate and adaptive immune responses.

CircRNAs in Innate Immunity

Innate immune response is mainly mediated by phagocytic cells and other cell types, such as macrophages, neutrophils, dendritic cells (DCs), and natural killer cells (NKs). In which, macrophages are one of the most important cell types in innate immune response. Through recognition of evolutionarily conserved structures on pathogens, macrophages become activated, and can engulf and destroy the invaders. Furthermore, macrophages can serve as antigen-presenting cells (APCs) to process and present foreign antigens during the adaptive immune response. According to the activation states and functions, macrophages can be divided into two subsets, i.e. classically activated macrophage (M1) and alternatively activated macrophage (M2). By performing a circRNA microarray analysis, Zhang et al. showed a total of 189 circRNAs were differentially expressed between M1 and M2 macrophages, indicating a role of circRNAs in macrophage polarization (70). Ng et al. reported that circ-RasGEF1B may play a regulatory role in macrophage activation by lipopolysaccharide (LPS) and protection against microbial infections (71). By comparing expression patterns of circRNAs in non-treated and RANKL/CSF1-treated bone marrow macrophage (BMM) cells, Chen et al. found that circRNA_28313 was significantly upregulated in RANK + CSF1-induced osteoclast differentiation by forming a ceRNA network of circRNA_28313/miR-195a/CSF1 (72). Circ-ASAP1 was reported to facilitate tumor-related macrophage infiltration by regulating miR-326/miR-532-5p-CSF-1 signaling pathway and may serve as a prognostic predict marker for hepatocellular carcinoma (73). By microarray analysis of circRNA expression profile in neutrophils derived from patients with asymptomatic moyamoya disease (MMD) and healthy individuals, 123 differentially expressed circRNAs were identified between the two groups. These differentially expressed circRNAs were mainly involved in immune responses, angiogenesis and metabolism in MMD (74). CircUHRF1 expression was elevated in human HCC tissues compared to adjacent non-tumor tissues. CircARSP91 may increase the susceptibility of HCC cells to NK cell cytotoxicity by upregulating UL16 binding protein 1 expression in HCC cells (75). More recently, Zhang et al. reported that tumor cell-derived exosomal circUHRF1 can induce NK cell exhaustion by inhibiting NK cell-derived IFN-γ and TNF-α secretion and may induce resistance to anti-PD1 therapy in human HCC (76). Expression of circRNA_001937 was significantly increased in PBMCs from patients with active tuberculosis and was positively correlated with disease severity (77). CircRNA-chr19 may function as a ceRNA by targeting miR-30b-3p/claudin-18 (CLDN18) axis in Ebola virus infection (78). Overexpression of a dsRNA-forming circRNA inhibited PKR activation and increased viral replication in encephalomyocarditis virus (EMCV) infection (79).

CircRNAs in Adaptive Immunity

Adaptive immunity is characterized by T cells specific for antigens derived from the invading pathogens, and by B cells producing antibodies that bind to these antigens. T cells and B cells, once primed, initiate a highly efficient response to the pathogens and develop immunologic memories to the encountered antigens. The adaptive immune response is meant to defense foreign pathogens but sometimes it can mistakenly turn against our own body, leading to the autoimmune diseases.

Wang et al. reported that circRNA_100783 was involved in the regulation of $CD8^+$ T cell ageing process by targeting a large number of miRNA-mRNA networks (80). Exosome-derived circRNA_002178 could be transferred into $CD8^+$ T cells and promoted PD1 expression by sponging miR-28-5p, leading to $CD8^+$ T cell exhaustion in lung adenocarcinoma (81). Huang et al. observed that circ_0005519 increased IL-13 and IL-6 expression *via* negatively regulating let-7a-5p in $CD4^+$ T cells from patients with asthma (82). The same group also reported an increased expression of circ_0002594 in $CD4^+$ T cells and might be a potential diagnostic marker for Th2-mediated allergic asthma (83). Gaffo et al. found that circRNAs displayed a cell type-specific expression pattern in healthy individuals, such as circRNAs specific for B-cells (circPAX5, circAFF3, circIL4R, and circSETBP1) and T-ceslls (circIKZF1, circTNIK, circTXK, and circFBXW7). The B cell-specific circRNAs circPAX5 and circAFF3 were highly overexpressed in pediatric B-precursor acute lymphoblastic leukemia (84). CircANKRD36 was significantly upregulated in peripheral blood and was correlated with chronic inflammation from patients with type 2 diabetes mellitus (T2DM) (85). Circ_402458 was significantly elevated in patients with primary biliary cholangitis (PBC). Circ_402458 may function as sponge for miR-522 and miR-943 and involved in the regulation of PBC (86).

CIRCRNAS IN SLE

In the past three years, increasing evidence has linked circRNAs to SLE, with main focus on identification and characterization of circRNAs in blood samples, renal biopsies and skin tissues. These data suggest that circRNAs may be involved in the pathogenesis of SLE and could be potential diagnostic markers or therapeutic targets for SLE (**Figure 3** and **Table 1**).

Peripheral Blood circRNAs in SLE

To date, the majority studies of circRNA in SLE were performed in blood samples, including plasma, whole blood, peripheral blood mononuclear cells (PBMCs), and T cells.

Plasma Derived circRNAs in SLE

As the high structural stability, the circRNAs are proposed to be promising biomarkers for diagnosis of diseases. By using circRNA microarray, Li et al. analyzed the circRNA expression profiling in plasma samples from patients with SLE and identified a number of circRNAs which were differentially expressed between SLE patients and healthy controls (87). By qPCR validation, four significantly dysregulated circRNAs, i.e., hsa_circ_400011, hsa_circ_102584, hsa_circ_101471, and hsa_circ_100226, were validated and predicted to be potential biomarkers for SLE diagnosis (87). Subsequently, Ouyang et al. reported that circRNA_002453 was markedly increased in plasma from patients with lupus nephritis (LN) compared with non-LN SLE patients, RA patients and healthy individuals (88). Although the expression level of circRNA_002453 had no significant association with C3, C4, and SLEDAI score, it was positively correlated with 24-hour proteinuria and renal SLEDAI score, which suggesting that this circRNA might severe as a novel biomarker for diagnosis of LN. Another research group has shown that hsa_circRNA_407176 and hsa_circRNA_001308 were underexpressed in both plasma and PBMCs of SLE patients (89). Furthermore, by the receiver operating characteristic (ROC) curve analysis, these two circRNAs could distinguish SLE patients from healthy controls, indicating their potential diagnostic value for SLE.

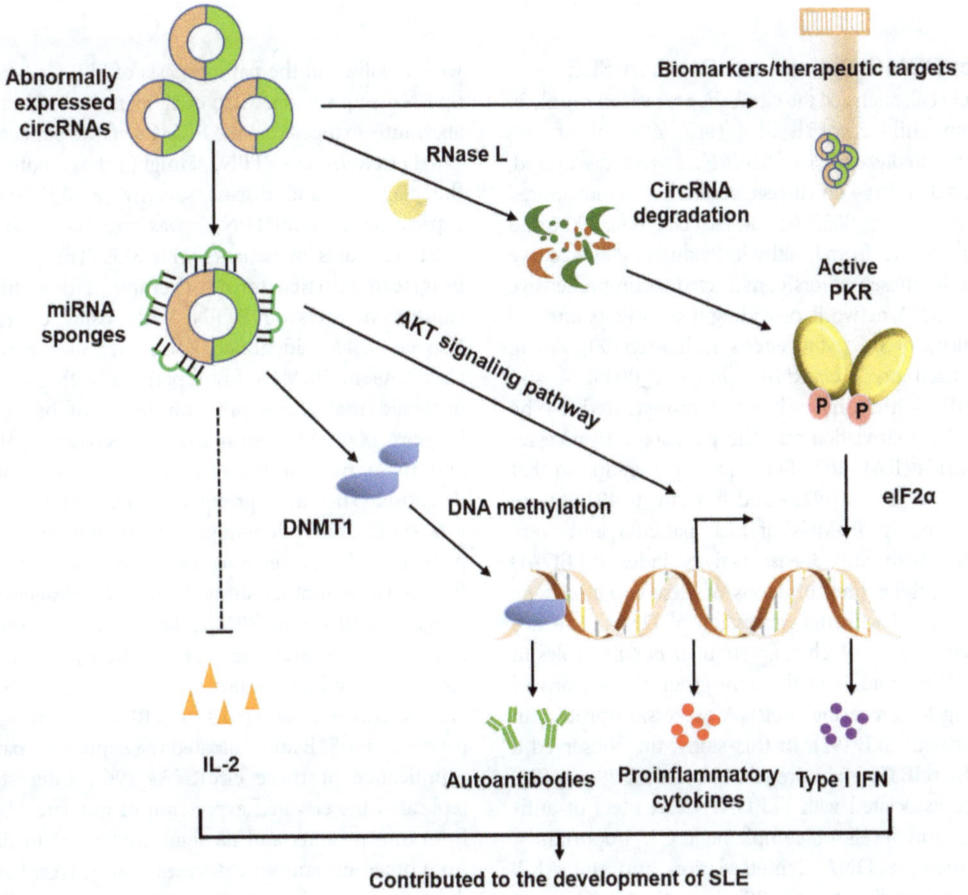

FIGURE 3 | Possible roles of circRNAs in SLE. CircRANs may be involved in the pathogenesis of SLE by regulating various biological processes, such as DNA methylation, activation of AKT signaling pathway, and aberrant PKR activation. Furthermore, circRNAs may serve as biomarkers for the diagnosis and severity of SLE.

TABLE 1 | Summary of circRNAs implicated in SLE.

CircRNAs	Source/Detection Methods	CircRNA_types	Tissues	Dysregulation	Potential Functions/Applications	Refs
hsa_circRNA_400011	CircRNA microarray	Intronic	Plasma	Up	Possibly involved in the development of SLE by acting as miRNA sponges, may serve as potential biomarkers	(87)
hsa_circRNA_102584		Exonic		Up		
hsa_circRNA_101471		Exonic		Up		
hsa_circRNA_100226		Exonic		Down		
hsa_circRNA_002453	CircRNA microarray	Not mentioned	Plasma	Up	Correlated with 24-hour proteinuria and renal SLEDAI score	(88)
hsa_circRNA_407176	CircRNA microarray	Not mentioned	Plasma	Down	Served as potential diagnostic biomarkers for SLE	(89)
hsa_circRNA_001308				Down		
hsa_circ_0057762	CircRNA microarray	Not mentioned	Whole blood	Up	Served as potential diagnostic biomarkers for SLE	(90)
hsa_circ_0003090				Up		
hsa_circ_0049224	Selected from other studies	Not mentioned	PBMCs	Down	Negatively associated with SLEDAI and the degree of SLE severity	(91)
hsa_circ_0049220				Down		
circIBTK	RNA-seq	Exonic	PBMCs	Down	Inhibited DNA demethylation and activation of AKT signaling pathway by binding to miR-29b, may serve as biomarkers and therapeutic targets for SLE	(92)
circPTPN22	RNA-seq	Exonic	PBMCs	Down	Acted as a biomarker for the diagnosis and severity of SLE	(93)
hsa_circ_0044235	CircRNA microarray	Not mentioned	PBMCs	Up	Served as potential biomarkers for SLE diagnosis	(94)
hsa_circ_0068367				Up		
hsa_circ_0000479	RNA-seq	Exonic	PBMCs	Up	Served as a novel diagnostic biomarker for SLE	(95)
hsa_circ_0000479	Selected from other studies	Exonic	PBMCs	Up	Served as a potential diagnostic biomarker for SLE	(96)
hsa_circ_0045272	CircRNA microarray	Not mentioned	T cells	Down	Upregulated the early apoptosis of Jurkat cells and promoted the production of IL-2 in activated Jurkat cells	(97)
hsa_circ_0012919	CircRNA microarray	Not mentioned	CD4+ T cells	Up	Inhibited DNA demethylation of CD11a and CD70 in CD4+ T cells, regulated the expression of RANTES and KLF13 *via* miR-125a-3p	(98)
circHLA-C	RNA-seq	Exonic	kidney	Up	Involved in the pathogenesis of lupus nephritis by sponging miR-150	(99)

Whole Blood or PBMC Derived circRNAs in SLE

In a recent study, Li et al. analyzed the circRNA expression profile in whole blood from children with SLE (90). A total of 348 differentially and markedly expressed circRNAs were discovered, with 184 up-regulated and 164 down-regulated. They demonstrated that the levels of the hsa_circ_0057762 and hsa_circ_0003090 could distinguish the SLE patients from healthy individuals by ROC curve analysis. In the study, these authors constructed a comprehensive circRNA-miRNA-mRNA network, providing new insights into the molecular mechanisms of SLE pathogenesis in children (90). Zhang et al. initially focused on 2 circRNAs (hsa_circ_0049224 and hsa_circ_0049220), which have been demonstrated to be correlated with DNA methylation and the pathological processes of rheumatoid arthritis (RA) (100). Subsequently, they found that expression levels of hsa_circ_0049224 and hsa_circ_0049220 were significantly decreased in PBMCs of SLE patients and were negatively correlated with SLE disease activity index (SLEDAI) score (91). Moreover, the expression levels of these two circRNAs were positively correlated with the expression of DNMT1, a key factor of DNA methylation, which suggests their possible roles in the pathogenesis of SLE. In addition, the same group also performed circRNA sequencing to screen the circRNA expression profiles in PBMCs of patients with SLE (92). In this study, they observed a downregulation of circIBTK and upregulation of miR-29b in SLE patients, both were associated with SLEDAI score, titers of anti-dsDNA antibodies and levels of complement C3. Importantly, circIBTK could regulate DNA demethylation and the AKT signaling pathway by binding to miR-29b in SLE (92). Of note, numerous studies have demonstrated that aberrant DNA methylation and abnormal activation of AKT signaling pathway were involved in the pathogenesis of SLE (101–103). Furthermore, by RNA sequencing, Miao et al. identified 128 circRNAs that were aberrantly expressed in the PBMCs of SLE patients and discovered a novel circRNA, circPTPN22, might act as a potential biomarker for the diagnosis and disease severity of SLE (93). The decreased expression of circPTPN22 was negatively correlated with the SLEDAI scores in patients with SLE. The patients who received long-term corticosteroid therapy had significant increased expression levels circPTPN22. By using circRNAs microarray, Luo et al. also identified a number of differentially expressed circRNAs in PBMCs from patients with SLE (94). This study observed that the expression levels of hsa_circ_0044235 and hsa_circ_0068367 were markedly decreased in patients with SLE and these two circRNAs could be novel biomarkers for SLE diagnosis. The same group also reported that hsa_circ_0044235 was significantly downregulated in peripheral blood from RA patients and may serve as a potential biomarker for diagnosis of RA (104). In another study, Guo and colleagues reported that the hsa_circ_0000479 in PBMCs has a great potential as a diagnostic biomarker for SLE (95). However, the results from different circRNA profiling studies were inconsistent. Based on previous studies, Luo et al. selected 11 circRNAs which were upregulated in patients with SLE and validated the expression patterns and clinical significance of these circRNAs (96). Interestingly, the study replicated the elevated expression of hsa_circ_0000479 in PBMCs from SLE patients and its significant value in distinguishing SLE from other autoimmune diseases (96). A recent study has reported that a number of circRNAs were downregulated in PBMCs from patients with SLE. Meanwhile, the author also observed a spontaneous RNase L activation in PBMCs derived from SLE patients (79). The RNase L activation led to circRNA degradation and this RNase L-mediated circRNA degradation was required for protein kinase (PKR) activation. The aberrant PKR activation further augmented type I IFN signature through eIF2α phosphorylation and therefore involved in the pathogenesis of SLE (79).

T-Cell Derived circRNAs in SLE

T cells play a key role in lupus pathogenesis, especially the CD4 T helper (Th) cells (105). Li et al. recently reported 127 differentially expressed circRNAs in T cells from SLE patients, and further validated a downregulated circRNA, hsa_circ_0045272 (97). Further functional data indicated that knockdown of hsa_circ_0045272 resulted in an enhanced early apoptosis and increased IL-2 production in activated Jurkat cells (97). In another report, 12 up-regulated and two down-regulated circRNAs were discovered in $CD4^+$ T cells of patients with SLE. Of which, three aberrantly up-regulated circRNAs, including hsa_circ_0012919, hsa_circ_0006239 and hsa_circ_0002227, were validated by qPCR (98). Of note, the hsa_circ_0012919 could be considered as a diagnostic potential for SLE. Downregulation of hsa_circ_0012919 led to an enhanced expression of DNA methyltransferase 1 and decreased expression of CD11a and CD70 on $CD4^+$ T cells from both inactive and active SLE patients (98). Notably, the overexpression of CD11a and CD70 in $CD4^+$ T cells in SLE may promote the production of autoantibodies (106). More recently, Zhang and colleagues analyzed 29 differentially expressed circRNAs obtained from the GSE84655 of GEO database (107). By statistical analysis and bioinformatic interpretation, the author predicted the circRNA-miRNA-mRNA regulatory networks for these circRNAs. These regulatory networks might be involved in the pathological process of SLE (107).

Renal circRNAs in SLE

Lupus nephritis (LN) is one of the most serious complications of SLE. Patients with lupus nephritis are at risk for kidney failure and premature death. Through RNA deep sequencing, a total of 171 circRNAs with 2-fold differential expression, including 142 upregulated and 29 downregulated circRNAs, were discovered in renal biopsies from LN patients compared with normal kidney specimens (99). The correlations between seven validated circRNAs and clinical features were analyzed, and the circHLA-C was found to be positively associated with proteinuria, serum creatinine, renal activity index and crescentic glomeruli. Bioinformatic analysis predicted that circHLA-C plays important roles in the pathogenesis of lupus nephritis by serving as sponges for miR-150 and regulating its expression. The renal-derived miR-150 showed a tendency of negative correlation with circHLA-C in LN patients (99).

Cutaneous circRNAs in SLE

Skin involvement is a common clinical manifestation in SLE patients. Of which, the discoid lupus erythematosus (DLE) is the most common form (108). By using RNA sequencing, Xuan and colleagues recently identified a number of differently expressed lncRNAs and circRNAs in the lesional lower lips from patients with DLE (109). In this study, a total of 161 circRNAs, including 57 up-regulated and 104 down-regulated circRNAs, showed remarkable differential expression in lesional skin compared with matched adjacent tissues. The principal roles of these markedly deregulated circRNAs were predicted using bioinformatics methods. These results suggested that certain circRNAs may have potential value in diagnosis and therapy of DLE.

CONCLUSIONS AND PERSPECTIVES

Recent advances in the circRNA research field have not only revealed a previously unexpected structure of eukaryotic transcriptomes but have also uncovered multiple aspects of circRNA biological function. CircRNAs generated by the non-canonical backsplicing can play important roles in biology and pathobiology by regulating gene expression at multiple molecular levels and interacting with proteins. These findings have been surprising and exciting, but there are still unrevealed answers concerning the biogenesis of these molecules. First, the complete set of elements that control the expression and localization of circRNAs remains unknown. For example, are there any factors that are indispensable for backsplicing but not for canonical splicing reactions? Second, the mechanisms involved in metabolic processing or degradation of circRNAs, particular in normal or unstressed cells, remain unclear. In addition, given the relatively low expression level of most circRNAs, how many circRNAs could truly act as miRNA sponges or competitors for protein binding?

The role of circRNAs in SLE has been in the spotlight in recent years. Several studies have shown that some aberrantly expressed circRNAs in SLE patients were implicated in DNA demethylation by acting as miRNA sponges (92, 98). However, the results were inconsistent from circRNA expression profiling studies of SLE PBMCs. These inconsistent results may be due to the disease heterogeneity and heterogeneous cell subsets in PBMCs such as monocytes, T cells and B cells. Therefore, it is important to stratify SLE patients by their clinical features and focus on certain cell subtypes. SLE is characterized by the production of a range of autoantibodies, indicating a critical role of B cells in the pathogenesis of SLE (2, 110). Therefore, it is worthy to functionally characterize the B cell-derived circRNAs involved in SLE pathogenesis. Additionally, a number of studies have shown that several circRNAs may serve as potential biomarkers for SLE. Nonetheless, the sample sizes in these studies were relatively small (95, 96). The results need to be further validated in larger sample sizes. More recently, an important study showed that overexpression of circPOLR2A, a double-stranded RNA (dsRNA)-containing circRNA, could remarkably attenuate the aberrant dsRNA-activated protein kinase activation cascade in PBMCs or T cells derived from SLE patients, suggesting that this type of circRNAs may serve as potential therapeutic modalities for SLE (79).

In conclusion, emerging evidence indicates that circRNAs are involved in the pathogenesis of SLE and may serve as novel biomarkers or therapeutics for SLE in the future. However, although the existing data support the potential value of circRNAs in diagnosis and treatment of SLE, the feasibility of circRNAs in clinical utility needs to be further studied.

AUTHOR CONTRIBUTIONS

LH wrote the manuscript. JG provided guidance, edited and revised the manuscript. ZY, CC, and YT helped in collecting the references and designed the figures. All authors contributed to the article and approved the submitted version.

REFERENCES

1. Lisnevskaia L, Murphy G, Isenberg D. Systemic lupus erythematosus. *Lancet* (2014) 384:1878–88. doi: 10.1016/s0140-6736(14)60128-8
2. Tsokos GC. Systemic lupus erythematosus. *N Engl J Med* (2011) 365:2110–21. doi: 10.1056/NEJMra1100359
3. Xia X, Tang X, Wang S. Roles of CircRNAs in Autoimmune Diseases. *Front Immunol* (2019) 10:639. doi: 10.3389/fimmu.2019.00639
4. Imamura K, Akimitsu N. Long Non-Coding RNAs Involved in Immune Responses. *Front Immunol* (2014) 5:573:573. doi: 10.3389/fimmu.2014.00573
5. Kristensen LS, Andersen MS, Stagsted LVW, Ebbesen KK, Hansen TB, Kjems J. The biogenesis, biology and characterization of circular RNAs. *Nat Rev Genet* (2019) 20:675–91. doi: 10.1038/s41576-019-0158-7
6. Suzuki H, Zuo Y, Wang J, Zhang MQ, Malhotra A, Mayeda A. Characterization of RNase R-digested cellular RNA source that consists of lariat and circular RNAs from pre-mRNA splicing. *Nucleic Acids Res* (2006) 34:e63. doi: 10.1093/nar/gkl151
7. Enuka Y, Lauriola M, Feldman ME, Sas-Chen A, Ulitsky I, Yarden Y. Circular RNAs are long-lived and display only minimal early alterations in response to a growth factor. *Nucleic Acids Res* (2016) 44:1370–83. doi: 10.1093/nar/gkv1367
8. Sanger HL, Klotz G, Riesner D, Gross HJ, Kleinschmidt AK. Viroids are single-stranded covalently closed circular RNA molecules existing as highly base-paired rod-like structures. *Proc Natl Acad Sci USA* (1976) 73:3852–6. doi: 10.1073/pnas.73.11.3852
9. Hsu MT, Coca-Prados M. Electron microscopic evidence for the circular form of RNA in the cytoplasm of eukaryotic cells. *Nature* (1979) 280:339–40. doi: 10.1038/280339a0
10. Nigro JM, Cho KR, Fearon ER, Kern SE, Ruppert JM, Oliner JD, et al. Scrambled exons. *Cell* (1991) 64:607–13. doi: 10.1016/0092-8674(91)90244-s
11. Cocquerelle C, Daubersies P, Majérus MA, Kerckaert JP, Bailleul B. Splicing with inverted order of exons occurs proximal to large introns. *EMBO J* (1992) 11:1095–8.
12. Capel B, Swain A, Nicolis S, Hacker A, Walter M, Koopman P, et al. Circular transcripts of the testis-determining gene Sry in adult mouse testis. *Cell* (1993) 73:1019–30. doi: 10.1016/0092-8674(93)90279-y
13. Cocquerelle C, Mascrez B, Hétuin D, Bailleul B. Mis-splicing yields circular RNA molecules. *FASEB J* (1993) 7:155–60. doi: 10.1096/fasebj.7.1.7678559
14. Wang PL, Bao Y, Yee MC, Barrett SP, Hogan GJ, Olsen MN, et al. Circular RNA is expressed across the eukaryotic tree of life. *PloS One* (2014) 9:e90859. doi: 10.1371/journal.pone.0090859
15. Jeck WR, Sorrentino JA, Wang K, Slevin MK, Burd CE, Liu J, et al. Circular RNAs are abundant, conserved, and associated with ALU repeats. *RNA* (2013) 19:141–57. doi: 10.1261/rna.035667.112
16. Salzman J, Chen RE, Olsen MN, Wang PL, Brown PO. Cell-type specific features of circular RNA expression. *PloS Genet* (2013) 9:e1003777. doi: 10.1371/journal.pgen.1003777
17. Hansen TB, Jensen TI, Clausen BH, Bramsen JB, Finsen B, Damgaard CK, et al. Natural RNA circles function as efficient microRNA sponges. *Nature* (2013) 495:384–8. doi: 10.1038/nature11993
18. Memczak S, Jens M, Elefsinioti A, Torti F, Krueger J, Rybak A, et al. Circular RNAs are a large class of animal RNAs with regulatory potency. *Nature* (2013) 495:333–8. doi: 10.1038/nature11928
19. Qu S, Yang X, Li X, Wang J, Gao Y, Shang R, et al. Circular RNA: A new star of noncoding RNAs. *Cancer Lett* (2015) 365:141–8. doi: 10.1016/j.canlet.2015.06.003
20. Nicolet BP, Engels S, Aglialoro F, van den Akker E, von Lindern M, Wolkers MC. Circular RNA expression in human hematopoietic cells is widespread and cell-type specific. *Nucleic Acids Res* (2018) 46:8168–80. doi: 10.1093/nar/gky721
21. Maass PG, Glažar P, Memczak S, Dittmar G, Hollfinger I, Schreyer L, et al. A map of human circular RNAs in clinically relevant tissues. *J Mol Med (Berl)* (2017) 95:1179–89. doi: 10.1007/s00109-017-1582-9
22. Xia S, Feng J, Lei L, Hu J, Xia L, Wang J, et al. Comprehensive characterization of tissue-specific circular RNAs in the human and mouse genomes. *Brief Bioinform* (2017) 18:984–92. doi: 10.1093/bib/bbw081
23. Hanan M, Soreq H, Kadener S. CircRNAs in the brain. *RNA Biol* (2017) 14:1028–34. doi: 10.1080/15476286.2016.1255398
24. Aufiero S, Reckman YJ, Pinto YM, Creemers EE. Circular RNAs open a new chapter in cardiovascular biology. *Nat Rev Cardiol* (2019) 16:503–14. doi: 10.1038/s41569-019-0185-2
25. Vo JN, Cieslik M, Zhang Y, Shukla S, Xiao L, Zhang Y, et al. The Landscape of Circular RNA in Cancer. *Cell* (2019) 176:869–81.e13. doi: 10.1016/j.cell.2018.12.021
26. Chen X, Yang T, Wang W, Xi W, Zhang T, Li Q, et al. Circular RNAs in immune responses and immune diseases. *Theranostics* (2019) 9:588–607. doi: 10.7150/thno.29678
27. Salzman J, Gawad C, Wang PL, Lacayo N, Brown PO. Circular RNAs are the predominant transcript isoform from hundreds of human genes in diverse cell types. *PloS One* (2012) 7:e30733. doi: 10.1371/journal.pone.0030733
28. Liang D, Tatomer DC, Luo Z, Wu H, Yang L, Chen LL, et al. The Output of Protein-Coding Genes Shifts to Circular RNAs When the Pre-mRNA Processing Machinery Is Limiting. *Mol Cell* (2017) 68:940–54.e3. doi: 10.1016/j.molcel.2017.10.034
29. Jeck WR, Sharpless NE. Detecting and characterizing circular RNAs. *Nat Biotechnol* (2014) 32:453–61. doi: 10.1038/nbt.2890
30. Lasda E, Parker R. Circular RNAs: diversity of form and function. *RNA* (2014) 20:1829–42. doi: 10.1261/rna.047126.114
31. Zhang Y, Zhang XO, Chen T, Xiang JF, Yin QF, Xing YH, et al. Circular intronic long noncoding RNAs. *Mol Cell* (2013) 51:792–806. doi: 10.1016/j.molcel.2013.08.017
32. Li Z, Huang C, Bao C, Chen L, Lin M, Wang X, et al. Exon-intron circular RNAs regulate transcription in the nucleus. *Nat Struct Mol Biol* (2015) 22:256–64. doi: 10.1038/nsmb.2959
33. Conn SJ, Pillman KA, Toubia J, Conn VM, Salmanidis M, Phillips CA, et al. The RNA binding protein quaking regulates formation of circRNAs. *Cell* (2015) 160:1125–34. doi: 10.1016/j.cell.2015.02.014
34. Ashwal-Fluss R, Meyer M, Pamudurti NR, Ivanov A, Bartok O, Hanan M, et al. circRNA biogenesis competes with pre-mRNA splicing. *Mol Cell* (2014) 56:55–66. doi: 10.1016/j.molcel.2014.08.019
35. Rybak-Wolf A, Stottmeister C, Glazar P, Jens M, Pino N, Giusti S, et al. Circular RNAs in the Mammalian Brain Are Highly Abundant, Conserved, and Dynamically Expressed. *Mol Cell* (2015) 58:870–85. doi: 10.1016/j.molcel.2015.03.027

36. Errichelli L, Dini Modigliani S, Laneve P, Colantoni A, Legnini I, Capauto D, et al. FUS affects circular RNA expression in murine embryonic stem cell-derived motor neurons. *Nat Commun* (2017) 8:14741. doi: 10.1038/ncomms14741
37. Zaiou M. Circular RNAs as Potential Biomarkers and Therapeutic Targets for Metabolic Diseases. *Adv Exp Med Biol* (2019) 1134:177–91. doi: 10.1007/978-3-030-12668-1_10
38. Lu Z, Filonov GS, Noto JJ, Schmidt CA, Hatkevich TL, Wen Y, et al. Metazoan tRNA introns generate stable circular RNAs in vivo. *Rna* (2015) 21:1554–65. doi: 10.1261/rna.052944.115
39. Zhang M, Zhao K, Xu X, Yang Y, Yan S, Wei P, et al. A peptide encoded by circular form of LINC-PINT suppresses oncogenic transcriptional elongation in glioblastoma. *Nat Commun* (2018) 9:4475. doi: 10.1038/s41467-018-06862-2
40. Bartel DP. MicroRNAs: genomics, biogenesis, mechanism, and function. *Cell* (2004) 116:281–97. doi: 10.1016/s0092-8674(04)00045-5
41. Salmena L, Poliseno L, Tay Y, Kats L, Pandolfi PP. A ceRNA hypothesis: the Rosetta Stone of a hidden RNA language? *Cell* (2011) 146:353–8. doi: 10.1016/j.cell.2011.07.014
42. Poliseno L, Salmena L, Zhang J, Carver B, Haveman WJ, Pandolfi PP. A coding-independent function of gene and pseudogene mRNAs regulates tumour biology. *Nature* (2010) 465:1033–8. doi: 10.1038/nature09144
43. Cesana M, Cacchiarelli D, Legnini I, Santini T, Sthandier O, Chinappi M, et al. A long noncoding RNA controls muscle differentiation by functioning as a competing endogenous RNA. *Cell* (2011) 147:358–69. doi: 10.1016/j.cell.2011.09.028
44. Li RC, Ke S, Meng FK, Lu J, Zou XJ, He ZG, et al. CiRS-7 promotes growth and metastasis of esophageal squamous cell carcinoma via regulation of miR-7/HOXB13. *Cell Death Dis* (2018) 9:838. doi: 10.1038/s41419-018-0852-y
45. Huang R, Zhang Y, Han B, Bai Y, Zhou R, Gan G, et al. Circular RNA HIPK2 regulates astrocyte activation via cooperation of autophagy and ER stress by targeting MIR124-2HG. *Autophagy* (2017) 13:1722–41. doi: 10.1080/15548627.2017.1356975
46. Zheng Q, Bao C, Guo W, Li S, Chen J, Chen B, et al. Circular RNA profiling reveals an abundant circHIPK3 that regulates cell growth by sponging multiple miRNAs. *Nat Commun* (2016) 7:11215. doi: 10.1038/ncomms11215
47. Hsiao K-Y, Lin Y-C, Gupta SK, Chang N, Yen L, Sun HS, et al. Noncoding Effects of Circular RNA CCDC66 Promote Colon Cancer Growth and Metastasis. *Cancer Res* (2017) 77:2339–50. doi: 10.1158/0008-5472.CAN-16-1883
48. Verduci L, Ferraiuolo M, Sacconi A, Ganci F, Vitale J, Colombo T, et al. The oncogenic role of circPVT1 in head and neck squamous cell carcinoma is mediated through the mutant p53/YAP/TEAD transcription-competent complex. *Genome Biol* (2017) 18:237. doi: 10.1186/s13059-017-1368-y
49. Guo JU, Agarwal V, Guo H, Bartel DP. Expanded identification and characterization of mammalian circular RNAs. *Genome Biol* (2014) 15:409. doi: 10.1186/s13059-014-0409-z
50. Holdt LM, Stahringer A, Sass K, Pichler G, Kulak NA, Wilfert W, et al. Circular non-coding RNA ANRIL modulates ribosomal RNA maturation and atherosclerosis in humans. *Nat Commun* (2016) 7:12429. doi: 10.1038/ncomms12429
51. Abdelmohsen K, Panda AC, Munk R, Grammatikakis I, Dudekula DB, De S, et al. Identification of HuR target circular RNAs uncovers suppression of PABPN1 translation by CircPABPN1. *RNA Biol* (2017) 14:361–9. doi: 10.1080/15476286.2017.1279788
52. Du WW, Yang W, Liu E, Yang Z, Dhaliwal P, Yang BB. Foxo3 circular RNA retards cell cycle progression via forming ternary complexes with p21 and CDK2. *Nucleic Acids Res* (2016) 44:2846–58. doi: 10.1093/nar/gkw027
53. Du WW, Yang W, Chen Y, Wu ZK, Foster FS, Yang Z, et al. Foxo3 circular RNA promotes cardiac senescence by modulating multiple factors associated with stress and senescence responses. *Eur Heart J* (2017) 38:1402–12. doi: 10.1093/eurheartj/ehw001
54. Zeng Y, Du WW, Wu Y, Yang Z, Awan FM, Li X, et al. A Circular RNA Binds To and Activates AKT Phosphorylation and Nuclear Localization Reducing Apoptosis and Enhancing Cardiac Repair. *Theranostics* (2017) 7:3842–55. doi: 10.7150/thno.19764
55. Huang A, Zheng H, Wu Z, Chen M, Huang Y. Circular RNA-protein interactions: functions, mechanisms, and identification. *Theranostics* (2020) 10:3503–17. doi: 10.7150/thno.42174
56. Abe N, Matsumoto K, Nishihara M, Nakano Y, Shibata A, Maruyama H, et al. Rolling Circle Translation of Circular RNA in Living Human Cells. *Sci Rep* (2015) 5:16435. doi: 10.1038/srep16435
57. Wang Y, Wang Z. Efficient backsplicing produces translatable circular mRNAs. *Rna* (2015) 21:172–9. doi: 10.1261/rna.048272.114
58. Wesselhoeft RA, Kowalski PS, Anderson DG. Engineering circular RNA for potent and stable translation in eukaryotic cells. *Nat Commun* (2018) 9:2629. doi: 10.1038/s41467-018-05096-6
59. Meyer KD, Patil DP, Zhou J, Zinoviev A, Skabkin MA, Elemento O, et al. 5' UTR m(6)A Promotes Cap-Independent Translation. *Cell* (2015) 163:999–1010. doi: 10.1016/j.cell.2015.10.012
60. Zhou J, Wan J, Gao X, Zhang X, Jaffrey SR, Qian SB. Dynamic m(6)A mRNA methylation directs translational control of heat shock response. *Nature* (2015) 526:591–4. doi: 10.1038/nature15377
61. Yang Y, Fan X, Mao M, Song X, Wu P, Zhang Y, et al. Extensive translation of circular RNAs driven by N(6)-methyladenosine. *Cell Res* (2017) 27:626–41. doi: 10.1038/cr.2017.31
62. Chen CY, Sarnow P. Initiation of protein synthesis by the eukaryotic translational apparatus on circular RNAs. *Science* (1995) 268:415–7. doi: 10.1126/science.7536344
63. Legnini I, Di Timoteo G, Rossi F, Morlando M, Briganti F, Sthandier O, et al. Circ-ZNF609 Is a Circular RNA that Can Be Translated and Functions in Myogenesis. *Mol Cell* (2017) 66:22–37 e9. doi: 10.1016/j.molcel.2017.02.017
64. Pamudurti NR, Bartok O, Jens M, Ashwal-Fluss R, Stottmeister C, Ruhe L, et al. Translation of CircRNAs. *Mol Cell* (2017) 66:9–21.e7. doi: 10.1016/j.molcel.2017.02.021
65. Yang Y, Gao X, Zhang M, Yan S, Sun C, Xiao F, et al. Novel Role of FBXW7 Circular RNA in Repressing Glioma Tumorigenesis. *J Natl Cancer Inst* (2018) 110:304–15. doi: 10.1093/jnci/djx166
66. Zhang M, Huang N, Yang X, Luo J, Yan S, Xiao F, et al. A novel protein encoded by the circular form of the SHPRH gene suppresses glioma tumorigenesis. *Oncogene* (2018) 37:1805–14. doi: 10.1038/s41388-017-0019-9
67. Xia X, Li X, Li F, Wu X, Zhang M, Zhou H, et al. A novel tumor suppressor protein encoded by circular AKT3 RNA inhibits glioblastoma tumorigenicity by competing with active phosphoinositide-dependent Kinase-1. *Mol Cancer* (2019) 18:131. doi: 10.1186/s12943-019-1056-5
68. Chen X, Han P, Zhou T, Guo X, Song X, Li Y. circRNADb: A comprehensive database for human circular RNAs with protein-coding annotations. *Sci Rep* (2016) 6:34985. doi: 10.1038/srep34985
69. Conn VM, Hugouvieux V, Nayak A, Conos SA, Capovilla G, Cildir G, et al. A circRNA from SEPALLATA3 regulates splicing of its cognate mRNA through R-loop formation. *Nat Plants* (2017) 3:17053. doi: 10.1038/nplants.2017.53
70. Zhang Y, Zhang Y, Li X, Zhang M, Lv K. Microarray analysis of circular RNA expression patterns in polarized macrophages. *Int J Mol Med* (2017) 39:373–9. doi: 10.3892/ijmm.2017.2852
71. Ng WL, Marinov GK, Chin YM, Lim YY, Ea CK. Transcriptomic analysis of the role of RasGEF1B circular RNA in the TLR4/LPS pathway. *Sci Rep* (2017) 7:12227. doi: 10.1038/s41598-017-12550-w
72. Chen X, Ouyang Z, Shen Y, Liu B, Zhang Q, Wan L, et al. CircRNA_28313/miR-195a/CSF1 axis modulates osteoclast differentiation to affect OVX-induced bone absorption in mice. *RNA Biol* (2019) 16:1249–62. doi: 10.1080/15476286.2019.1624470
73. Hu ZQ, Zhou SL, Li J, Zhou ZJ, Wang PC, Xin HY, et al. Circular RNA Sequencing Identifies CircASAP1 as a Key Regulator in Hepatocellular Carcinoma Metastasis. *Hepatology* (2020) 72:906–22. doi: 10.1002/hep.31068
74. Ma Q, Li L, Yu B, Jiao L, Han Z, Zhao H, et al. Circular RNA profiling of neutrophil transcriptome provides insights into asymptomatic Moyamoya disease. *Brain Res* (2019) 1719:104–12. doi: 10.1016/j.brainres.2019.05.033
75. Ma Y, Zhang C, Zhang B, Yu H, Yu Q. circRNA of AR-suppressed PABPC1 91 bp enhances the cytotoxicity of natural killer cells against hepatocellular carcinoma via upregulating UL16 binding protein 1. *Oncol Lett* (2019) 17:388–97. doi: 10.3892/ol.2018.9606
76. Zhang PF, Gao C, Huang XY, Lu JC, Guo XJ, Shi GM, et al. Cancer cell-derived exosomal circUHRF1 induces natural killer cell exhaustion and may cause resistance to anti-PD1 therapy in hepatocellular carcinoma. *Mol Cancer* (2020) 19:110. doi: 10.1186/s12943-020-01222-5

77. Huang ZK, Yao FY, Xu JQ, Deng Z, Su RG, Peng YP, et al. Microarray Expression Profile of Circular RNAs in Peripheral Blood Mononuclear Cells from Active Tuberculosis Patients. *Cell Physiol Biochem* (2018) 45:1230–40. doi: 10.1159/000487454
78. Wang ZY, Guo ZD, Li JM, Zhao ZZ, Fu YY, Zhang CM, et al. Genome-Wide Search for Competing Endogenous RNAs Responsible for the Effects Induced by Ebola Virus Replication and Transcription Using a trVLP System. *Front Cell Infect Microbiol* (2017) 7:479:479. doi: 10.3389/fcimb.2017.00479
79. Liu CX, Li X, Nan F, Jiang S, Gao X, Guo SK, et al. Structure and Degradation of Circular RNAs Regulate PKR Activation in Innate Immunity. *Cell* (2019) 177:865–80.e21. doi: 10.1016/j.cell.2019.03.046
80. Wang YH, Yu XH, Luo SS, Han H. Comprehensive circular RNA profiling reveals that circular RNA100783 is involved in chronic CD28-associated CD8 (+)T cell ageing. *Immun Ageing* (2015) 12:17. doi: 10.1186/s12979-015-0042-z
81. Wang J, Zhao X, Wang Y, Ren F, Sun D, Yan Y, et al. circRNA-002178 act as a ceRNA to promote PDL1/PD1 expression in lung adenocarcinoma. *Cell Death Dis* (2020) 11:32. doi: 10.1038/s41419-020-2230-9
82. Huang Z, Cao Y, Zhou M, Qi X, Fu B, Mou Y, et al. Hsa_circ_0005519 increases IL-13/IL-6 by regulating hsa-let-7a-5p in CD4(+) T cells to affect asthma. *Clin Exp Allergy* (2019) 49:1116–27. doi: 10.1111/cea.13445
83. Huang Z, Fu B, Qi X, Xu Y, Mou Y, Zhou M, et al. Diagnostic and Therapeutic Value of Hsa_circ_0002594 for T Helper 2-Mediated Allergic Asthma. *Int Arch Allergy Immunol* (2020) 1–11. doi: 10.1159/000511612
84. Gaffo E, Boldrin E, Dal Molin A, Bresolin S, Bonizzato A, Trentin L, et al. Circular RNA differential expression in blood cell populations and exploration of circRNA deregulation in pediatric acute lymphoblastic leukemia. *Sci Rep* (2019) 9:14670. doi: 10.1038/s41598-019-50864-z
85. Fang Y, Wang X, Li W, Han J, Jin J, Su F, et al. Screening of circular RNAs and validation of circANKRD36 associated with inflammation in patients with type 2 diabetes mellitus. *Int J Mol Med* (2018) 42:1865–74. doi: 10.3892/ijmm.2018.3783
86. Zheng J, Li Z, Wang T, Zhao Y, Wang Y. Microarray Expression Profile of Circular RNAs in Plasma from Primary Biliary Cholangitis Patients. *Cell Physiol Biochem* (2017) 44:1271–81. doi: 10.1159/000485487
87. Li H, Li K, Lai W, Li X, Wang H, Yang J, et al. Comprehensive circular RNA profiles in plasma reveals that circular RNAs can be used as novel biomarkers for systemic lupus erythematosus. *Clin Chim Acta* (2018) 480:17–25. doi: 10.1016/j.cca.2018.01.026
88. Ouyang Q, Huang Q, Jiang Z, Zhao J, Shi GP, Yang M. Using plasma circRNA_002453 as a novel biomarker in the diagnosis of lupus nephritis. *Mol Immunol* (2018) 101:531–8. doi: 10.1016/j.molimm.2018.07.029
89. Zhang MY, Wang JB, Zhu ZW, Li LJ, Liu RS, Yang XK, et al. Differentially expressed circular RNAs in systemic lupus erythematosus and their clinical significance. *BioMed Pharmacother* (2018) 107:1720–7. doi: 10.1016/j.biopha.2018.08.161
90. Li S, Zhang J, Tan X, Deng J, Li Y, Piao Y, et al. Microarray expression profile of circular RNAs and mRNAs in children with systemic lupus erythematosus. *Clin Rheumatol* (2019) 38:1339–50. doi: 10.1007/s10067-018-4392-8
91. Zhang C, Huang J, Chen Y, Shi W. Low Expression and Clinical Value of hsa_circ_0049224 and has_circ_0049220 in Systemic Lupus Erythematous Patients. *Med Sci Monit* (2018) 24:1930–5. doi: 10.12659/msm.906507
92. Wang X, Zhang C, Wu Z, Chen Y, Shi W. CircIBTK inhibits DNA demethylation and activation of AKT signaling pathway via miR-29b in peripheral blood mononuclear cells in systemic lupus erythematosus. *Arthritis Res Ther* (2018) 20:118. doi: 10.1186/s13075-018-1618-8
93. Miao Q, Zhong Z, Jiang Z, Lin Y, Ni B, Yang W, et al. RNA-seq of circular RNAs identified circPTPN22 as a potential new activity indicator in systemic lupus erythematosus. *Lupus* (2019) 28:520–8. doi: 10.1177/0961203319830493
94. Luo Q, Zhang L, Li X, Fu B, Guo Y, Huang Z, et al. Identification of circular RNAs hsa_circ_0044235 and hsa_circ_0068367 as novel biomarkers for systemic lupus erythematosus. *Int J Mol Med* (2019) 44:1462–72. doi: 10.3892/ijmm.2019.4302
95. Guo G, Wang H, Ye L, Shi X, Yan K, Lin K, et al. Hsa_circ_0000479 as a Novel Diagnostic Biomarker of Systemic Lupus Erythematosus. *Front Immunol* (2019) 10:2281:2281. doi: 10.3389/fimmu.2019.02281
96. Luo Q, Zhang L, Fang L, Fu B, Guo Y, Huang Z, et al. Circular RNAs hsa_circ_0000479 in peripheral blood mononuclear cells as novel biomarkers for systemic lupus erythematosus. *Autoimmunity* (2020) 53:167–76. doi: 10.1080/08916934.2020.1728529
97. Li LJ, Zhu ZW, Zhao W, Tao SS, Li BZ, Xu SZ, et al. Circular RNA expression profile and potential function of hsa_circ_0045272 in systemic lupus erythematosus. *Immunology* (2018) 155:137–49. doi: 10.1111/imm.12940
98. Zhang C, Wang X, Chen Y, Wu Z, Zhang C, Shi W. The down-regulation of hsa_circ_0012919, the sponge for miR-125a-3p, contributes to DNA methylation of CD11a and CD70 in CD4(+) T cells of systemic lupus erythematous. *Clin Sci (Lond)* (2018) 132:2285–98. doi: 10.1042/CS20180403
99. Luan J, Jiao C, Kong W, Fu J, Qu W, Chen Y, et al. circHLA-C Plays an Important Role in Lupus Nephritis by Sponging miR-150. *Mol Ther Nucleic Acids* (2018) 10:245–53. doi: 10.1016/j.omtn.2017.12.006
100. Song X, Zhang L, Zhao S, Wang X, Wang L, Chen L, et al. Peripheral blood circRNA expression profile analysis in patients with rheumatoid arthritis. *Chin J Rheumatol* (2016) 20:541–6.
101. Wu H, Zhao M, Tan L, Lu Q. The key culprit in the pathogenesis of systemic lupus erythematosus: Aberrant DNA methylation. *Autoimmun Rev* (2016) 15:684–9. doi: 10.1016/j.autrev.2016.03.002
102. Tang H, Tan G, Guo Q, Pang R, Zeng F. Abnormal activation of the Akt-GSK3beta signaling pathway in peripheral blood T cells from patients with systemic lupus erythematosus. *Cell Cycle* (2009) 8:2789–93. doi: 10.4161/cc.8.17.9446
103. Taher TE, Parikh K, Flores-Borja F, Mletzko S, Isenberg DA, Peppelenbosch MP, et al. Protein phosphorylation and kinome profiling reveal altered regulation of multiple signaling pathways in B lymphocytes from patients with systemic lupus erythematosus. *Arthritis Rheumatol* (2010) 62:2412–23. doi: 10.1002/art.27505
104. Luo Q, Zhang L, Li X, Fu B, Deng Z, Qing C, et al. Identification of circular RNAs hsa_circ_0044235 in peripheral blood as novel biomarkers for rheumatoid arthritis. *Clin Exp Immunol* (2018) 194:118–24. doi: 10.1111/cei.13181
105. Crispín JC, Kyttaris VC, Terhorst C, Tsokos GC. T cells as therapeutic targets in SLE. *Nat Rev Rheumatol* (2010) 6:317–25. doi: 10.1038/nrrheum.2010.60
106. Zhao M, Sun Y, Gao F, Wu X, Tang J, Yin H, et al. Epigenetics and SLE: RFX1 downregulation causes CD11a and CD70 overexpression by altering epigenetic modifications in lupus CD4+ T cells. *J Autoimmun* (2010) 35:58–69. doi: 10.1016/j.jaut.2010.02.002
107. Zhang J, Liu Y, Shi G. The circRNA-miRNA-mRNA regulatory network in systemic lupus erythematosus. *Clin Rheumatol* (2020) 40:331–39. doi: 10.1007/s10067-020-05212-2
108. Okon LG, Werth VP. Cutaneous lupus erythematosus: diagnosis and treatment. *Best Pract Res Clin Rheumatol* (2013) 27:391–404. doi: 10.1016/j.berh.2013.07.008
109. Xuan J, Xiong Y, Shi L, Aramini B, Wang H. Do lncRNAs and circRNAs expression profiles influence discoid lupus erythematosus progression?-a comprehensive analysis. *Ann Transl Med* (2019) 7:728. doi: 10.21037/atm.2019.12.10
110. Scharer CD, Blalock EL, Mi T, Barwick BG, Jenks SA, Deguchi T, et al. Epigenetic programming underpins B cell dysfunction in human SLE. *Nat Immunol* (2019) 20:1071–82. doi: 10.1038/s41590-019-0419-9

4

In Rheumatoid Arthritis Patients, HLA-DRB1*04:01 and Rheumatoid Nodules are Associated with ACPA to a Particular Fibrin Epitope

*Guillaume Larid[1], Mikael Pancarte[2], Géraldine Offer[2], Cyril Clavel[2], Marielle Martin[3], Vincent Pradel[4], Isabelle Auger[3], Pierre Lafforgue[1], Jean Roudier[1,3], Guy Serre[2] and Nathalie Balandraud[1,3]**

[1] Rhumatologie, Institut du Mouvement et de l'appareil Locomoteur (IML), Assistance Publique - Hôpitaux de Marseille (AP-HM), Marseille, France, [2] Université de Toulouse, INSERM, UMRs 1056, UDEAR, Hôpital Purpan, Toulouse, France, [3] Aix Marseille Université, INSERM UMRs 1097, Arthrites autoimmunes, Marseille, France, [4] CEIP de Marseille (PACA-Corse, Centre Associé), Laboratoire de Santé Publique, Faculté de Médecine, Marseille, France

***Correspondence:**
Nathalie Balandraud
Nathalie.balandraud@ap-hm.fr

Objectives: Rheumatoid arthritis (RA) is associated with HLA-DRB1 genes encoding the shared epitope (SE), a 5-amino acid motive. RA is usually preceded by the emergence of anti-citrullinated protein/peptide antibodies (ACPAs). Citrulline is a neutral amino acid resulting from post-translational modification of arginine involved in peptidic bounds (arginyl residue) by PeptidylArginine Deiminases (PADs). ACPAs recognize epitopes from citrullinated human fibrin(ogen) (hFib) and can be specifically detected by the AhFibA assay. Five citrullinated peptides derived from hFib together represent almost all of the epitopes recognized by patients with ACPA-positive RA, namely: α36–50cit, α171–185cit, α501–515cit, α621–635cit, and β60–74cit. The use of antibody fine specificities as markers of clinical phenotypes has become a major challenge. Our objective was to study whether RA clinical characteristics and HLA-DRB1 genetic background were associated with a specific reactivity against the epitopes borne by the five peptides.

Methods: 184 ACPA-positive RA patients fulfilling the 2010 ACR/EULAR criteria were studied. Patient characteristics including HLA-DRB1 genotype, were collected from their medical files. Anti-CCP2 antibodies, AhFibA, and antibodies against the five citrullinated hFib (hFib-cit) peptides were analyzed by ELISA.

Results: Anti-α505-515cit antibodies were associated with HLA-DRB1*04:01 (OR = 5.52 [2.00 – 13.64]; p = 0.0003). High level anti-α505-515cit antibodies were associated with rheumatoid nodules (OR = 2.71 [1.00 – 7.16], p= 0.044).

Conclusion: Immune complexes containing anti-α501-515cit antibodies and rheumatoid factors might be involved in the development of rheumatoid nodules on the HLA-DRB1*04:01 background. Apheresis of these epitope-specific antibodies might be a new therapeutic opportunity for patients with rheumatoid nodules.

Keywords: ACPA, rheumatoid arthritis, HLA-DRB1, AhFibA, citrullinated peptides 2

INTRODUCTION

Rheumatoid arthritis (RA) is the most severe type of chronic autoimmune arthritis. Its prevalence ranges from 0.5% to 1.1% in North America and northern Europe, and between 0.3 and 0.7% in southern Europe (1).

RA features symmetrical bilateral polyarthritis of the small joints. Extra-articular manifestations such as rheumatoid nodules, lung damage, or vasculitis can also be present (2).

RA is usually preceded by the emergence of anti-citrullinated protein/peptide antibodies (ACPAs) and rheumatoid factors of various isotypes. Citrullyl is a neutral residue resulting from post-translational modification of an arginyl residue in the peptidic sequence by PeptidylArginine Deiminases (PADs). The deiminated protein/peptide is said citrullinated.

In ACPA-positive RA, the genetic risk is mostly carried by shared epitope (SE)-positive HLA-DR molecules. The SE (a five-amino acid motif encompassing positions 70 to 74 of the HLA-DRB1 chain) encoded in the major histocompatibility complex (MHC) is present in approximately 70% of patients with ACPA-positive RA (3). Different combinations of HLA-DR alleles (genotypes) confer different relative risks of developing ACPA-positive RA, with highest risks for genotypes encoding two copies of the SE (4).

ACPA present in patients with RA recognize citrullinated epitopes on various proteins (5). A major citrullinated autoantigen expressed in the rheumatoid joint is fibrin, both its alpha and beta chain being recognized by ACPA (6). ACPA are likely to play a role in the pathophysiology of the disease. Indeed, ACPAs have been shown to predict progression of undifferentiated arthritis to RA and are associated with severe disease (7). However, given the heterogeneity of the disease's clinical features, more reliable prognostic and phenotypic markers are missing.

The discovery of ACPA led to the development of diagnostic tests based on a first synthetic cyclic citrullinated peptides (CCP) (8). Since then, several generations of anti-CCP tests have been commercialized (9). ACPAs have become one of the 2010 American College of Rheumatology (ACR)/EULAR RA classification criteria (10).

Besides anti-CCP tests, a test for autoantibodies to human citrullinated fibrinogen (AhFibA) can be used for the serological diagnosis of early RA (11).

Five peptides from human citrullinated fibrinogen (hFib-cit) together contain almost all of the epitopes recognized by patient's sera with ACPA-positive RA. These immunodominant epitopes are borne by the peptides $\alpha 36\text{–}50cit_{38,42}$, $\alpha 171\text{–}185cit_{178,181}$, $\alpha 501\text{–}515cit_{510,512}$, $\alpha 621\text{–}635cit_{621,627,630}$ and $\beta 60\text{–}74cit_{60,72,74}$ (6, 12, 13). Whether reactivity of sera toward these five peptides might allow definition of subgroups among RA patients that might have different disease phenotypes, is an important question.

Previous studies analyzed the recognition by various samples of patients of only 3 (α36–50cit, β60–74cit and FibCit α621-635) out of the 5 major peptides, and only studied early RA defined by the 1987 ACR criteria (14) and not the 2010 ACR/EULAR criteria.

The primary objective of this work was to study whether, in a cohort of 184 patients with ACPA-positive RA fulfilling the 2010 ACR/EULAR criteria, a particular HLA-DR background or original clinical patterns, were associated with antibodies to the epitopes from the 5 major hFib-cit peptides α36–50cit, α171–185cit, α501–515cit, α621–635cit, and β60–74cit.

MATERIAL AND METHODS

Patients

We undertook a prospective study on 184 patients followed at the rheumatology department of Sainte Marguerite Hospital in Marseille. Patients included were considered ACPA-positive RA based on previous results of anti-CCP2 antibodies obtained with various commercial assays, and fulfilled the 2010 ACR/EULAR criteria. Patients treated with Rituximab were excluded due to its potential effect on ACPA levels.

Patient characteristics were collected from their medical files: presence of rheumatoid nodules, smoking habits, age at diagnosis, HLA-DR genotype, IgM rheumatoid factor (RF), activity and erosive characteristics of the disease, treatment response, dry eye syndrome, cardiovascular event, osteoporosis.

- In order to state the presence or absence of rheumatoid nodules, patients medical files and all available chest CT scans were analyzed.
- Disease activity was measured using the Disease Activity Score calculated with the level of C-reactive protein (DAS28-CRP) on the day of the sample.
- Treatment response was evaluated according to the EULAR response criteria. Patients were considered to have shown a good response if their DAS28 was ≤3.2 or has decreased by >1.2 (15) according to the 2019 update of EULAR recommendations for the management of RA, the time needed to achieve treatment target has been set at 6 months before concluding to treatment failure (16).
- Patient personal history of a cerebrovascular accident, myocardial infarction or heart failure was defined as a major cardiovascular event.
- Patients were categorized as smokers (active or previous smokers) or non-smokers.
- Erosive RA was defined according to the EULAR definition of erosive RA (17).
- Dry eye syndrome was defined as a Schirmer's test value ≤ 5 mm/5 min, or an Ocular Staining Score ≥ 5. Dry mouth was defined as an unstimulated salivary flow rate of ≤ 0,1 mL/min.
- Osteoporosis was defined either by personal history of osteoporosis fracture, or by bone mineral density with a T-score below – 2,5 for at least one of the testing sites.

Samples

Patients gave a single blood sample from which plasma was isolated. Samples were stored at -80°C. AhFibA and ACPA fine specificities were assayed and anti-CCP2 were re-assayed with a same test in all patients.

Ethics

All patients gave informed written consent for this study. Patient data was pseudo-anonymized. Sample collection was approved by the ethics committee under the number DC-2008-327. This study was declared to the Assistance Publique – Hôpitaux de Marseille (AP-HM) under the number PADS19-332.

ACPA Testing

For all the ACPA tests, we used the positivity threshold (N) corresponding to 95% diagnostic specificity.

Plasma anti-CCP2 assays were performed using the ELISA CCPlus® IMMUNOSCAN kit (Euro Diagnostica, Arnhem, The Netherlands) according to the manufacturer's recommendations. Antibody titers expressed in arbitrary units (AU/mL) were considered positive above 25 AU/mL.

Anti-human citrullinated fibrinogen IgG autoantibodies were detected with a previously described ELISA (AhFibA). Antibody "titers" (ELISA optical density) above 0.056 were considered positive (6, 18).

Rheumatoid Factor Testing

IgM Rheumatoid Factor (RF) was assayed with the RF ELISA from Orgentec and considered positive if >20 UI/mL.

Antibodies to Human Fibrin(ogen) Citrullinated Peptides

Peptides with the following sequences were synthetized with either arginines (R) in control peptides or citrullines ($\underline{R}$) in target peptides, and used as immunosorbents:

-α36-50: GP$\underline{R}$VVE$\underline{R}$HQSACKDS
-α171-185: biotin-ahx*-VDIDIKI$\underline{R}$SC$\underline{R}$GSCS
-α501-515: biotin-ahx*-SGIGTLDGF$\underline{R}$H$\underline{R}$HPD
-α621-635: $\underline{R}$GHAKS$\underline{R}$PV$\underline{R}$GIHTS
-β60-74: $\underline{R}$PAPPPISGGGY$\underline{R}$A$\underline{R}$

*: ahx: aminohexanoic acid

IgG autoantibodies to the fibrinogen-derived citrullinated peptides α36-50cit, α621-635cit and β60-74cit were tested by ELISA according to a previously described method in which peptides are passively adsorbed on polystyrene microtitration plates (6, 18). IgG autoantibodies to the peptides α171-185cit and α501-515cit were tested by ELISA with biotinylated peptides linked to previously adsorbed Avidin. Briefly, plates (Maxisorp; NUNC, VWR International, Fontenay-sous-Bois, France) were incubated overnight with Avidin at 5 µg/mL. After washing with PBS 0.1% Tween-20 (PBS-T) biotinylated peptides were incubated for 1 hour at 1µg/mL in PBS 2% BSA (PBS-BSA). After 3 washings the plates were incubated for 1 hour with patient plasma diluted to 1/100 in PBS-BSA then washed 3 times in PBS-T. A peroxidase-conjugated goat anti-human IgG antibody (Southern Biotechnology) diluted to 1/2500 in PBS-BSA was incubated for 1h and, after 3 washings, reactivity was revealed by ortho-phenylenediamine dihydrochloride and hydrogen peroxide in a pH5 citrate buffer. The reaction was stopped after 5 min with H_2SO_4 and optical density (OD) read at 492 nm. All the steps were performed at room temperature around 20°C (6). The specific antibody reactivity was defined as the OD difference between the citrullinated and the non-citrullinated related control peptide. Interassay variations were corrected by linear regression analysis using reference peptide and plasma, tested on each plate. ΔOD below the cut-off value of 0.25 were considered negative. Patients with ΔOD over the cut-off were divided into 3 equal groups (tertiles) with weak (T1), medium (T2) or high titers (T3). Patients from the medium and high-titer groups (T2-T3 combined) were considered together to have a "high level" reactivity.

Statistical Analysis

Association studies were carried out with contingency tables using the Chi2 test and Fisher's exact test when Chi2 was not applicable.

The Baptista-Pike method was used to obtain the 95% confidence interval for Odds Ratio (OR).

Spearman's rank correlation coefficient rho was used to measure the correlations between anti-CCP2 antibodies, AhFibA, and antibodies to the 5 peptides and tested against the null hypothesis of rho =0.

Statistical analysis was carried out using PRISM software for Windows (GraphPad Software, 169 San Diego, California, USA) and IBM®SPSS® Statistics version 20. The significance threshold was set at $p < 0.05$.

RESULTS

Clinical Description of the Population

The clinical characteristics of the 184 patients with ACPA-positive RA are shown in **Table 1** (see details in **Supplementary Data File 1**). Half of patients were treated with methotrexate, 24% in monotherapy, and 76% in association with a bDMARD. Among

TABLE 1 | Clinical characteristics of patients.

Number of patients	184
Age (years, mean)	62
Women (%)	75.5
Symptoms duration (mean, years)	15.5
Age at diagnosis (mean, years)	46.4
Rheumatoid nodules	30/180 (16.6%)
Smoker (active or previous)	90/180 (50%)
DAS28 at inclusion	2.44
Major cardiovascular event	15/180 (8.3%)
Erosive rheumatoid arthritis	64/180 (35.5%)
Dry eye syndrome	11/167 (6.6%)
Rheumatoid Factor	121/161 (75%)
Methotrexate treated	96/184 (52.2%)
Monotherapy	23/96 (24.0%)
Associated with other DMARDs	73/96 (76.0%)
Treatment	**Good responders/number treated**
TNF-alpha inhibitors	90/137 (65.6%)
Tocilizumab	37/53 (69.8%)
Abatacept	24/46 (52.1%)

30 patients with rheumatoid nodules, 15/93 had methotrexate, 15/97 had not (p = 0.841, OR = 0.923 [0.44 - 1.941]).

Serological Profile of the 184 Patients With ACPA-Positive RA

The biological characteristics of the 184 patients recruited as ACPA-positive RA based on their anti-CCP2 status are shown in **Table 2** (see details in **Supplementary Data File 1**). When re-assayed with the same reference assay, 98.51% of patients had anti-CCP2 antibodies. On the other hand, 83.23% had AhFibA, and 69.98% had IgM RF.

Among the Citrullinated Peptides

Among the citrullinated peptides, 76.13% of patients recognized biotin-α171-185cit, 67.10% recognized biotin-α501-515cit, 58.06% recognized β60-74cit, 45.16% recognized α621-635cit, and 14.84% recognized α36-50cit.

Epitopic Profiles of ACPA

Analysis of the profiles of epitope recognition in the 184 patients showed that 19% of patients recognized the 4 peptides α171-185cit, α501-515cit, α621-635cit, and β60-74cit, 15% of patients recognized the 3 peptides α171-185cit, α501-515cit, and β60-74cit, and 6% of patients recognized a single peptide (4%: α171-185cit, 1%: α501–515cit, and 1%: β60–74cit) (see **Figure 1**).

Correlations of the Titers of Anti-CCP2 and Anti-Citrullinated Fibrin Peptide Antibodies

The titers of anti-CCP2 and AhFibA were strongly correlated (Spearman's rank correlation coefficient rho (rs): 0.706; p= $4.06x10^{-29}$).

The titers of anti-CCP2 and anti-citrullinated fibrin peptides antibodies were also significantly correlated for 4 of the 5 peptides: α171-185cit (rs: 0.647; p = $3.2x10^{-23}$), α501-515cit (rs: 0.299; p = $3.7x10^{-5}$), α621-635cit (rs: 0.271; p= 0.0002), β60-74cit (rs: 0.517; p = $5.5x10^{-14}$).

By contrast there was no correlation of anti-CCP2 antibodies titers with those of anti-α36-50cit antibodies (rs: -0.010; p = 0.894) (see **Figure 2**).

HLA-DRB1 Background

Among the 184 patients with ACPA-positive RA, 155 were genotyped for HLA-DRB1: 67.1% of patients were SE-positive (49% of patients expressed one copy of the SE, 18.1% expressed two copies). Their clinical characteristics were not different from those in the total 184 patients (see **Supplementary Tables 1, 2, Supplementary Data File 1**).

TABLE 2 | AhFibA and five major citrullinated Fibrin peptides antibodies.

	Negative	Positive
AhFibA	27/184 (14.67%)	157/184 (85.33%)
β60–74cit	76/184 (41.30%)	108/184 (58.70%)
α36–50cit	157/184 (85.33%)	27/184 (14.67%)
α621–635cit	103/184 (55.98%)	81/184 (44.02%)
α501–515cit	62/184 (33.70%)	122/184 (66.3%)
α171–185cit	45/184 (24.46%)	139/184 (75.54%)

HLA-DR Status Association With Clinical Characteristics

HLA-DRB1*04:01 was weakly associated with rheumatoid nodules. Indeed, 44/155 patients expressed HLA-DRB1*04:01 of whom 11 (25%) had rheumatoid nodules, 111/155 patients did not express HLA-DRB1*04:01 of whom 19 (17%) had rheumatoid nodules (Chi2, OR = 2.15 [0.91 - 5.25]; p = 0.081). Other clinical characteristics were not associated with any HLA-DRB1 allele.

HLA-DRB1 Status Association With the Recognition of Citrullinated Peptides

SE Dose Effect on the Number of Peptides Recognized

Patients with two copies of the SE were more likely to recognize more than 3 peptides (OR = 3.02 [1.12 - 8.74]; p = 0.034) (see **Table 3**).

HLA-DRB1 Alleles and Epitopic Specificity

HLA-DRB1*04:01 was associated with antibodies to α501-515 (OR = 5.52 [2.00 - 13.64]; p = $3x10^{-4}$). Conversely, HLA-DRB1*04:01 was associated with absence of antibody to α621-625 (OR=0.46 [0.23 - 0.95]; p=0.036) (see **Table 3**).

Epitopic Specificity of Anti-Citrullinated Fibrin Peptide Antibodies and Clinical Characteristics

Multiple Peptide Recognition

42 of 184 patients recognized more than 3 citrullinated peptides. The 142 remaining patients recognized 3 peptides or less. Patients who recognized more than 3 peptides showed better responses to TNF-alpha inhibitors (OR = 2.93 [1.16 - 7.48]; p = 0.025) and had less often erosive RA (OR = 0.45 [0.19 - 1.04]; p = 0.051) (see **Supplementary Table 3**).

Recognition of the α501-515 Citrullinated Peptide Was Associated With Rheumatoid Nodules and With RF

Rheumatoid nodules were present in 30/180 patients, absent in 130 patients, data being unknown for 20 patients. On the whole group of patients, reactivity against α501-515cit tended to be associated with rheumatoid nodules (OR= 2.32 [0.95 -5.80], p = 0.08) but high level reactivity against the peptide was significantly associated with rheumatoid nodules (see **Table 4**). Indeed, 79/184 (43%) patients had high level reactivity against α501-515cit and among them 18/184 (10%) patients had rheumatoid nodules whereas 61/184 (33%) patients had low level reactivity against α501-515cit of whom only 6/184 (3%) patients had rheumatoid nodules (OR=2.71 [1.00 - 7.16], p=0.044).

Anti-α501-515cit antibodies were also associated with RF (OR=2.31 [1.10 - 4.78], p= 0.026).

DISCUSSION

We studied the associations between HLA-DR background, specificity of ACPAs to epitopes borne by citrullinated fibrin

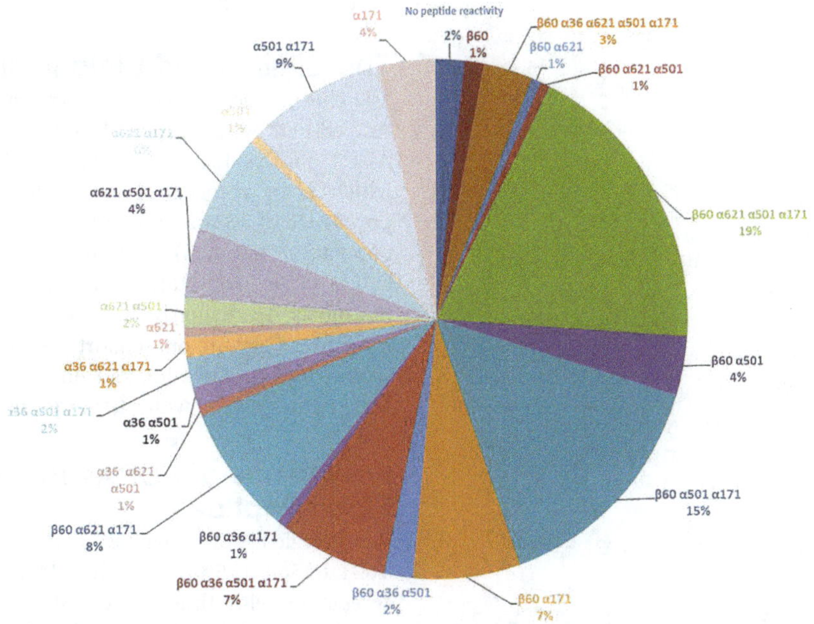

FIGURE 1 | Different profiles of epitopic reactivity in the cohort of 184 patients.

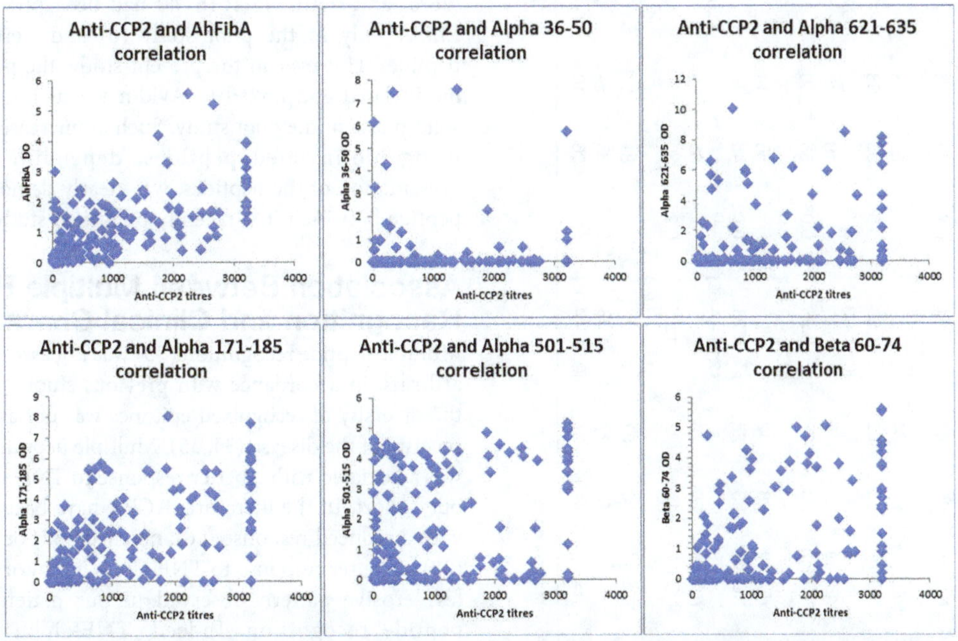

FIGURE 2 | Correlations of anti-CCP2 titers and anti-citrullinated fibrin peptides antibodies (Spearman's rank correlation coefficient rho (rs). OD , optical density; AhFibA , anti-citrullinated human fibrinogen antibodies; anti-CCP2, anti-cyclic citrullinated peptides. There was a positive correlation between anti-CCP2 and AhFibA (r_s : 0.706; p = 4.06x10^{-29}), between anti-CCP2 and anti-α171-185cit (rs: 0.647; p = 3.2x10^{-23}), anti-α501-515cit (rs: 0.299; p = 3.7x10^{-5}),anti-α621-635cit (rs: 0.271; p= 0.0002), and anti-β60-74cit antibodies (rs: 0.517; p = 5.5x10^{-14}). There was no correlation between anti-CCP2 and anti α36–50 (rs: -0.010; p = 0.894) antibodies.

TABLE 3 | Association between epitopic specificity of ACPAs and HLA-DRB1 alleles.

		Shared Epitope N=104/155				HLA-DRB1*04:01 N=44/155				HLADRB1*04:04,*04:05, *04:08,*01 N=69/155				HLADRB1*10:01 N=14/155			
		NO (n)	YES (n)	Odds Ratio [CI 95%]	p	NO (n)	YES (n)	Odds Ratio [CI 95%]	p	NO (n)	YES (n)	Odds Ratio [CI 95%]	p	NO (n)	YES (n)	Odds Ratio [CI 95%]	p
β60-74cit	NO (n)	25	40	1.54 [0.80 – 2.98]	0.21	49	16	1.38 [0.68 – 2.84]	0.37	37	28	1.11 [0.58 – 2.13]	0.76	61	4	1.91 [0.60 – 5.72]	0.29
	YES (n)	26	64			62	28			49	41			80	10		
α36-50cit	NO (n)	45	88	1.36 [0.54 – 3.68]	0.54	95	38	0.93 [0.34 – 2.41]	0.90	77	56	1.99 [0.804 – 4.69]	0.14	120	13	0.44 [0.04 – 2.68]	0.42
	YES (n)	6	16			16	6			9	13			21	1		
α621-635cit	NO (n)	23	62	0.55 [0.28 – 1.06]	0.08	55	30	0.46 [0.23 – 0.95]	**0.04**	45	40	0.80 [0.42 – 1.50]	0.48	79	6	1.70 [0.53 – 5.27]	0.34
	YES (n)	28	42			56	14			41	29			62	8		
α501-515cit	NO (n)	23	28	2.23 [1.10 – 4.55]	**0.02**	46	5	5.52 [2.00 – 13.64]	**0.0003**	31	20	1.38 [0.71 – 2.77]	0.35	45	6	0.63 [0.19 – 1.97]	0.40
	YES (n)	28	76			65	39			55	49			96	8		
α171-185cit	NO (n)	15	22	1.55 [0.74 – 3.28]	0.26	30	7	1.96 [0.78 – 5.00]	0.14	22	15	1.24 [0.60 – 2.71]	0.58	35	2	1.65 [0.41 – 7.81]	0.52
	YES (n)	36	82			81	37			64	54			106	10		
Number of specificities	≤3	42	77	1.63 [0.71 – 4.01]	0.25	85	34	0.96 [0.42 – 2.20]	0.92	69	50	1.54 [0.74 – 3.28]	0.25	111	8	2.78 [0.85 – 8.31]	0.07
	>3	9	27			26	10			17	19			30	6		

N, number. Bold values are the significant ones.

peptides and clinical characteristics in 184 patients with ACPA-positive RA fulfilling the ACR/EULAR 2010 criteria.

The Clinical and Biological Characteristics

The clinical and biological characteristics of the RA population studied here were classical. In our population of patients with ACPA-positive RA, 17% of patients had rheumatoid nodules which is in accordance with other European populations prevalence of 18%-22.4% and less than in northern European population (30-40%) (19). It was previously reported that cvDMARDs or bDMARDs could accelerate rheumatoid nodulosis, particularly methotrexate (20) and TNF-alpha inhibitors (21). In our cohort we could not find any over-representation of rheumatoid nodules in patients treated with DMARDs, specially with methotrexate.

Prevalence of ACPAs to the Citrullinated Fibrin Peptides

The prevalence of antibodies to the peptides α36-50cit (15%), α621-635cit (45%), and β60-74cit (58%), were in close agreement with those previously described with the same ELISAs (11, 13, 22–26) and also those recently described in very large cohorts of patients with a multiplex peptide chip (27–32). The pilot study (6) which identified the peptides bearing the immunodominant epitopes, only used sera selected for highest titers of ACPA, therefore leading to prevalences which are not representative of patient population.

The prevalence of antibodies to the peptides α171-185cit (76%) and α501-515cit (67%) had been previously studied by ELISA only in the pilot study (6) and were 45% for the 2 peptides. However in the present study, the peptides were used biotinylated and linked to Avidin versus immunoadsorbed on solid phase in the pilot study. Such an increased reactivity when using biotinylated peptides, depending on a different presentation of the peptides, was clearly demonstrated with the peptide β60-74cit in a recently published study (33).

Association Between Multiple Peptide Recognition and Clinical Characteristics

Multiple peptide recognition (>3) was not associated with erosive arthritis, in accordance with previous studies that showed that the diversity of recognized epitopes was not associated with the severity of the disease (34, 35). Multiple peptide recognition (>3) was associated with a better response to TNF-alpha inhibitors in our cohort. In the literature, ACPA have been associated either with a reduced response (36), no effect (37) or a better response (38). A better response to TNF-alpha inhibitors may explain the less erosive pattern observed in our patients with multiple peptide recognition. Indeed, TNF-alpha inhibitors limit radiographic progression in patients with RA as already demonstrated (39).

A study of van Beers et al. (40) failed to find association between ACPA fine-specificity profiles in early rheumatoid arthritis patients and clinical features at baseline or with disease progression, however, the citrullinated peptides used in our study were not analyzed, neither rheumatoid nodules.

TABLE 4 | Rheumatoid nodules and Rheumatoid factor association with peptide reactivity.

		Rheumatoid Nodules (n = 30/180)				**Rheumatoid Factor (n = 122/161)**			
		NO (n)	**YES (n)**	**Odds Ratio [CI 95%]**	**p**	**NO (n)**	**YES (n)**	**Odds Ratio [CI 95%]**	**p**
Rheumatoid Factor (n=122/161)	NO (n)	35	3	**2.89 [0.88 – 9.52]**	**0.08**				
	YES (n)	97	24						
β60-74cit	NO (n)	63	11	1.25 [0.55 – 2.69]	0.59	15	54	0.79 [0.37 – 1.68]	0.52
	YES (n)	87	19			24	68		
α36-50cit	NO (n)	130	26	0.23 [0.33 – 2.89]	0.99	36	102	2.35 [0.70 – 7.83]	0.17
	YES (n)	20	4			3	20		
α621-635cit	NO (n)	81	19	0.68 [0.32 – 1.53]	0.35	25	68	1.42 [0.66 – 2.88]	0.36
	YES (n)	69	11			14	54		
α501-515cit**	NO (n)	55	6	**2.32 [0.95 – 5.80]**	**0.08****	18	33	2.31 [1.10 – 4.78]	**0.026**
	YES (n)	95	24			21	89		
α171-185cit	NO (n)	37	7	1.08 [0.45 – 2.75]	0.88	11	30	1.21 [0.56 – 2.68]	0.65
	YES (n)	113	23			28	92		
Number of specificity	≤ 3	119	21	1.65 [0.69 – 3.78]	0.26	35	93	2.73 [0.91 – 7.61]	**0.07**
	> 3	31	9			4	29		

N, number of patients; NS, not significant.
High level anti-α501–515cit (T2-T3 tertiles combined) was significantly associated with rheumatoid nodules,* ***OR =2.71 [1.00 – 7.16], p= 0.044. *79/184 patients had high level anti-α501–515cit, among them 18 patients had rheumatoid nodules, 61/184 patients did not have high level anti- α501–515cit, of whom 6 patients had rheumatoid nodules.*
Bold values are the one which are important regarding the text of the article.

Recently, Manca et al. studied the clinico-serological association of ACPA detected using VCP1 and VCP2 (EBV-derived citrullinated peptides) and HCP1 and HCP2 (histone-H4-derived citrullinated peptides) in 413 established RA. Higher number/levels of ACPA subtypes were associated with lung involvement but not with erosive disease (41).

In Joshua and al. association between ACPA fine specificities and lung abnormalities were studied. Three out of our 5 antibodies (FibCit α36-50, FibCit β60-74, and FibCit α621-635) were used in the study. There was no association between reactivity to any of them and lung abnormalities studied by HR-CT scan but in contrast a significant correlation when reactivity to the various fibrin peptides was considered as a whole (42).

Here, CT scanners were not available for the whole population studied, so we could not confirm any association between number of specificities and lung involvement.

Association Between Particular Anti-Citrullinated Fibrin Peptide Antibodies, HLA Background, and Clinical Characteristics

We found that: 1/HLA-DRB1*04:01 was associated with anti-α501-515cit antibodies, 2/Rheumatoid nodules were associated with HLA-DRB1*04:01, 3/"High level" anti-α501–515cit antibodies were associated with rheumatoid nodules and with IgM rheumatoid factor.

HLA-DRB1*04:01 Was Associated With Anti-α501–515cit Antibodies

Associations between fine-specificity antibodies and the presence of the SE have been already analyzed.

Pratesi et al. studied viral citrullinated peptides (VCP) derived from Epstein-Barr virus nuclear proteins EBNA-1 and EBNA-2. Analyzing the contribution of individual SE alleles, the *0401 allele conferred an increased risk to produce anti-VCP2 ($p = 0.007$) and anti-CCP2 ($p = 0.02$) antibodies whereas *0404 was associated with the production of anti-VCP1 ($p = 0.05$) and anti-VCP2 ($p = 0.04$) antibodies (43).

The C. Terao et al. study (29) investigated whether subtle differences in ACPA serological profiles might be connected to different driving HLA alleles, by analyzing 18 ACPA fine-specificities in RA-affected individuals. A clustering of the peptide reactivities led to divide the patients as having "non-canonical" (including CCP2-negative) or "canonical" serologies (including CCP2-positive). When associations with HLA-A, B, and DR alleles were analyzed, a significant association with aspartic acid residue at Bpos-9 was found between patients with non canonical serologies and an inverse correlation with the canonical ones. In the multiplex peptide array used in that study, 7 peptides from Fibrinogen were present among the 18 tested but only 3 of our 5 peptides, namely α36–50cit, α621–635cit, and β60–74cit. Thus, our study appears as the first correlation analysis of HLA-DR and reactivities to α171–185cit and α501–515cit.

Here, HLA-DRB1*04:01 was associated with anti-α501-515cit antibodies.

In the development of IgG antibody responses, HLA-DR molecules intervene by presenting antigenic peptides to T follicular helper (Tfh) lymphocytes that provide help to B lymphocytes with surface IgM of a given specificity. Specificity of the antibody response relies on the IgM molecule on the B lymphocyte, not on the antigenic peptide presented by-HLA-DR. Thus, association of HLA-DRB1*04:01 with anti-α501-515cit antibodies does not indicate that this RA-associated allele is capable to choose between different B cell epitopes. Rather it suggests that HLA-DRB1*04:01 can provide help to B lymphocytes specific for the α501-515cit peptide and that others HLA-DR alleles can't. This suggests special efficacy of HLA-DRB1*04:01 as a peptide processor and presentator which in turn allows the development of a more efficient Tfh response. HLA-DR molecules encoded by HLA-DRB1*04:01 have been shown to undergo a shortcut from endoplasmic reticulum to lysosomes which allows association with better processed antigenic peptide (44, 45).

HLA-DRB1*04:01 Was Associated With Rheumatoid Nodules

Association of HLA-DRB1*04:01 with rheumatoid nodules is classical. More, in a studied population, rheumatoid nodule frequency correlates directly with the prevalence of HLA-DRB1*04:01 of this population (19).

"High Level" Anti-α501-515cit Antibodies Were Associated With Rheumatoid Nodules and With IgM Rheumatoid Factor

Association between high level anti-α501-515cit antibodies, RF and rheumatoid nodules refers to rheumatoid nodules nature. As previously described, they contain fibrin and IgG but nothing is known about the specificity of those IgG. Necrotic centers were shown to contain citrullinated proteins and RF (46, 47). Our data suggests that at least some of the IgG are anti-α501-515cit antibodies. They might form immune complexes with citrullinated fibrin secondarily transformed in macroimmune complexes by rheumatoid factors (48 49) and be at the origin of rheumatoid nodules.

That link of reactivity to a particular fibrinogen peptide and the presence of rheumatoid nodules needs to be further examined and replication studies must be performed. Moreover, while these findings raise new hypothesis about the pathogenesis of rheumatoid nodules, no study of antigen specificity of the IgG present in the nodules has been performed to date. It could be the purpose of further investigations.

In this cohort we analyzed the epitopic specificity of ACPAs using five major citrullinated fibrin peptides which bear the immunodominant ACPA epitopes and checked whether the specificity was associated with particular clinical, biological, or genetic patterns. Our main finding is the association of antibodies to the epitope borne by the citrullinated peptide α501–515 on the alpha chain of fibrin, with HLA-DRB1*04:01 and with rheumatoid nodules. This unexpected epitope specificity of ACPAs in HLA-DRB1*04:01 patients may relate to the original intracellular route of HLA-DRB1*04:01. The association of anti-α501-515cit antibodies with rheumatoid nodules may suggest that the antibodies to the epitope borne by the α501-515cit peptide particularly contribute to the immune complexes in rheumatoid nodules. This finding pave the way of a potential treatment of rheumatoid nodules by purifying patient's serum from this particular ACPA subtype.

ETHICS STATEMENT

The studies involving human participants were reviewed and approved by Comité d'éthique Aix Marseille Université - DC-2008-327. The patients/participants provided their written informed consent to participate in this study.

AUTHOR CONTRIBUTIONS

NB, GS, and GL designed research and analyzed data. MM, NB, and IA collected samples. MP, GO, and CC tested and analyzed ne specificities. VP performed statistical analysis. GL, NB, and PL analyzed patients files. GL, NB, and JR wrote the manuscript. NB, JR, and GS corrected the manuscript. All authors contributed to the article and approved the submitted version.

ACKNOWLEDGMENTS

The authors would like to thank all physicians who participated in the diagnostics and therapy of the presented patients.

REFERENCES

1. Alamanos Y, Drosos A. Epidemiology of Adult Rheumatoid Arthritis. *Autoimmun Rev* (2005) 4:130–6. doi: 10.1016/j.autrev.2004.09.002
2. Smolen JS, Aletaha D, McInnes IB. Rheumatoid Arthritis. *Lancet* (2016) 388:2023–38. doi: 10.1016/S0140-6736(16)30173-8
3. Gregersen PK, Silver J, Winchester RJ. The Shared Epitope Hypothesis. An Approach to Understanding the Molecular Genetics of Susceptibility to Rheumatoid Arthritis. *Arthritis Rheum* (1987) 30:1205–13. doi: 10.1002/art.1780301102
4. Balandraud N, Picard C, Reviron D, Landais C, Toussirot E, Lambert N, et al. Hla-Drb1 Genotypes and the Risk of Developing Anti Citrullinated Protein Antibody (Acpa) Positive Rheumatoid Arthritis. *PloS One* (2013) 8:e64108. doi: 10.1371/journal.pone.0064108
5. Schellekens GA, de Jong BA, van den Hoogen FH, van de Putte LB, van Venrooij WJ. Citrulline Is an Essential Constituent of Antigenic Determinants Recognized by Rheumatoid Arthritis-Specific Autoantibodies. *J Clin Invest* (1998) 101:273–81. doi: 10.1172/JCI1316
6. Sebbag M, Moinard N, Auger I, Clavel C, Arnaud J, Nogueira L, et al. Epitopes of Human Fibrin Recognized by the Rheumatoid Arthritis-Specific Autoantibodies to Citrullinated Proteins. *Eur J Immunol* (2006) 36:2250–63. doi: 10.1002/eji.200535790
7. Meyer O, Nicaise-Roland P, Santos M, Labarre C, Dougados M, Goupille P, et al. Serial Determination of Cyclic Citrullinated Peptide Autoantibodies Predicted Five-Year Radiological Outcomes in a Prospective Cohort of Patients With Early Rheumatoid Arthritis. *Arthritis Res Ther* (2006) 8:R40. doi: 10.1186/ar1896
8. Schellekens GA, Visser H, de Jong BA, van den Hoogen FH, Hazes JM, Breedveld FC, et al. The Diagnostic Properties of Rheumatoid Arthritis Antibodies Recognizing a Cyclic Citrullinated Peptide. *Arthritis Rheum* (2000) 43:155–63. doi: 10.1002/1529-0131(200001)43:1<155::AID-ANR20>3.0.CO;2-3
9. Ji M, Hur M, Moon H-W, Park M, Yun Y-M, Lee S-H. Comparison of Second- and Third-Generation Immunoassays for Detection of Anti-Cyclic Citrullinated Peptide Antibodies. *Scand J Clin Lab Invest* (2018) 78:477–82. doi: 10.1080/00365513.2018.1499957
10. Aletaha D, Neogi T, Silman AJ, Funovits J, Felson DT, Bingham CO, et al. 2010 Rheumatoid Arthritis Classification Criteria: An American College of Rheumatology/European League Against Rheumatism Collaborative Initiative. *Arthritis Rheumatism* (2010) 62:2569–81. doi: 10.1002/art.27584
11. Nicaise-Roland P, Nogueira L, Demattei C, de Chaisemartin L, Rincheval N, Cornillet M, et al. Autoantibodies to Citrullinated Fibrinogen Compared With Anti-MCV and Anti-CCP2 Antibodies in Diagnosing Rheumatoid Arthritis at an Early Stage: Data From the French ESPOIR Cohort. *Ann Rheum Dis* (2013) 72:357–62. doi: 10.1136/annrheumdis-2011-201056
12. Iobagiu C, Magyar A, Nogueira L, Cornillet M, Sebbag M, Arnaud J, et al. The Antigen Specificity of the Rheumatoid Arthritis-Associated ACPA Directed to Citrullinated Fibrin Is Very Closely Restricted. *J Autoimmun* (2011) 37:263–72. doi: 10.1016/j.jaut.2011.07.003
13. Nogueira L, Cornillet M, Singwe-Ngandeu M, Viatte S, Bas S, Gabay C, et al. In Black Africans With Rheumatoid Arthritis, ACPA Recognize Citrullinated Fibrinogen and the Derived Peptides α36-50Cit38,42 and β60-74Cit60,72,74, Like in Caucasians. *Clin Immunol* (2014) 152:58–64. doi: 10.1016/j.clim.2014.02.011
14. Arnett FC, Edworthy SM, Bloch DA, Mcshane DJ, Fries JF, Cooper NS, et al. The American Rheumatism Association 1987 Revised Criteria for the Classification of Rheumatoid Arthritis. *Arthritis Rheumatism* (1988) 31:315–24. doi: 10.1002/art.1780310302
15. van Gestel AM, Haagsma CJ, van Riel PL. Validation of Rheumatoid Arthritis Improvement Criteria That Include Simplified Joint Counts. *Arthritis Rheum* (1998) 41:1845–50. doi: 10.1002/1529-0131(199810)41:10<1845::AID-ART17>3.0.CO;2-K
16. Smolen JS, Landewé RBM, Bijlsma JWJ, Burmester GR, Dougados M, Kerschbaumer A, et al. EULAR Recommendations for the Management of Rheumatoid Arthritis With Synthetic and Biological Disease-Modifying Antirheumatic Drugs: 2019 Update. *Ann Rheum Dis.* (2020) 79(6):685–99. doi: 10.1136/annrheumdis-2019-216655. annrheumdis-2019-216655.
17. van der Heijde D, van der Helm-van Mil AHM, Aletaha D, Bingham CO, Burmester GR, Dougados M, et al. EULAR Definition of Erosive Disease in Light of the 2010 ACR/EULAR Rheumatoid Arthritis Classification Criteria. *Ann Rheum Dis* (2013) 72:479–81. doi: 10.1136/annrheumdis-2012-202779
18. Chapuy-Regaud S, Nogueira L, Clavel C, Sebbag M, Vincent C, Serre G. Igg Subclass Distribution of the Rheumatoid Arthritis-Specific Autoantibodies to Citrullinated Fibrin. *Clin Exp Immunol* (2005) 139:542–50. doi: 10.1111/j.1365-2249.2004.02708.x
19. Turesson C, Jacobsson L. Epidemiology of Extra-Articular Manifestations in Rheumatoid Arthritis. *Scand J Rheumatol* (2004) 33:65–73. doi: 10.1080/03009740310004621
20. Nakamura T, Higashi S, Tomoda K, Tsukano M, Iyama K. Cutaneous Nodules in Patients With Rheumatoid Arthritis: A Case Report and Review of Literatures. *Clin Rheumatol* (2011) 30:719–22. doi: 10.1007/s10067-010-1602-4
21. Toussirot E, Berthelot JM, Pertuiset E, Bouvard B, Gaudin P, Wendling D, et al. Pulmonary Nodulosis and Aseptic Granulomatous Lung Disease Occurring in Patients With Rheumatoid Arthritis Receiving Tumor Necrosis Factor-α-Blocking Agent: A Case Series. *J Rheumatol* (2009) 36:2421–7. doi: 10.3899/jrheum.090030
22. Cornillet M, Sebbag M, Verrouil E, Magyar A, Babos F, Ruyssen-Witrand A, et al. The Fibrin-Derived Citrullinated Peptide β60-74Cit$_{60,72,74}$ Bears the Major ACPA Epitope Recognised by the Rheumatoid Arthritis-Specific Anticitrullinated Fibrinogen Autoantibodies and Anti-CCP2 Antibodies. *Ann Rheum Dis* (2014) 73:1246–52. doi: 10.1136/annrheumdis-2012-202868
23. Degboé Y, Constantin A, Nigon D, Tobon G, Cornillet M, Schaeverbeke T, et al. Predictive Value of Autoantibodies From Anti-CCP2, Anti-MCV and Anti-Human Citrullinated Fibrinogen Tests, in Early Rheumatoid Arthritis Patients With Rapid Radiographic Progression at 1 Year: Results From the ESPOIR Cohort. *RMD Open* (2015) 1:e000180. doi: 10.1136/rmdopen-2015-000180
24. Cornillet M, Verrouil E, Cantagrel A, Serre G, Nogueira L. In ACPA-Positive RA Patients, Antibodies to EBNA35-58Cit, a Citrullinated Peptide From the Epstein-Barr Nuclear Antigen-1, Strongly Cross-React With the Peptide β60-74Cit Which Bears the Immunodominant Epitope of Citrullinated Fibrin. *Immunol Res* (2015) 61:117–25. doi: 10.1007/s12026-014-8584-2
25. Cornillet M, Ajana S, Ruyssen-Witrand A, Constantin A, Degboé Y, Cantagrel A, et al. Autoantibodies to Human Citrullinated Fibrinogen and Their Subfamilies to the α36-50Cit and β60-74Cit Fibrin Peptides Similarly Predict Radiographic Damages: A Prospective Study in the French ESPOIR Cohort of Very Early Arthritides. *Rheumatology* (2016) 55:1859–70. doi: 10.1093/rheumatology/kew014
26. Rönnelid J, Hansson M, Mathsson-Alm L, Cornillet M, Reed E, Jakobsson P-J, et al. Anticitrullinated Protein/Peptide Antibody Multiplexing Defines an Extended Group of ACPA-positive Rheumatoid Arthritis Patients With Distinct Genetic and Environmental Determinants. *Ann Rheum Dis* (2018) 77:203–11. doi: 10.1136/annrheumdis-2017-211782
27. Sohrabian A, Mathsson-Alm L, Hansson M, Knight A, Lysholm J, Cornillet M, et al. Number of Individual ACPA Reactivities in Synovial Fluid Immune Complexes, But Not Serum Anti-CCP2 Levels, Associate With Inflammation and Joint Destruction in Rheumatoid Arthritis. *Ann Rheum Dis* (2018) 77:1345–53. doi: 10.1136/annrheumdis-2017-212627
28. Jonsson MK, Hensvold AH, Hansson M, Aga A-B, Sexton J, Mathsson-Alm L, et al. The Role of Anti-Citrullinated Protein Antibody Reactivities in An Inception Cohort of Patients With Rheumatoid Arthritis Receiving Treat-to-Target Therapy. *Arthritis Res Ther* (2018) 20:146. doi: 10.1186/s13075-018-1635-7
29. Terao C, Brynedal B, Chen Z, Jiang X, Westerlind H, Hansson M, et al. Distinct HLA Associations With Rheumatoid Arthritis Subsets Defined by Serological Subphenotype. *Am J Hum Genet* (2019) 105:616–24. doi: 10.1016/j.ajhg.2019.08.002
30. Boman A, Brink M, Lundquist A, Hansson M, Mathsson-Alm L, Rönnelid J, et al. Antibodies Against Citrullinated Peptides Are Associated With Clinical and Radiological Outcomes in Patients With Early Rheumatoid Arthritis: A Prospective Longitudinal Inception Cohort Study. *RMD Open* (2019) 5:e000946. doi: 10.1136/rmdopen-2019-000946
31. Reed E, Hedström AK, Hansson M, Mathsson-Alm L, Brynedal B, Saevarsdottir S, et al. Presence of Autoantibodies in "Seronegative" Rheumatoid Arthritis Associates With Classical Risk Factors and High Disease Activity. *Arthritis Res Ther* (2020) 22:170. doi: 10.1186/s13075-020-02191-2

32. Westerlind H, Rönnelid J, Hansson M, Alfredsson L, Mathsson-Alm L, Serre G, et al. Anti-Citrullinated Protein Antibody Specificities, Rheumatoid Factor Isotypes, and Incident Cardiovascular Events in Patients With Rheumatoid Arthritis. *Arthritis Rheumatol* (2020) 72:1658–67. doi: 10.1002/art.41381
33. Cornillet M, Babos F, Magyar A, Sebbag M, Verrouil E, Hudecz F, et al. Seropositivity and Antibody Profiling of Patients Are Dramatically Impacted by the Features of Peptides Used as Immunosorbents: A Lesson From Anti–Citrullinated Protein/Peptide Antibody. *JI* (2018) 201:3211–7. doi: 10.4049/jimmunol.1800330
34. Joo YB, Park Y-J, Park K-S, Kim K-J. Association of Cumulative Anti-Cyclic Citrullinated Protein Antibodies With Radiographic Progression in Patients With Rheumatoid Arthritis. *Clin Rheumatol* (2019) 38:2423–32. doi: 10.1007/s10067-019-04554-w
35. Scherer HU, van der Woude D, Willemze A, Trouw LA, Knevel R, Syversen SW, et al. Distinct ACPA Fine Specificities, Formed Under the Influence of HLA Shared Epitope Alleles, Have No Effect on Radiographic Joint Damage in Rheumatoid Arthritis. *Ann Rheum Dis* (2011) 70:1461–4. doi: 10.1136/ard.2010.146506
36. Potter C, Hyrich KL, Tracey A, Lunt M, Plant D, Symmons DPM, et al. Association of Rheumatoid Factor and Anti-Cyclic Citrullinated Peptide Positivity, But Not Carriage of Shared Epitope or *PTPN22* Susceptibility Variants, With Anti-Tumour Necrosis Factor Response in Rheumatoid Arthritis. *Ann Rheum Dis* (2009) 68:69–74. doi: 10.1136/ard.2007.084715
37. Lv Q, Yin Y, Li X, Shan G, Wu X, Liang D, et al. The Status of Rheumatoid Factor and Anti-Cyclic Citrullinated Peptide Antibody Are Not Associated With the Effect of Anti-Tnfα Agent Treatment in Patients With Rheumatoid Arthritis: A Meta-Analysis. *PloS One* (2014) 9:e89442. doi: 10.1371/journal.pone.0089442
38. Sokolove J, Schiff M, Fleischmann R, Weinblatt ME, Connolly SE, Johnsen A, et al. Impact of Baseline Anti-Cyclic Citrullinated Peptide-2 Antibody Concentration on Efficacy Outcomes Following Treatment With Subcutaneous Abatacept or Adalimumab: 2-Year Results From the AMPLE Trial. *Ann Rheum Dis* (2016) 75:709–14. doi: 10.1136/annrheumdis-2015-207942
39. Murray E, Ellis A, Butylkova Y, Skup M, Kalabic J, Garg V. Systematic Review and Network Meta-Analysis: Effect of Biologics on Radiographic Progression in Rheumatoid Arthritis. *J Comp Eff Res* (2018) 7:959–74. doi: 10.2217/cer-2017-0106
40. van Beers JJ, Willemze A, Stammen-Vogelzangs J, Drijfhout JW, Toes RE, M Pruijn GJ. Anti-Citrullinated Fibronectin Antibodies in Rheumatoid Arthritis Are Associated With Human Leukocyte Antigen-DRB1 Shared Epitope Alleles. *Arthritis Res Ther* (2012) 14:R35. doi: 10.1186/ar3744
41. Manca ML, Alunno A, D'Amato C, Bistoni O, Puxeddu I, Gerli R, et al. Anti - Citrullinated Peptide Antibodies Profiling in Established Rheumatoid Arthritis. *Joint Bone Spine* (2018) 85:441–5. doi: 10.1016/j.jbspin.2017.07.009
42. Joshua V, Hensvold AH, Reynisdottir G, Hansson M, Cornillet M, Nogueira L, et al. Association Between Number and Type of Different ACPA Fine Specificities With Lung Abnormalities in Early, Untreated Rheumatoid Arthritis. *RMD Open* (2020) 6:e001278. doi: 10.1136/rmdopen-2020-001278
43. Pratesi F, Petit-Teixeira E, Sidney J, Teixeira VH, Puxeddu I, Sette A, et al. Effect of Rheumatoid Arthritis (Ra) Susceptibility Genes on the Immune Response to Viral Citrullinated Peptides in RA. *J Rheumatol* (2012) 39:1490–3. doi: 10.3899/jrheum.111548
44. Auger I, Escola JM, Gorvel JP, Roudier J. Hla-DR4 and HLA-DR10 Motifs That Carry Susceptibility to Rheumatoid Arthritis Bind 70-Kd Heat Shock Proteins. *Nat Med* (1996) 2:306–10. doi: 10.1038/nm0396-306
45. Roth S, Willcox N, Rzepka R, Mayer MP, Melchers I. Major Differences in Antigen-Processing Correlate With a Single Arg ^{71} ↔Lys Substitution in HLA-DR Molecules Predisposing to Rheumatoid Arthritis and With Their Selective Interactions With 70-Kda Heat Shock Protein Chaperones. *J Immunol* (2002) 169:3015–20. doi: 10.4049/jimmunol.169.6.3015
46. Turunen S, Huhtakangas J, Nousiainen T, Valkealahti M, Melkko J, Risteli J, et al. Rheumatoid Arthritis Antigens Homocitrulline and Citrulline are Generated by Local Myeloperoxidase and Peptidyl Arginine Deiminases 2, 3 and 4 in Rheumatoid Nodule and Synovial Tissue. *Arthritis Res Ther* (2016) 18:239. doi: 10.1186/s13075-016-1140-9
47. Athanasou NA, Quinn J, Woods CG, Mcgee JO. Immunohistology of Rheumatoid Nodules and Rheumatoid Synovium. *Ann Rheum Dis* (1988) 47:398–403. doi: 10.1136/ard.47.5.398
48. Anquetil F, Clavel C, Offer G, Serre G, Sebbag M. Igm and IgA Rheumatoid Factors Purified From Rheumatoid Arthritis Sera Boost the Fc Receptor- and Complement-Dependent Effector Functions of the Disease-Specific Anti-Citrullinated Protein Autoantibodies. *J Immunol* (2015) 194:3664–74. doi: 10.4049/jimmunol.1402334
49. Laurent L, Anquetil F, Clavel C, Ndongo-Thiam N, Offer G, Miossec P, et al. Igm Rheumatoid Factor Amplifies the Inflammatory Response of Macrophages Induced by the Rheumatoid Arthritis-Specific Immune Complexes Containing Anticitrullinated Protein Antibodies. *Ann Rheum Dis* (2015) 74:1425–31. doi: 10.1136/annrheumdis-2013-204543

5

Cartilage Oligomeric Matrix Protein Induced Arthritis—A New Model for Rheumatoid Arthritis in the C57BL/6 Mouse

Yunjuan Zhao[1,2], Vilma Urbonaviciute[2], Bingze Xu[2], Weiwei Cai[2], Zeynep Sener[2], Changrong Ge[2] and Rikard Holmdahl[2]*

[1] *Department of Endocrinology, The Second Affiliated Hospital of Guangzhou Medical University, Guangzhou, China,*
[2] *Medical Inflammation Research, Department of Medical Biochemistry and Biophysics, Karolinska Institute, Stockholm, Sweden*

Correspondence:
Rikard Holmdahl
rikard.holmdahl@ki.se

The most commonly used strains in experimental research, including genetically modified strains, are C57BL/6 mice. However, so far, no reliable model for rheumatoid arthritis is available, mainly due to the restriction by the MHC class II haplotype H-2^b. Collagen-induced arthritis (CIA) is the most widely used animal model of rheumatoid arthritis, but C57BL/6 strain is resistant to CIA because there is no collagen II peptide associated with H-2^b. To establish a rheumatoid arthritis model in C57BL/6 mice, we immunized C57BL/6NJ (B6N) mice with human cartilage oligomeric matrix protein (COMP), which induced severe arthritis with high incidence, accompanied by a strong auto-antibody response. Native COMP was required, as denatured COMP lost its ability to induce arthritis in B6N mice. An immunodominant COMP peptide was identified as the key T cell epitope, with a perfect fit into the A^b class II peptide binding pocket. A critical amino acid in this peptide was found to be phenylalanine at position 95. Recombinant COMP mutated at position 95 (COMP_F95S) lost its ability to induce arthritis or a strong immune response in the B6N mice. In conclusion, A new model for RA has been established using C57BL/6 mice through immunization with COMP, which is dependent on a COMP specific peptide binding A^b, thus in similarity with CIA in A^q expressing strains.

Keywords: rheumatoid arthritis, cartilage oligomeric matrix protein, C57BL/6 mice, T cell epitope, B cell epitope

Abbreviations: CIA, collagen-induced arthritis; COMP, cartilage oligomeric matrix protein; RA, rheumatoid arthritis; CII, type II collagen; SPF, specific pathogen-free; CFA, complete Freund adjuvant; IFA, in incomplete Freund's adjuvant.

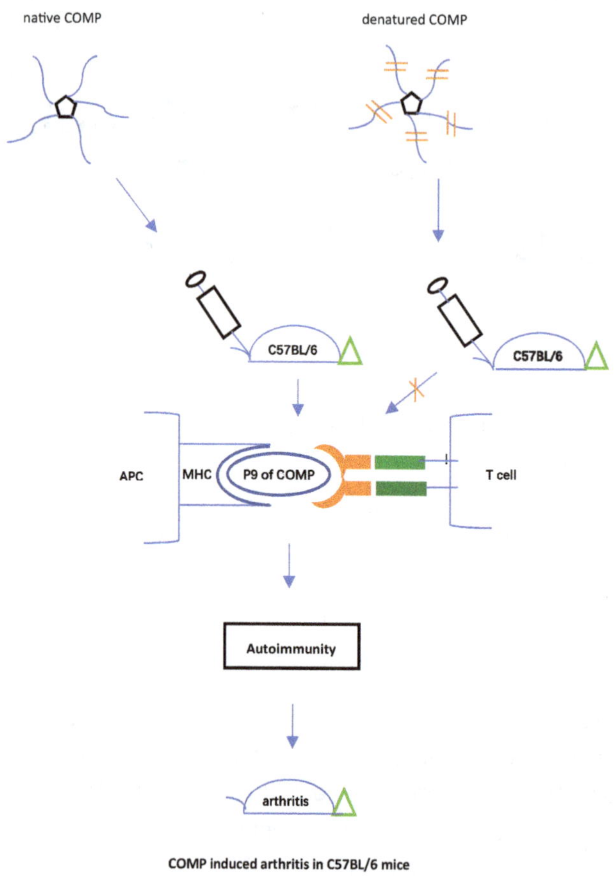

GRAPHICAL ABSTRACT |

HIGHLIGHTS

1. A new model of rheumatoid arthritis in C57BL/6 mice, the COMP induced arthritis (COMPIA), was established.
2. The major T and B cell epitopes on COMP critically involved in the arthritis development were defined.

INTRODUCTION

Rheumatoid arthritis (RA) is a chronic inflammatory disease, which is characterized by leucocyte infiltration into synovial tissue and leads to cartilage and bone damage (1). It is a disease induced by not yet defined environmental factors but it also has a genetic component. The major histocompatibility complex (MHC) region class II shows the by far strongest association, strongly implicating peptide binding to an MHC class II molecule to be a critical bottleneck for the development of RA (2–5). Disease-associated risk alleles in DRB1 may share common amino acid sequences in the peptide-binding groove, suggesting peptide presentation to T cells in disease susceptibility (6, 7). To study the pathogenesis of RA, it is important to use animal models which mimic RA genetically, through an induced autoimmune response associated with the MHC class II locus.

Collagen-induced arthritis (CIA) is the most widely used animal model of RA. The susceptibility to arthritis after immunization with heterologous type II collagen (CII) is strongly associated with MHC class II genes, more precisely the A^q beta gene (8) due to binding of the immunodominant CII-derived glycosylated peptide 260-271 (9). In a screen of different MHC congenic strains only mice expressing A^q and A^r developed arthritis whereas mice with the A^b (H-2^b) haplotype, as in commonly used C57BL/6 strains, were resistant to CIA (10–12). However, the most commonly used mouse strains in research are based on C57BL/6 (H-2^b) (13–15), in particular in genetic research as it is often the reference standard. The discovery that immunization with various collagen preparations together with high content of mycobacteria adjuvant could induce arthritis also in B6 mice (13), has therefore been very popular and is today the most commonly used model for RA. However, despite its name, it does not represent collagen induced arthritis, as the disease develops in response to contaminants in the CII preparations (13). One contaminant is pepsin used for the cleavage of CII during the preparation and others are non-self-matrix proteins when derived from cows or chicken. It means that the T cell response binds to non-collagen proteins forming complexes with CII, enabling interaction with CII specific B cells, and thereby a specific pathogenic antibody response to CII could be elicited (16).

To establish a model for RA in C57BL/6 mice we turned our interest to other proteins that have earlier been shown to induce arthritis in mice, i.e. glucose-6-phosphoisomerase (GPI) (17) and cartilage oligomeric matrix protein (COMP) (18). We found that immunization with COMP led to severe arthritis in C57BL/6 mice.

COMP, also known as thrombospondin 5, is a pentameric glycoprotein of 524 kD (19) with five identical subunits (19). It is primarily found in cartilage, tendon, synovium and meniscus. COMP stabilizes the matrix and acts as a catalyst in the fibril formation of collagens I and II (20). It is also considered to be involved in pathological changes of cartilage during the pathogenesis of osteoarthritis (21). Immunization with COMP induces severe arthritis mimicking RA in both rats and mice (COMPIA) (18, 22). In similarity with CIA, the induction of COMPIA requires break of self-tolerance, and recognition of peptides on non-self-COMP by T cells, although the immunogenic epitopes have not been defined. Previously, the COMP induced arthritis was shown to be associated with MHC class II haplotypes, H-2^q, H-2^p, and also with transgenic human DR*0401 (18). However, in these studies the responsiveness of B6 mice with H-2^b was not included and there are no other studies describing COMPIA in C57BL/6 mice.

In the present study, we describe arthritis induced in C57BL/6 mice and identify the key COMP peptide recognized by T cells.

MATERIALS AND METHODS

Mice

Male C57BL/6NJ (denoted B6N) mice, which carry the H-2^b haplotype, originally obtained from Jackson Laboratory, were used in the experiments. Animals were bred and maintained in the animal facility of Medical Inflammation Research, Karolinska Institute, with specific pathogen-free (SPF) conditions and individually ventilated cages contained wood shavings and folded paper strips. The cages were kept in the same room with a climate-controlled environment in a 12-h light-dark cycle. All of the experiments were carried out when the mice were 9–12 weeks old. Experimental mice were divided randomly, blinded and age-matched. Clinical evaluation of arthritis was performed blindly and double-checked for each experiment. All experiments were approved by Stockholm regional ethics committee for animal research, Sweden (N35/16).

Antigens

Native Recombinant Human COMP

The COMP sequence was obtained from UniProtKB with accession number P49747. The construct contains the native leader sequence and the full-length COMP sequence and the C-terminal his-tag. The gene was synthesized at Eurofins with KpnI and XhoI restriction sites at the 5' and 3' ends. The synthesized gene was restriction enzyme digested using FastDigestTM enzymes (ThermoFisher Scientific). The digested DNA fragment was cloned into a mammalian expression vector pCEP4 (Life technologies) that was digested using the same restriction enzymes. After sequence verification, the recombinant plasmid was transfected into Expi393FTM cells (Life technologies) using the FectoPROTM DNA transfection reagent (Polyplus transfection). The supernatants were harvested 6 days post transfection. The recombinant protein was first captured using a 5 ml HisTrap Excel (GE Healthcare Life Sciences) affinity column followed by size exclusion chromatography on a HiLoad Superdex 200 pg column (GE Healthcare life Sciences) equilibrated in PBS. The purified recombinant protein (**Supplement Figure 1**) was obtained as a single peak and was concentrated using an Amicon centrifuge device with MWCO of 30 kD. The protein concentration was determined using absorbance at 280 nm.

Denatured COMP

Denatured COMP was prepared by incubating native human COMP in a high concentration of guanidinium chloride as previously described (23).

Synthetic Peptide Library of Human COMP

Overlapping peptide libraries consisting of 18-aa-long peptides (totally 76 peptides) were generated using the sequence of human COMP. Synthetic peptides containing interest sequences were synthesized by Biomatik Corporation (Ontario, CA).

Synthetic Peptides (P9, P9-1, P9-2, P9-3, P9-4, mP9)

Synthetic peptides (P9, P9-1, P9-2, P9-3, P9-4, mP9) were synthesized by Hangzhou Taijia Biotech Co., Ltd (Hangzhou, China). Further details are given in **Table 1**.

Synthetic Cyclic Peptides

Synthetic cyclic peptides were synthesized as previously described (24).

Mutated COMP_F95S

For the expression of a single amino acid mutated COMP_F95S, two primers were designed with forward primer: 5'-AGGTTCCTGCTTTCCCGGAGTAGCG-3' and reverse primer: 5'-GGTGCACAGTGCAGCAGAGGCC-3'. A Q5 site-directed mutagenesis kit (E0554S, New England BioLabs) was used according to the manufacturer's instruction. After transformation, several colonies were selected and the sequences verified. The plasmid with the right sequence was transfected into the Expi393FTM cells as described above.

TABLE 1 | Amino acid sequence of mutated COMP P9 peptides.

Peptide	Amino acid sequence
P9-human	**APGFCFPGVACIQTESGA**
P9-1	**APGSCFPGVACIQTESGA**
P9-2	**APGFCFPGVVCIQTESGA**
P9-3	**APGFCFPGVACSETESGA**
P9-4	**APGFCFPGVACIQTASGA**

Red font means the mutated amino acid site compared with P9-human.

Induction of Experimental Arthritis

Mice were immunized intradermally (i.d.) at the base of the tail with 100 ug of native COMP emulsified 1:1 in Freund,s complete adjuvant (CFA, #263810, Difco, BD) or in Freund,s incomplete adjuvant (IFA, #263910, Difco, BD) containing Mycobacterium Tuberculosis H37Ra (M.T., #231141, Difco, 0.5 mg/ml) in a total volume of 100 ul on day 0. All the mice were boosted on day 35 with 50 ug of native COMP in IFA in a total volume of 50 ul. Mice were double blind scored 3 times per week for the peripheral joint inflammation, starting 2 weeks after the first immunization. The evaluation of arthritis was conducted in a blinded manner according to an extended scoring protocol (25), using 0–15 scale for each paw (0 = normal joint; 1 = each swollen toe or joint; 5= one swollen ankle). The total maximum score per mouse was 60 points.

To evaluate the requirement of the native structure of COMP for the arthritis induction, mice were immunized with 100 ug of native COMP (group 1), denatured COMP (group 2) emulsified 1:1 in Freund's complete adjuvant (CFA, #263810, Difco, BD) or CFA only (group 3) separately on day 0. On day 35, all the mice were boosted with or without COMP in IFA (#263910, Difco, BD) in a total volume of 50ul (group 1 = 50 ug of native COMP in IFA; group 2=50ug of denatured COMP in IFA; group 3 = IFA only). The evaluation of arthritis was conducted as described above.

To prove the importance of phenylalanine at position 95 for the T cell epitope recognition and arthritis development, mice were immunized i.d. at the base of the tail with 100ug of COMP_F95S or native COMP emulsified 1:1 in Freund's complete adjuvant (CFA, #263810, Difco, BD) on day 0. On day 35, the mice were boosted with 50ug of COMP_F95S or native COMP in IFA (#263910, Difco, BD) in a total volume of 50ul. The evaluation of arthritis was conducted as described above.

Detection of Autoantibodies

Detection of serum levels of antibodies against COMP and CII: Serum antibody levels against COMP were analyzed in 96-well plate (Nunc, Thermo Fisher Scientific, Denmark) by ELISA using recombinant human COMP. Recombinant human COMP (50uL/well; 10ug/ml in phosphate buffer saline (PBS), PH 7.4) was precoated overnight at 4. Then the plates were blocked with 3% milk in PBS to decrease background disturbance. The plates were washed for 5 times with ELISA buffer (PBS with 0.1% Tween 20). The serum was diluted (*500) in PBS (5*time titration, 5 wells for each sample), and incubated for 2 h. Serum from COMP- induced arthritis mice were used as positive control. 50ul of secondary antibody was added and incubated for 1 h. The secondary antibodies were as following: Rat Anti-Mouse Kappa- Horseradish peroxidase (HRP) (Southern Biotech, #117-05), Goat Anti-Mouse IgG(H +L) (Southern Biotech, #1031-05), Goat Anti-Mouse IgG_1 (Southern Biotech, #1070-05) and Goat Anti-Mouse IgG_{2b}-HRP (Southern Biotech, #1091-05). After washing for 5 times, ExtrAvidin® -Peroxidase (1:5000 dilution, Sigma E-2886) was added and incubated for 45 mins. 5mg ABTS substrate (ABTS tablets, Boehringer Mannheim) was diluted in 5 ml of freshly prepared buffer (ABTS buffer, Boehringer Mannheim). After 20 min-incubation in the dark at 20, absorbance was measured at 405nm (OD405). Serum antibody against CII were analyzed by sandwich ELISA, as previously described (26).

Immune Assays

Peptide-Based ELISA

In the first experiment, we performed epitope mapping of whole human COMP by ELISA to identify linear B cell epitopes with serum from COMPIA B6N model. Maxisorb plates were coated with COMP peptides or native COMP at a concentration of 5 ug/ml in PBS overnight at 4. The second day the plates were washed with PBST for 3 times and then blocked with 1% bovine serum albumin (BSA) in PBS. Different dilutions (1:100 to 1:2500) of mice serum (B6N mice immunized with COMP+CFA) were added to the wells and incubated for 1 h at room temperature. Then the plates were washed with PBST for 3 times. HRP-conjugated anti-mouse second antibody was added for further incubation of 1 h followed by the detection using ABTS-HRP system as previous description. Absorbance was measured at 405nm (OD405).

ELISpot Assay

The 96-well ELISpot plates (MSIPS4W10, Millipore) were prewetted with 70% EtOH and then precoated with anti-mouse IFN-γ capture antibody R46A2 (15 ug/ml, 50 ul/well) overnight at 4. The second day the plates were washed with PBS for twice and then blocked with 1% BSA in PBS. Splenocytes or cells from draining lymph nodes were obtained from the immunized B6N mice and added to the plates ($1x10^6$ cells per well for splenocytes, $0.5x10^6$ cells per well for lymph node cells). The cells were stimulated with 50 ug/ml different peptides (peptides from human COMP library; P9; P9-1, P9-2, P9-3, P9-4) in triplicates at 37for 24 h. Concanavalin A (Con A, 1 ug/ml) used as a positive control. The plates were washed with PBS twice and a washing buffer (PBS containing 0.01% Tween 20) for 4 times followed by incubation with 50ul/well of biotinylated anti-IFN-γ (clone An18, 4 ug/ml in PBS/BSA 0.5%) at room temperature for 2 h. After washing the plates with the washing buffer for 5 times, streptavidin-alkaline phosphatase (50 ul/well, 1:2500 in PBS) was added to each well and incubated for 45 min at room temperature. After washing with the washing buffer for 3 times and PBS for 3 times, cytokine spots were visualized using Sigma Fast BCIP/nitroblue tetrazolium (100 ul/well) and enumerated using an ImmunoScan ELISpot Analyzer (CTL Europe).

Histological Analyses

Mice were sacrificed at the end time point, and the hind paws were dissected and subsequently fixed in 10% buffer formalin solution. Fixed tissues were decalcified for 30 days in EDTA-solution (100g EDTA, 75 g polyvinylpyrrolidone, Tris 0.1M in 1L H_2O, add KOH to PH = 6.95) for decalcification, followed by dehydration and paraffin embedding. Tissue sections (7 μm) were then stained with hematoxylin and eosin (HE). HE-stained sections were blindly assessed in naive B6N mice or B6N mice immunized with native COMP.

Molecular Modeling

The homology model of the MHC class II molecule A^b in complex with COMP (92–109) was constructed using the SWISS-MODEL (27), and the crystal structure of A^b with an PADI4 peptide (PDB code: 6MNM) was selected as a template due to high sequence similarity (28). The potential core binding residues (FCFPGVACI) of COMP (92–109) was predicted using Consensus algorithm (29). For modeling the COMP (92–109) peptide in the binding groove of A^b, the PADI4 peptide from crystal structure of A^b in complex with PADI4 peptide (PDB code: 6MNM) was used as a basis, then several residues were modeled by FoldX program (30), then the side chains were optimized by Swrl4 program (31).

Statistical Analyses

All data are expressed as the mean ± SEM. Mann-Whitney test and Kruskal-Wallis test were used for statistical analyses (GraphPad Prism version 8.0.2). $p<0.05$ was considered as significant $^*p<0.05$, ** $p<0.01$.

RESULTS

Immunization With COMP Induces Severe Arthritis With High Incidence in B6N Mice

To test the potential of COMP for the induction of arthritis, we immunized B6N mice with COMP emulsified in complete Freund, adjuvant (CFA, #263810, Difco, BD) or in incomplete Freund's adjuvant (IFA, #263910, Difco, BD) containing Mycobacterium Tuberculosis strain H37Ra (M.T., #231141, Difco, 0.5 mg/ml). Both groups immunized with COMP developed severe arthritis with high incidence (**Figures 1A, B**).

The arthritic joints from arthritic B6N mice revealed prominent synovial hyperplasia, inflammatory cells infiltration and cartilage and bone destruction in both group of mice immunized with native COMP+CFA or native COMP + IFA + 0.5 mg/ml M.T. at the end time point of the experiment, similarly to human RA (**Figure 1C**).

Native COMP Induces Antibody Responses and Specific B Cell Epitopes Are Recognized in B6N Mice

Next, we compared anti-COMP autoantibody responses between three groups. Mice in both immunized groups (immunized with native COMP+CFA or native COMP + 0.5 mg/ml M.T.+IFA) developed a prominent IgG anti-COMP autoantibody response, compared with naïve B6N mice ($^*p<0.05$). There was no difference between mice immunized with native COMP+CFA and mice immunized with native COMP + 0.5 mg/ml M.T.+IFA ($p>0.05$) (**Figure 2A**). Similar trends were observed in values of IgG1 and IgG2b between three groups (**Figure 2A**).

To test whether an immune response to CII was triggered, we analyzed anti-CII Ig levels. Anti-CII Ig levels, as detected with antibodies to kappa, showed no significant difference between immunized and naïve B6N mice (**Figure 2B**).

To confirm that the B cell response is specific for COMP and to identify peptide B cell epitopes, we first screened an overlapping peptide library of COMP with serum from COMP-immunized B6N mice by ELISA. Serum samples were taken at the end point. Results indicated five potential B cell epitopes (peptide 7, 29, 30, 37, 39). We selected 15 peptides (including the five potential epitopes) to repeat the experiment at different serum dilution (n=4), which confirmed the result (**Figure 2C**). We subsequently selected six cyclic COMP peptides with the same sequences as the candidate peptides and used them for testing the serum response. It confirmed that these peptides had positive reaction with immunized mice serum (**Figure 2D**), showing that these are peptide sequential epitopes. In conclusion, a peptide specific antibody response to COMP is induced after immunization of COMP in the B6 mouse.

Induction of Arthritis Is Dependent on the Native Structure of COMP

To investigate if the conformational structure of COMP has an effect on arthritogenicity, we immunized B6N mice with native COMP + CFA, denatured COMP + CFA or CFA separately. All B6N mice immunized with native COMP developed severe arthritis whereas mice immunized with denatured COMP developed only very mild arthritis with low incidence (14%). As expected, B6N mice immunized with CFA did not develop arthritis (**Figure 3A**).

To test whether the native conformational of COMP is recognized by antibodies developed after the immunization with both COMP preparations, we analyzed the sera at different time points during COMPIA (at days 35 and 88 post-immunization). Both native COMP immunized group and denatured COMP group developed an anti-COMP antibody response at both time points ($^*p<0.05$) (**Figure 3B**). However, the immunization with native COMP induced stronger IgG, IgG1, and IgG2b anti-COMP responses than immunization with denatured COMP ($^*p<0.05$). We conclude that antibodies to conformational epitopes are pathogenic and need for the induction of arthritis and that these antibodies are likely triggered by help from COMP specific T cell.

Identification of a Major T Cell Epitope, of Critical Importance for Development of Arthritis

A library of overlapping human COMP peptides (Fig 4A) were tested for their ability to activate T cells after immunization with human COMP. IFN-γ secretion by $CD4^+$ T cells was used as a read-out and ConA was used as a positive control. Spleen cells from mice immunized with COMP showed strong IFN-γ T cell recognition of peptide P9 (APGFCFPGVACIQTESGA) (**Figure 4A**). Out of 76 pairs of peptides tested, only P9 was able to significantly active CD4+T cells from H-2^b mice (**Figures 4B–D**). Additionally, splenocytes from naïve B6N mice were tested, which shows negative reaction to P9 (**Figures 4B–D**).

To determine how the P9 peptide is located in the Ab MHC class II molecule we compared with earlier published

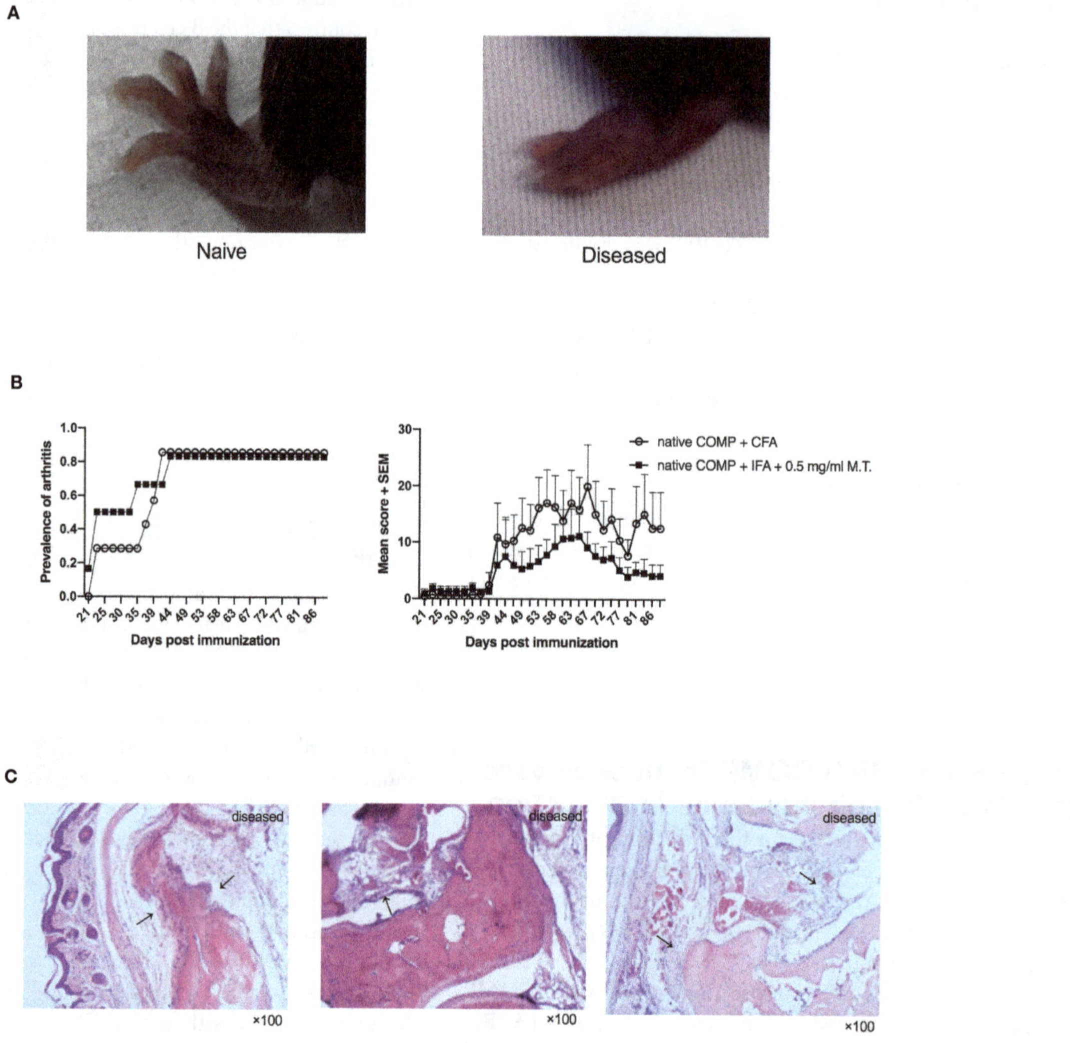

FIGURE 1 | Native COMP induces arthritis in B6N mice with high incidence and severe arthritis. **(A)** The arthritis joint phenotype of B6N mice. **(B)** B6N mice were immunized with native COMP emulsified in CFA (n=7) or IFA+0.5 mg/ml M.T. (n=6), and monitored for prevalence and clinical score of arthritis. **(C)** Histological analysis of ankle joint of B6N mice with COMP-induced arthritis at the end of the experiment. Sections were stained with H&E staining. Prominent synovial hyperplasia, inflammatory cells infiltration and cartilage and bone destruction in mice immunized with native COMP+CFA. All images were taken at ×100 magnification.

structural data (32). The topological structure of the binding of the P9 peptide fitted will molecular modeling and docking onto the Ab molecule (**Figure 4E**). On the A^b structure, COMP-P9 fits into the most regions of the A^b groove (**Figures 4F, G**). We conclude that the A^b can accommodate the P9 peptide which adopts an MHC class II-binding conformation.

Identification of Critical Amino Acids Within the Immunodominant COMP Epitope

To make a strong T cell recall response to human COMP the targeted peptide must differ from the endogenous peptide, to avoid tolerance. To identify the critical amino acids, we compared the sequence of mouse COMP with human COMP and found differences at several positions. New peptides varying at these positions were synthesized (**Table 1**) and tested in the IFN-γ ELISpot assay using splenocytes of human COMP immunized B6N mice (**Supplement Figure 2**). We observed that P9-2, P9-3, P9-4 and P9 induced IFN-γ secretion, but not P9-1 (**Figures 5A–C**). This suggest that the phenylalanine at position 95 is critical for the immunogenicity of human COMP. Imaging analysis of the peptide interaction with MHC class II showed that this amino acid is most likely filling the P1 position on the A^b molecule (**Figure 4E**).

Phenylalanine at Position 95 of COMP Is Critical for Induction of Arthritis

To determine whether phenylalanine at position 95 is critical for the development of arthritis we made a new recombinant COMP protein replacing phenylalanine with serine at position

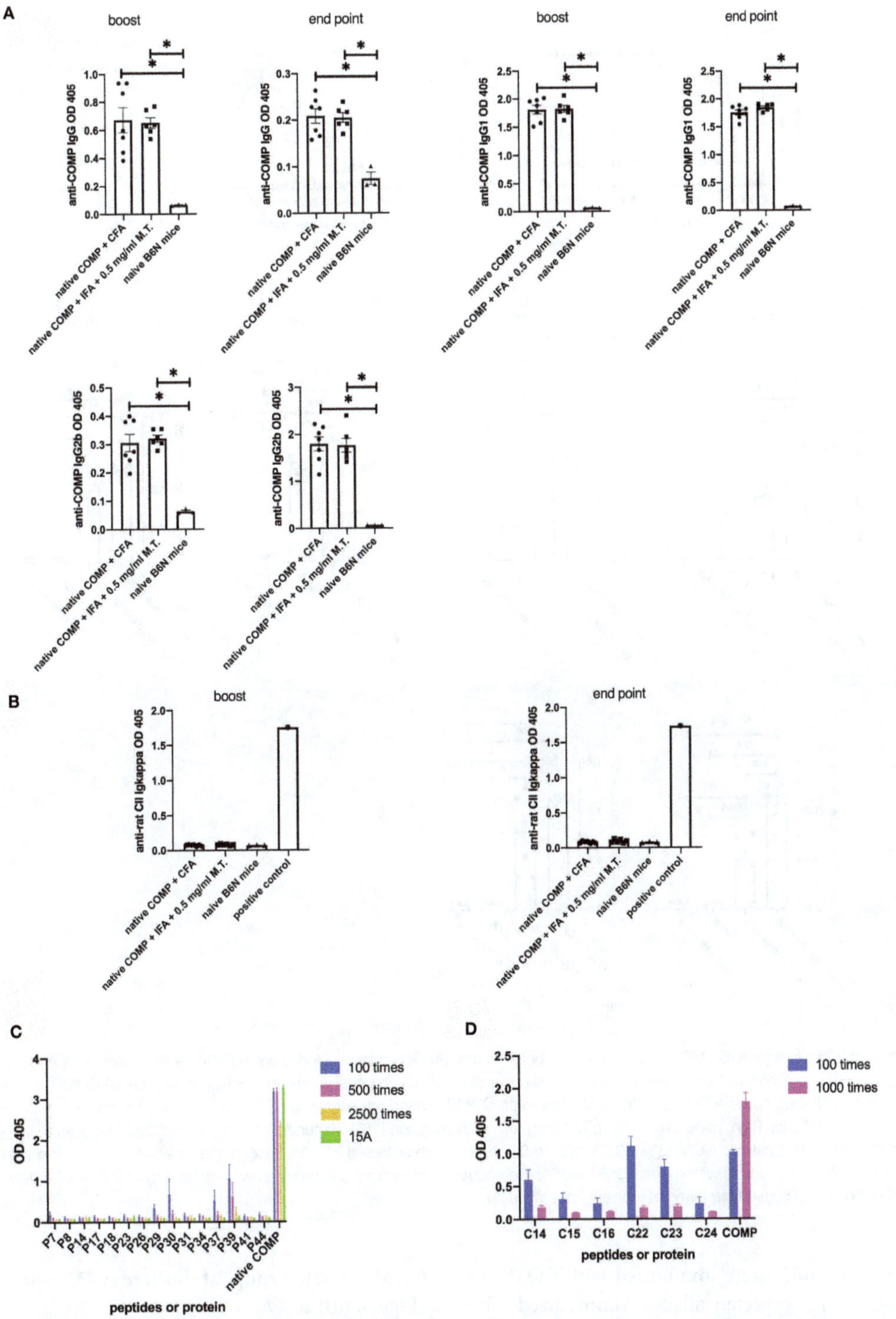

FIGURE 2 | Native COMP induces antibody responses and specific B cell epitopes are characterized in B6N mice. **(A, B)** Native COMP induced anti-COMP antibodies but no anti-CII antibodies in B6N mice. **(A)** Both native COMP+CFA group (n=7) and native COMP+IFA+0.5 mg/ml M.T. group (n=6) have anti-COMP IgG, gG1 and IgG2b production throughout the experiment (*$p < 0.05$). There are no differences of anti-COMP IgG, IgG1, and IgG2b levels between the two groups (p>0.05). **(B)** No response to rat CII could be detected in COMP immunized mice (p>0.05) (A B6N mouse immunized with rat CII was chosen as positive control). **(C)** Mapping of human COMP linear B-cell epitopes using overlapping peptide library of COMP protein (n=6) **(D)** According to the results of experiment A **(C)**, We choose six cyclic COMP peptides (C14, C15, C16, C22, C23 and C24) in a cyclic COMP library, which are similar to the sequences of the candidate peptides (peptide 7, 29, 30, 37, 39). We precoated the plate with these cyclic peptides and added two dilutions of serum of B6N mice immunized with COMP with 2 dilute (diluted 100 times and 1000 times) to test the OD value by ELISA. Positive binding was defined as 3SD from the mean of naïve mice (n=4). Antibody binding was measured by ELISA. The results presented as absorbance at nm 405.

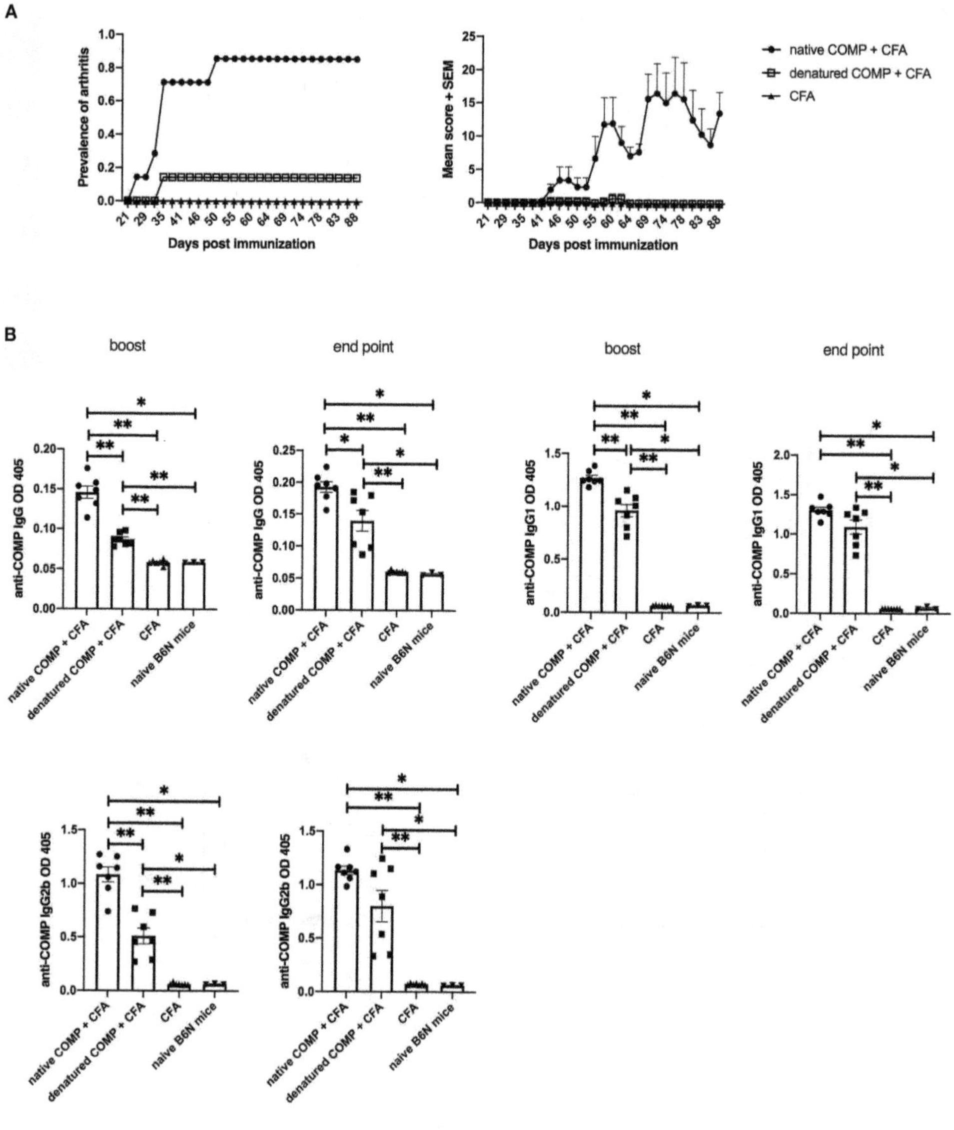

FIGURE 3 | Induction of arthritis requires COMP to be in its native conformation. **(A)** B6N mice were immunized with native COMP + CFA (n=7), denatured COMP + CFA (n=7) or CFA only (n=7) and monitored for prevalence and clinical score of arthritis. Left panel shows immunization with native COMP can induce arthritis in B6N mice with high incident rate (100%); however, immunization with denatured COMP can induce arthritis in B6N mice with very low incident rate (14.3%); immunization with CFA only do not induce arthritis. Right panel shows the clinic score of the three groups. **(B)** Immunization with native COMP induces a stronger specific IgG response than immunization with denatured COMP (*$p < 0.05$, **$p < 0.01$). Blood were collected 35 days (boost) after the immunization and the end point from B6N mice. Filled circles indicate mice immunized with native COMP + CFA; filled squares indicate mice immunized with denatured COMP + CFA; filled triangles indicate mice immunized with CFA only; inverted filled triangles indicate naïve mice.

95 (COMP_F95S). B6N mice were immunized with COMP or COMP_F95S in CFA. As expected all mice immunized with COMP developed severe arthritis. Only 1 out of 8 B6N mice immunized with COMP_F95S developed arthritis, with very low scores (**Figure 6A**).

To test whether COMP_F95S immunization induces anti-COMP antibodies, we determined the production of anti-COMP antibodies during the disease progression. The antibody levels (IgG, IgG1, and IgG2b) were clearly higher in mice immunized with native COMP group compared with those immunized with COMP_F95S group at both day 35 and at the endpoint (**Figure 6B**).

We tested the T cell response specificity in a recall IFN-γ ELISpot assay (**Supplement Figure 3**). As expected the COMP immunized mice showed a response to the P9 peptide but not the COMP_F95S immunized mice. Interestingly, mice immunized with COMP_F95S could still make a detectable T cell response to COMP protein indicating that the F95S mutation did not abolish all T cell responses, only the T cell response of importance for arthritis development (**Figure 6C**).

A

MVPDTACVLLLTLAALGASGQGQSPLGSDLGPQMLRELQETNAALQDVRELLRQQ
VREITFLKNTVMECDACGMQQSVRTGLPSVRPLLHC**APGFCFPGVACIQTESGA**RC
GPCPAGFTGNGSHCTDVNECNAHPCFPRVRCINTSPGFRCEACPPGYSGPTHQGVGL
AFAKANKQVCTDINECETGQHNCVPNSVCINTRGSFQCGPCQPGFVGDQASGCQRR
AQRFCPDGSPSECHEHADCVLERDGSRSCVCAVGWAGNGILCGRDTDLDGFPDEKL
RCPERQCRKDNCVTVPNSGQEDVDRDGIGDACDPDADGDGVPNEKDNCPLVRNPD
QRNTDEDKWGDACDNCRSQKNDDQKDTDQDGRGDACDDDIDGDRIRNQADNCPR
VPNSDQKDSDGDGIGDACDNCPQKSNPDQADVDHDFVGDACDSDQDQDGDGHQD
SRDNCPTVPNSAQEDSDHDGQGDACDDDDDNDGVPDSRDNCRLVPNPGQEDADR
DGVGDVCQDDFDADKVVDKIDVCPENAEVTLTDFRAFQTVVLDPEGDAQIDPNWV
VLNQGREIVQTMNSDPGLAVGYTAFNGVDFEGTFHVNTVTDDDYAGFIFGYQDSSS
FYVVMWKQMEQTYWQANPFRAVAEPGIQLKAVKSSTGPGEQLRNALWHTGDTESQ
VRLLWKDPRNVGWKDKKSYRWFLQHRPQVGYIRVRFYEGPELVADSNVVLDTTMR
GGRLGVFCFSQENIIWANLRYRCNDTIPEDYETHQLRQA

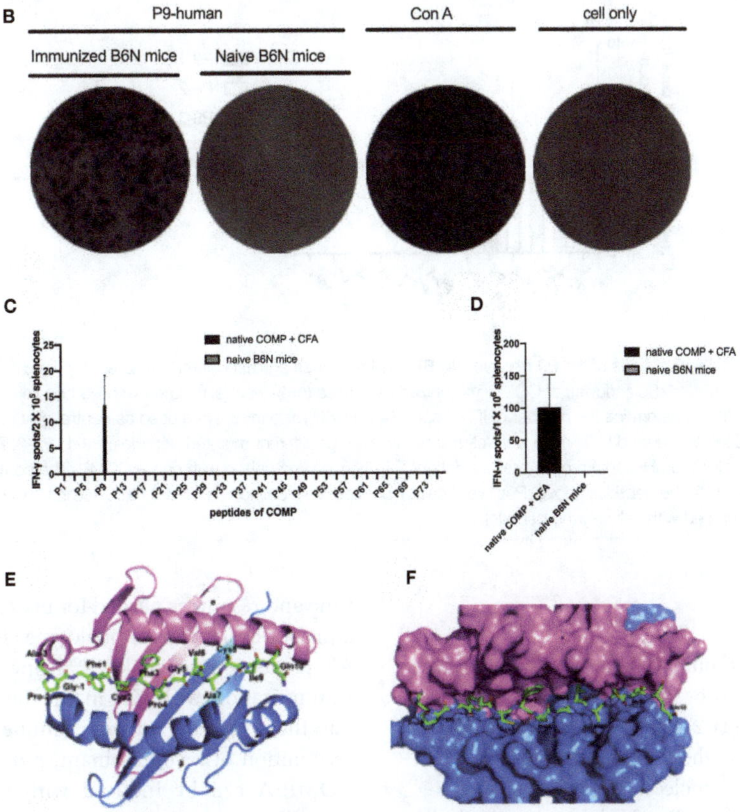

G

```
CLUSTAL O(1.2.4) multiple sequence alignment


COMP       APGFCFPGVACIQTESGA   18
PADI4      RVSYYGPKTSPVQ-----   13
             .:  * .: :*
```

FIGURE 4 | P9 (human COMP peptide 92-109) is identified as the key T cell epitope, which induces arthritis in COMP-immunized B6N mice. We build an overlapping peptides library of human COMP, which includes 76 peptides. **(A)** shows the human COMP sequence and the red sequence is the candidate T cell epitope. **(B)** shows that P9 of human COMP shows positive T-cell reaction in COMP-immunized B6N mice. **(C)** peptides screening: B6N mice were immunized with native COMP + CFA (n=3), and naïve B6N mice (n=3) were chosen as control. 14 days later, splenocytes were harvested, 2×10^5 cells were added to each well (50 ug/ml for peptide, 76 peptides for each well separately) for 24 h in an IFN-γ ELISpot assay to screen the COMP library. P9 shows positive T-cell reaction in COMP-immunized B6N mice, which suggests it should be the candidate T cell epitope. **(D)** P9 identification: B6N mice were immunized with native COMP + CFA (n=3), and naïve B6N mice (n=3) were chosen as control. 14 days later, splenocytes were harvested, 1×10^6 cells were incubated with P9 (50 ug/ml) for 24 h in an IFN-γ ELISpot assay. The peptide with spots >10 with PP/control ratio ≥ 3 is considered as the positive peptides. Graph shows the mean number of spots ± SEM from 3 individual B6N mice. **(E)** Top view of COMP- P9 - H-2^b shown in cartoon presentation with the peptide (P9) shown in stick representation. α, β of H-2^b and COMP-P9 are colored with pink, blue and green, respectively. **(F)** Proposed model of overall crystal structure of H-2^b/P9 peptide complex: P9 peptide recognition by the H-2^b loop. α, β of H-2^b and COMP-P9 are colored with pink, blue and green, respectively. **(G)** The P9 peptide structure modeled based on PADI4 structure.

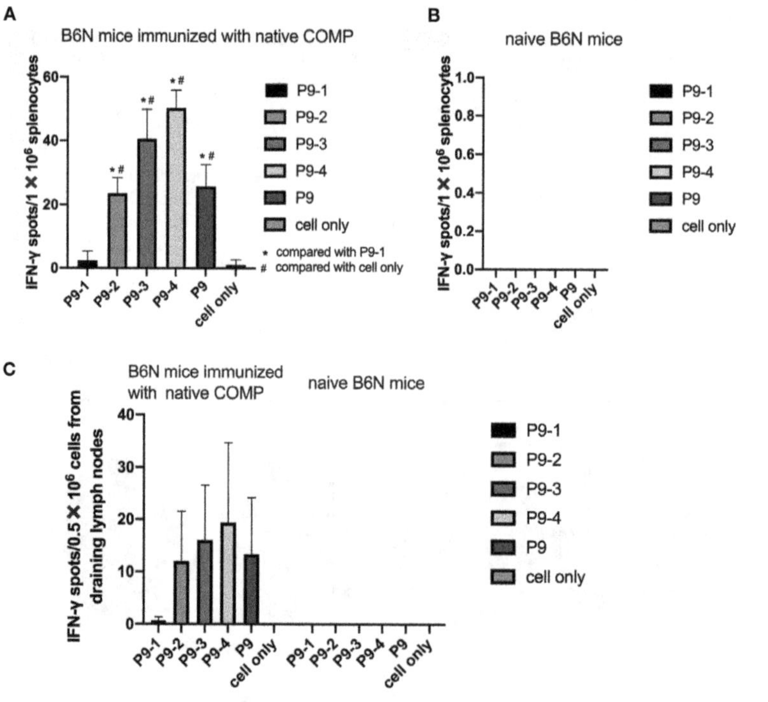

FIGURE 5 | Identification of the critical amino acids of the P9 peptide. **(A, B)** T cell response against different mutated peptides or control as detected in IFN-γ ELISpot assay after 14-day recall stimulation. Splenocytes of COMP immunized B6N mice (n=3) were stimulated with P9 or different mutated peptides (P9-1, P9-2, P9-3, P9-4), followed by ELISpot assay to determine the number of IFN-γ spot. Naïve B6N mice (n=3) were used as control group. Con A were included as positive control. **(C)** Lymph node cells of COMP immunized H-2^b mice were stimulated with P9 or different mutated peptides (P9-1, P9-2, P9-3, P9-4), followed by ELISpot assay to determine the number of IFN-γ spot. Histogram plots present data of 3 B6N mice immunized with native COMP. The control conditions are lymph node cells from naïve B6N mice stimulated with the peptides above. Positive T cell responses were defined as SPU/0.5×10^6 cells ≥ 10 with PP/control ratio ≥ 3. $^*p < 0.05$ compared with P9-1, $^{\#}p < 0.05$ compared with cell only (no peptide).

DISCUSSION

In this study, we show that human COMP, a non-collagen glycoprotein primarily produced by cartilage, can induce arthritis in C57BL/6 mice that carry the H-2^b haplotype, which is useful as a model for human RA. It requires the T cell recognition of a COMP derived peptide bound to the A^b molecule.

The new COMPIA model in B6N mice has many similarities with the well-known CIA model. It induces a severe polyarthritis in diarthrodial joints. It is MHC class II associated and the COMP-derived peptide recognized by T cells is defined. In similarity with CIA the induction of arthritis is facilitated by a T cell response to non-self -COMP, due to that the immunodominant peptide is not binding well to the MHC class II molecule and is thus likely to be ignored for development of tolerance (33). The COMP immunization also induces a strong antibody response, which likely contributes to the development of arthritis (34). Importantly, the COMPIA model has a major advantage as compared with the CIA model, it is inducible in C57BL/6 mice, carrying the H-2^b haplotype. This is important as C57BL/6 mice is regarded as a standard background in immunology research and is a background commonly used for genetically modified mouse strains. Thus, to use the novel COMPIA model in B6 mice does not require the time and resources needed for backcrossing of mice to introgress a proper MHC class II haplotype, as the MHC class II molecule A^q is needed to make a proper CIA experiment (8, 13). Immunization with CII in the B6 mice may lead to arthritis, but the triggering of an immune response is due to T cell recognition of a contaminant, most likely complexed with CII. COMPIA can be induced with recombinant COMP and is dependent on a specific T cell response to COMP. Interestingly, in similarity with CII, COMP induces arthritis in mice expressing the murine A^q and the human DR*0401 MHC class II molecules (18). Thus, the COMPIA model is useful in many strains developed for arthritis research and the immune response is directly comparable with human RA.

Systemic delivery of nanoparticles coated with antigens (autoimmune-relative peptides) bound to MHC class II molecules trigger autoimmune reaction in different mouse models (35), which confirms the core role of peptide recognition by MHC class II in the pathogenesis of autoimmune diseases. Recognition of peptide by an H-2^b derived MHC class II molecule has not earlier been reported to be of relevance in a RA model. To understand the detailed molecular basis of the interaction of COMP-P9 with H-2^b, we mutated the amino acids of COMP-P9 and produced the mutated protein by refolding Escherichia coli, we demonstrated a direct interaction between COMP-P9 with the A^b molecule. The

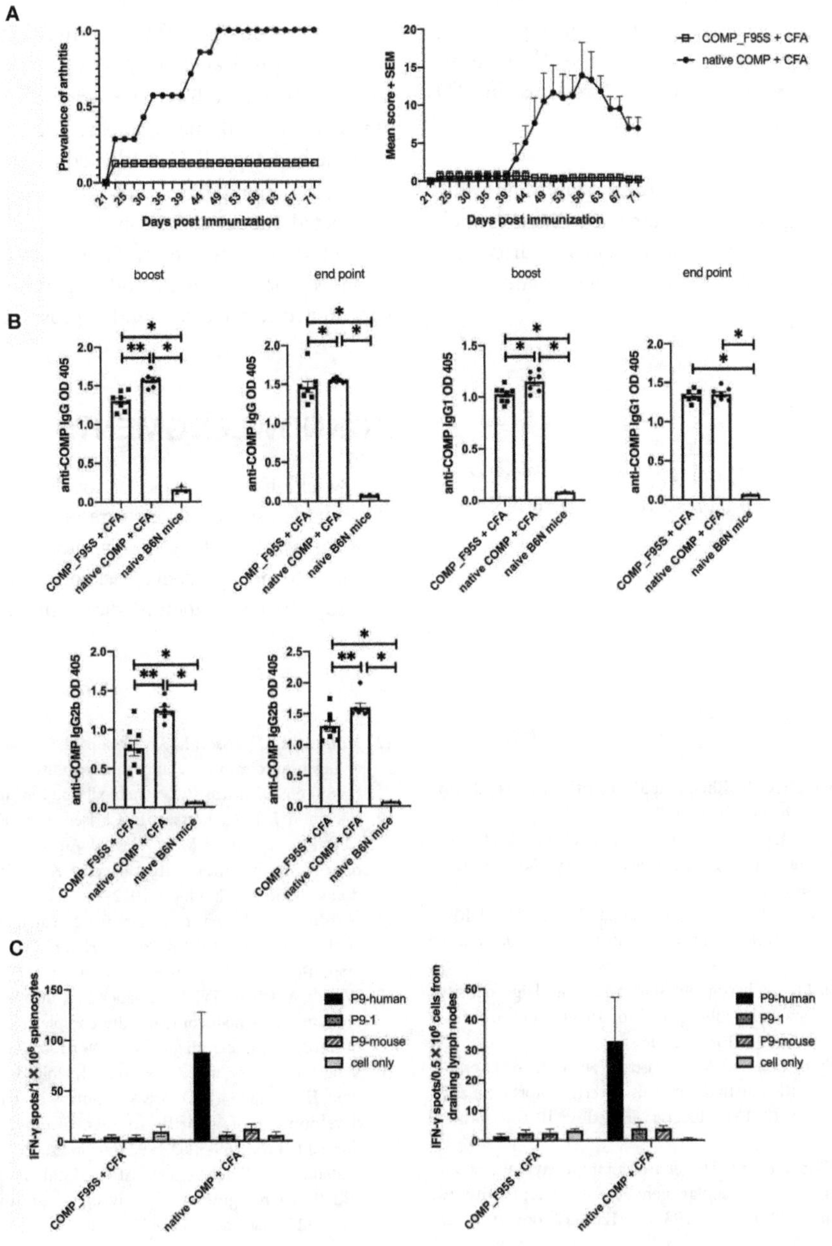

FIGURE 6 | Only COMP, and not COMP_F95S, induces severe arthritis. **(A)** B6N mice were immunized with native COMP (n=7) or COMP_F95S (n=8) emulsified in CFA and monitored for development of arthritis. Left panel shows the prevalence of arthritis; Right panel shows clinical scores of arthritis. The figures show that immunization with native COMP induce severe arthritis in 7 out of 7 B6N mice whereas only 1 out of 8 mice immunized with COMP_F95S developed arthritis. **(B)** B6N mice were immunized with native COMP + CFA (n=7) or COMP_F95S + CFA (n=8). Blood were collected 35 days after the immunization and at the end point. Filled circles indicate mice immunized with native COMP + CFA; filled squares indicate mice immunized with COMP_F95S + CFA; filled triangles indicate naïve mice. The antibody levels (IgG, IgG1 and IgG2b) are higher in native COMP + CFA group than COMP_F95S + CFA mice (*$P < 0.05$, **$P < 0.01$). **(C)** Mice immunized with COMP_F95S have no reaction with P9 of COMP in T cell recall assay. Left panel: 14 days later, splenocytes of COMP_F95S (n=3) or native COMP (n=3) immunized mice were stimulated with peptide (P9-human, P9-1 and P9-mouse) or protein (COMP_F95S and native COMP), followed by ELISpot assay to determine the number of IFN-γ spot. It shows that splenocytes of mice immunized with native COMP has strong T cell reaction with P9 of human COMP, however, splenocytes of mice immunized with COMP_F95S has no reaction with P9 of human COMP. Right panel: 14 days later, cells from draining lymph nodes of COMP_F95S (n=3) or native COMP (n=3) immunized mice were stimulated with peptide (P9-human, P9-1 and P9-mouse) or protein (COMP_F95S and native COMP), followed by ELISpot assay to determine the number of IFN-γ spot. It shows that cells from draining lymph nodes of mice immunized with native COMP has strong T cell reaction with P9 of human COMP, however, cells from draining lymph nodes of mice immunized with COMP_F95S show no reaction with P9 of human COMP. Positive T cell responses were defined as SPU/0.5 × 10^6 cells ≥ 10 with PP/control ratio ≥ 3.

mutational experiment resulted in a different profile of arthritis susceptibility, as the mutants COMP (COMP-F95S) resulted in eight-time reduction of incidence of arthritis. Our experiments provide a conclusive biochemical evidence that the A^b molecule binds COMP-P9 leading to COMP-specific T cell response in B6N mice, that is a key step for induction of arthritis.

In summary, a new model for RA has been established using C57BL/6 (H-2^b) mice through immunization with COMP, which is dependent on a COMP specific peptide, thus in similarity with collagen induced arthritis in H-2^q (A^q) expressing strains.

ETHICS STATEMENT

The animal study was reviewed and approved by Stockholm regional ethics committee for animal research, Sweden (N35/16).

AUTHOR CONTRIBUTIONS

YZ was in charge of the animal experiments, methodology, software, formal analysis, resources, investigation, data collection, and wrote and edited the original draft. VU conducted the investigation and methodology. BX conducted the investigation and methodology. WC conducted the investigation. CG conducted the investigation, and provided the methodology and software. ZS conducted the investigation. RH conceptualized the study and subject design, wrote, reviewed, and edited the manuscript, provided the resources, and supervised the study. All authors contributed to the article and approved the submitted version.

ACKNOWLEDGMENTS

We would like to thank Carlos Palestro, Kristina Palestro, and Veronika Jansson for taking care of the animals in the KMA facility of Karolinska Institute. YZ is supported by the "Jingying Plan" scholarship and "Academic-backbone training program of high-level university" of Guangzhou Medical University to study in Sweden.

REFERENCES

1. Smolen JS, Aletaha D, McInnes IB. Rheumatoid arthritis. *Lancet* (2016) 388:2023–38. doi: 10.1016/S0140-6736(16)30173-8
2. Okada Y, Wu D, Trynka G, Raj T, Terao C, Ikari K, et al. Genetics of rheumatoid arthritis contributes to biology and drug discovery. *Nature* (2014) 506:376–81. doi: 10.1038/nature12873
3. Meyer JM, Evans TI, Small RE, Redford TW, Han J, Singh R, et al. HLA-DRB1 genotype influences risk for and severity of rheumatoid arthritis. *J Rheumatol* (1999) 26:1024–34.
4. Eyre S, Bowes J, Diogo D, Lee A, Barton A, Martin P, et al. High density genetic mapping identifies new susceptibility loci for rheumatoid arthritis. *Nat Genet* (2012) 44:1336–40. doi: 10.1038/ng.2462
5. Viatte S, Plant D, Han B, Fu B, Yarwood A, Thomson W, et al. Association of HLA-DRB1 Haplotypes with Rheumatoid Arthritis Severity, Mortality, and Treatment Response. *JAMA* (2015) 313:1645–56. doi: 10.1001/jama.2015.3435
6. Gregersen PK, Silver J, Winchester RJ. The Shared Epitope Hypothesis. an approach to understanding the molecular genetics of susceptibility to rheumatoid arthritis. *Arthritis Rheumatol* (1987) 30:1205–12. doi: 10.1002/art.1780301102
7. McInnes IB, Schett G. The pathogenesis of rheumatoid arthritis. *N Engl J Med* (2011) 365:2205–19. doi: 10.1056/NEJMra1004965
8. Brunsberg U, Gustafsson K, Jansson L, Michaëlsson E, Ahrlund-Richter L, Pettersson S, et al. Expression of a transgenic class II Ab gene confers susceptibility to collagen-induced arthritis. *Eur J Immunol* (1994) 24:1698–702. doi: 10.1002/eji.1830240736
9. Michaëlsson E, Andersson M, Engström A, Holmdahl R. Identification of an immunodominant type-II collagen peptide recognized by T cells in H-2q mice: self tolerance at the level of determinant selection. *Eur J Immunol* (1992) 22:1819–25. doi: 10.1002/eji.1830220722
10. Wooley PH, Luthra HS, Stuart JM, David CS. Type II collagen-induced arthritis in mice. I. Major histocompatibility complex (I region) linkage and antibody correlates. *J Exp Med* (1981) 154:688–700. doi: 10.1084/jem.154.3.688
11. Wooley P, Dillon A, Luthra H, Stuart J, David C. Genetic control of type ii collagen-induced arthritis in mice: factors influencing disease susceptibility and evidence for multiple mhc-associated gene control. *Subj Strain Bibliogr 1983* (1983), 180–5. https://mouseion.jax.org/ssbb1983/343.
12. Holmdahl R, Jansson L, Andersson M, Larsson E. Immunogenetics of type II collagen autoimmunity and susceptibility to collagen arthritis. *Immunology* (1988) 65:305. https://www.ncbi.xilesou.top/pmc/articles/PMC1384929/.
13. Bäcklund J, Li C, Jansson E, Carlsen S, Merky P, Nandakumar K-S, et al. C57BL/6 mice need MHC class II Aq to develop collagen-induced arthritis dependent on autoreactive T cells. *Ann Rheum Dis* (2013) 72:1225–32. doi: 10.1136/annrheumdis-2012-202055
14. Nishimura Y, Iwanaga T, Inamitsu T, Yanagawa Y, Yasunami M, Kimura A, et al. Expression of the human MHC, HLA-DQW6 genes alters the immune response in C57BL/6 mice. *J Immunol* (1990) 145:353–60.
15. Woods A, Chen HY, Trumbauer ME, Sirotina A, Cummings R, Zaller DM. Human major histocompatibility complex class II-restricted T cell responses in transgenic mice. *J Exp Med* (1994) 180:173–81. doi: 10.1084/jem.180.1.173
16. Vingsbo C, Larsson P, Andersson M, Holmdahl R. Association of pepsin with type II collagen (CII) breaks control of CII autoimmunity and triggers development of arthritis in rats. *Scand J Immunol* (1993) 37:337–42. doi: 10.1111/j.1365-3083.1993.tb02562.x
17. Matsumoto I, Staub A, Benoist C, Mathis D. Arthritis provoked by linked T and B cell recognition of a glycolytic enzyme. *Science* (1999) 286:1732–5. doi: 10.1126/science.286.5445.1732
18. Carlsen S, Nandakumar KS, Bäcklund J, Holmberg J, Hultqvist M, Vestberg M, et al. Cartilage oligomeric matrix protein induction of chronic arthritis in mice. *Arthritis Rheumatol* (2008) 58:2000–11. doi: 10.1002/art.23554
19. Hedbom E, Antonsson P, Hjerpe A, Aeschlimann D, Paulsson M, Rosa-Pimentel E, et al. Cartilage matrix proteins. An acidic oligomeric protein (COMP) detected only in cartilage. *J Biol Chem* (1992) 267:6132–6.
20. Halász K, Kassner A, Mörgelin M, Heinegård D. COMP Acts as a Catalyst in Collagen Fibrillogenesis. *J Biol Chem* (2007) 282:31166–73. doi: 10.1074/jbc.M705735200
21. Lorenzo P, Bayliss MT, Heinegård D. Altered patterns and synthesis of extracellular matrix macromolecules in early osteoarthritis. *Matrix Biol* (2004) 23:381–91. doi: 10.1016/j.matbio.2004.07.007
22. Carlsén S, Hansson AS, Olsson H, Heinegård D, Holmdahl R. Cartilage oligomeric matrix protein (COMP)-induced arthritis in rats. *Clin Exp Immunol* (1998) 114:477–84. doi: 10.1046/j.1365-2249.1998.00739.x

23. Guo Y, Kammerer R, Engel J. The unusually stable coiled-coil domain of COMP exhibits cold and heat denaturation in 4-6 M guanidinium chloride. *Biophys Chem* (2000) 85:179–86. doi: 10.1016/s0301-4622(00)00119-8
24. Ge C, Tong D, Liang B, Lönnblom E, Schneider N, Hagert C, et al. Anti-citrullinated protein antibodies cause arthritis by cross-reactivity to joint cartilage. *JCI Insight* (2017) 2:e93688. doi: 10.1172/jci.insight.93688
25. Hagert C, Sareila O, Kelkka T, Nandakumar KS, Collin M, Xu B, et al. Chronic Active Arthritis Driven by Macrophages Without Involvement of T Cells. *Arthritis Rheumatol* (2018) 70:1343–53. doi: 10.1002/art.40482
26. Hultqvist M, Olofsson P, Holmberg J, Bäckström BT, Tordsson J, Holmdahl R. Enhanced autoimmunity, arthritis, and encephalomyelitis in mice with a reduced oxidative burst due to a mutation in the Ncf1 gene. *Proc Natl Acad Sci U S A* (2004) 101:12646. doi: 10.1073/pnas.0403831101
27. Biasini M, Bienert S, Waterhouse A, Arnold K, Studer G, Schmidt T, et al. SWISS-MODEL: modelling protein tertiary and quaternary structure using evolutionary information. *Nucleic Acids Res* (2014) 42:W252–258. doi: 10.1093/nar/gku340
28. Stern LJ, Brown JH, Jardetzky TS, Gorga JC, Urban RG, Strominger JL, et al. Crystal structure of the human class II MHC protein HLA-DR1 complexed with an influenza virus peptide. *Nature* (1994) 368:215–21. doi: 10.1038/368215a0
29. Wang P, Sidney J, Kim Y, Sette A, Lund O, Nielsen M, et al. Peptide binding predictions for HLA DR, DP and DQ molecules. *BMC Bioinf* (2010) 11:568. doi: 10.1186/1471-2105-11-568
30. Schymkowitz J, Borg J, Stricher F, Nys R, Rousseau F, Serrano L. The FoldX web server: an online force field. *Nucleic Acids Res* (2005) 33:W382–8. doi: 10.1093/nar/gki387
31. Dunbrack RL, Cohen FE. Bayesian statistical analysis of protein side-chain rotamer preferences. *Protein Sci* (1997) 6:1661–81. doi: 10.1002/pro.5560060807
32. Jones EY, Fugger L, Strominger JL, Siebold C. MHC class II proteins and disease: a structural perspective. *Nat Rev Immunol* (2006) 6:271–82. doi: 10.1038/nri1805
33. Malmström V, Michaëlsson E, Burkhardt H, Mattsson R, Vuorio E, Holmdahl R. Systemic versus cartilage-specific expression of a type II collagen-specific T-cell epitope determines the level of tolerance and susceptibility to arthritis. *Proc Natl Acad Sci U S A* (1996) 93:4480–5. doi: 10.1073/pnas.93.9.4480
34. Geng H, Nandakumar KS, Pramhed A, Aspberg A, Mattsson R, Holmdahl R. Cartilage oligomeric matrix protein specific antibodies are pathogenic. *Arthritis Res Ther* (2012) 14:R191. doi: 10.1186/ar4022
35. Clemente-Casares X, Blanco J, Ambalavanan P, Yamanouchi J, Singha S, Fandos C, et al. Expanding antigen-specific regulatory networks to treat autoimmunity. *Nature* (2016) 530:434–40. doi: 10.1038/nature16962

6

The Administration of Apoptotic Cells for Treating Rheumatoid Arthritis: Current Knowledge and Clinical Perspectives

Eric Toussirot[1,2,3,4,5*†], *Francis Bonnefoy*[5,6], *Charline Vauchy*[1,5], *Sylvain Perruche*[2,5,6] *and Philippe Saas*[1,2,5†]

[1] INSERM CIC-1431, Centre d'Investigation Clinique Biothérapie, Pôle Recherche, CHU de Besançon, Besançon, France, [2] Fédération Hospitalo-Universitaire INCREASE, CHU de Besançon, Besançon, France, [3] Rhumatologie, Pôle PACTE (Pathologies Aiguës Chroniques Transplantation Éducation), CHU de Besançon, Besançon, France, [4] Département Universitaire de Thérapeutique, Université de Bourgogne Franche-Comté, Besançon, France, [5] Univ. Bourgogne Franche-Comté, INSERM, EFS BFC, UMR1098, Interactions Hôte-Greffon-Tumeur/Ingénierie Cellulaire et Génique, LabEx LipSTIC, Besançon, France, [6] MED'INN'Pharma, Besançon, France

***Correspondence:**
Eric Toussirot
etoussirot@chu-besancon.fr

Rheumatoid arthritis (RA) is a chronic immune-mediated disease managed by conventional synthetic drugs, such as methotrexate (MTX), and targeted drugs including biological agents. Cell-based therapeutic approaches are currently developed in RA, mainly mesenchymal stroma cell-based approaches. Early-stage apoptotic cells possess direct and indirect anti-inflammatory properties. During the elimination of dying cells (a process called efferocytosis), specific mechanisms operate to control immune responses. There are compelling evidences in experimental models of arthritis indicating that apoptotic cell administration may benefit joint inflammation, and may even have therapeutic effects on arthritis. Additionally, it has been demonstrated that apoptotic cells could be administered with standard treatments of RA, such as MTX or TNF inhibitors (TNFi), given even a synergistic response with TNFi. Interestingly, apoptotic cell infusion has been successfully experienced to prevent acute graft-vs.-host disease after hematopoietic cell transplantation in patients with hematologic malignancies, with a good safety profile. In this mini-review, the apoptotic cell-based therapy development in arthritis is discussed, as well as its transfer in the short-term to an innovative treatment for patients with RA. The use of apoptotic cell-derived factors, including secretome or phosphatidylserine-containing liposomes, in RA are also discussed.

Keywords: rheumatoid arthritis, cell-based therapy, apoptotic cells, efferocytosis, inflammation

INTRODUCTION

Rheumatoid arthritis (RA) is a chronic immune-mediated disease that primarily affects the peripheral joints. This inflammatory rheumatic disease is responsible for joint inflammation, cartilage, and bone destruction that progressively lead to joint deformations, structural damage, and disability (1). Rheumatoid arthritis is associated with specific comorbidities, such as an enhanced cardiovascular risk (2), but also systemic complications and premature death (1). Dramatic improvements have been done these past 20 years in the diagnosis and management of RA. Indeed, new classification criteria have been proposed, and new treatment paradigms together with the development of novel therapeutics have considerably improved the prognosis of the disease (3, 4). Currently, the treatment of RA is based on conventional synthetic drugs [conventional synthetic disease modifying antirheumatic drugs (csDMARDs)] or targeted drugs, including targeted synthetic and biological drugs (tsDMARDs and bDMARDs, respectively) (5). The treatment strategy of RA has been now clarified, and specific international recommendations help the physician in the drug choice and the therapeutic management, taking into account disease activity and severity (6). However, a substantial proportion of patients does not respond adequately to these drugs and, some of them do not achieve remission or low disease activity (7), the therapeutic goals in RA. In addition, the long-term use of these drugs could lead to severe adverse events (8).

Cell-based therapies have been developed in the treatment of RA (9). Administration of cells that can modulate or even dampen the inflammatory process of RA is an exciting therapeutic challenge. Preliminary data with the administration of hematopoietic or mesenchymal stem cells in phase 1/2 clinical trials are currently available in patients with RA (9). In these approaches, the mode of action of hematopoietic or mesenchymal stem cells is still under debate. Administration of apoptotic cells could represent another relevant cell-based therapy for the treatment of RA (10). This cell therapy—developed in different experimental indications, such as transplantation or immune-mediated diseases—has been shown to modulate the immune response and to control, at least partially, the inflammatory process in experimental models of arthritis (10, 11). Thus, in this review, we will comment the current knowledge of apoptotic cell-based treatment in arthritis, and discuss the potential use of this cellular therapy in patients with RA.

RHEUMATOID ARTHRITIS: A BRIEF OVERVIEW OF ITS PATHOPHYSIOLOGY

The exact cause of RA remains currently unknown. Its development results from the complex interplay between genetic, environmental, hormonal, and psychological factors (12). Rheumatoid arthritis is characterized by inflammation and hyperplasia of the synovium, leading to the so-called rheumatoid "pannus." Joint inflammation in RA is related to an immune activation with the participation of both innate immune cells [i.e., neutrophils, monocytes and macrophages, NK cells, dendritic cells (DC), mast cells, and innate lymphoid cells], and adaptive immune cells (Th1 and Th17 cells, B cells, and plasma cells). A strong cellular response has been initiated within the synovium with the activation of local synovial cells, including fibroblast- and macrophage-like synoviocytes (13). These resident synovial cells exhibit an aggressive phenotype with the production, together with immune cells, of a complex network of soluble factors, i.e., cytokines and chemokines, perpetuating the cellular activation and inflammatory reaction (14). Resident synoviocytes also produce metalloproteases that degrade the extra-cellular matrix components, i.e., cartilage and subchondral bone, ultimately promoting joint destruction (15). Rheumatoid arthritis is characterized by the production of well-described autoantibodies, of which rheumatoid factors (RF) and anti-citrullinated protein antibodies (ACPA) are the most common (16). ACPA can bind citrullinated motifs expressed by several self-proteins, including vimentin, fibrinogen, fibronectin, α-enolase, or type II collagen. The presence of RF and/or ACPA is associated with a more severe disease. Post-translational protein modifications explain the reaction of citrullination under the influence of the peptidyl-arginine deiminase enzymatic activity, with subsequent immunization and the production of ACPA (17). Other post-translational reactions have been described in RA, such as the formation of carbamylated residues promoting the synthesis of anti-carbamylated antibodies (18).

The treatment of RA is now well-defined, and has profoundly changed over the past 20 years (4). Methotrexate (MTX) is used as first line csDMARDs, and is considered as the reference treatment in RA (19). Targeted drugs (such as tsDMARDs or bDMARDs) are proposed as second line therapy in the case of inadequate response to csDMARDs (20). Among bDMARDs, TNFi have been available on the market for more than 20 years, and are widely used in clinical practice. Other bDMARDs include IL-6 blocking agents, a T cell costimulation blocker (abatacept) and a B cell depleting agent (rituximab) (21). Janus kinase inhibitors (tofacitinib, baricitinib, upadacitinib and filgotinib) correspond to tsDMARDs. These agents interfere with signal transduction involved in T cell activation (22).

CELL-BASED THERAPIES IN RHEUMATOID ARTHRITIS

Cell-based therapeutic approaches have been recently developed in RA. The rationale is based on the administration of cells exhibiting direct or indirect anti-inflammatory properties targeting inflammatory cells involved in the RA pathophysiology (9). The cells used in RA are mainly stem cells from the hematopoietic or the mesenchymal lineage. Hematopoietic stem cells (HSC) possess the property of multilineage differentiation, resulting in all blood cell types. They are isolated from bone marrow, peripheral blood after G-CSF mobilization, or umbilical cord. The curative effect of hematopoietic cell transplantation (HCT) is based on the conditioning regimen that eliminates pathogenic immune cells and the re-establishment of the host immune system. This procedure has been performed in a limited number of RA patients [reviewed in (9)]. In this setting, allogeneic HCT is tolerated and can improve disease activity and/or maintain remission for the short term. However, these patients received a cytotoxic regimen before transplantation with potential immunologic or infectious complications, and are at risk of developing severe acute graft-vs.-host disease (GvHD). Another approach is the administration of mesenchymal stem/stroma cells (MSC). These cells are multipotent stromal cells that can differentiate into different cellular lineages. They derive from bone marrow, adipose tissue, umbilical cord, or other organs including the synovium. They exhibit several immunomodulatory effects, including: inhibition of T cell activation/proliferation, suppression of B cell activation and antibody production, reduction of NK cell activity, generation of regulatory T (Treg) cells, and polarization of macrophages toward an anti-inflammatory phenotype (9). In a large cohort of patients who had inadequate response to csDMARDs, MSCs were administrated intravenously together with csDMARDs and compared to patients who received only csDMARDs. A significant improvement of RA was observed in the MSC group, with a remission sustained up to 3–6 months (23). Another phase 1/2 clinical trial evaluated the safety and efficacy of allogeneic expanded adipose tissue-derived MSCs administered intravenously. That dose escalation, placebo controlled study consisted of 3 infusions over 2 weeks. The treatment was well-tolerated and yielded clinical improvement after 1 month. However, the efficacy was not sustained and the clinical response was mitigated at month 3 (24). Other cellular therapies have been tried in patients with RA, including the intra-articular (IA) administration of autologous tolerogenic DC, leading to promising results (25).

THE IMMUNOMODULARY PROPERTIES OF APOPTOTIC CELLS

Apoptosis is a physiological cell death process that occurs during the development, and throughout the life in all tissues. Every day, a billion of cells die and are eliminated without deleterious consequences as inflammation or inadequate immune response (26). Apoptosis is followed by the efficient clearance of dead cells by professional phagocytes, a mechanism called efferocytosis. Efferocytosis is a key mechanism for tissue homeostasis (26). The appropriate efferocytosis of apoptotic neutrophils is a major event in the resolution of inflammation (27). Conversely, a defective efferocytosis may contribute to impaired tissue homeostasis, delayed tissue repair, and non-resolving inflammation. In this context, inadequate clearance of apoptotic cells may promote auto-inflammatory and/or autoimmune diseases (28). Altered efferocytosis has been reported in RA (28, 29).

Apoptotic cells display immunomodulatory properties that can be harnessed for therapeutic use (10, 11). Indeed, both apoptotic cells themselves and the interaction of apoptotic cells with professional phagocytes are associated with immune regulation mechanisms (**Figures 1A–C**). Before being removed, apoptotic cells create a local transient suppressive microenvironment (30–34) (**Figure 1A**). In response to specific signals released by apoptotic cells, called "find me" signals, professional phagocytes move toward the sites where cells are dying (37–39). Professional phagocytes correspond mainly to tissue-resident and monocyte-derived macrophages, as well as specific DC subsets (10). Apoptotic cell engulfment is then driven by specific signals expressed on apoptotic cells or fragments of apoptotic cells [collectively called "don't eat me" and "eat me" (i.e., phosphatidylserine; Ptdser) signals] (40). While "don't eat me" signals prevent the uptake of viable cells, "eat me" signals stimulates the engulfment and modulate the immune responses. Thus, liposomes expressing Ptdser have been shown to mimic some immunomodulatory effects of apoptotic cells (41). Apoptotic cells may cooperate with macrophages to induce an immunosuppressive environment (**Figure 1B**) (35). After efferocytosis, an anti-inflammatory reprogramming of macrophages is initiated (26, 27), leading to a sustained immunosuppressive environment (**Figure 1C**) through the release of several anti-inflammatory cytokines [e.g., TGF-β, IL-10 (42, 43)], and other regulatory factors (44, 45), such as pro-resolving mediators (10, 11, 46). Reprogramming of macrophages also includes a decreased capacity to produce pro-inflammatory cytokines (e.g., TNF-α, IL-1β, IL-12, or IL-23) (10). Phagocyting dendritic cells are also maintained in an immature stage and/or developed a tolerogenic profile, contributing to the generation of regulatory immune cells, including IL-10-producing T cells, $CD4^+$ Treg, $CD8^+$ Treg or regulatory B (Breg) cells (**Figure 1C**). This tolerogenic microenvironment participates in the inhibition of Th1 and Th17 responses (10, 11). Overall, the administration of apoptotic cells may control an ongoing pro-inflammatory process by different regulatory mechanisms and by inhibiting pathogenic cells. All these mechanisms support the rationale to use apoptotic cell administration in chronic systemic inflammation, like in arthritis (46). We thus reviewed the effects of apoptotic cells, apoptotic cell-derived factors, approaches mimicking apoptotic cell injection, or factors released during efferocytosis in animal models of arthritis. A systematic literature search was performed in PUBMED Medline database until November 2020, using the following keywords: [apoptotic cells] OR [apoptotic cell factors] OR [efferocytosis factors] AND [arthritis] AND [animal models]. After title and abstracts selection, duplicate elimination and manual search, 10 articles were finally selected for analysis (34, 47–55) (**Table 1**).

THE EFFECTS OF APOPTOTIC CELLS IN PRECLINICAL MODEL OF ARTHRITIS

Six articles were selected (47–52). Apoptotic cell-based therapies have been evaluated through intravenous (IV), intraperitoneal (IP), or IA administration of early stage apoptotic cells in the main arthritis models. The main results are summarized in **Table 1**. According to the experimental model used and to the time of apoptotic cell injection (i.e., at the time of arthritis induction, before clinical symptom occurrence, or during ongoing arthritis), one may distinguish preventive vs. curative effects. A preventive effect of apoptotic cell administration on clinical scores has been observed in all the arthritis models tested (47–50), except in the serum transfer-induced arthritis (STIA) model (47). This negative result may be explained by the experimental model used, lacking the adaptive immune response (46). Indeed, implication of IL-10-producing T cells [T regulatory 1 (Tr1) cells], Treg and/or IL-10-secreting Breg cells has been shown to be triggered by apoptotic cell infusion in arthritis models and associated with the reduction of joint inflammation (47–49) (**Table 1**). In streptococcal cell wall (SCW)-induced arthritis, IP injection of apoptotic cells along

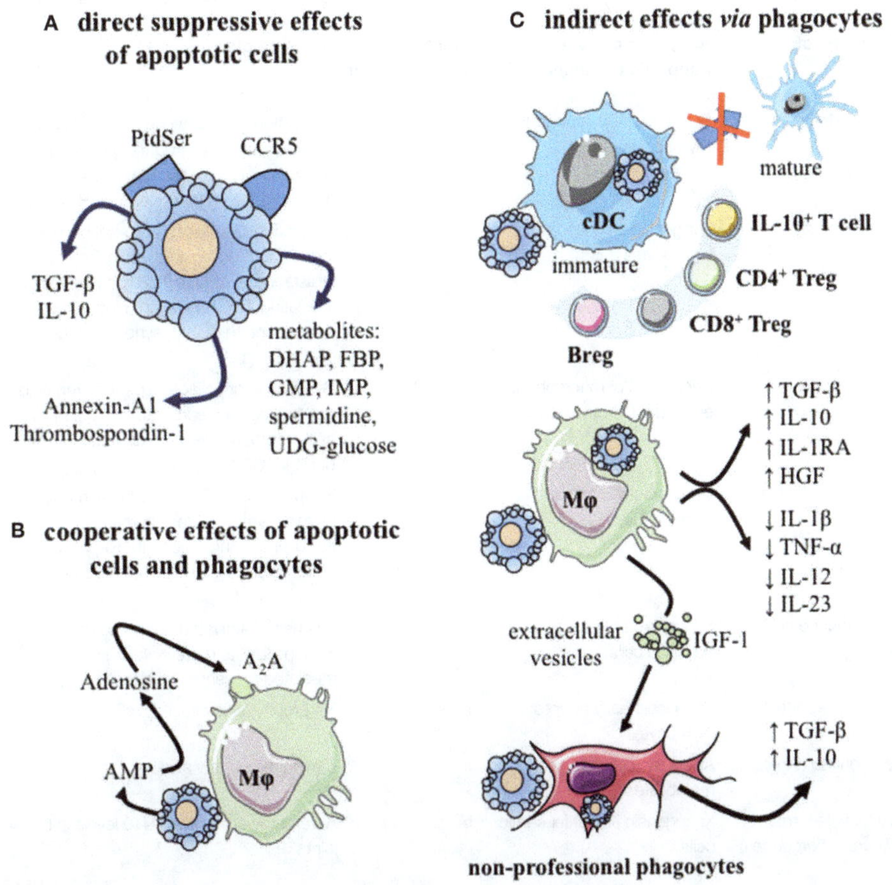

FIGURE 1 | The immunomodulatory effects of apoptotic cells. **(A)** Apoptotic cells exert direct anti-inflammatory effects by: (i) neutralizing inflammatory chemokines, via CCR5 expression (30), and (ii) releasing different factors, including: anti-inflammatory cytokines [e.g., TGF-β (31)], mediators [i.e., annexin-A1 (32) or thrombospondin-1 (33)], as well as cellular metabolites [e.g., spermidine, guanosine monophosphate, inosine monophosphate (34)]. **(B)** Cooperation between apoptotic cells and their phagocytes may mediate immunosuppression. Apoptotic cells release adenosine monophosphate (AMP) which is then converted into adenosine by phagocyting macrophages. This factor interacts with macrophage adenosine A_{2A} receptors and stimulates anti-inflammatory gene expression (35). **(C)** Different phagocytes propagate the immunomodulatory effects of apoptotic cells after efferocytosis. Professional phagocytes (immature cDC and macrophages), as well as amateur phagocytes (e.g., fibroblasts, epithelial cells) may participate to efferocytosis (10). The consequences for phagocytes differ depending on the considered phagocytes. Efferocytosis by cDC blocks them in an immature stage or induces a tolerogenic profile that generates regulatory adaptive immune cells: IL-10-secreting cells, $CD4^+$ Treg, $CD8^+$ Treg, and/or IL-10-producing Breg cells. After efferocytosis, macrophages secrete anti-inflammatory factors (e.g., TGF-β, IL-10, IL-1RA, and HGF) and reduce their production of inflammatory cytokines (e.g., TNF-α, IL-1β, IL-12, and IL-23). Efferocytosis triggers macrophage reprogramming toward a pro-resolving profile (26, 27). Moreover, macrophages may stimulate via extracellular vesicles factors and IGF-1 the efferocytic capacity of amateur phagocytes (36). Finally, these amateur phagocytes may secrete immunosuppressive cytokines, such as TGF-β or IL-10. A_2A, Adenosine 2A receptor; AMP, adenosine-monophosphate; Breg, regulatory B cells; cDC, conventional dendritic cell; DHAP, dihydroxyacetone phosphate; FBP, fructose-1,6-biphosphate; GMP, guanosine-5′-monophosphate; HGF, hepatocyte growth factor; IGF-1, insulin-like growth factor; IL-, interleukin; IMP, Inosine-5′-monophosphate; Mϕ, macrophage; Ptdser, phosphatidylserine; TGF-β, transforming growth factor-beta; Treg, regulatory T cells. This figure was depicted, in part, by using Servier Medical Art, https://smart.servier.com/.

with arthritis induction induced a significant improvement of joint inflammation and limited joint destruction (48). In this rat model, the results are more impressive on the chronic stage of the disease (48). A therapeutic effect of IV apoptotic cell administration has been reported in ongoing arthritis using the collagen-induced arthritis (CIA) model (51). In this model, co-administration of MTX with apoptotic cells induces arthritis reduction that was similar to apoptotic cell injection alone, thus demonstrating that MTX does not interfere with apoptotic cell infusion (51). The concomitant administration of a TNFi together with apoptotic cells induces better arthritis reduction (51), indicating a synergistic effect between the mode of action of both therapies. Finally, IA apoptotic cell injection has exerted also a therapeutic effect in a mouse Lyme arthritis model (52). Altogether, these different experimental results well illustrate the beneficial consequences of apoptotic cell administration in acute and chronic arthritis, with both preventive and curative effects. Apoptotic cell-based therapy may thus be potentially able to control ongoing clinical arthritis, to dampen inflammation and attenuate destructive articular changes. This strongly supports the therapeutic use of apoptotic cells in patients with RA.

TABLE 1 | Experimental studies evaluating the effects of apoptotic cell administration or apoptotic cell-derived factors in animal models of arthritis.

Reference	Experimental model of arthritis	Apoptotic cell source or apoptotic cell mimetic	Route of administration	Main effects	Final result and duration of the effect
(47)	Collagen-induced arthritis (DBA/1 mice)	Syngeneic early apoptotic thymocytes	IV or IP	Reduction of collagen auto-antibodies; induction of IL-10-producing $CD4^{+}$ T cells; reduction of IFN-γ secreting $CD4^{+}$ T cells; IL-10-producing marginal zone B cells	Prophylactic effect on arthritis
(51)	Collagen-induced arthritis (DBA/1 mice)	Syngeneic early apoptotic thymocytes	IV	Reduction of collagen auto-antibodies; induction of collagen-specific Treg cells; resistance of APC to TLR ligand activation, indicating APC reprogramming; effects dependent on TGF-β; synergic results with TNFi	Transient therapeutic effect on arthritis
(55)	Collagen-induced arthritis (DBA/1 mice)	Secretome of macrophages eliminating apoptotic cells	IV or IP	Generation of collagen-specific Treg cells; pro-tolerogenic reprogramming of pDC and macrophages; mediated at least in part by TGF-β	Therapeutic effect on arthritis up to 60 days following secretome administration
(49)	Methylated BSA-induced arthritis (C57BL/6 mice)	Syngeneic early apoptotic thymocytes	IV	Suppression of Th17 response in the draining lymph nodes; increase of IL-10-producing T cells; IL-10-producing marginal zone B cells; effects dependent on natural IgM	Prophylactic effect on arthritis
(50)	Methylated BSA-induced arthritis (C57BL/6 mice)	Syngeneic apoptotic dendritic cells	IV	The use of activated apoptotic cells induces IL-6 and prevents TGF-β mediated prevention of arthritis	Prophylactic effect on arthritis
(47)	Serum transfer-induced arthritis (C57BL/6 mice)	Syngeneic early apoptotic thymocytes	IV or IP	No prophylactic effect	No improvement of arthritis
(34)	Serum transfer-induced arthritis (C57BL/6 mice)	Apoptotic cell-derived metabolites*	IP	Diminution of paw swelling	Prophylactic effect on arthritis
(52)	Lyme arthritis (C3H/HeJ mice infected with *Borrelia burgdorferi*)	Xenogeneic Jurkat leukemic cells	IA	A trend toward higher IL-10 levels in the joints	Therapeutic effect on arthritis (accelerated disease resolution)
(53)	Adjuvant arthritis (Lewis rat)	Phosphatidylserine-containing liposomes	IM	Reduction of *RANK* and *RANKL* mRNA; inhibitory effect on osteoclast formation; increased production of TGF-β and PGE2	Therapeutic effect on arthritis (reduction of paw volume at day 28, then rat sacrifice)
(54)	Adjuvant arthritis (Lewis rat)	Phosphatidylserine-containing liposomes	IM	Reduction of *RANK* and *RANKL* mRNA; Increased IL-10 and decreased IL-1β and IL-17 in the ankle joint; shift from IL-1β- to IL-10-producing infiltrated macrophages	Therapeutic effect on arthritis (reduction of paw volume at day 28, then rat sacrifice)
(48)	Streptococcal wall-induced arthritis (Lewis rat)	Xenogeneic early apoptotic thymocytes	IP	Decrease in the pro-inflammatory response of peritoneal macrophages; induction of Treg cells in the draining lymph node; effects dependent on TGF-β	Prophylactic effect on arthritis

APC, antigen presenting cells; BSA, bovine serum albumin; IA, intra-articular ankle injection; IM, intramuscular (in the hind limbs); IP, intraperitoneal; IV, intravenous; pDC, plasmacytoid dendritic cell; PGE2, prostaglandin-E2; TNFi, TNF inhibitors; Treg, $CD4^{+}$ $FoxP^{+}$ regulatory T cells.

**Two cocktails were tested: one with six metabolites [dihydroxyacetone phosphate (DHAP), fructose-1,6-biphosphate (FBP), guanosine-5′-monophosphate (GMP), Inosine-5′-monophosphate (IMP), spermidine, UDG-glucose] and the other with 3 metabolites (GMP, IMP, and spermidine).*

THE EFFECTS OF APOPTOTIC CELL-DERIVED FACTORS IN PRECLINICAL MODEL OF ARTHRITIS

Four articles were selected for this review (34, 53–55) (**Table 1**). It has been shown that the intramuscular (IM) administration of Ptdser-containing liposomes in adjuvant arthritis (AA) is able to inhibit AA-induced trabecular bone loss (53). The same group demonstrated that this approach induced macrophage reprogramming with the reduction of IL-1β release and an increase in IL-10 production (54). This confirms that Ptdser-containing liposomes can mimic some effects of apoptotic cells (41). Recently, the administration of a mixture of 3 or 6 metabolites identified in apoptotic cell secretome has been shown to diminish paw swelling in the STIA model (34) (**Table 1**). These apoptotic cell-derived metabolites are able to control macrophage reprogramming toward a pro-resolving profile (34). Thus, selective apoptotic cell-derived factors may also be considered as innovative therapeutic approaches in arthritis. Furthermore, the secretome of macrophages eliminating apoptotic leukocytes has been shown to exert a therapeutic effect on arthritic clinical score in CIA by inducing collagen-specific $CD4^{+}$ Treg cells and reprogramming plasmacytoid dendritic cells (pDC) and macrophages toward a tolerogenic state (55). This treatment of arthritis has been associated with a restored functional resolution of inflammation (47). This confirms the main role of efferocytosis in the control of inflammation (27), as well as the importance of the macrophage/pDC/Treg cell crosstalk in apoptotic cell-induced tolerance (56). Overall, apoptotic cell "derivatives" can be an alternative to apoptotic cell-based therapy.

APOPTOTIC CELLS IN THE TREATMENT OF ARTHRITIS: TOWARD A CLINICAL USE

Results from experimental studies detailed above support the rational for a clinical perspective in RA. This is based on the preclinical data, but also on an extensive research in the fields of cancer and transplantation (10, 11, 46). However, there are several concerns before translating these results to a clinical trial in humans. First, in most of the experimental models used to evaluate the apoptotic cell-based approach, arthritis is induced by a known and specific auto-antigen, which is not the case in patients. Second, certain models are self-resolving, without a chronic phase after the acute peak of the disease. This does not mimic the clinical situation. Third, most of the data have been obtained with a therapy given at the initiation of the disease, even before the onset of arthritic clinical symptoms. This is not feasible in clinic. Despite the fact that a mouse is not human and that regulatory mechanisms may differ between these two species (57), the feasibility must be discussed. What type of cell has to be used as apoptotic cells? Indeed, peripheral blood leukocytes are the easiest cell source to consider in human, contrary to apoptotic cells used in experimental models that are from the thymus, the spleen, DCs, and even leukemic cells (**Table 1**). As observed in experimental settings, apoptotic leukocytes would need to be at an early apoptotic stage, i.e., annexin-V$^+$, 7-aminoactinomycin D or propidium iodide negative. These cells may be collected using cytapheresis. Different procedures may render the cells apoptotic and the different stimuli include γ-, X-ray, or UV-irradiation, Fas-mediated cell death, as well as corticosteroid treatment. The appropriate route of administration for the patients is the IV route, since this approach seems appropriate for a systemic disease, such as RA. This allows a quick diffusion of apoptotic cells through the body. To summarize, one may propose the following procedure for the apoptotic cell preparation in a clinical trial: a cytapheresis collecting peripheral blood leukocytes that are then exposed to a 35-Gy dose of γ- or X-ray irradiation to induce apoptosis. In these irradiation settings, one may obtain around 40–50% of cells in an early apoptotic stage, with a limited number of cells (<10%) in a necrotic stage. The concomitant use of csDMARDs (such as MTX) and of bDMARDs (TNFi) is not a limit, since MTX does not alter the therapeutic effects of apoptotic cells (51), whereas TNFi displays a synergistic effect (51). Glucocorticoids (GCs) are still used in clinical practice for the treatment of RA, and this medication may be administered with apoptotic cells. Indeed, GCs enhance apoptotic cell removal during the different phases of apoptotic cell clearance (40). The safety of apoptotic cell infusion is another concern. This cell-based therapy has been previously used in a clinical trial in the setting of HCT (58). In this phase 1/2a trial, donor early apoptotic cells have been administered intravenously the day before allogeneic HCT in order to prevent acute GvHD in 13 patients with hematological malignancies. The administered cells have been obtained from hematopoietic cell donors after cytapheresis. This cell-based therapy has been well-tolerated without related serious adverse events. The overall incidence of stage II to IV GvHD was 25% while in the group of patients who received the highest dose of apoptotic cells, this rate was 0% (58). The conclusion of this trial was that apoptotic cell infusion during HCT is a safe procedure and potentially effective in the prevention of GvHD. This illustrates the feasibility of this cell therapy approach. Considering these results, we plan to start a clinical trial on apoptotic cell infusion in RA patients who do not respond adequately to at least one bDMARD. The APO-RA project is a phase 1/2 trial that proposes one infusion of peripheral blood leukocytes rendered apoptotic cells by X-ray irradiation (ClinicalTrials.gov identifier: NCT02903212).

CONCLUSION AND PERSPECTIVES

The use of dying cell or their byproducts as a therapeutic approach in the treatment of RA, or other forms of arthritis, still represents an exciting and innovative therapeutic opportunity. Besides cell-targeted therapies that are currently used in RA (e.g., abatacept or rituximab), and besides MSC or tolerogenic DC administration, apoptotic cells represent another cellular approach with an attractive mode of action. There are compelling evidences demonstrating that apoptotic cell administration may dampen the inflammatory process of RA. Preliminary data in the setting of HCT indicate the feasibility of this approach with a good safety profile. It is, thus, now time to translate all these preclinical data in clinical settings. Some questions persist such as the exact therapeutic protocol to use (number of cells to administer, stimulus to generate early apoptotic cells without high a rate of necrotic cells), and whether a single infusion of apoptotic cells will give a sustained response.

AUTHOR CONTRIBUTIONS

ET performed the bibliographic search, wrote the first version of the manuscript, and made the table. PS completed the bibliographic search, edited the first version of the manuscript, and made the figure. All authors reviewed and edited the manuscript.

ACKNOWLEDGMENTS

We would like to thank Sarah Odrion for her help in editing our manuscript, and the members of our laboratory for their work.

REFERENCES

1. Smolen JS, Aletaha D, Mcinnes IB. Rheumatoid arthritis. *Lancet.* (2016) 388:2023–38. doi: 10.1016/S0140-6736(16)30173-8
2. Castaneda S, Nurmohamed MT, Gonzalez-Gay MA. Cardiovascular disease in inflammatory rheumatic diseases. *Best Pract Res Clin Rheumatol.* (2016) 30:851–69. doi: 10.1016/j.berh.2016.10.006
3. Aletaha D, Neogi T, Silman AJ, Funovits J, Felson DT, Bingham CO, et al. 2010 Rheumatoid arthritis classification criteria: an American College of Rheumatology/European League Against Rheumatism collaborative initiative. *Arthritis Rheum.* (2010) 62:2569–81. doi: 10.1002/art.27584
4. Smolen JS, Breedveld FC, Burmester GR, Bykerk V, Dougados M, Emery P, et al. Treating rheumatoid arthritis to target: 2014 update of the recommendations of an international task force. *Ann Rheum Dis.* (2016) 75:3–15. doi: 10.1136/annrheumdis-2015-207524
5. Smolen JS, Van Der Heijde D, Machold KP, Aletaha D, Landewe R. Proposal for a new nomenclature of disease-modifying antirheumatic drugs. *Ann Rheum Dis.* (2014) 73:3–5. doi: 10.1136/annrheumdis-2013-204317
6. Smolen JS, Landewe RBM, Bijlsma JWJ, Burmester GR, Dougados M, Kerschbaumer A, et al. EULAR recommendations for the management of rheumatoid arthritis with synthetic and biological disease-modifying antirheumatic drugs: 2019 update. *Ann Rheum Dis.* (2020) 79:685–99. doi: 10.1136/annrheumdis-2019-216655
7. Radner H, Smolen JS, Aletaha D. Remission in rheumatoid arthritis: benefit over low disease activity in patient-reported outcomes and costs. *Arthritis Res Ther.* (2014) 16:R56. doi: 10.1186/ar4491
8. Listing J, Strangfeld A, Kary S, Rau R, Von Hinueber U, Stoyanova-Scholz M, et al. Infections in patients with rheumatoid arthritis treated with biologic agents. *Arthritis Rheum.* (2005) 52:3403–3412. doi: 10.1002/art.21386
9. Liu R, Zhao P, Tan W, Zhang M. Cell therapies for refractory rheumatoid arthritis. *Clin Exp Rheumatol.* (2018) 36:911–9.
10. Saas P, Kaminski S, Perruche S. Prospects of apoptotic cell-based therapies for transplantation and inflammatory diseases. *Immunotherapy.* (2013) 5:1055–73. doi: 10.2217/imt.13.103
11. Saas P, Daguindau E, Perruche S. Concise review: apoptotic cell-based therapies-rationale, preclinical results and future clinical developments. *Stem Cells.* (2016) 34:1464–73. doi: 10.1002/stem.2361
12. Mcinnes IB, Schett G. The pathogenesis of rheumatoid arthritis. *N Engl J Med.* (2011) 365:2205–19. doi: 10.1056/NEJMra1004965
13. Croft AP, Campos J, Jansen K, Turner JD, Marshall J, Attar M, et al. Distinct fibroblast subsets drive inflammation and damage in arthritis. *Nature.* (2019) 570:246–51. doi: 10.1038/s41586-019-1263-7
14. Szekanecz Z, Pakozdi A, Szentpetery A, Besenyei T, Koch AE. Chemokines and angiogenesis in rheumatoid arthritis. *Front Biosci. (Elite Ed).* (2009) 1:44–51.
15. Mcinnes IB, Leung BP, Liew FY. Cell-cell interactions in synovitis. Interactions between T lymphocytes and synovial cells. *Arthritis Res.* (2000) 2:374–8. doi: 10.1186/ar128
16. De Rycke L, Peene I, Hoffman IE, Kruithof E, Union A, Meheus L, et al. Rheumatoid factor and anticitrullinated protein antibodies in rheumatoid arthritis: diagnostic value, associations with radiological progression rate, extra-articular manifestations. *Ann Rheum Dis.* (2004) 63:1587–93. doi: 10.1136/ard.2003.017574
17. Wegner N, Wait R, Sroka A, Eick S, Nguyen KA, Lundberg K, et al. Peptidylarginine deiminase from Porphyromonas gingivalis citrullinates human fibrinogen and alpha-enolase: implications for autoimmunity in rheumatoid arthritis. *Arthritis Rheum.* (2010) 62:2662–72. doi: 10.1002/art.27552
18. Shi J, Van Veelen PA, Mahler M, Janssen GM, Drijfhout JW, Huizinga TW, et al. Carbamylation and antibodies against carbamylated proteins in autoimmunity and other pathologies. *Autoimmun Rev.* (2014) 13:225–30. doi: 10.1016/j.autrev.2013.10.008
19. Gaujoux-Viala C, Nam J, Ramiro S, Landewe R, Buch MH, Smolen JS, et al. Efficacy of conventional synthetic disease-modifying antirheumatic drugs, glucocorticoids and tofacitinib: a systematic literature review informing the 2013 update of the EULAR recommendations for management of rheumatoid arthritis. *Ann Rheum Dis.* (2014) 73:510–5. doi: 10.1136/annrheumdis-2013-204588
20. Nam JL, Ramiro S, Gaujoux-Viala C, Takase K, Leon-Garcia M, Emery P, et al. Efficacy of biological disease-modifying antirheumatic drugs: a systematic literature review informing the 2013 update of the EULAR recommendations for the management of rheumatoid arthritis. *Ann Rheum Dis.* (2014) 73:516–28. doi: 10.1136/annrheumdis-2013-204577
21. Kerschbaumer A, Sepriano A, Smolen JS, Van Der Heijde D, Dougados M, Van Vollenhoven R, et al. Efficacy of pharmacological treatment in rheumatoid arthritis: a systematic literature research informing the 2019 update of the EULAR recommendations for management of rheumatoid arthritis. *Ann Rheum Dis.* (2020) 79:744–59. doi: 10.1136/annrheumdis-2019-216656
22. O'shea JJ, Kontzias A, Yamaoka K, Tanaka Y, Laurence A. Janus kinase inhibitors in autoimmune diseases. *Ann Rheum Dis.* (2013) 72(Suppl. 2): ii111–5. doi: 10.1136/annrheumdis-2012-202576
23. Wang L, Wang L, Cong X, Liu G, Zhou J, Bai B, et al. Human umbilical cord mesenchymal stem cell therapy for patients with active rheumatoid arthritis: safety and efficacy. *Stem Cells Dev.* (2013) 22:3192–202. doi: 10.1089/scd.2013.0023
24. Alvaro-Gracia JM, Jover JA, Garcia-Vicuna R, Carreno L, Alonso A, Marsal S, et al. Intravenous administration of expanded allogeneic adipose-derived mesenchymal stem cells in refractory rheumatoid arthritis. (Cx611): results of a multicentre, dose escalation, randomised, single-blind, placebo-controlled phase Ib/IIa clinical trial. *Ann Rheum Dis.* (2017) 76:196–202. doi: 10.1136/annrheumdis-2015-208918
25. Bell GM, Anderson AE, Diboll J, Reece R, Eltherington O, Harry RA, et al. Autologous tolerogenic dendritic cells for rheumatoid and inflammatory arthritis. *Ann Rheum Dis.* (2017) 76:227–34. doi: 10.1136/annrheumdis-2015-208456
26. Doran AC, Yurdagul A Jr, Tabas I. Efferocytosis in health and disease. *Nat Rev Immunol.* (2020) 20:254–67. doi: 10.1038/s41577-019-0240-6
27. Kourtzelis I, Hajishengallis G, Chavakis T. Phagocytosis of apoptotic cells in resolution of inflammation. *Front Immunol.* (2020) 11:553. doi: 10.3389/fimmu.2020.00553
28. Abdolmaleki F, Farahani N, Gheibi Hayat SM, Pirro M, Bianconi V, Barreto GE, et al. The role of efferocytosis in autoimmune diseases. *Front Immunol.* (2018) 9:1645. doi: 10.3389/fimmu.2018.01645
29. Lu Q, Lemke G. Homeostatic regulation of the immune system by receptor tyrosine kinases of the Tyro 3 family. *Science.* (2001) 293:306–11. doi: 10.1126/science.1061663
30. Ariel A, Fredman G, Sun YP, Kantarci A, Van Dyke TE, Luster AD, et al. Apoptotic neutrophils and T cells sequester chemokines during immune response resolution through modulation of CCR5 expression. *Nat Immunol.* (2006) 7:1209–16. doi: 10.1038/ni1392
31. Chen W, Frank ME, Jin W, Wahl SM. TGF-beta released by apoptotic T cells contributes to an immunosuppressive milieu. *Immunity.* (2001) 14:715–25. doi: 10.1016/S1074-7613(01)00147-9
32. Pupjalis D, Goetsch J, Kottas DJ, Gerke V, Rescher U. Annexin A1 released from apoptotic cells acts through formyl peptide receptors to dampen inflammatory monocyte activation via JAK/STAT/SOCS signalling. *EMBO Mol Med.* (2011) 3:102–14. doi: 10.1002/emmm.201000113
33. Krispin A, Bledi Y, Atallah M, Trahtemberg U, Verbovetski I, Nahari E, et al. Apoptotic cell thrombospondin-1 and heparin-binding domain lead to dendritic-cell phagocytic and tolerizing states. *Blood.* (2006) 108:3580–9. doi: 10.1182/blood-2006-03-013334
34. Medina CB, Mehrotra P, Arandjelovic S, Perry JSA, Guo Y, Morioka S, et al. Metabolites released from apoptotic cells act as tissue messengers. *Nature.* (2020) 580:130–5. doi: 10.1038/s41586-020-2121-3
35. Yamaguchi H, Maruyama T, Urade Y, Nagata S. Immunosuppression via adenosine receptor activation by adenosine monophosphate released from apoptotic cells. *Elife.* (2014) 3:e02172. doi: 10.7554/eLife.02172

36. Han CZ, Juncadella IJ, Kinchen JM, Buckley MW, Klibanov AL, Dryden K, et al. Macrophages redirect phagocytosis by non-professional phagocytes and influence inflammation. *Nature.* (2016) 539:570–4. doi: 10.1038/nature20141
37. Lauber K, Bohn E, Krober SM, Xiao YJ, Blumenthal SG, Lindemann RK, et al. Apoptotic cells induce migration of phagocytes via caspase-3-mediated release of a lipid attraction signal. *Cell.* (2003) 113:717–30. doi: 10.1016/S0092-8674(03)00422-7
38. Truman LA, Ford CA, Pasikowska M, Pound JD, Wilkinson SJ, Dumitriu IE, et al. CX3CL1/fractalkine is released from apoptotic lymphocytes to stimulate macrophage chemotaxis. *Blood.* (2008) 112:5026–36. doi: 10.1182/blood-2008-06-162404
39. Chekeni FB, Elliott MR, Sandilos JK, Walk SF, Kinchen JM, Lazarowski ER, et al. Pannexin 1 channels mediate 'find-me' signal release and membrane permeability during apoptosis. *Nature.* (2010) 467:863–7. doi: 10.1038/nature09413
40. Poon IK, Lucas CD, Rossi AG, Ravichandran KS. Apoptotic cell clearance: basic biology and therapeutic potential. *Nat Rev Immunol.* (2014) 14:166–80. doi: 10.1038/nri3607
41. Huynh ML, Fadok VA, Henson PM. Phosphatidylserine-dependent ingestion of apoptotic cells promotes TGF-beta1 secretion and the resolution of inflammation. *J Clin Invest.* (2002) 109:41–50. doi: 10.1172/JCI0211638
42. Voll RE, Herrmann M, Roth EA, Stach C, Kalden JR, Girkontaite I. Immunosuppressive effects of apoptotic cells. *Nature.* (1997) 390:350–1. doi: 10.1038/37022
43. Fadok VA, Bratton DL, Konowal A, Freed PW, Westcott JY, Henson PM. Macrophages that have ingested apoptotic cells *in vitro* inhibit proinflammatory cytokine production through autocrine/paracrine mechanisms involving TGF-beta, PGE2, and PAF. *J Clin Invest.* (1998) 101:890–8. doi: 10.1172/JCI1112
44. Craciun LI, Digiambattista M, Schandene L, Laub R, Goldman M, Dupont E. Anti-inflammatory effects of UV-irradiated lymphocytes: induction of IL-1Ra upon phagocytosis by monocyte/macrophages. *Clin Immunol.* (2005) 114:320–6. doi: 10.1016/j.clim.2004.11.006
45. Lee YJ, Moon C, Lee SH, Park HJ, Seoh JY, Cho MS, et al. Apoptotic cell instillation after bleomycin attenuates lung injury through hepatocyte growth factor induction. *Eur Respir J.* (2012) 40:424–35. doi: 10.1183/09031936.00096711
46. Saas P, Bonnefoy F, Toussirot E, Perruche S. Harnessing apoptotic cell clearance to treat autoimmune arthritis. *Front Immunol.* (2017) 8:1191. doi: 10.3389/fimmu.2017.01191
47. Gray M, Miles K, Salter D, Gray D, Savill J. Apoptotic cells protect mice from autoimmune inflammation by the induction of regulatory B cells. *Proc Natl Acad Sci U S A.* (2007) 104:14080–5. doi: 10.1073/pnas.0700326104
48. Perruche S, Saas P, Chen W. Apoptotic cell-mediated suppression of streptococcal cell wall-induced arthritis is associated with alteration of macrophage function and local regulatory T-cell increase: a potential cell-based therapy? *Arthritis Res Ther.* (2009) 11:R104. doi: 10.1186/ar2750
49. Notley CA, Brown MA, Wright GP, Ehrenstein MR. Natural IgM is required for suppression of inflammatory arthritis by apoptotic cells. *J Immunol.* (2011) 186:4967–72. doi: 10.4049/jimmunol.1003021
50. Notley CA, Brown MA, Mcgovern JL, Jordan CK, Ehrenstein MR. Engulfment of activated apoptotic cells abolishes TGF-beta-mediated immunoregulation via the induction of IL-6. *J Immunol.* (2015) 194:1621–7. doi: 10.4049/jimmunol.1401256
51. Bonnefoy F, Daoui A, Valmary-Degano S, Toussirot E, Saas P, Perruche S. Apoptotic cell infusion treats ongoing collagen-induced arthritis, even in the presence of methotrexate, and is synergic with anti-TNF therapy. *Arthritis Res Ther.* (2016) 18:184. doi: 10.1186/s13075-016-1084-0
52. Hilliard KA, Brown CR. Treatment of Borrelia burgdorferi-infected mice with apoptotic cells attenuates lyme arthritis via PPAR-gamma. *J Immunol.* (2019) 202:1798–806. doi: 10.4049/jimmunol.1801179
53. Wu Z, Ma HM, Kukita T, Nakanishi Y, Nakanishi H. Phosphatidylserine-containing liposomes inhibit the differentiation of osteoclasts and trabecular bone loss. *J Immunol.* (2010) 184:3191–201. doi: 10.4049/jimmunol.0803609
54. Ma HM, Wu Z, Nakanishi H. Phosphatidylserine-containing liposomes suppress inflammatory bone loss by ameliorating the cytokine imbalance provoked by infiltrated macrophages. *Lab Invest.* (2011) 91:921–31. doi: 10.1038/labinvest.2011.54
55. Bonnefoy F, Gauthier T, Vallion R, Martin-Rodriguez O, Missey A, Daoui A, et al. Factors produced by macrophages eliminating apoptotic cells demonstrate pro-resolutive properties and terminate ongoing inflammation. *Front Immunol.* (2018) 9:2586. doi: 10.3389/fimmu.2018.02586
56. Bonnefoy F, Perruche S, Couturier M, Sedrati A, Sun Y, Tiberghien P, et al. Plasmacytoid dendritic cells play a major role in apoptotic leukocyte-induced immune modulation. *J Immunol.* (2011) 186:5696–705. doi: 10.4049/jimmunol.1001523
57. Saas P, Chague C, Maraux M, Cherrier T. Towards the characterization of human pro-resolving macrophages? *Front Immunol.* (2020) 11:593300. doi: 10.3389/fimmu.2020.593300
58. Mevorach D, Zuckerman T, Reiner I, Shimoni A, Samuel S, Nagler A, et al. Single infusion of donor mononuclear early apoptotic cells as prophylaxis for graft-versus-host disease in myeloablative HLA-matched allogeneic bone marrow transplantation: a phase I/IIa clinical trial. *Biol Blood Marrow Transplant.* (2014) 20:58–65. doi: 10.1016/j.bbmt.2013.10.010

7

Serum Amyloid A in Inflammatory Rheumatic Diseases: A Compendious Review of a Renowned Biomarker

Iva Sorić Hosman[1], *Ivanka Kos*[2] *and Lovro Lamot*[2,3*]

[1] Department of Pediatrics, Zadar General Hospital, Zadar, Croatia, [2] Division of Nephrology, Dialysis and Transplantation, Department of Pediatrics, University Hospital Centre Zagreb, Zagreb, Croatia, [3] Department of Pediatrics, University of Zagreb School of Medicine, Zagreb, Croatia

***Correspondence:**
Lovro Lamot
lovro.lamot@gmail.com

Serum amyloid A (SAA) is an acute phase protein with a significant importance for patients with inflammatory rheumatic diseases (IRD). The central role of SAA in pathogenesis of IRD has been confirmed by recent discoveries, including its involvement in the activation of the inflammasome cascade and recruitment of interleukin 17 producing T helper cells. Clinical utility of SAA in IRD was originally evaluated nearly half a century ago. From the first findings, it was clear that SAA could be used for evaluating disease severity and monitoring disease activity in patients with rheumatoid arthritis and secondary amyloidosis. However, cost-effective and more easily applicable markers, such as C-reactive protein (CRP) and erythrocyte sedimentation rate (ESR), overwhelmed its use in clinical practice. In the light of emerging evidences, SAA has been discerned as a more sensitive biomarker in a wide spectrum of IRD, especially in case of subclinical inflammation. Furthermore, a growing number of studies are confirming the advantages of SAA over many other biomarkers in predicting and monitoring response to biological immunotherapy in IRD patients. Arising scientific discoveries regarding the role of SAA, as well as delineating SAA and its isoforms as the most sensitive biomarkers in various IRD by recently developing proteomic techniques are encouraging the revival of its clinical use. Finally, the most recent findings have shown that SAA is a biomarker of severe Coronavirus disease 2019 (COVID-19). The aim of this review is to discuss the SAA-involving immune system network with emphasis on mechanisms relevant for IRD, as well as usefulness of SAA as a biomarker in various IRD. Therefore, over a hundred original papers were collected through an extensive PubMed and Scopus databases search. These recently arising insights will hopefully lead to a better management of IRD patients and might even inspire the development of new therapeutic strategies with SAA as a target.

Keywords: serum amyloid A, biomarkers, markers of inflammation, rheumatic inflammatory disease, autoinflammatory disease, amyloidosis, biological therapy, COVID-19

INTRODUCTION

Serum amyloid A (SAA) is the most prominent acute phase reactant as its serum levels in acute phase response demonstrate the most notable increase. In healthy individuals, SAA is present at the blood concentration below 3 mg/L. During the acute phase of the inflammatory response, SAA increases up to 1,000-fold in 24 h by stimulation of the pro-inflammatory cytokines. This effect is followed by a rapid decline which implies a remarkable feedback regulation (1). SAA shares many similarities with the C-reactive protein (CRP), the most commonly used serum biomarker for assessing disease severity in inflammatory rheumatic diseases (IRD). Both SAA and CRP concentration increases rapidly following an inflammatory stimuli, mostly as a result of the increased synthesis in hepatocytes (1, 2). Moreover, they share some intracellular signaling pathways. In fact, both are induced by interleukin (IL)-6 and addition of IL-1 to IL-6 has a synergistic effect on their synthesis (3). Serum levels of SAA and CRP show a close relationship and are usually significantly positively correlated with each other in a wide range of clinical conditions (4). SAA is significantly elevated in patients with IRD and is commonly used for evaluating disease severity and monitoring disease activity (5). However, the non-superiority of SAA to the other commercially available inflammatory markers, such as CRP and the erythrocyte sedimentation rate (ESR), as well as technical difficulties in measuring the SAA levels have led to neglection of SAA in everyday clinical practice of not IRD specialized centres.

Lately, arising scientific discoveries regarding the role of SAA in IRD as well as the development of proteomic techniques for serum biomarker analysis encouraged a revival of clinical use of SAA. There are more than few arguments in favor of using SAA over CRP in several clinical scenarios associated with inflammation. Firstly, increased concentrations of SAA despite normal levels of CRP and ESR are frequently observed in IRD patients with mild disease activity, while increased CRP or ESR levels with normal SAA concentration are extremely rarely observed. Moreover, the low-grade inflammation with persistent elevated SAA values is associated with the development of life-threatening complications – secondary amyloidosis and coronary heart disease (6, 7). Furthermore, unlike CRP, SAA is locally expressed in inflamed synovial tissue and is directly involved in the pathogenesis of IRD by multiple immunomodulatory and cytokine-like properties, making SAA a potential therapeutic target. Therefore, it is not surprising that accumulating evidences suggests SAA as a more reliable biomarker than CRP or ESR for monitoring disease activity in various rheumatic and autoinflammatory diseases, including rheumatoid arthritis (RA), ankylosing spondylitis (AS), juvenile idiopathic arthritis (JIA), systemic lupus erythematosus (SLE), different types of vasculitis, sarcoidosis, familial Mediterranean fever (FMF), secondary amyloidosis, etc., especially in the era of biologic immunosuppressive therapy.

The aim of this review is to give a brief insight into the complex network of the multiple SAA roles in the pathogenesis of inflammation, as well as to summarize and discuss the current evidences of its clinical utility in assessing an early diagnosis and monitoring the disease activity and response to therapy in a wide range of IRD.

LITERATURE REVIEW

A comprehensive literature review was conducted using PubMed and Scopus databases to identify articles exploring the role and utility of SAA in IRD, according to the published guidance on narrative reviews (8). We used search terms of "serum amyloid A", "serum biomarkers", "markers of inflammation", "rheumatic disease", "autoinflammatory disease" and "COVID-19" in different combinations. The latter term was added since we are currently experiencing a pandemic of Coronavirus disease 2019 (COVID-19). Search terms were used as key words and as MeSH terms to maximize the output from the literature. Only available full-text articles in English published until September 2020 were included. Additional exclusion criteria were studies on non-human species, case reports, reviews, commentaries and studies not concerning rheumatic diseases or not discussing SAA. The reference lists of the selected articles were reviewed to identify additional articles meeting the eligibility criteria. The database search resulted in 2675 articles of which 300 remained after the removal of duplicates and title/abstract screening. Finally, after assessing the full-text articles for eligibility and screening of the reference lists, a total of 180 full-text articles were included in the present review. The included articles were divided in two groups: articles reporting on the role of the SAA-related genes and proteins in the pathogenesis of IRD (n=72) and articles reporting on correlations between SAA and clinical features of various IRD (n=102) or COVID-19 (n=6) (**Figure 1**). Results from the first group are summarized in the "SAA-related genes and proteins" and "SAA in rheumatic diseases" sections, while results from the latter group are summarized in a narrative manner in each relevant section of this review. Summary tables with characteristics of each article included in each section are provided (**Tables 1–9**).

SAA-RELATED GENES AND PROTEINS

The SAA gene family is located on the short arm of chromosome 11 (11p15.1). It contains four genes, namely *SAA1*, *SAA2*, *SAA3* and *SAA4* (115). All the genes consist of 4 exons and 3 introns, and their initial transcripts have 18 aa signal sequence that is removed in the serum proteins. Within the SAA gene cluster, only the *SAA1* and *SAA2* genes encode an acute phase serum proteins (SAA1 and SAA2 isotypes) with approximately 95% sequence identity, which are coordinately induced in response to inflammation (116). *SAA3* contains an early stop codon suggesting it is a non-translated pseudogene (117). The corresponding protein of the *SAA4* gene is constitutively synthesized, meaning it is not induced in the acute phase response (118). The inducible SAA isoforms, SAA1 and SAA2, are termed acute-phase SAA.

SAA has several allelic variants (α, β, γ in *SAA1* and α, β in *SAA2*). Two single nucleotide polymorphisms (SNPs) within the exon 3 of the *SAA1* gene generate three common isoformes: SAA1α (52Valine/57 Alanine), SAA1β (52Alanine/57 Alanine)

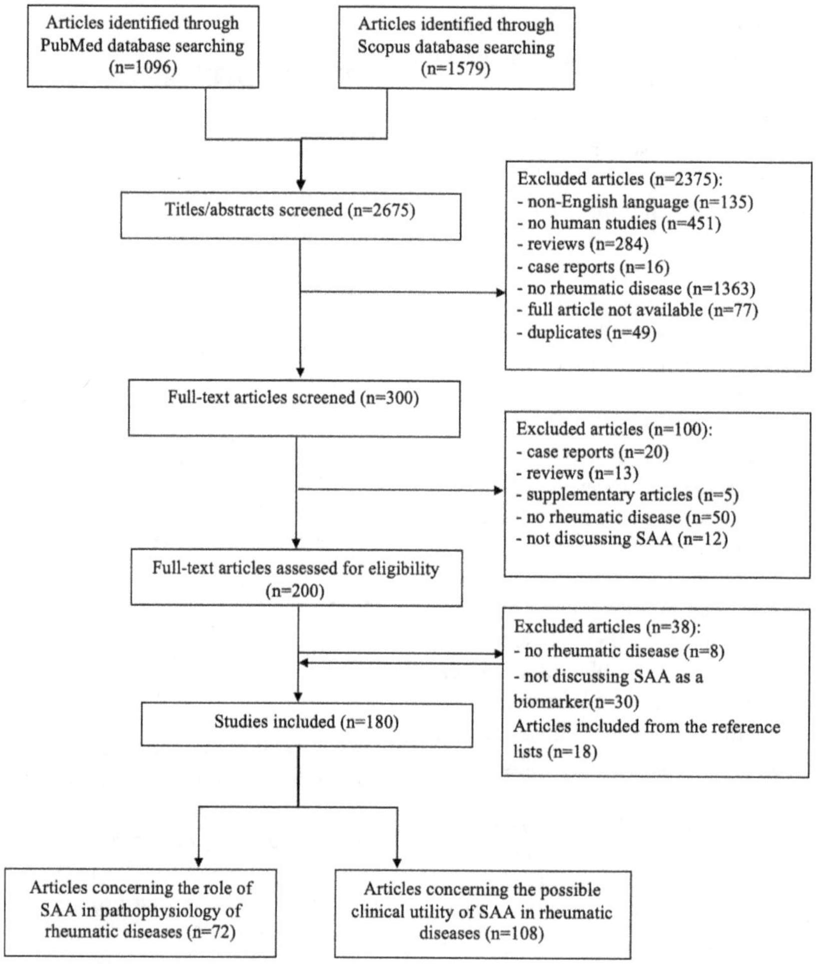

FIGURE 1 | Flow chart illustrating the literature search and study selection process.

and SAA1γ (52Alanine/57 Valine). Some of these variants contribute to the susceptibility to AA amyloidosis. In particular, *SAA1α* allele is a risk factor for developing AA amyloidosis in Caucasian (119–121). Contrarily, in the Japanese population this allelic variant has protective properties, while *SAA1γ*allele carries a higher risk of developing AA amyloidosis (122–124). Blank et al. (119) reported a 100% incidence of *SAA1α/α* genotype among patients with idiopathic AA amyloidsosis. Moreover, another SNP in the *SAA1* gene at position -13 in the 5' regulatory region (promoter region), is associated with the AA amyloidosis occurrence in both Japanese and Caucasian rheumatoid arthritisnbsp;patients, which might explain the discrepancy between previous reports (125, 126). The latter SNP also affects the SAA transcription with the -13T allele having greater activity (127).

SAA transcription can be up-regulated by several cytokines including the tumor necrosis factor alpha (TNFα), IL-1β and IL-6 (128). TNFα and IL-1β activate the nuclear factor-kappa B (NF-κB) site. IL-6 binds to a transmembrane G-coupled protein 130 (gp130) leading to the activation of Janus kinase 2 (JAK-2), which results in the recruitment of the signal transducer and activator of transcription 3 (STAT3), finally resulting in an impressive SAA gene transcription (129, 130). However, a weak expression of SAA messenger RNA (mRNA) is induced by the stimulation with IL-6 alone, whereas almost no expression is induced by the stimulation with TNFα or IL-1β alone. On the other hand, the synergistic induction of SAA mRNA has been observed by a co-stimulation with IL-6 and TNFα or IL-1β (131). It seems that the activation of STAT3 by an IL-6 stimulated JAK is essential for the production of SAA and the supplementation of NF-κB activity stimulated by TNFα or IL-1β strengthens the SAA expression (132). This evidence is important for the therapeutic effects of monoclonal antibodies: JAK inhibitors (tofacitinib) and anti-IL-6 receptor antibodies (tocilizumab and sarilumab) almost completely inhibit the expression of the SAA mRNA, whereas the IL-1 antagonists (anakinra) and TNFα antibodies (infliximab, adalimumab, etanercept) achieve only a partial inhibition (108, 130). However, SAA mRNA translation is 10-fold lower than the rate of mRNA synthesis due to post-transcriptional regulation. SAA mRNA undergoes poly(A) tail shortening over time, a

TABLE 1 | Characteristics and results of articles investigating clinical utility of SAA in patients with rheumatoid arthritis.

First author (reference number)	The aim of the study regarding the clinical utility of SAA	Number of patients	Diagnosis (number of patients)	Method used for SAA measuring	Results / Comments
Benson and Cohen (5)	To investigate the possible uses of SAA in rheumatic diseases	277	RA (n=65) JIA (n=26) SLE (n=25) OA (n=23) HC (n=138)	Radioimmuno-assay	➢ SAA is significantly elevated in RA, JIA and SLE patients compared to HC and patients with degenerative joint disease ➢ SAA is significantly correlated with ESR and with disease activity in RA
De Beer et al. (9)	To evaluate SAA as a marker of diagnosis and severity in rheumatic diseases	266	RA (n=99) JIA (n=24) SLE (n=43) HC (n=100)	Radioimmuno-assay	➢ SAA is significantly elevated in RA, JIA and SLE patients compared to HC ➢ SAA is a marker of disease activity in RA and JIA, but is not significantly correlated with disease activity in SLE patients
Maury et al. (10)	To evaluate SAA and CRP levels in RA and SLE patients	65	RA (n=48) SLE (n=17)	Radioimmuno-assay	➢ SAA is significantly correlated with disease activity in RA patients, but not in SLE patients ➢ SAA levels are strongly correlated with CRP levels in RA and SLE patients
Shen et al. (11)	To evaluate possible uses of SAA in patients with RA	265	RA (n=88) OA (n=54) SLE (n=43) Other AID (n=30) HC (n=50)	ELISA and western blot analysis	➢ SAA can be used as a marker for diagnosis of RA (among patients with other autoimmune diseases or osteoarthritis) ➢ SAA significantly correlates with RA disease activity (measured as DAS28-ESR)
Kumon et al. (12)	To compare SAA levels in serum and synovial fluid between OA and RA patients	55	RA (n=34) OA (n=21)	ELISA	➢ SAA levels are significantly higher in both serum and synovial fluid in RA patients compared to OA patients and therefore can be used as a marker for RA diagnosis
Targonska-Stepniak et al. (13)	To assess SAA level in RA patients and its correlation with cardiovascular and renal involvement	140	RA (98 high activity + 42 low activity)	ELISA	➢ SAA is a sensitive marker of RA and is significantly correlated with disease activity ➢ SAA is an indicator of cardiovascular and renal involvement in RA patients
Chambers et al. (14)	To assess SAA as a marker of disease activity in RA patients	385	RA (n=185) HC (n=200)	Radioimmuno-assay	➢ SAA is a more sensitive marker of disease activity in RA than CRP
Cunnane et al. (15)	To compare SAA with CRP and ESR in relation to diagnosis and disease activity in early inflammatory arthritis	140	RA (n=64) PsA (n=19) UA (n=57)	ELISA	➢ Compared with CRP and ESR, SAA correlates best with disease activity ➢ SAA, unlike CRP or ESR, can be used for distinguishing patients with a final diagnosis of RA in early inflammatory arthritis
Yoo et al. (16)	To evaluate serum and exosomal AA levels in RA patients	60	RA (30 with active disease + 30 with inactive disease)	ELISA	➢ both serum and exosomal AA may be used as a RA disease activity biomarker
Ostensen et al. (17)	To evaluate SAA as a marker of disease activity during pregnancy in RA and AS patients	52	RA (n=11) AS (n=13) HC (n=28)	Radioimmuno-assay	➢ SAA is a reliable marker of disease activity in RA and AS even during pregnancy
Hwang et al. (18)	To evaluate use of SAA in monitoring disease activity and therapy response in RA patients	594	RA	Immunonephelo-metric assay	➢ SAA correlates better than CRP with RA disease activity, especially during treatment with TNFα antagonists
Wild et al. (19)	To compare the utility of different biomarkers as diagnostic indicators of RA	645	RA (n=364) OA (n=281)	ELISA	➢ SAA is the only biomarker (among 131 initially considered in the study) that increases sensitivity of anti-CCP for RA diagnosis ➢ sensitivity and specificity of SAA are higher than those of CRP for diagnosing RA
De Seny et al. (20)	To compare SAA levels in serum and synovial fluid between OA and RA patients	91	RA (n=27) OA (n=29) HC (n=35)	ELISA	➢ SAA levels are significantly higher in both serum and synovial fluid in RA patients compared to OA patients and healthy controls and therefore can be used as a marker for RA diagnosis
Ally et al. (21)	To evaluate serum biomarkers as markers of disease activity in early RA	128	RA	Immunonephelo-metric assay	➢ SAA is significantly correlated with disease activity in DMARD-naive patients with early RA
Targonska-Stepniak et al. (22)	To investigate effects of leflunomide therapy on SAA concentrations and disease activity in RA patients	50	RA (13 with SAA<50 mg/L + 37 with SAA> 50mg/L)	ELISA	➢ Baseline SAA can be used for predicting response to leflunomide (cut off value 50 mg/L) ➢ In spite of a significant reduction in ESR and CRP in RA patients receiving leflunomide, high SAA levels may persist and can be used for detecting subclinical inflammation and adjusting treatment

(Continued)

TABLE 1 | Continued

First author (reference number)	The aim of the study regarding the clinical utility of SAA	Number of patients	Diagnosis (number of patients)	Method used for SAA measuring	Results / Comments
Connolly et al. (23)	To investigate the relationship between SAA and disease progression in RA and PsA patients undergoing biologic therapy	62	RA (n=45) PsA (n=17)	ELISA	➢ SAA significantly correlates with RA and PsA disease activity ➢ SAA is independently associated with 1-year radiographic progression in RA ➢ SAA is a more accurate predictor of radiographic progression and a more sensitive biomarker of disease activity in patients receiving biologic therapy compared with CRP or ESR
Centola et al. (24)	To develop a multi-biomarker disease activity (MBDA) test for RA	702	RA	ND	➢ SAA is a marker of disease activity incorporated in MBDA test
Ma et al. (25)	To explore the utility of serum biomarkers incorporated in MBDA for predicting remission in RA patients	148	RA	ELISA	➢ baseline SAA levels are significantly correlated with remission at 1 year in RA patients ➢ SAA levels are significantly higher in RA patients with low disease activity compared to those in remission and therefore can be used for detecting minimal inflammation
Wong et al. (26)	To relate serum biomarkers to vascular elasticity in RA patients	106	RA (n=53: 15 with + 38 without coronary artery disease) HC (n=53)	Immunonephelometric assay	➢ SAA levels are significantly inversely correlated with arterial elasticity in RA patients, indicating cardiovascular disease
Rho et al. (27)	To evaluate SAA as a marker of atherosclerosis severity in RA patients	261	RA (n=169) HC (n=92)	ELISA	➢ SAA shows a trend of association with the severity of coronary atherosclerosis in RA patients
Kullich et al. (28)	To evaluate effect of leflunomide on serum biomarker levels	36	RA	ELISA	➢ SAA is a sensitive marker of response to leflunomide (DMARD) therapy in RA patients
Momohara et al. (29)	To evaluate SAA as a marker of disease activity in RA	140	RA	ELISA	➢ SAA is a more sensitive marker of RA disease activity than CRP or ESR ➢ SAA is highly expressed in chondrocytes from RA patients
Boeters et al. (30)	To identify biomarkers for predicting sustained DMARD-free remission in RA patients	299	RA	ELISA	➢ SAA level at disease onset may be used as a predictor of achieving DMARD-free remission in ACPA-negative RA patients
Migita et al. (31)	To explore effects of tofacitinib on inflammatory biomarkers in RA patients	14	RA	Immunonephelometric assay	➢ SAA is a sensitive indicator of response to tofacitinib in RA patients
Visvanathan et al. (32)	To evaluate the effect of golimumab on SAA levels in RA patients	137	RA	ELISA	➢ SAA may be used for monitoring response to golimumab in RA patients ➢ Measuring SAA level at week 4 after initiation of golimumab therapy can be used to predict clinical response at week 16
Doyle et al. (33)	To investigate effects of golimumab on inflammatory biomarkers in RA patients	49	RA	ND	➢ SAA is a sensitive biomarker of response to golimumab in RA patients
Kobayashi et al. (34)	To analyze effects of adalimumab on inflammatory biomarkers in RA patients	20	RA	2DE + MS	➢ SAA is a sensitive biomarker for response to adalimumab in RA patients
Berner Hammer et al. (35)	To examine effects of adalimumab on inflammatory biomarkers in RA patients	20	RA	Immunonephelometric assay	➢ SAA is a sensitive biomarker for monitoring response to adalimumab in RA patients
Gabay et al. (36)	To evaluate effects of adalimumab and sarilumab on inflammatory biomarkers in RA patients	307	RA	ND	➢ SAA is a marker of disease activity in RA ➢ SAA is a sensitive biomarker of response to both anti-IL-6 and anti-TNFα therapy in RA ➢ High baseline SAA levels may be used for distinguishing non-responders to anti-TNFα therapy
Nissinen et al. (37)	To analyze changes in inflammatory biomarkers in RA patients receiving infliximab	25	RA	ELISA	➢ SAA is a marker of response to infliximab treatment in RA patients
Xu et al. (38)	To explore SAA isoforms in sera from RA patients	169	RA (n=85) HC (n=84)	ELISA	➢ Both SAA1 and total SAA are significantly elevated in RA compared to HC ➢ SAA1/SAA ratio is not significantly different between RA patients and HC

(Continued)

TABLE 1 | Continued

First author (reference number)	The aim of the study regarding the clinical utility of SAA	Number of patients	Diagnosis (number of patients)	Method used for SAA measuring	Results / Comments
De Seny et al. (39)	To identify RA serum biomarkers by a proteomic approach	103	RA (n=34) AS (n=19) PsA (n=22) OA (n=20) HC (n=16)	SELDI-TOF MS, Western blot	➢ SAA and its truncated forms are significantly elevated in sera from RA patients compared to healthy controls and patients with osteoarthritis
Li et al. (40)	To screen candidate RA associated serum proteins by comparative proteomics	76	RA (n=38) HC (n=38)	2-DE, MS, ELISA	➢ SAA serum concentration is significantly higher in RA patients compared to HC
Seok et al. (41)	To identify biomarkers for improving the accuracy of RA prescreening	80	RA (n=40) HC (n=40)	LC-MS/MS, ELISA	➢ SAA4 is significantly higher in sera with high rheumatoid factor values and may represent a novel prescreening marker for RA diagnosis
Nys et al. (42)	To explore SAA isoforms in different rheumatic diseases	224	RA (n=46: 14 early onset + 20 low activity + 12 high activity) AS (n=30) SLE (n=23) SSc (n=20) OA (n=43) HC (n=62)	LC-MS/MS	➢ SAA2 and SAA1β isoforms are potential RA diagnostic biomarkers prior the onset of symptomatic RA ➢ SAA1α/SAA1β ratio could be used as a marker of disease severity and response to treatment

TABLE 2 | Characteristics and results of articles investigating clinical utility of SAA in patients with juvenile idiopathic arthritis.

First author (reference number)	The aim of the study regarding the clinical utility of SAA	Number of patients	Diagnosis (number of patients)	Method used for SAA measuring	Results / Comments
Filipowicz-Sonowska et al. (43)	To investigate SAA levels and its correlations in Polish and American children with JIA and secondary amyloidosis	86	JIA (21 with secondary amyloidosis, 45 without) HC (n=20 with mild infections)	Radioimmuno-assay	➢ SAA is significantly elevated in patients with JIA, especially in polyarticular and systemic forms in which amyloidosis occurs more frequently ➢ SAA is not significantly higher in JIA patients with amyloidosis than in those without, therefore is not useful for detecting amyloidosis
Scheinberg et al. (44)	To evaluate clinical utility of measuring SAA levels in JIA	90	JIA (4 with secondary amyloidosis, 96 without)	Radioimmuno-assay	➢ SAA levels are significantly correlated with polyarticular and systemic forms as well as with disease activity in patients with JIA, but not with the presence of secondary amyloidosis
Kutulculer et al. (45)	To investigate several biomarkers in assessing disease stage in JIA patients	147	JIA (n=82) FMF (n=35) HC(n=30)	Immunonephelo-metric assay	➢ SAA levels show significant difference between active and remission stages in individuals with JIA or FMF
Cantarini et al. (46)	To investigate SAA as a marker of disease activity in JIA	67	JIA (n=41: 16 polyarticular + 25 oligoarticular) HC(n=26)	ELISA	➢ SAA is a more sensitive marker than ESR and CRP in assessing disease activity in JIA (evaluated as presence and number of active joints- clinically)
Dev et al. (47)	To investigate SAA as a marker of disease activity in JIA	90	JIA (n=50) HC (n=40)	ELISA	➢ SAA is a more sensitive marker than ESR and CRP in assessing disease activity in JIA (evaluated as presence and number of active joints- clinically and USG score)
Miyamae et al. (48)	To explore biomarkers for monitoring and predicting response to therapy in JIA	23	Systemic JIA	SELDI-TOF MS, Immunonephelo-metric assay	➢ SAA is significantly correlated with response to both conventional and biologic therapy ➢ Baseline SAA level may be used for predicting response to therapy

posttranscriptional event that has been functionally coupled to gene expression and translation. These post-transcriptional mechanisms are only partially explained, suggesting possible epigenetic modifications (133, 134). The half-life time of SAA (~35h) is significantly shorter than that of CRP (~47h) (4). Interestingly, half-life time of their mRNAs (SAA mRNA~8.5h, CRP mRNA~2.5h) indicate that SAA mRNA stability is substantially greater than the CRP mRNA. Taken all together, it seems that CRP expression is regulated mainly at the transcriptional level, while post-transcriptional mechanisms are involved in the regulation of SAA (133, 135). This is somewhat in line with the notion that SAAcan be readily produced locally by

TABLE 3 | Characteristics and results of articles investigating clinical utility of SAA in patients with ankylosing spondylitis.

First author (reference number)	The aim of the study regarding the clinical utility of SAA	Number of patients	Diagnosis (number of patients)	Method used for SAA measuring	Results / Comments
Lange et al. (49)	To evaluate SAA as marker of inflammation in AS	72	AS	ELISA	➢ SAA correlates significantly with disease activity in AS patients (assessed by BASDAI score), but is not superior to CRP or ESR
Jung et al. (50)	To evaluate SAA as marker of disease activity in AS patients	76	AS (n=38) HC (n=38)	Immunonephelo-metric assay	➢ SAA is a more sensitive marker than ESR and CRP in assessing disease activity in AS (evaluated by BASDAI score)
De Vries et al. (51)	To evaluate SAA as disease activity marker in AS patients receiving anti-TNF therapy	155	AS	ELISA	➢ SAA correlates significantly with disease activity, response to anti-TNF therapy, and has high predictive value for response to anti-TNF therapy ➢ SAA may be indicator of anti-drug antibodies development
Li et al. (52)	To find a diagnostic marker for AS by proteomic approach	76	AS (n=38) HC (n=38)	2-DE+MALDI-TOF MS, ELISA	➢ SAA may be used as a diagnostic indicator of AS , since it is over-expressed by more than 3-fold in the sera of AS patients compared to healthy controls
Rademacher et al. (53)	To find biomarkers for predicting radiographic progression of AS	117	AS (28 progressors + 89 nonprogressors)	ELISA	➢ SAA levels are significantly elevated in AS patients, but do not correlate with future radiographic progression
Wu et al. (54)	To find serum biomarkers for assessing response to adalimumab in AS patients by proteomic approach	151	AS (n=82) HC (n=69)	Human antibody array, ELISA	➢ SAA1 is significantly correlated with disease activity in AS patients treated with adalimumab ➢ SAA1 significantly correlates with peripheral joint involvement in AS
Liu et al. (55)	To explore serum biomarkers in AS patients by proteomic approach	410	AS (n=192: 164 active + 28 inactive) HC (n=218)	Tandem Mass Tag Proteomics, ELISA	➢ SAA is a sensitive marker for diagnosis and assessing disease activity in AS ➢ SAA1 is even more sensitive marker than total SAA ➢ Combination of CRP and SAA1 increases sensitivity and specificity of CRP alone for diagnosis and assessing disease activity in AS

synovial cells in joints of RA patients (20, 136). Moreover, Thorn et al. (128, 137) detected a putative glucocorticoid response element (GRE) functionally active in the *SAA1* gene, whereas it was disrupted in the *SAA2* gene. A paradox of an anti-inflammatory drug inducing the pro-inflammatory mediator was confirmed by De Seny et al. (20) who demonstrated glucocorticoid-induced SAA secretion in human primary joint cells.

SAA IN RHEUMATIC DISEASES

The role of SAA in pathogenesis of rheumatic diseases has been most extensively investigated in RA, a IRD prototype, characterized by synovial inflammation leading to a cartilage destruction. The finding that the SAA concentration might be even higher in synovial fluid than plasma, led to discovery of local SAA production by rheumatoid synovial cells (20, 29, 138). Connolly et al. demonstrated a SAA-induced leukocyte migration and tissue infiltration, angiogenesis and inflammation in synovial cells in rheumatoid arthritis (98, 139). Moreover, SAA exhibits cytokine-like properties and can induce synthesis and secretion of several proinflammatory cytokines, including TNFα, IL-6 and IL-1ß (140, 141). SAA plays a pathogenic role in joint leading to the cartilage destruction by activating multiple receptors, including N-formyl peptide receptor-like 1 (FPRL1, also called lipoxin A4 receptor) (142, 143), scavenger receptor class B type 1 (SR-B1) (144, 145), Toll-like receptor 4 (TLR4) (146, 147), Toll-like receptor 2 (TLR2) (148–151) and receptors of advanced glycation end products (RAGE) (147, 152). The expression of these receptors is increased in RA synovial tissue and mediates SAA-induced proinflammatory and angiogenic effects by the activation of MAPKs and NF-κB (153). Moreover, SAA stimulates the production of matrix metalloproteinases (MMPs) by chondrocytes and synovial fibroblasts (154–156). Stimulation of these cartilage-degrading proteinases contributes to the chronic tissue injury in arthritis. Matrix metalloproteinase-3 (MMP-3) is found highly concentrated in the synovial fluid as well as in the serum of RA patients and correlates with progression of erosion in RA (21, 157). MMP-3 production is simultaneously up-regulated by the proinflammatory cytokines IL-1β, TNFα and IL-17. Cytokine- and SAA-driven production of MMP-3 in the rheumatoid joint appears to be a key mediator of the cartilage destruction. Furthermore, SAA induces pentraxin 3 (PTX3) in rheumatoid synoviocytes. PTX3 is also an acute-phase reactant involved in amplification of the inflammatory response. This loop seems to involve N-formyl peptide receptor ligand-1 (FRLP-1) (158).

A new subset of interleukin 17 (IL-17) producing T helper cells (Th17 cells) has been recently reported to play a critical role in inflammatory joint diseases including RA, AS and psoriatic arthritis (PsA) (159–165). In contrast to the other effector T-cell

TABLE 4 | Characteristics and results of articles investigating clinical utility of SAA in patients with different types of vasculitis.

First author (reference number)	The aim of the study regarding the clinical utility of SAA	Diagnosis (number of patients)	Method used for SAA measuring	Results / Comments
Ma et al. (56)	To find a potential biomarker for assessing TA activity	TA (n=43: 18 active + 25 inactive), HC (n=20)	ELISA	➢ SAA is significantly higher in patients with active TA than in those with inactive disease, and is significantly higher in both groups compared to HC
Nair et al. (57)	To evaluate SAA as a marker of disease activity and treatment response in TA	TA (n=99: 43 active + 48 inactive + 8 indeterminate), HC (n=40)	ELISA	➢ SAA is a more sensitive biomarker of disease activity and treatment response than CRP or ESR in TA patients
Hocevar et al. (58)	To explore serum biomarkers utility for predicting relapse in GCA patients receiving GCs	GCA (n=68: 31 relapsed + 37 nonrelapsed)	ND	➢ High baseline SAA values are predictors of early relapse in GCA patients treated with GCs ➢ Baseline SAA is better correlated with future relapses than CRP or ESR
Burja et al. (59)	To identify serum biomarkers for monitoring disease activity in patients with GCA	GCA (n=82: 35 relapsed + 47 nonrelapsed), HC (n=46)	Immuno-nephelometric assay	➢ SAA may be used as a marker for GCA diagnosis and disease activity (more sensitive than CRP or ESR)
Dartavel et al. (60)	To evaluate SAA as a marker of disease activity in GCA	GCA (n=80: 21 active + 59 inactive), microbial infections (n=8)	ND	➢ SAA is significantly different between GCA patients with active and inactive disease ➢ SAA levels are not different between patients with active GCA and microbial infections
Van Sleen et al. (61)	To find biomarkers for predicting disease course in GCA and for monitoring response too therapy	GCA (n=41) HC (n=33) microbial infections (n=13)	ELISA	➢ SAA is significantly elevated in GCA compared to HCs, but not compared to patients with infection ➢ SAA correlates with disease activity in GCA patients receiving GCs ➢ Baseline SAA levels do not have a predictive value for disease course in GCA
Mitani et al. (62)	To find potential biomarkers of coronary artery lesions late after KD	KD (n=65: 20 with coronary artery lesions, 45 without)	Immuno-nephelometric assay	➢ SAA is significantly higher in patients with coronary artery lesion persistence late after KD than in patients with regressed or without lesions
Whitin et al. (63)	To find a serum biomarker for diagnosis of KD	KD (n=68) Febrile controls (n=61)	SELDI-TOF MS + hybrid MS immunoassay	➢ A truncated form of SAA (7860 Da) may be a diagnostic marker for KD
Purevdorj et al. (64)	To find a serum biomarker for diagnosis of HSP	HSP (n=127), Infections (n=110), HC (n=121)	ELISA	➢ SAA is a sensitive and specific diagnostic biomarker for HSP (better than CRP)
Kuret et al. (65)	To evaluate serum biomarkers for diagnosis of IgA vasculitis	IgA vasculitis (n=62) HC (n=53)	Immuno-nephelometric assay	➢ SAA is significantly increased in adult IgA vasculitis and may be used as a diagnostic marker

subsets, Th17 cells express the IL-23 receptor (IL-23R) on their membrane and are dependent on IL-23 for their survival, expansion and cytokine production (159). In addition, Th17 cells express the chemokine receptor 6 (CCR6) on their membrane which can be activated by the chemokine ligand 20 (CLC20) (160). CLC20 acts as a chemo-attractant on Th17 cells and stimulates IL-17 production. SAA is a potent inducer of both IL-23 and CCL20 in synovium and, consequently, induces Th17 polarization from CD4 + T cells and IL-17 production (161, 162). Furthermore, IL-17 also up-regulates the expression of CCL20 (166). Taken together, SAA sustains the chronic inflammation by contributing to the recruitment of Th17 cells to the inflamed synovium. Although serum and synovial fluid IL-17 levels in RA patients are significantly elevated (163, 164), results of clinical trials with anti-IL-17 antibodies have been discouraging. On the other hand, IL17 blockade is highly effective in AS and PsA (166, 167). This may be due to a non-IL-23 dependent IL-17 production in innate immune cells, which can contribute to the pathogenesis of these diseases (166). **Figure 2** summarizes the described SAA signal transduction and feedback pathways.

Recent studies (168–170) have shown that SAA also induces the synthesis of pro-IL-1β and activation of the NOD-like receptor family, pyrin domain containing 3 (NLRP3) inflammasome and subsequent activation of caspase-1 which converts pro-IL-1β to its active form IL-1β, suggesting a further link between SAA and systemic autoinflammatory disease. Activation of the inflammasome cascade has one of the key roles in initiation of the whole immune system. This recently discovered connection, in addition to the above mentioned SAA immunomodulatory pathways, emphasizes the importance of SAA in the pathogenesis of rheumatic diseases. Proteins that are mutated in autoinflammatory diseases mediate the regulation of NF-κB activation, cell apoptosis, and IL-1β secretion through cross-regulated signaling pathways. Since almost all clinical manifestations associated with inflammasome dysregulation are due to an inappropriate and/or excessive release of IL-1β,

TABLE 5 | Characteristics and results of articles investigating clinical utility of SAA in patients with sarcoidosis.

First author (reference number)	The aim of the study regarding the clinical utility of SAA	Diagnosis (number of patients)	Method used for SAA measuring	Results /Comments
Rothkrantz-Kos et al. (66)	To evaluate the clinical usefulness of SAA for assessing sarcoidosis severity	Sarcoidosis (n=144: 73 untreated + 71 treated) HC (n=282)	Immunonephelometric assay	➢ SAA does not correlate with the disease severity in sarcoidosis
Miyoshi et al. (67)	To identify marker predictive of increased parenchymal infiltration in sarcoidosis	Sarcoidosis (n=43)	Immunoturbidimetric assay	➢ SAA concentration at diagnosis is not predictive of increased parenchymal infiltration later in sarcoidosis
Salazar et al. (68)	To evaluate SAA as a marker of disease activity in patients with sarcoidosis	Sarcoidosis (n=85: 40 active + 45 inactive)	ELISA	➢ SAA is significantly higher in sarcoidosis patients with active disease than in those with inactive disease
Bargagli et al. (69)	To investigate possible benefits of SAA as a biomarker in sarcoidosis	sarcoidosis (n=55) HC (n=24)	2-DE+western blot, ELISA	➢ SAA and SAA1 may be used as a diagnostic marker for sarcoidosis, marker of disease activity and a predictor of severe disease (requiring steroid therapy)
Gungor et al. (70)	To find a sensitive marker of sarcoidosis disease activity	Sarcoidosis (n=48: 37 active + 11 inactive) HC (n=20)	ELISA	➢ SAA can be used as a marker of sarcoidosis activity since it correlates with disease activity (better than CRP)
Zhang et al. (71)	To find a serum marker for differential diagnosis of sarcoidosis from other lung diseases	Sarcoidosis (n=37) Tuberculosis (N=20) Other pulmonary diseases(n=20) HC (n=20)	MALDI-TOF MS, ELISA	➢ SAA levels are significantly higher in sarcoidosis patients compared to other lung diseases and can be used as a diagnostic marker for sarcoidosis ➢ Truncated SAA forms might be an even more specific diagnostic marker for sarcoidosis
Enyedi et al. (72)	To evaluate markers for differential diagnosis of sarcoidosis from other lung diseases	Sarcoidosis (n=69) Other lung diseases (n=35)	Immunonephelometric assay	➢ SAA does not significantly differ between patients with biopsy-proven sarcoidosis and biopsy negative patients

TABLE 6 | Characteristics and results of articles investigating clinical utility of SAA in patients with systemic sclerosis, systemic lupus erythematosus or psoriatic arthritis.

First author (reference number)	The aim of the study regarding the clinical utility of SAA	Number of patients	Diagnosis (number of patients)	Method used for SAA measuring	Results / Comments
Brandwein et al. (73)	To explore SAA as a marker of SSc severity	74	SSc (n=62) HC (n=12)	Radioimmuno-assay	➢ SAA is significantly correlated with SSc severity (assessed by extension of skin thickening)
Lakota et al. (74)	To determine clinical correlations of SAA in patients with SSc	227	SSc (n=129) HC (n=98)	ELISA	➢ SAA significantly correlates with pulmonary function and is a sensitive marker of pulmonary involvement in SSc
Lis Swiety et al. (75)	To evaluate SAA in SSc patients in relation to skin and pulmonary involvement	48	SSc (n=33: 18 early dSSc + 15 late dSSc) HC (n=15)	ELISA	➢ SAA is superior to CRP as a biomarker of pulmonary involvement in SSc
Wang et al. (76)	To investigate correlation between SAA levels and disease activity in SLE	284	SLE (n=135: 52 active + 83 inactive disease) HC (n=149)	Immunonephelometric assay	➢ SAA is independently significantly correlated with SLE disease activity (assessed by SLEDAI score)
Boyd et al. (77)	To evaluate correlations between serum biomarkers and disease activity in psoriatic arthritis	45	PsA (n=45)	ELISA	➢ SAA is the marker with the highest correlation to the disease activity in PsA patients (compared to 15 measured biomarkers including CRP)

targeted IL-1β blockade is the mainstay of treatment, and its remarkable efficacy is well established. Biological therapies such as anakinra (recombinant IL-1 receptor antagonist) and canakinumab (monoclonal anti-IL-1β antibody) are both licensed for several autoinflammatory diseases.

In 1974, Husby et al. identified amyloid protein A as a proteolytic derivate of SAA by a sequence analysis of the protein purified from amyloid deposits. Amyloid protein A is a 76 amino acids N-terminal derivate of SAA (171). The aberrant processing of SAA in macrophage lysosomes leads to accumulation of newly formed AA amyloid fibrils and development of AA amyloidosis (172, 173). The generation of SAA N-terminal fragments has been related to the activity of MMPs (174). MMP1 has a putative cleavage site next to the site of SAA1 amino acid substitutions at positions 52 and 57 (175). SAA1α has a higher affinity for cleavage by MMP1 than SAA1β or SAA1γ consequently leading to a larger amounts of amyloidogenic truncated SAA forms (175). These data indicate

TABLE 7 | Characteristics and results of articles investigating clinical utility of SAA in patients with systemic autoinflammatory diseases.

First author (reference number)	The aim of the study regarding the clinical utility of SAA	Diagnosis (number of patients)	Method used for SAA measuring	Results / Comments
Duzova et al. (78)	To evaluate SAA in detecting subclinical activity in FMF and for guiding colchicine therapy	FMF (n=183, attack-free period)	ND	➢ SAA level remains high even between attacks in children with FMF, therefore can be used for detecting subclinical inflammation ➢ SAA monitoring should be used as a guidance for therapy adjustment
Lachmann et al. (79)	To evaluate inflammatory activity in FMF patients	FMF (n=43) MEFV mutation carriers (n=67) HC (n=50)	Immunonephelometric assay	➢ SAA is significantly elevated during FMF attacks and remains increased between attacks ➢ SAA is higher among asymptomatic heterozygous carriers of MEFV mutations compared to HC, potentially leading to development of amyloidosis (phenotype II) ➢ SAA level monitoring should be used for assessment of and reinforcing patients compliance for therapy
Berkun et al. (80)	To evaluate SAA as a marker for diagnosis and therapy adjustment in FMF	FMF (n=204)	Immunonephelometric assay	➢ SAA level is an indicator of subclinical inflammation in FMF patients, a guidance for colchicine adjustment and a marker for differentiating noncompliance and nonresponse to colchicine
Yalcinkaya et al. (81)	To evaluate the clinical utility of SAA in FMF patients with amyloidosis	FMF (n=51: 36 without amyloidosis + 15 with amyloidosis) MEFV mutation carriers (n=39) Other chronic inflammatory diseases (n=39) Infections (n=20) HC (n=19)	ELISA	➢ SAA is elevated during acute attacks and remains above reference range even during attack-free periods in FMF patients ➢ SAA is not significantly higher in FMF patients with a higher potential for developing amyloidosis than in those without, so cannot be used for predicting amyloidosis
Kallinich et al. (82)	To find biomarkers of inflammation in FMF	FMF (n=52: 28 without attack, 19 during attack, 5 mutation carriers)	Immunonephelometric assay	➢ SAA concentration is significantly elevated in FMF patients at diagnosis, during attacks, in between the attacks and in MEFV mutation carriers
Lofty et al. (83)	To investigate the clinical utility of monitoring SAA levels in FMF	FMF (n=71)	ELISA	➢ SAA is elevated even during attack-free periods in FMF and, therefore, should be used for detecting subclinical inflammation
Cakan et al. (84)	To determine the capability of SAA in differentiating attacks of FMF from acute febrile infections	FMF (n=28) Acute respiratory infection (n=28)	Immunonephelometric assay	➢ SAA is significantly higher in acute FMF attack than in acute febrile respiratory infection
Bilginer et al. (85)	To find biomarkers for predicting atherosclerosis in FMF patients	FMF (n=70, attack-free period) HC (n=50)	ELISA	➢ SAA is significantly higher in FMF patients even in attack-free periods compared to HC ➢ SAA is significantly correlated with CIMT (an early predictor of atherosclerosis)
Mohamed et al. (86)	To explore relationship between SAA and CIMT in FMF patients	FMF (n=45, attack-free period) HC (n=40)	ELISA	➢ SAA is significantly elevated in FMF patients compared to HC ➢ SAA is significantly correlated with attack severity and CIMT in FMF patients
Sargsyan et al. (87)	To find biomarkers of vascular involvement in FMF patients	FMF (n=102: 50 with vascular disease, 52 without)	ELISA	➢ SAA is significantly higher in FMF patients with vascular involvement than in those without
Aygunduz et al. (88)	To evaluate SAA as a marker of disease activity in BD	BD (n=43: active 20 + inactive 23) HC (n=27)	ELISA	➢ SAA is significantly elevated in patients with BD and correlates with disease activity
Cantarini et al. (89)	To evaluate potential correlations between circulating biomarkers and clinical activity of BD	BD (n=27) HC (n=35)	ELISA	➢ SAA is not significantly correlated with disease activity in BD ➢ SAA is an indicator of skin involvement in BD
Vitale et al. (90)	To evaluate SAA as a marker of disease activity in BD	BD (n=26)	ELISA	➢ SAA serum levels higher than 30, 50 and 150 mg/L are significantly associated with the occurence of oral aphthosis, neurological and ocular involvement, respectively
Sota et al. (91)	To explore potential values of SAA as a biomarker in patients with BD	BD (n=64)	ELISA	➢ SAA levels do not correlate with disease activity in BD ➢ SAA levels >200 mg/L are significantly associated with major organ involvement

(Continued)

TABLE 7 | Continued

First author (reference number)	The aim of the study regarding the clinical utility of SAA	Diagnosis (number of patients)	Method used for SAA measuring	Results / Comments
				➢ SAA levels >150mg/L are associated with ocular, skin and mucosal involvement in BD
Lee et al. (92)	To evaluate SAA as a biomarker in intestinal BD by proteomic analysis	Intestinal BD (n=64: 9 mild + 35 moderate + 20 severe) HC (n=56)	2-DE + MALDI-TOF/TOF MS, ELISA	➢ SAA is significantly elevated, but is not correlated with disease severity in patients with intestinal BD
Hawkins et al. (93)	To evaluate SAA in monitoring response to anakinra (anti-IL-1R antibody) in MWS patients	MWS (n=3)	Immunonephelometric assay	➢ SAA is significantly reduced after initiation of anakinra treatment in MWS as well as the clinical symptoms, therefore can be used for monitoring response to biologic therapy
Scarpioni et al. (94)	To evaluate SAA in monitoring response to canakinumab in MWS patients	MWS (n=2)	Immunonephelometric assay	➢ SAA is significantly reduced after initiation of canakinumab treatment in MWS as well as the clinical symptoms, therefore can be used for monitoring response to therapy
Hoffman et al. (95)	To evaluate SAA in monitoring response to rilonacept in patients with CAPS	FCAS (n=95) MWS (n=3) FCAS/MWS (n=3)	ND	➢ SAA levels are significantly reduced after initiation of rilonacept therapy and remain low during long-term follow-up
Goldbach-Mansky et al. (96)	To evaluate SAA in monitoring response to rilonacept (anti-IL-1R therapy) in patients with CAPS	FCAS (n=5)	ND	➢ SAA significantly correlates with disease activity and response to anti-IL-1 therapy in FCAS patients
Wiken et al. (97)	To evaluate SAA in monitoring response to anakinra in patients with CAPS	NOMID (98) MWS (7)	Immunonephelometric assay	➢ SAA is significantly reduced after initiation of anakinra treatment in CAPS as well as the clinical symptoms and the development of anti-drug antibodies does not effect either

that susceptibility to N-terminal cleavage at residue 57 might be related to a higher risk of developing amyloidosis.

In blood circulation SAA associates with high density lipoproteins (HDL), where it replaces apolipoprotein A1. During the acute phase response, SAA constitutes up to 87% of the apolipoprotein content of HDL particles. Incorporation of SAA into the HDL particle leads to a structural modification with a consequent functional deficiency. These so-called proinflammatory HDLs (piHDLs) are characterized by reduced capacity for reverse cholesterol transport, increased oxidation of low density lipoproteins (LDLs) and reduced inhibition of monocyte chemoattractant protein 1 (MCP-1) production in vascular smooth muscle cells. These changes result in an increased atherogenic potential (176, 177). Recent studies (178, 179) have proposed piHDLs as biomarkers of disease activity in IRD. Additionally, high expression of SAA mRNA by several cell types in atherosclerotic lesions suggests a role in the pathogenesis of atherosclerotic plaques (180). The earliest phase of atherogenesis involves vascular endothelial cell (EC) dysfunction. The SAA-induced pro-inflammatory cytokine TNFα stimulates the expression of adhesion molecules on ECs and stimulates the production of tissue factor (TF) which promotes the formation of atherosclerotic plaque (181, 182). SAA-treated ECs show a significantly increased expression of TNFα, TF and vascular endothelial growth factor (VEGF) (183). Pharmacological blockade of SAA receptors, including FPRL1, TLR2/4 and RAGE, inhibits SAA-mediated pro-atherogenic effects in ECs. However, the pharmacological inhibition is only partial in contrast to adding isolated human HDL which almost completely abrogates SAA-induced pro-atherogenic activity (183, 184). HDL reduces SAA's bioavailability, but other mechanisms for modulating SAA pro-atherogenic activities in EC are also possible. For instance, circulating HDL may indirectly inactivate membrane SAA receptors by membrane cholesterol level modulation (185). Therefore, SAA:HDL blood ratio may be of a critical importance for HDL's ability to protect ECs from SAA pro-atherogenic activities. Furthermore, SAA up-regulates the expression of TLR2 in EC, suggesting a positive feedback loop (186). On top of all that, SAA significantly decreases endothelial nitric oxide (NO) synthase levels, NO bioavailability and the activity of internal antioxidant enzymes catalase and superoxide dismutase in ECs, leading to an increased superoxide radical anion production, impaired NO activity and, consequently, endothelial dysfunction and atherosclerotic plaque formation (187). Intriguingly, atherosclerotic cardiovascular diseases are the primary cause of premature death in patients with rheumatic diseases.

SAA IN RHEUMATOID ARTHRITIS

SAA can be used as a diagnostic marker for RA since its serum levels are significantly elevated in RA patients compared to healthy controls and patients with osteoarthritis (OA) (5, 9–11). SAA levels are increased in RA compared to OA patients not only in the serum, but also in synovial fluid, as a result of a local production (12, 20, 29). A number of researches demonstrated a significant correlation between SAA serum concentration and RA disease activity (9, 10, 13). SAA is a more sensitive marker of disease activity in RA than CRP or ESR (11, 14–16, 21), even during pregnancy (17). Chambers et al. were the first to report an increased SAA level in RA patients with normal CRP levels in

TABLE 8 | Characteristics and results of articles investigating clinical utility of SAA in patients with AA amyloidosis.

First author (reference number)	The aim of the study regarding the clinical utility of SAA	Diagnosis (number of patients)	Method used for SAA measuring	Results / Comments
Falck et al. (6)	To investigate the role of monitoring SAA levels in RA patients with secondary amyloidosis	RA with AA amyloidosis (n=20)	Radioimmuno-assay	➢ Mean SAA levels are significantly correlated with the change in renal function (creatinine clearance), therefore can be used for predicting renal deterioriation in amyloidosis
Ishii et al. (99)	To investigate SAA serum levels and SAA genotype in RA patients with amyloidosis	RA (n=217: 200 without + 17 with amyloidosis)	ND	➢ SAA levels are significantly higher in RA patients with amyloidosis than in those without ➢ SAA1.3 allel is a risk factor for developing amyloidosis in Japanese population
Migita et al. (100)	To investigate correlation between SAA concentrations and the presence of amyloidosis in RA patients	RA (n=56: 18 with amyloidosis + 38 without)	Immuno-nephelometric assay	➢ SAA concentration is not correlated with the presence of amylodiosis in RA patients ➢ The ratio of SAA-derived fragments to total SAA is significantly higher in patients with amyloidosis
Gorlier et al. (101)	To find a diagnostic marker for AA amyloidosis in FMF patients	FMF (n=56: 50 without + 6 with amyloidosis)	ND	➢ Mean SAA is not significantly correlated with the presence of AA amyloidosis, therefore is not clinically useful for detecting amyloidosis in FMF
Lachmann et al. (102)	To evaluate potential benefits from monitorig SAA levels in AA amyloidosis	AA amyloidosis (n=374, different underlying diseases)	Immuno-nephelometric assay	➢ Median SAA level is an indicator of changes in renal function, prognostic factor and indicator of death risk in AA amyloidosis ➢ SAA monitoring should be used for therapy guidance in patients with AA amyloidosis
Gilmore et al. (103)	To assess amyloid load in relation to SAA levels in amyloidosis	AA amyloidosis (n=80, different underlying diseases)	ELISA	➢ Median SAA level is significantly correlated with changes in amyloid load and long-term survival in patients with secondary amyloidosis
Perry et al. (104)	To investigate the effect of etanercept on SAA levels in patients with amyloidosis	AA amyloidosis (n=9, different underlying diseases)	ND	➢ SAA serum levels may be used for monitoring response to etanercept in patients with AA amyloidosis
Nakamura et al. (105)	To investigate etanercept effects on SAA levels and disease activity in amyloidosis	RA with amyloidosis (n=14)	ND	➢ Etanercept induced SAA decrease is followed by decrease in disease activity in amyloidosis patients, therefore SAA may be used for monitoring response to etanercept
Mijagawa et al. (106)	To assess effects of tocilizumab on SAA levels in AA amyloidosis	RA with amyloidosis(n=5)	ND	➢ Tocilizumab induced SAA decrease is associated with clinical improvement in amyloidosis, therefore SAA may be used for monitoring response to tocilizumab
Lane et al. (107)	To study efficacy of tocilizumab in AA amyloidosis	AA amyloidosis (n=14, different underlying diseases)	Immunonephelo-metric assay	➢ Decrease in SAA levels in amyloidosis patients receiving tocilizumab is associated with decreased proteinuria and amyloid regression, therefore SAA can be used as a marker of response to tocilizumab
Okuda et al. (108)	To compare the effects of anti-IL-6 and anti-TNFα therapy on SAA levels in AA amyloidosis	AA amyloidosis (n=42, different underlying diseases)	ND	➢ Decrease in SAA levels and disease activity is significantly greater in patients receiving anti-IL-6 than in those receiving anti-TNFα therapy

TABLE 9 | Characteristics and results of articles investigating clinical utility of SAA in patients with COVID-19.

First author (reference number)	The aim of the study regarding the clinical utility of SAA	Number of patients (n)	Results / Comments
Xu et al. (109)	To explore changes in serum biomarkers in COVID-19 patients	187	➢ SAA levels are significantly increased in COVID-19 patients and may be used as a diagnostic marker ➢ The mean SAA concentration in critically-ill patients is significantly higher than in mild-ill patients, therefore may be used as a marker of disease severity in COVID-19
Shi et al. (110)	To find serum biomarkers of disease severity in COVID-19	114	➢ SAA may be used as a marker of disease severity in COVID-19 patients
Wang et al. (111)	To evaluate biomarkers in assessing COVID-19 severity	143	➢ SAA is significantly associated with COVID-19 severity ➢ SAA levels above 100 mg/L are indicative of disease progress to the critical stage
Li H et al. (112)	To evaluate SAA as a marker of COVID-19 severity and prognosis	132	➢ SAA is a sensitive marker of COVID-19 severity ➢ Dynamic changes in SAA level are significantly correlated with clinical outcome of COVID-19
Li X et al. (113)	To reveal a predictor of fatal outcome in COVID-19	25	➢ SAA might be a predictor of fatal outcome in patients with COVID-19
Mo et al. (114)	To find a serum biomarker with a predictive value for COVID-19 prognosis	118	➢ SAA levels correlate with COVID-19 severity ➢ SAA is an independent predictor of severe COVID-19 with accuracy of 89.1% at the cut-off value of 122.9 mg/L

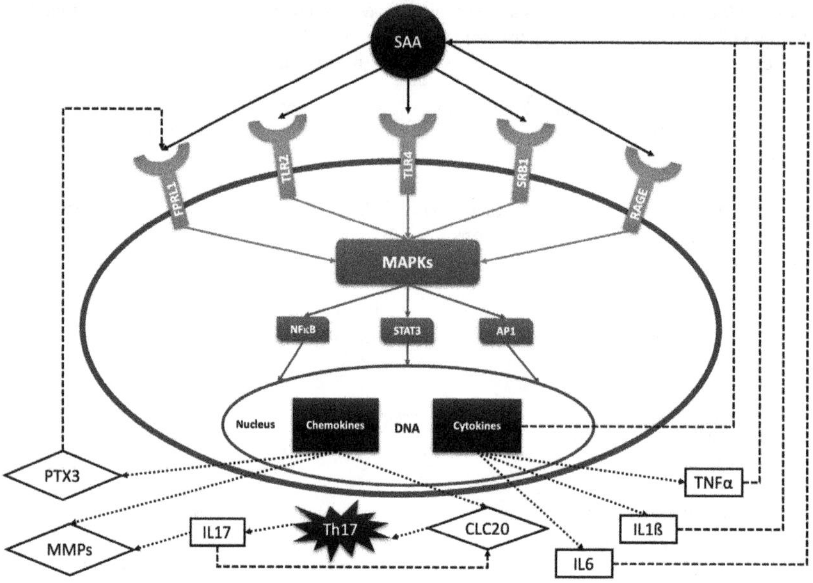

FIGURE 2 | SAA signal transduction pathways and feedback loops with relevance for rheumatic diseases. SAA activates several cell receptors including Toll-like receptors 2 and 4 (TLR2, TLR4), formyl peptide receptor -like 1 (FPRL1), scavenger receptor class B type 1 (SRB1) and receptors of advanced glycation end products (RAGE). SAA receptors share common properties in activating protein kinases (MAPKs) and transcription factors such as nuclear factor kappa B (NF-kB), signal transducer and activator of transcription 3 (STAT-3) and activator protein 1 (AP-1). These factors promote transcription of interleukin 6 (IL-6), interleukin 1ß (IL-1ß), tumor necrosis factor α (TNFα), matrix metalloproteinases (MMPs), chemokine ligand 20 (CLC20), pentraxin 3 (PTX3), etc. IL-6, IL-1ß and TNFα stimulate SAA production, while PTX3 promotes inflammation by activating FPRL-1. CLC20 recruits Th17 cells which stimulate transcription of cartilage-degrading MMPs and CLC20 chemokine by producing IL-17.

40% of the patients included in their study (14). Authors considered sex, age, disease duration as well as therapy differences between groups in consideration, but did not find a significant divergence that could influence results. Subsequent studies confirmed the usefulness of SAA for detecting subclinical inflammation, even in patients with CRP within the reference values (18, 19, 22, 29). Hwang et al. (18) and Connolly et al. (23) proposed SAA for monitoring RA disease activity in patients receiving anti-TNFα therapy, since anti-TNFα therapy reduced CRP even without reduction in disease activity, while SAA was less affected. This may be a result of synthesis under the influence of different cytokine combinations.

Furthermore, considerably increased SAA levels (>520 mg/L) in patients with recent onset arthritis can distinguish patients with a final diagnosis of RA from those with persistent undifferentiated arthritis (15). In addition, baseline SAA levels, contrarily to CRP or ESR, are independently correlated with RA radiographic progression at 1-year (23). Wild et al. (19) performed a multivariate analysis of 32 biomarkers (including SAA and CRP), out of 131 initially considered, which were subjected to three inclusion criteria: discrimination between RA patients and healthy controls, ability to identify anti-cyclic citrullinated peptide antibody (anti-CCP) negative RA patients and specificity for RA. Among the tested biomarkers, only the combination of SAA and anti-CCP increased the sensitivity of anti-CCP alone (80.1% vs. 75.8%, respectively), although this was followed by a drop in specificity (94% for anti-CCP alone vs. 86.6% for SAA+ anti-CCP). Moreover, SAA is incorporated in the widely used multi-biomarker disease activity (MBDA) test developed by Centola et al. (24) for RA activity assessment and discrimination of patients with a low disease activity from those with a moderate or high disease activity. The group tested 130 biomarkers for estimating RA activity in samples obtained from 702 patients and finally included only 12 biomarkers in MBDA score. While most of the MBDA score biomarkers can predict either Swollen Joint Count (SJC28), Tender Joint Count (TJC28) or Patient Global Assessment (PGA), SAA predicts all of them. Recently, Ma et al. (25) investigated the utility of the MBDA score and its individual components for predicting outcomes in patients who are in a stable low disease activity. They found that the baseline SAA level can be used for predicting remission over 12 months. The average of 3 measurements obtained over the first 6 months had an even better predictive value. Moreover, baseline SAA concentrations were significantly higher in patients with low disease activity than patients in total remission. Therefore, SAA may be used for detecting subclinical inflammation and for predicting remission at 1 year in patients with RA.

SAA has also been correlated with cardiovascular disease in RA patients. Wong et al. (26) found that the decreased arterial elasticity in RA patients, which may precede atherosclerosis, is significantly inversely correlated with SAA concentration. Another study reported a trend of association between SAA levels and severity of coronary atherosclerosis in patients with

RA (27). Along with a significant correlation between SAA and cardiovascular involvement, Targonska-Stepniak et al. found a significant correlation with renal involvement (assessed by serum levels of cystatin C—an early marker of chronic kidney disease) (13).

Numerous researches verified SAA as an indicator of response to therapy in RA patients. Kullich et al. investigated the effects of leflunomide, a conventional disease-modifying antirheumatic drug (DMARD) therapy in RA (28). Their *in vivo* results with significant reduction of SAA and MMP levels after 6 months of leflunomide therapy confirmed a previously reported suppressive effects of leflunomide *in vitro* (188). Targonska-Stepniak et al. (22) also investigated the influence of leflunomide and found that, in spite of a reduction in disease activity and other laboratory inflammatory markers including CRP and ESR, the mean SAA concentration at 12 months of leflunomide treatment did not significantly differ from the SAA level at the start of treatment, revealing an ongoing subclinical inflammation. More recently, Boeters et al. (30) revealed a significant association between higher SAA levels (>3 ug/ml) at disease onset and achievement of sustained-DMARD-free remission (defined as the absence of synovitis that sustained after discontinuation of all DMARD therapy to at least 1 year) suggesting a predictive value of SAA. Migita et al. (130) demonstrated that Janus kinase inhibition down-regulates IL-6 induced SAA expression in rheumatoid synovium. In the subsequent study (31) they validated SAA as a sensitive biomarker of response to tofacitinib (Janus kinase inhibitor) in patients with active RA. Tofacitinib reduced both IL-6 and SAA serum levels. In patients who experienced a post-treatment SAA normalization, the decrease of disease activity was greater compared to those with persistently high levels. This finding suggests that SAA may be used for monitoring response to tofacitinib in RA patients, although the caution is needed when interpreting the results, since only 14 patients were included in the study, and only 4 received tofacitinib as monotherapy. Finally, many researchers investigated response to anti-TNFα antibodies in RA patients by monitoring SAA levels. Visvanathan et al. (32) reported that the reduction in serum level of SAA at week 4 after initiation of golimumab therapy in RA patients correlates significantly with clinical improvement at week 16, suggesting the use of SAA for predicting the clinical response. Doyle et al. (33) validated SAA as a potential biomarker for evaluating response to golimumab in RA patients but did not found clinically relevant correlation between baseline SAA levels and clinical improvement at week 24 of golimumab therapy. Furthermore, the clinical utility of SAA for assessing response to adalimumab in RA patients has been validated by Kobayashi et al., Berner Hammer et al. and Gabay et al. (34–36), while Nissinen et al. (37) reported SAA levels to be significantly correlated with clinical improvement in RA patients treated with infliximab. In addition, Gabay et al. (36) compared effects of adalimumab and sarilumabon serum biomarkers in a large cohort (n=307) of RA patients. They found a significant greater decrease of SAA at week 24 in responders than non-responders in adalimumab group. Although total SAA reduction was greater in sarilumab group, the association between clinical efficacy and SAA reduction was not found in this group, suggesting that a direct effect of IL-6 blockade on SAA production is independent of its effect on disease activity. In addition, this research reported a significant predictive value of high baseline SAA levels for a better clinical response to sarilumab than adalimumab. Further studies with a longer follow-up are needed for validating and expanding these results.

Lately, quantitative methods for measuring different SAA isoforms and proteomic techniques for exploring clinical relevance of these isoforms are being developed. Xu et al. (38) developed ELISA for SAA1 and investigated levels and ratios of SAA1 in total SAA in healthy subjects and RA patients. They found that both SAA1 and total SAA are significantly elevated in RA patients compared to healthy subjects, although the SAA1/SAA ratio did not differ between the two groups. De Seny et al. (39) used SELDI-TOF MS (surface-enhanced laser desorption/ionization time-of-flight mass spectrometry) for finding proteins that are significantly elevated in RA patients. Interestingly, along with SAA of 11,682 Da, two truncated and probably post-translationally modified SAA proteins were also identified: SAA without its first N-terminal Arg residue of 11,526 Da (SAA des-Arg) and SAA truncated at the N-terminal end by 2 residues, Arg and Ser, of 11,439 Da (SAA des-Arg/des-Ser). Li et al. (40) confirmed the differential expression of SAA in the serum of RA patients compared to healthy controls by proteomics. Seok et al. (41) used a nanoliquid chromatography-tandem mass spectrometry (LC-MS/MS) to identify candidate biomarkers for RA pre-screening. They found the concentration of SAA4 in the serum of clinically healthy individuals with high rheumatoid factor (RF) values significantly higher compared to sera with normal RF values. Furthermore, by using ELISA, they validated a significantly up-regulated SAA4 in RA patients. Therefore, SAA4 may represent a novel prescreening marker for early RA detection. Remarkably, SAA4 was found to be superior to CRP as RA biomarker, and the combination of SAA4 and CRP had even higher pre-screening efficacy. Nys et al. (42) investigated SAA1 and SAA2 isoforms and their allelic variants in patients with early-onset, weak/moderate and severe RA, AS, SLE, OA and healthy controls. They found SAA2 levels significantly higher in all the RA patients compared to controls and other pathologies (SLE; OA), while SAA1β levels were increased only in early-onset RA and SAA1α in severe RA. The weights of SAA1α and SAA1β levels in the total SAA response were different according to the studied pathologies and RA severity. In particular, SAA1α made up to 80% of total SAA in RA while SAA1β made up to 69% in SLE. This leads to the conclusion that SAA2 and SAA1β isoforms can serve as RA biomarkers before the symptoms onset (along with RF and anti-CCP), while the SAA1α/SAA1β ratio is useful for evaluating disease severity and response to treatment. Furthermore, this study demonstrated that SAA is not only quantitatively different among various inflammatory pathologies, but also qualitatively by different representation of isoforms.

In conclusion, described observations (as summarized in **Table 1**) indicate that assessment of the commonly used markers of disease activity (CRP or ESR) is insufficient for evaluation of the disease activity in RA. Moreover, persistent elevated SAA levels represent subclinical inflammation and a risk for developing amyloidosis. Subsequent determinations of SAA serum levels could therefore be useful for recognizing patients in a need of a more intensive treatment with biologic immunotherapy. Additionally, the identification of various SAA truncated isoforms by proteomics, which is not possible by ELISA, may be of importance because of their possibly different pathophysiological roles. For the time being, only SAA forms with a role for diagnosis have been investigated, while further studies should explore the specificity of these SAA forms for different rheumatic diseases and their value in monitoring disease activity and predicting disease course.

SAA IN JUVENILE IDIOPATHIC ARTHRITIS

Filipowicz-Sosnowska et al. (43) and Scheinberg et al. (44) were the first to report a significant correlation between SAA concentration and disease activity in JIA patients. Moreover, both groups noticed significantly higher levels of SAA in systemic and polyarticular forms of JIA than in the oligoarticular type. Intriguingly, the first two forms have higher incidence of amyloidosis. However, in both studies, SAA levels were not different between JIA patients with secondary amyloidosis and those without, indicating that SAA levels cannot be used for detecting amyloid deposits in JIA patients. Kutulculer et al., Cantarini et al. and Dev et al. (45–47) discerned SAA as a more sensitive marker than CRP or ESR for assessing JIA disease activity defied by the presence and number of active joints assessed by clinical and ultrasonographic examination. In addition, SAA was elevated in 18% of patients with normal ESR and 28% of patients with normal CRP (47). This suggests that SAA should be used as a marker of disease activity in JIA patients, especially in terms of low disease activity.

Miyamae et al. (48) explored differentially expressed proteins in systemic JIA patients. Paired sera from each patient were analyzed prior to and after the treatment with conventional or biologicDMARDs, using the SELDI-TOF MS proteomic analysis. Despite the small number of patients (n=23), highly significant and consistent changes were observed, with SAA (11.6 kDa) showing the biggest decrease in expression upon the treatment. In addition, responders and non-responders to conventional therapy had significant differences in baseline SAA expression, suggesting clinical utility of SAA for both predicting and monitoring response to therapy in JIA patients. Articles concerning utility of SAA in JIA patients are summarized in **Table 2**.

SAA IN ANKYLOSING SPONDYLITIS

Many studies have shown that SAA can be used as a marker of disease activity and response to therapy in AS patients (**Table 3**). Lange et al. (49) evaluated SAA as a marker of disease activity in AS and found a significant correlation with Bath Ankylosing Spondylitis Disease Activity Index (BASDAI), the established disease activity score. Moreover, Jung et al. (50) reported that SAA is superior to CRP and ESR in the detection of AS inflammatory activity. SAA and BASDAI score were elevated and positively correlated even in AS patients with normal ESR (42% of all patients) and CRP levels (24% of all patients included in the study).

De Vries et al. investigated the usefulness of SAA for predicting and monitoring response to anti-TNFα therapy (infliximab or etanercept) in AS patients (51). They found that normal baseline levels of both CRP and SAA were significantly associated with nonresponse to therapy, while elevated baselines of each of these acute phase proteins had a high predictive value for response. The combination of elevated baseline CRP and SAA levels was the strongest predictor of response to anti-TNFα therapy, suggesting these baseline values should be added to anti-TNFα response criteria in order to facilitate selection of AS patients who are likely to respond to this kind of treatment. Interestingly, a secondary increase of SAA levels after initial normalization was associated with developing antibodies against infliximab. Therefore, monitoring SAA levels might be used for detecting anti-drug antibodies even before the loss of response to adalimumab and clinical deterioration. This intriguing finding was recently verified in a large cohort of IBD patients (n=805) receiving adalimumab by Rubin et al. (189). SAA concentrations were significantly decreased after introducing adalimumab to therapy. After initial normalization, SAA levels significantly increased in patients who developed anti-adalimumab antibodies. High titter of these antibodies were associated with 4.8-fold increase in the SAA expression.

Li et al. (52) confirmed SAA as a diagnostic indicator of AS by a proteomic approach (MALDI-TOF MS). Rademacher et al. (53) validated increased SAA levels in AS patients but did not found a significant correlation between baseline SAA levels and radiographic spinal progression after two years. However, baseline SAA was measured in a cohort of patients with advanced AS (mean disease duration was 15 years). Therefore, before reaching the final conclusion, the further studies evaluating SAA as a predictor of the radiographic progression in early-stage AS patients is needed.

Recently, Wu et al. (54) discovered 7 over-expressed proteins in the sera from AS patients compared to healthy controls by using an human antibody array. In this study, a protein with the highest differential expression was SAA1, even in patients receiving adalimumab. Moreover, SAA1 was significantly higher in patients with peripheral joint involvement and significantly decreased after 24-weaks of adalimumab therapy. Liu et al. (55) also performed a proteomic analysis of AS patient's sera and found that the combination of CRP and SAA1 has the highest sensitivity and specificity for AS diagnosis and disease activity. They confirmed that SAA1 is more sensitive than total SAA in differentiating active from stable AS as well as AS from healthy controls. All participants in this study were treatment naïve and without comorbidities, making the results highly reliable and worth of further exploration.

SAA IN DIFFERENT TYPES OF VASCULITIS

As in other IRD, studies have shown that SAA is a potentially good biomarker of diseases activity and response to therapy in patients with Takayasu arteritis (TA) and other types of vasculitis (**Table 4**). Ma et al. (56) and Nair et al. (57) found circulating SAA levels significantly higher in TA patients with active disease compared to those with inactive disease. Nevertheless, SAA levels in the inactive group were still higher than in healthy controls, suggesting an ongoing subclinical inflammation, which was occasionally confirmed by a FDG PET-CT (fluorodeoxiglucose positron-emission computed tomography) and led to therapy adjustment. In the same manner, no significant differences were found for CRP. Furthermore, Nair et al. (57) analyzed changes in biomarker levels and disease activity as a response to therapy (mycophenolate mofetil, azathioprine or methotrexate). SAA levels significantly decreased during the follow-up of mean duration of 7.5 months in treatment responders, while there were no significant changes in non-responders. The relative changes in SAA values during follow-up reflected the response to treatment more accurately than the same changes in CRP or ESR values. These results are limited by a small cohort size, hence further studies with a longer follow-up and in a larger cohort should ascertain the utility of monitoring SAA levels in the management of TA patients.

Lately, an important role of SAA in the pathogenesis of giant cell arteritis (GCA) has been recognized. Along with proangiogenic properties and the induction of cell growth and angiogenesis mediated by TLR2, O'Neil et al. (190) proved that SAA is directly secreted in inflammatory temporal arteries. Hocevar et al. (58) reported a predictive value of high baseline SAA levels (measured at diagnosis) for an early relapse in patients with GCA receiving corticosteroids, indicating a clinical utility of SAA in an early identification of non-responders to corticosteroid therapy. The correlation of baseline SAA with relapse was more significant than that of CRP or ESR. The reported correlations are limited by a small cohort size and potential selection bias since the study was performed at one department in a single centre. Burja et al. (59) identified SAA as the most differentially expressed serum biomarker between patients with GCA and HC (83-fold increase in patients) out of 48 tested laboratory parameters (including CRP and ESR). All patients included in the study were in early disease stage, treatment naïve and were followed up for at least 1 year. Changes in SAA levels were better correlated with disease activity than changes in CRP or ESR levels. Considering the large proportion of smokers (38%), type II diabetes (14%) and hypertensive patients (53%) in the study cohort, as well as the fact that healthy controls significantly differed in age (median age of 74.1 in patients vs. 50.8 in healthy controls), future research should corroborate the observed correlations. Dartevel et al. (60) confirmed clinical utility of SAA in distinguishing GCA patients with active from those with inactive disease. Despite tendency to higher SAA concentrations in microbial infections, they observed no statistically significant difference between active disease and infection, similarly to Van Sleen et al. (61). Intriguingly, SAA was significantly correlated with serum IL-6 levels only in GCA but not in infection group, suggesting pathophysiological differences. The latter group also confirmed SAA expression at the tissue level (temporal artery biopsy), emphasizing its important role in GCA.

The clinical applicability of SAA has also been investigated in Kawasaki disease (KD). Mitani et al. (62) revealed a significant association of elevated SAA concentration and persistence of coronary artery lesions (aneurysms, stenosis or occlusion) late after KD (mean time after onset was 10 years). This association was supported by logistic regression analysis (adjusting for age, smoking, BMI, blood pressure, total cholesterol/HDL ratio) and was stronger for SAA than for CRP. When interpreting the results, a caution is needed since the study was cross-sectional and the number of patients was relatively small, so large cohort corroboration is required. Whitin et al. (63) published an intriguing report on a novel truncated SAA form in patients in Kawasaki disease. By using a proteomic approach (SELDI-TOF MS), the group investigated differences in serum protein expression between children with KD and febrile children with at least 3 day-long fever and at least one of the clinical criteria for KD. One mass spectrometry peak (7,860 Da) had significantly higher intensity in children with KD than controls, along with a significant difference among acute and subacute KD patients. Noteworthy, the peak, which was identified as truncated form of SAA with N-terminal at Lys-34, disappeared when the symptoms resolved. Moreover, the possibility of ex vivo SAA proteolysis was excluded by the presence of the truncated form even when the blood samples were collected in tubes containing protease inhibitors. Nevertheless, the relevance of this SAA form as a diagnostic biomarker in KD and possibly in other types of vasculitis as well as its place in pathogenesis is yet to be discovered. Moreover, it is important to underline that for the peptide identity confirmation the hybrid mass spectrometry immunoassay technique was used, since a conventional ELISA would not have detected the truncated SAA peptide because its signal would have been a minor contributor to the overall plasma SAA content.

Finally, Purevdorj et al. (64) identified SAA as the most sensitive biomarker for diagnosis of Henoch-Schonlein purpura (HSP) among 12 tested biomarkers (including CRP), however no significant difference was found between SAA levels in HSP and sepsis. In a cross-sectional study by Kuret et al. (65). SAA levels were significantly increased (12-fold) in the sera of adult patients with IgA vasculitis compared to healthy controls. Based on these reports, the potential clinical utility of SAA in IgA vasculitis in both children and adults is worth of further studies.

SAA IN SARCOIDOSIS

SAA has been evaluated as a marker of sarcoidosis in many reports (summarized in **Table 5**). Chen et al. (191) demonstrated a more intense SAA expression in the sarcoidosis granuloma compared to other granulomatous diseases, suggesting it as a diagnostic biomarker for sarcoidosis. SAA also emerged as a key protein regulating granulomatous inflammation through TLR-2. Serum levels of SAA are increased in all sarcoidosis patients but reports regarding SAA correlation with sarcoidosis severity are non-consistent. Rothenkrantz-Kos et al. (66) defined disease severity by chest radiographs and lung function test results and found no correlation with SAA levels. They characterized SAA as a sensitive (96%), but not specific (37%) diagnostic marker for sarcoidosis (cut-off level of 2.5 mg/L). However, the control samples in this cross-sectional study came from a cohort of a not well-defined ostensibly healthy donors and the treatment administered to patients was not reported. In a study by Miyoshi et al. (67) baseline SAA levels were not predictive for an increased lung infiltration in patients with sarcoidosis, although SAA was not influenced by immunosuppressive therapy unlike the commonly used ACE (angiotensine-coverting enzyme). On the other hand, Salazar et al., Bargagli et al. and Gungor et al. (68–70) reported significantly higher SAA levels in patients with active sarcodiosis than in patients with inactive disease. Moreover, Bargagli et al. (69) found a predictive value of SAA for prolonged steroid requirement. Interestingly, proteomic analysis revealed two highly expressed SAA1 isoforms in all of the sarcoidosis sera and in none of the sera from healthy controls. These SAA1 isoforms could match the unidentified biomarker of sarcoidosis previously reported in a proteomic study by Bons et al. (192). The latter group used SELDI-TOF MS and reported two unidentified serum proteins that were up-regulated in the sarcoidosis sera. The molecular weights of those proteins (11,995 and 11,734 Da) correspond to those of the two SAA1 isoforms in the study by Bargagli et al. (69). and Bons et al. reported the high sensitivity and specificity of these proteins for sarcoidosis (192). Zhang et al. (71) confirmed that SAA was significantly higher in the sera from sarcoidosis patients compared to patients with other pulmonary diseases including tuberculosis (the sensitivity of 96.3% and specificity of 52.3% at the cutoff value of 101.98 mg/L). Furthermore, by a proteomic analysis, a unique protein peak of 3210 Da with the highest expression in sarcoidosis sera was revealed. The peak was identified as the N-terminal peptide of 29 amino acids of SAA. Additionally, immunohistochemical staining showed more intense SAA depositions in lung tissue in sarcoidosis than in other groups, suggesting SAA to be used in differential diagnosis of sarcoidosis from other pulmonary diseases. Contrarily, Enyedi et al. (72) reported no differences in SAA or CRP levels between patients with biopsy-proven sarcoidosis and biopsy negative patients. Nevertheless, it must be noticed that the latter group had histological diagnoses of lymphoma, carcinoma, histiocytosis, anthracosis, etc, all of which are associated with increased markers of inflammation.

In light of these findings, the utilization of SAA1 as well as truncated SAA forms as markers for diagnosis, assessing disease activity and response to therapy in patients with sarcoidosis requires additional research.

SAA IN OTHER INFLAMMATORY RHEUMATIC DISEASES

SAA has been investigated in other rheumatic diseases as well, as shown in **Table 6**.

In patients with systemic sclerosis (SSc), SAA levels are elevated and correlate with disease severity. Brandwein et al. (73) were first to investigate SAA as a marker of disease activity in SSc. The group reported elevated SAA concentrations in 98% of their patients and a significant correlation with disease severity (determined by extension of skin thickening). Lakota et al. (74) included patients with limited and diffuse SSc in the study and found elevated SAA levels in 25% of patients, while Lis Swiety et al. (75) included only patients with diffuse SSc and detected increased SAA levels in 66%. The discrepancy between these results may be explained by inclusion or exclusion of limited SSc patients and different SAA cut-off values between the studies. Furthermore, both of these studies found a significant correlation between SAA levels and deterioration of lung function (assessed by forced vital capacity, diffusion capacity for carbon monoxide or reticulation pattern on chest CT). According to these studies, SAA is superior to CRP as a marker of pulmonary involvement in SSc. Still, longitudinal studies are needed to validate SAA as a marker of disease activity, predictor of disease progression and response to therapy in SSc.

The only article reporting on SAA in SLE patients that was found through comprehensive literature search is the study by Wang et al. (76). The group revealed a significant correlation between SAA levels and SLE disease activity (determined by SLE disease activity score—SLEDAI). Although SAA was significantly correlated with serum levels of hs-CRP (high sensitivity CRP) and ESR, a binary logistic regression analysis showed that SAA values are independently associated with active SLE. Since this research was retrospective and cross-sectional, a prospective, longitudinal, large cohort study is necessary to confirm the clinical utility of SAA for monitoring SLE patients.

Boyd et al. (77) reported that among 15 biomarkers (including CRP), SAA levels were most significantly correlated with disease activity in patients with psoriatic arthritis (PsA). However, the study was cross sectional in a small cohort (45 patients) and included patients receiving different therapies (including conventional and biological DMARDs). Moreover, disease activity assessment did not include ankle and feet involvement that are frequently seen in PsA. Future studies should therefore validate the utility of SAA in monitoring PsA patients.

SAA IN SYSTEMIC AUTOINFLAMMATORY DISEASES

Amongst the systemic autoinflammatory diseases (SAID), the clinical utility of SAA has been most extensively investigated in patients with FMF. SAA levels are elevated in FMF patients not only during attacks, but also in the attack-free period revealing a sustained subclinical inflammation. Furthermore, asymptomatic MEFV mutation carriers also have an increased SAA concentration potentially leading to the development of amyloidosis.

Duzova et al. (78) found SAA levels above the reference range in more than 95% of the FMF children in between the attacks, even though 50% of them had not experienced attacks within the last 12 months. SAA was shown to be the best biomarker of subclinical inflammation in FMF (compared to CRP, ESR, ferritin and fibrinogen). An increase in the colchicine dose resulted in a dramatic decrease of SAA concentration advocating the use of SAA for therapy guidance. Lachmann et al. (79) reported significantly elevated SAA levels (>3 mg/L) in MEFV mutation carriers and in the attack-free period in more than 70% of their patients, even though all patients were under colchicine therapy. Moreover, a remarkable degree of acute-phase activity (measured monthly by SAA and CRP levels) led the authors to question about the participants compliance. This suspicion was eventually confirmed in a considerable number of the patients. Therefore, they suggested to measure frequently SAA in patients with FMF for reinforcing their therapy compliance. Berkun et al. (80) confirmed elevated SAA levels in the attack-free period and in MEFV mutation carriers. However, in this report SAA was increased (>6 mg/L) in only 25% of FMF patients between attacks compared to 70% reported by Lachmann et al. (79). The discrepancy between the results may be due to the different definition of elevated SAA levels as well as the difference in therapy doses and perhaps compliance to colchicine therapy. In 30% of patients SAA measurement led to a change in colchicine dose and, consequently, SAA level normalization. Another interesting finding was significantly higher SAA in noncompliant patients than in nonresponders to therapy, therefore supporting suggestion of Lachmann et al. for frequent SAA measuring for distinguishing these two groups and reinforcing compliance.

Yalcinkaya et al. (81) validated SAA level above reference range in FMF patients during the attack and the attack-free period in the same patients. Similarly, increased SAA levels were observed in clinically healthy FMF heterozygotes. In patients that suffered from chronic inflammatory diseases or chronic infections with a high potential for developing secondary amyloidosis, SAA concentrations were not higher than in those with acute infections with an almost zero chance for developing amyloidosis, implying SAA has no predictive value for amyloid formation. Another important observation was lack of significant difference between SAA levels in children with FMF exacerbation and those with acute infections, although in both groups SAA was significantly increased. Nevertheless, it must be noticed that all FMF patients were receiving colchicine at the time of the study, which is known for reducing SAA levels. Kallinich et al. (82) validated elevated SAA levels in FMF patients at diagnosis, during attacks, in between the attacks and in MEFV mutation carriers. Lofty et al. (83) found increased SAA (>30 mg/L) in 79% of FMF patients two weeks after the last attack. Only 31% had elevated CRP concentration, indicating that SAA can persist elevated after FMF attacks more than CRP. More recently, Cakan et al. (84) reported that SAA is significantly higher in children with acute FMF attacks than in children with acute febrile respiratory infection and therefore can be used for differentiating those two clinical entities. Again, of note is that all FMF patients were treated with colchicine. At the cut-off value of 111.5 mg/L, the SAA sensitivity for discriminating FMF attack from acute infection was 100%, and the specificity was 65.1%. Since these results are opposite to those of Yalcinkaya et al. (81), further research with a larger sample size and before introducing colchicine to therapy are necessary to determine whether SAA provides additional value compared to CRP in suspected acute FMF attacks.

Since SAA is considered to be involved in the pathogenesis of atherosclerosis, some of the research investigated a potential value of SAA for predicting atherosclerosis in patients with FMF. Bilinger et al. (85) and Mohamed et al. (86) found a significant correlation between SAA levels and intima media thickness of the common carotid artery (CIMT)—an early marker of atherosclerosis. The patients studied were receiving NSAIDS and colchicine, so SAA levels were suppressed, but still higher than normal. Possibly an even stronger correlation would have been found if the patients were untreated. Sargsyan (87) found SAA significantly higher in FMF patients with any kind of vascular involvement than in those without. The role of SAA in atherosclerosis needs to be further explored, on both molecular and clinical level.

Taken all together, measurement of SAA in FMF patients should be used in evaluating disease activity, risk of amyloidosis and atherosclerosis, as well as response to therapy. Moreover, determination of SAA level may serve as a screening test for asymptomatic family members to determine the need for genotyping. However, further studies are required to determine the clinical benefits of SAA normalization by increasing colchicine dose in the asymptomatic patients. Furthermore, the target SAA level for colchicine dose modification should be defined as well as the needed frequency and time of longitudinal monitoring of SAA levels in the asymptomatic FMF individuals before making adjustments.

Except in FMF, benefits of SAA level monitoring have been explored in other SAIDs. In Behçet's disease (BD), a multifactorial SAID, SAA might not be useful for assessing disease activity, but is positively correlated with major organ involvement and can be used for identifying patients at higher risk of life-threatening complications. Aygunduz et al. (88) reported SAA as a more sensitive and specific marker for BD than CRP, advocating the use of SAA as diagnostic marker and indicator of subclinical inflammation in BD. Contrarily, Cantarini et al. (89) and Vitale et al. (90) reported no significant difference of SAA levels between patients with active and inactive BD (assessed by Behcets disease current activity form—BDCAF), but they found SAA levels associated with skin involvement. Vitale et al. (90) suggested SAA as an indicator of oral aphthosis, neurological and ocular involvement in BD because of the strong correlation between these factors (SAA serum levels higher than 30, 50, and 150 mg/L, respectively). Interestingly, SAA was found to be significantly correlated with homocysteine serum levels (indicator of vascular involvement). This possible use of SAA for indicating vascular involvement and predicting thrombotic risk in BD patients should be of interest for future studies. Recently, Sota et al. (91) confirmed no association between SAA levels and BD activity (BDCAF) but found a significant association between SAA levels above

200 mg /L and a major organ involvement as well as between SAA levels above 150 mg/L and ocular, skin or mucosal manifestations. They suggested SAA as a predictor of major organ involvement and ocular disease relapse in BD. Lee et al. (92) validated a non-significant correlation between SAA and disease activity in BD patients by proteomic analysis. However, this study included BD patients with only intestinal involvement, so future studies should explore biomarkers of BD patients with multisystemic involvement by a proteomic approach. All of the abovementioned studies included a small number of patients, so large cohort studies are needed to confirm these potential advantages of monitoring SAA in patients with BD.

Monitoring SAA levels has also been incorporated in evaluating patients with Muckle-Wells syndrome (MWS). Hawkins et al. (93) and Scarpioni et al. (94) reported that SAA serum levels and clinical symptoms are concomitantly significantly increased after introducing biologic therapy in MWS patients (anakinra and canakinumab, respectively). Hoffman and co-workers (95) used SAA together with hs-CRP as serum biomarkers of efficacy of rilonacept in CAPS patients, as well as previously reported study by Goldbach-Mansky et al. (96). The latter study found that the change in SAA level as a response to rilonacept therapy is better correlated with improvement in clinical symptoms than CRP or ESR levels. In cases of reoccurrence of disease flare, SAA levels significantly increased despite the rilonacept treatment. Wiken and co-workers (97) confirmed utility of SAA as a marker of response to anakinra in MWS and neonatal onset multisystem inflammatory disease (NOMID) patients, as well as a high incidence of anti-drug antibodies development, but with no influence on efficacy of anakinra or SAA levels. These findings highlight the potential utility of SAA in assessing response to biologic therapy in MWS and NOMID patients. The articles discussed in this section are summarized in **Table 7**.

SAA IN SECONDARY (AA) AMYLOIDOSIS

The association between SAA and secondary (AA) amyloidosis was one of the first investigated roles of SAA, with many new studies still emerging (**Table 8**). Amyloidosis is a single- or multiorgan disease characterized by extracellular tissue deposition of low-molecular weight, insoluble and amorphous proteinaceous material, causing progressive organ dysfunction. Rheumatic and autoinflammatory diseases are associated with a high rate of secondary (AA) amyloidosis. As already mentioned, SAA gene polymorphisms have an influence on developing amyloidosis. The strong correlation between amyloid deposition and SAA1γ allele in Japanese RA patients was confirmed by Ishii et al. (99). Furthermore, the group reported significantly higher SAA levels in RA patients with amyloidosis than in those without. SAA showed a stronger correlation with the presence of amyloid deposits than CRP. However, according to the most of published reports, SAA serum levels are not correlated with the presence of amyloid deposits (43, 44, 100, 101). Therefore, contrary to expectations, high SAA levels are a prerequisite, but not a sufficient condition for developing amyloidosis and cannot be used as a diagnostic marker for amyloidosis. It is possible that increased proteolytic cleavage of SAA contributes to the development of amyloidosis. Indeed, Migita et al. (100) detected, in addition to the full-length SAA protein, 6 kDA and 4.5 kDa SAA-derived fragments in the sera of RA patients. The ratio of these fragments to total SAA was significantly higher in patients with than in those without amyloidosis, confirming the increased proteolysis hypothesis. The potential use of these truncated SAA forms as diagnostic markers for amyloidosis should be further investigated.

Subsequent studies in amyloidosis patients revealed some clinically important properties of SAA. Although SAA may not be a diagnostic or predictive marker of amyoidosis, once amyloidosis has developed, the SAA levels over the course of the disease represent the main factor affecting amyloidosis progression and survival. The kidney is one of the most frequent sites of amyloid deposition and, without treatment, amyloidosis-associated kidney disease usually progresses to end-stage renal disease (ESRD). Prognosis of renal amyloidosis significantly correlates with the SAA concentration. Falck et al. (6) and Lachmann et al. (102) reported a strong correlation between the mean SAA value and changes in renal function in patients with renal amyloidosis, suggesting SAA for predicting renal deterioration. Reportedly, renal improvement is expected when SAA median is less than 6 mg/ml and deterioration when SAA median is above 28 mg/L.

Furthermore, SAA levels are significantly connected to changes in amyloid load and long-term survival in amyloidosis. In a study by Gilmore et al. (103), SAA values were significantly higher among patients with further amyloid accumulation than in those with stable amyloid load in whom SAA levels were still higher than in patients with deposit regression. According to a large cohort prospective study of amyloidosis by Lachmann et al. (102), patients with SAA concentrations in the low-normal range (<4 mg/L) have relatively favorable outcome, while persistent elevation of SAA is a powerful risk factor for progression to ESRD and death. The risk of death is 17.7 times higher among patients with uppermost SAA concentrations (>155 mg/L) than in those with SAA concentrations below 4 mg/L. Even in the patients with slightly elevated SAA concentrations during follow-up (4–9 mg/L), the risk of death is 4 times increased. Interestingly, decrease in median SAA level below 10 mg/L is associated with the regression of amyloid deposits. Therefore, therapy that decreases SAA production to within the reference range prevents further accumulation of amyloid deposits and can stabilize or even reverse existing amyloid deposits leading to a better long-term survival. Based on these findings, frequent SAA measurements in patients with secondary amyloidosis should be used for therapy guidance. However, median SAA concentration and status of amyloid deposits varied substantially between individuals in these studies, possibly due to the differences in underlying diseases and anti-inflammatory treatment or comorbidities (obesity, diabetes, hypertension, tobacco consumption) that may influence SAA levels.

Finally, SAA can be used in monitoring response to biologic therapy in rheumatic patients with AA amyloidosis. A number of recent studies have verified that therapeutic strategies involving IL-6 inhibitors and TNFα inhibitors result in a decrease of serum SAA level and consequently represent an excellent therapeutic strategy for AA amyloidosis. Perry et al. (104) and Nakamura et al. (105) verified concomitant decrease in SAA concentration, disease activity and proteinuria in RA patients with AA amyloidosis receiving etanercept (anti-TNFα antibody). Miyagawa et al. (106) and Lane et al. (107) studied the efficacy of tocilizumab (TCZ, anti-IL-6 receptor antibody) in patients with AA amyloidosis. In all patients, SAA levels significantly decreased together with a remarkable decrease in proteinuria, regression of amyloid deposits and significant improvement in clinical symptoms. Okuda et al. (108) compared the effects of anti-TNFα (etanercept, infliximab and adalimumab) and anti-IL-6 (TCZ) therapy against AA amyloidosis by measuring SAA levels. Along with a more imposing improvement in eGFR and amyloid regression, SAA concentration decreased more significantly in the anti-IL-6 group than anti-TNFα group. Taken all together, SAA seems to be a reliable marker of response to biologic therapy in rheumatic patients with secondary amyloidosis.

SAA IN COVID-19

Since we are currently experiencing a pandemic of COVID-19, we summarized 6 articles reporting on SAA as a biomarker in patients with COVID-19 found in our research through PubMed and Scopus databases (**Table 9**). All of the articles were published in 2020.

In critically ill COVID-19 patients a cytokine storm with highly elevated IL-6 has been described (193). Since SAA is correlated with IL-6 and involved in the pathogenesis of the risk conditions for severe COVID-19 (obesity, diabetes and atherogenesis), it might also play a role in the pathogenesis of COVID-19 and therefore present a potential biomarker and therapeutic target.

SAA is increased in all COVID-19 patients with the mean SAA value 4 times higher in critically ill than in mild-ill patients (109). Moreover, Shi et al. (110) reported SAA levels were increased whereas CRP levels were normal in more than 20% of patients. While in patients with both SAA and CRP within the reference range no severe pneumonia occurred, in some of the patients with normal CRP but elevated SAA severe pneumonia was found, suggesting higher sensitivity of SAA for assessing COVID-19 severity. Wang and co-workers (111) validated more significant correlation between disease severity and SAA level than CRP or ESR. In addition, they found SAA value above 100 mg/L as an indicator of disease progress to the critical stage. Huan Li et al. (112) reported SAA and SAA to lymphocyte count ratio as sensitive indicators of COVID-19 severity and prognosis (more sensitive than CRP or PCT). The initial SAA level was correlated with future dynamic changes of CT scans meaning that patients with higher initial SAA levels are more likely to have worsening of CT scans. Interestingly, initial SAA was found to have a higher predictive value for disease progression than the initial CT scan. A retrospective study of COVID-19 death cases revealed that, among included serum biomarkers, only SAA was significantly elevated in all of the patients with fatal outcome (113). Mo et al. (114) showed by logistic regression analysis that SAA, but not CRP, can serve as an independent predictive factor of COVID-19 course. At the cut-off value of 122.9 mg/L, SAA can predict acute exacerbation with an accuracy of 89.1%.

To conclude, SAA might give additional information about COVID-19 severity and prognosis to more commonly used biomarkers. Therefore, SAA measurement should be included in managing COVID-19 patients. At the present moment, to our knowledge, there are no published data on SAA as a biomarker of COVID-19 severity in patients with IRD, so future studies should explore the clinical relevance of SAA as a biomarker in the new era of coexistence of IRD patients and SARS-CoV-2.

LIMITATIONS OF SAA AS A BIOMARKER OF INFLAMMATORY RHEUMATIC DISEASES

Despite many discussed advantages provided by the use of SAA as a biomarker in various rheumatic and autoinflammatory diseases, as with many other biomarkers, there are several limitations arising mostly from the different protein isoforms, genotype and measurement methods.

Firstly, most of the studies that investigated the role of SAA in disease pathogenesis used recombinant human SAA (rhSAA) that differs from the native SAA1 and SAA2 isoforms by 2 amino acids, resulting in a hybrid of SAA1 and SAA2. Some researchers reported differences between rhSAA and endogenous SAA proinflammatory functions (194, 195), thus further experiments should use isolated endogenous SAA from synovial fluid or explants models to identify the effects of SAA in the *in vivo* environment.

Although SAA has been described as the most suitable inflammatory marker for certain rheumatic diseases more than five decades ago, it is still not used as a common biomarker of disease activity in clinical practice. CRP has been widely used as a routine clinical test, while SAA is less popular mostly due to technical difficulties in large scale purification of SAA, stable production of antibodies with high titer, development of an assay system, and standardization of the assay. Various assay methods for SAA quantification have been used. Radioimmunoassay (RIA), radial immunodiffusion and enzyme-linked immunosorbent assay (ELISA) are highly sensitive (detection limit 0.2 μg/L) but time-consuming and therefore inconvenient for clinical use. On the other hand, immunonephelometric and immunoturbidimetric assay are rapid and fully automatic, but have relatively low sensitivity (detection limit >3mg/L). In addition, the commercially available kits for SAA are based on polyclonal antibodies which lack isotype specificity.

Furthermore, SAA genotype may also influence baseline SAA levels (99, 196–198), indicating the need for an individual approach when using SAA plasma levels for assessing disease activity. Unsurprisingly, there are significant variations in the absolute values of SAA among research groups. Even physiological SAA concentrations vary substantially among studies (0.1–10 mg/L) what might have led to critical errors because in some cases even 100-fold increase could not be detected. Additionally, comorbidities such as epilepsy, diabetes and other chronic inflammatory diseases, as well as drugs such as statins and dietary supplements including vitamins A and E and polyunsaturated fatty acids can influence SAA plasma levels along with alcohol use, smoking and obesity (199–203). Obese but otherwise healthy patients have elevated SAA plasma levels and diet-induced weight loss is associated with significant decrease in plasma SAA level. This effect is proportional to the amount of weight lost but independent of dietary macronutrient composition (199). Ethanol induces the SAA production in a dose-dependent manner (202). Tobacco smoking significantly increases serum SAA level and the increase is correlated to the degree of smoking (203). Therefore, all of these variables should be taken in consideration when analysing research results.

As a consequence of these limitations, reliable testing and laboratories that measure SAA levels are not widely available, and data about levels expected in diseases are limited. In time, the availability of assay methods and their wider use should corroborate variables that have a significant impact on SAA levels and provide a clearer picture when interpreting results.

CONCLUSION

Although SAA was sporadically used as a biomarker in many chronic diseases for the past five decades, the use of other inflammatory biomarkers, such as CRP and ESR, has overwhelmed its use in clinical practice. Advantages of these commonly used biomarkers for being cost-effective and easily applicable are also associated with limitations of sensitivity and specificity especially in settings of low-activity rheumatic disorders. In the era of biological therapy, the need for a new biomarker for predicting disease activity and monitoring remission and relapse for various rheumatic diseases has been emphasized. With the discovery of new disease mechanisms and development of proteomic techniques as the most effective methods for identifying molecular markers of disease activity and treatment response, SAA started to regain its importance. In such circumstances, we aimed to collect and summarize all the relevant articles on the clinical utility of SAA in a number of rheumatic and systemic autoinflammatory diseases.

Although articles included in this review are very heterogeneous in design, subjects, parameters measured and results, the general conclusion is that SAA plays an important role in the pathogenesis and clinical course of rheumatic diseases. SAA is involved in many processes important for initiation, perpetuation and resolution of chronic inflammation in IRD. Furthermore, SAA is a sensitive biomarker of disease activity and indicator of the disease prognosis and therapeutic response in a wide range of immune mediated IRD (**Table 10**). In plenty of studies SAA has been demonstrated to provide more information and higher sensitivity than CRP, especially in a state of subclinical inflammation, as well as in patients receiving glucocorticoids or conventional or biologic immunosuppressive therapy. According to the results of proteomic analyses, specific SAA forms have even higher sensitivity and specificity for certain diseases than the total serum SAA value.

TABLE 10 | Summary of possible uses of SAA concentration monitoring in different chronic inflammatory diseases and relevant studies.

Disease	Possible uses of SAA concentration follow-up	Relevant studies, reference number
Rheumatoid arthritis	Diagnostic marker;Biomarker of disease activity;Indicator of subclinical inflammation;Predictor of clinical outcome;Indicator of therapeutic response;Indicator of risk for amyloidosis;Indicator of cardiovascular risk;	(9–42)
Juvenile idiopathic arthritis	Biomarker of disease activity,Indicator of subclinical inflammation;Indicator of risk of developing amyloidosis;Indicator of therapeutic response;Predictor of response to therapy;	(43–48)
Ankylosing spondylitis	Biomarker of disease activity:Indicator of subclinical inflammation;Indicator of therapeutic response;Predictor of response to therapy;	(49–55)
Takayasu`s arteritis	Biomarker of disease activity;Indicator of subclinical inflammation; Indicator of therapeutic response;	(56, 57)
Giant cell arteritis	Biomarker of disease activity;Predictor of response to therapy;	(190–61)
Kawasaki disease	Indicator of persistence of coronary artery lesions;	(62, 63)
IgA vasculitis	Diagnostic marker;	(64, 65)
Sarcoidosis	Diagnostic marker;Biomarker of disease activity;Predictor of future prolonged steroid requirement;	(191–72)
Systemic sclerosis	Indicator of pulmonary involvement;	(73–75)
Systemic lupus erythematosus	Biomarker of disease activity;Indicator of cardiovascular risk;	(76, 178)
Psoriatic arthritis	Biomarker of disease activity;	(77)
Familial Mediterranean Fever	Biomarker of disease activity;Indicator of subclinical inflammation;Indicator of need for genetic testing;Indicator of risk for amyloidosis;Indicator of therapeutic response;Guide for therapy adjustment;	(78–86)
Behcet's disease	Predictor of major organ involvement:;Indicator of high risk for life- and sight-threatening complications;	(87–92)
Mucle-Wells syndrome	Biomarker of disease activity;Indicator of therapeutic response;	(93–97)
Amyloidosis	Indicator of renal function improvement/deterioration;Prognostic biomarker;Marker of therapeutic response;	(99–107)

In conclusion, we strongly advocate the use of SAA as a cheap and reliable biomarker for use in everyday clinical practice of a wide range of physicians dealing with rheumatic and other immune mediated inflammatory diseases in both children and adults, and propose exploration of clinical utility of specific SAA isoforms in future studies.

AUTHOR CONTRIBUTIONS

All authors discussed the contents. IS and LL wrote and edited this manuscript. LL supervised and oversaw the manuscript. All authors contributed to the article and approved the submitted version.

REFERENCES

1. Maury C. Comparative-study of serum amyloid-A protein and C-reactive protein in disease. *Clin Sci* (1985) 68:233–8. doi: 10.1042/cs0680233
2. Chambers R, Hutton C, Dieppe P, Whicher J. Comparative-study of C-reactive protein and serum amyloid-A protein in experimental inflammation. *Ann Rheum Dis* (1991) 50:677–9. doi: 10.1136/ard.50.10.677
3. Goldberger G, Bing DH, Sipe JD, Rits M, Colten HR. Transcriptional regulation of genes encoding the acute-phase proteins CRP, SAA, and C3. *J Immunol* (1987) 138(11):3967–71.
4. Takata S, Wada H, Tamura M, Koide T, Higaki M, Mikura SI, et al. Kinetics of C-reactive protein (CRP) and serum amyloid A protein (SAA) in patients with community-acquired pneumonia (CAP), as presented with biologic half-life times. *Biomarkers* (2011) 16(6):530–5. doi: 10.3109/1354750X.2011.607189
5. Benson MD, Cohen AS. Serum amyloid A protein in amyloidosis, rheumatic, and neoplastic diseases. *Arthritis Rheumatol* (1979) 22(1):36–42. doi: 10.1002/art.1780220106
6. Falck HM, Maury CPJ, Teppo AM, Wegelius O. Correlation of persistently high serum amyloid A protein and C-reactive protein concentrations with rapid progression of secondary amyloidosis. *Br Med J* (1983) 286 (6375):1391–3. doi: 10.1136/bmj.286.6375.1391
7. Danesh J, Whincup P, Walker M, Lennon L, Thomson A, Appleby P, et al. Low grade inflammation and coronary heart disease: Prospective study and updated meta-analyses. *Br Med J* (2000) 321:199–204. doi: 10.1136/bmj.321.7255.199
8. Gasparyan AY, Ayvazyan L, Blackmore H, Kitas GD. Writing a narrative biomedical review: considerations for authors, peer reviewers, and editors. *Rheumatol Int* (2011) 31(11):1409–17. doi: 10.1007/s00296-011-1999-3
9. De Beer FC, Mallya RK, Fagan EA, Lanham JG, Hughes GR, Pepys MB. Serum amyloid-A protein concentration in inflammatory diseases and its relationship to the incidence of reactive systemic amyloidosis. *Lancet* (1982) 2(8292):231–4. doi: 10.1016/s0140-6736(82)90321-x
10. Maury CPJ, Teppo AM, Wegelius O. Relationship between urinary sialylated saccharides, serum amyloid A protein and C-reactive protein in rheumatoid arthritis and systemic lupus erythematosus. *Ann Rheum Dis* (1982) 41 (3):268–71. doi: 10.1136/ard.41.3.268
11. Shen C, Sun XG, Liu N, Mu Y, Hong CC, Wei W, et al. Increased serum amyloid A and its association with autoantibodies, acute phase reactants and disease activity in patients with rheumatoid arthritis. *Mol Med Rep* (2014) 11:1528–34. doi: 10.3892/mmr.2014.2804
12. Kumon Y, Suehiro T, Hashimoto K, Nakatani K, Sipe JD. Local expression of acute phase serum amyloid A mRNA in rheumatoid arthritis synovial tissue and cells. *J Rheumatol* (1999) 26:785–90.
13. Targonska-Stepniak B, Majdan M. Serum amyloid A as a marker of persistent inflammation and an indicator of cardiovascular and renal involvement in patients with rheumatoid arthritis. *Mediators Inflamm* (2014) 2014:793628. doi: 10.1155/2014/793628
14. Chambers RE, MacFarlane DG, Whicher JT, Dieppe PA. Serum amyloid-A protein concentration in rheumatoid arthritis and its role in monitoring disease activity. *Ann Rheum Dis* (1983) 42(6):665–7. doi: 10.1136/ard.42.6.665
15. Cunnane G, Grehan S, Geoghegan S, McCormack C, Shields D, Whitehead AS, et al. Serum amyloid A in the assessment of early inflammatory arthritis. *J Rheumatol* (2000) 27(1):58–63.
16. Yoo J, Lee SK, Lim M, Sheen D, Choi EH, Kim SA. Exosomal amyloid A and lymphatic vessel endothelial hyaluronic acid receptor-1 proteins are associated with disease activity in rheumatoid arthritis. *Arthritis Res Ther* (2017) 19:119. doi: 10.1186/s13075-017-1334-9
17. Ostensen M, Marhaug G, Husby G. Amyloid-related serum protein (SAA) during and after pregnancy in healthy women and women with rheumatic disease. *APMIS Immunol* (1985) 93(1):1–5. doi: 10.1111/j.1699-0463.1985.tb02913.x
18. Hwang YG, Balasubramani GK, Metes ID, Levesque MC, Bridges SLJr, Moreland LW. Differential response of serum amyloid A to different therapies in early rheumatoid arthritis and its potential value as a disease activity biomarker. *Arthritis Res* (2016) 18:108. doi: 10.1186/s13075-016-1009-y
19. Wild N, Karl J, Grunert VP, Schmitt RI, Garczarek U, Krause F, et al. Diagnosis of rheumatoid arthritis: multivariate analysis of biomarkers. *Biomarkers* (2008) 13(1):88–105. doi: 10.1080/13547500701669410
20. De Seny D, Cobraiville G, Charlier E, Neuville S, Esser N, Malaise D, et al. Acute-phase serum amyloid a in osteoarthritis: regulatory mechanism and proinflammatory properties. *PloS One* (2013) 8(6):e66769. doi: 10.1371/journal.pone.0066769
21. Ally MM, Hodkinson B, Meyer PW, Musenge E, Tikly M, Anderson R. Serum matrix metalloproteinase-3 in comparison with acute phase proteins as a marker of disease activity and radiographic damage in early rheumatoid arthritis. *Mediators Inflamm* (2013) 2013:183653. doi: 10.1155/2013/183653
22. Targońska-Stępniak B, Dryglewska M, Majdan M. Influence of long-term leflunomide treatment on serum amyloid concentration in rheumatoid arthritis patients. *Pharmacol Rep* (2010) 62(4):719–25. doi: 10.1016/s1734-1140(10)70329-7
23. Connolly M, Mullan RH, McCormick J, Matthews C, Sullivan O, Kennedy A, et al. Acute-phase serum amyloid A regulates tumor necrosis factor alpha and matrix turnover and predicts disease progression in patients with inflammatory arthritis before and after biologic therapy. *Arthritis Rheumatol* (2012) 64(4):1035–45. doi: 10.1002/art.33455
24. Centola M, Cavet G, Shen Y, Ramanujan S, Knowlton N, Swan KA, et al. Development of a multi-biomarker disease activity test for rheumatoid arthritis. *PloS One* (2013) 8:e60635. doi: 10.1371/journal.pone.0060635
25. Ma MHY, Defranoux N, Li W, Sasso EH, Ibrahim F, Scott DL, et al. A multi-biomarker disease activity score can predict sustained remission in rheumatoid arthritis. *Arthritis Res Ther* (2020) 22(1):158. doi: 10.1186/s13075-020-02240-w
26. Wong M, Toh L, Wilson A, Rowley K, Karschimkus C, Prior D, et al. Reduced arterial elasticity in rheumatoid arthritis and the relationship to vascular disease risk factors and inflammation. *Arthritis Rheumatol* (2003) 48(1):81–9. doi: 10.1002/art.10748
27. Rho YH, Chung CP, Oeser A, Solus J, Asanuma Y, Sokka T, et al. Inflammatory mediators and premature coronary atherosclerosis in rheumatoid arthritis. *Arthritis Rheumatol* (2009) 61(11):1580–5. doi: 10.1002/art.25009
28. Kullich WC, Mur E, Aglas F, Niksic F, Czerwenka C. Inhibitory effects of leflunomide therapy on the activity of matrixmetalloproteinase-9 and the release of cartilage oligomeric matrix protein in patients with rheumatoid arthritis. *Clin Exp Rheumatol* (2006) 24(2):155–60.
29. Momohara S, Okamoto H, Yamanaka H. Chondrocyte of rheumatoid arthritis serve as a source of intra-articular acute-phase serum amyloid A protein. *Clin Chim Acta* (2008) 398(1-2):155–6. doi: 10.1016/j.cca.2008.07.034
30. Boeters DM, Burgers LE, Sasso EH, Huizinga TWJ, van der Helm-van Mil AHM. ACPA-negative RA consists of subgroups: patients with high likelihood of achieving sustained DMARD-free remission can be identified by serological markers at disease presentation. *Arthritis Res Ther* (2019) 21 (1):121. doi: 10.1186/s13075-019-1902-2
31. Migita K, Izumi Y, Jiuchi Y, Kozuru H, Kawahara C, Izumi M, et al. Effects of Janus kinase inhibitor tofacitinib on circulating serum amyloid A and

interleukin-6 during treatment for rheumatoid arthritis. *Clin Exp Immunol* (2014) 175(2):208–14. doi: 10.1111/cei.12234
32. Visvanathan S, Wagner C, Rojas J, Kay J, Dasgupta B, Matteson EL, et al. E-selectin, interleukin 18, serum amyloid A, and matrix metalloproteinase 9 are associated with clinical response to golimumab plus methotrexate in patients with active rheumatoid arthritis despite methotrexate therapy. *J Rheumatol* (2009) 36(7):1371–9. doi: 10.3899/jrheum.080755
33. Doyle MK, Rahman MU, Frederick B, Birbara CA, de Vries D, Toedter G, et al. Effects of subcutaneous and intravenous golimumab on inflammatory biomarkers in patients with rheumatoid arthritis: results of a phase 1, randomized, open-label trial. *Rheumatol (Oxford)* (2013) 52(7):1214–9. doi: 10.1093/rheumatology/kes381
34. Kobayashi T, Yokoyama T, Ito S, Kobayashi D, Yamagata A, Okada M, et al. Periodontal and serum protein profiles in patients with rheumatoid arthritis treated with tumor necrosis factor inhibitor adalimumab. *J Periodontol* (2014) 85(11):1480–8. doi: 10.1902/jop.2014.140194
35. Hammer HB, Fagerhol MK, Wien TN, Kvien TK. The soluble biomarker calprotectin (an S100 protein) is associated to ultrasonographic synovitis scores and is sensitive to change in patients with rheumatoid arthritis treated with adalimumab. *Arthritis Res Ther* (2011) 13(5):R178. doi: 10.1186/ar3503
36. Gabay C, Burmester GR, Strand V, Msihid J, Zilberstein M, Kimura T, et al. Sarilumab and adalimumab differential effects on bone remodelling and cardiovascular risk biomarkers, and predictions of treatment outcomes. *Arthritis Res Ther* (2020) 22(1):70. doi: 10.1186/s13075-020-02163-6
37. Nissinen R, Leirisalo-Repo M, Peltomaa R, Palosuo T, Vaarala O. Cytokine and chemokine receptor profile of peripheral blood mononuclear cells during treatment with infliximab in patients with active rheumatoid arthritis. *Ann Rheum Dis* (2004) 63(6):681–7. doi: 10.1136/ard.2003.008599
38. Xu Y, Yamada T, Satoh T, Okuda Y. Measurement of serum amyloid A1 (SAA1), a major isotype of acute phase SAA. *Clin Chem Lab Med* (2006) 44 (1):59–63. doi: 10.1515/CCLM.2006.012
39. De Seny D, Fillet M, Ribbens C, Marée R, Meuwis MA, Lutteri L. Monomeric calgranulins measured by SELDI-TOF mass spectrometry and calprotectin measured by ELISA as biomarkers in arthritis. *Clin Chem* (2008) 54 (6):1066–75. doi: 10.1373/clinchem.2007.099549
40. Li TW, Zheng BR, Huang ZX, Lin Q, Zhao LK, Liao ZT, et al. Screening disease-associated proteins from sera of patients with rheumatoid arthritis: a comparative proteomic study. *Chin Med J (Engl)* (2010) 123(5):537–43.
41. Seok A, Lee HJ, Lee S, Lee J, Mun S, Park A, et al. Identification and Validation of SAA4 as a Rheumatoid Arthritis Prescreening Marker by Liquid Chromatography Tandem-mass Spectrometry. *Molecules* (2017) 22 (5):805. doi: 10.3390/molecules22050805
42. Nys G, Cobraiville G, Servais AC, Malaise MG, de Seny D, Fillet M. Targeted proteomics reveals serum amyloid A variants and alarmins S100A8-S100A9 as key plasma biomarkers of rheumatoid arthritis. *Talanta* (2019) 204:507–17. doi: 10.1016/j.talanta.2019.06.044
43. Filipowicz-Sosnowska AM, Roztropowicz-Denisiewicz K, Rosenthal CJ, Baum J. The amyloidosis of juvenile rheumatoid arthritis–comparative studies in Polish and American children. I. Levels of serum SAA protein. *Arthritis Rheumatol* (1978) 21(6):699–703. doi: 10.1002/art.1780210615
44. Scheinberg MA, Hubscher O, Morteo OG, Benson MD. Serum amyloid protein levels in south american children with rheumatoid arthritis: A co-operative study. *Ann Rheum Dis* (1980) 39:228–30. doi: 10.1136/ard.39.3.228
45. Kutulculer N, Karaca NE, Azarsiz E, Aksu G, Gulez N. Immunoglobulin light chain levels can be used to determine disease stage in children with juvenile idiopathic arthritis. *Clin Lab Sci* (2011) 24(2):93–8.
46. Cantarini L, Giani T, Fioravanti A, Iacoponi F, Simonini G, Pagnini I, et al. Serum amyloid A circulating levels and disease activity in patients with juvenile idiopathic arthritis. *Yonsei Med J* (2012) 53(5):1045–8. doi: 10.3349/ymj.2012.53.5.1045
47. Dev S, Singh A. Study of role of serum amyloid A (SAA) as a marker of disease activity in juvenile idiopathic arthritis. *J Family Med Prim Care* (2019) 8(6):2129–33. doi: 10.4103/jfmpc.jfmpc_339_19
48. Miyamae T, Malehorn DE, Lemster B, Mori M, Imagawa T, Yokota S, et al. Serum protein profile in systemic-onset juvenile idiopathic arthritis differentiates response versus nonresponse to therapy. *Arthritis Res Ther* (2005) 7(4):R746–55. doi: 10.1186/ar1723
49. Lange U, Boss B, Teichmann J, Klör HU, Neeck G. Serum amyloid A–an indicator of inflammation in ankylosing spondylitis. *Rheumatol Int* (2000) 19:119–22. doi: 10.1007/s002960050114
50. Jung SY, Park MC, Park YB, Lee SK. Serum amyloid A as a useful indicator of disease activity in patients with ankylosing spondylitis. *Yonsei Med J* (2007) 48:218–24. doi: 10.3349/ymj.2007.48.2.218
51. De Vries MK, Eijk IC, Horst-Bruinsma IE, Peters MJL, Nurmohamed MT, Dijkmans BAC. Erythrocyte Sedimentation Rate, C-reactive Protein Level, and Serum Amyloid a Protein for Patient Selection and Monitoring of Anti-Tumor Necrosis Factor Treatment in Ankylosing Spondylitis. *Arthritis Rheumatol* (2009) 61(11):1484–90. doi: 10.1002/art.24838
52. Li T, Huang Z, Zheng B, Liao Z, Zhao L, Gu J. Serum disease-associated proteins of ankylosing spondylitis: results of a preliminary study by comparative proteomics. *Clin Exp Rheumatol* (2010) 28(2):201–7.
53. Rademacher J, Tietz LM, Le L, Hartl A, Hermann KA, Sieper J, et al. Added value of biomarkers compared with clinical parameters for the prediction of radiographic spinal progression in axial spondyloarthritis. *Rheumatol (Oxford)* (2019) 58(9):1556–64. doi: 10.1093/rheumatology/kez025
54. Wu J, Wu X, Chen Z, Lv Q, Yang M, Zheng X, et al. Circulating Retinol-Binding Protein 4 as a Possible Biomarker of Treatment Response for Ankylosing Spondylitis: An Array-Based Comparative Study. *Front Pharmacol* (2020) 11:231. doi: 10.3389/fphar.2020.00231
55. Liu S, Ji W, Lu J, Tang X, Guo Y, Ji M, et al. Discovery of Potential Serum Protein Biomarkers in Ankylosing Spondylitis Using Tandem Mass Tag-Based Quantitative Proteomics. *J Proteome Res* (2020) 19(2):864–72. doi: 10.1021/acs.jproteome.9b00676
56. Ma J, Luo X, Wu Q, Chen Z, Kou L, Wang H. Circulation levels of acute phase proteins in patients with Takayasu arteritis. *J Vasc Surg* (2010) 51 (3):700–6. doi: 10.1016/j.jvs.2009.09.038
57. Nair AM, Goel R, Hindhumati M, Jayakanthan K, Visalakshi J, Joseph G, et al. Serum amyloid A as a marker of disease activity and treatment response in Takayasu arteritis. *Rheumatol Int* (2017) 37(10):1643–9. doi: 10.1007/s00296-017-3786-2
58. Hocevar A, Rotar Z, Jese R, Semrl SS, Pizem J, Hawlina M, et al. Do Early Diagnosis and Glucocorticoid Treatment Decrease the Risk of Permanent Visual Loss and Early Relapses in Giant Cell Arteritis: A Prospective Longitudinal Study. *Med (Baltimore)* (2016) 95(14):e3210. doi: 10.1097/MD.0000000000003210
59. Burja B, Feichtinger J, Lakota K, Thallinger GG, Sodin-Semrl S, Kuret T, et al. Utility of serological biomarkers for giant cell arteritis in a large cohort of treatment-naïve patients. *Clin Rheumatol* (2019) 38(2):317–29. doi: 10.1007/s10067-018-4240-x
60. Dartevel A, Toussaint B, Trocme C, Arnaud M, Simon N, Faure P, et al. Serum amyloid A as a marker of disease activity in Giant cell arteritis. *Autoimmun Rev* (2020) 19(1):102428. doi: 10.1016/j.autrev.2019.102428
61. Van Sleen Y, Sandovici M, Abdulahad WH, Bijzet J, van der Geest SMK, Boots AMH, et al. Markers of angiogenesis and macrophage products for predicting disease course and monitoring vascular inflammation in giant cell arteritis. *Rheumatology* (2019) 58(8):1383–92. doi: 10.1093/rheumatology/kez034
62. Mitani Y, Sawada H, Hayakawa H, Aoki K, Ohashi H, Matsumura M, et al. Elevated levels of high-sensitivity C-reactive protein and serum amyloid-A late after Kawasaki disease: association between inflammation and late coronary sequelae in Kawasaki disease. *Circulation* (2005) 111(1):38–43. doi: 10.1161/01.CIR.0000151311.38708.29
63. Whitin JC, Yu TT, Ling XB, Kanegaye JT, Burns JC, Cohen HJ. A Novel Truncated Form of Serum Amyloid A in Kawasaki Disease. *PloS One* (2016) 11(6):e0157024. doi: 10.1371/journal.pone.0157024
64. Purevdorj N, Mu Y, Gu Y, Zheng F, Wang R, Yu J, et al. Clinical significance of the serum biomarker index detection in children with Henoch-Schonlein purpura. *Clin Biochem* (2018) 52:167–70. doi: 10.1016/j.clinbiochem.2017.11.006
65. Kuret T, Lakota K, Žigon P, Ogrič M, Sodin-Šemrl S, Čučnik S, et al. Insight into inflammatory cell and cytokine profiles in adult IgA vasculitis. *Clin Rheumatol* (2019) 38:331–8. doi: 10.1007/s10067-018-4234-8
66. Rothkrantz-Kos S, Van Dieijen-Visser MP, Mulder PGH, Drent M. Potential usefulness of inflammatory markers to monitor respiratory functional

impairment in sarcoidosis. *Clin Chem* (2003) 49(9):1510–17. doi: 10.1373/49.9.1510

67. Miyoshi S, Hamada H, Kadowaki T, Hamaguchi N, Ito R, Irifune K, et al. Comparative evaluation of serum markers in pulmonary sarcoidosis. *Chest* (2010) 137(6):1391–7. doi: 10.1378/chest.09-1975
68. Salazar A, Pinto X, Mana J, Serum amyloid A. and high-density lipoprotein cholesterol: serum markers of inflammation in sarcoidosis and other systemic disorders. *Eur J Clin Invest* (2001) 31(12):1070–7. doi: 10.1046/j.1365-2362.2001.00913.x
69. Bargagli E, Magi B, Olivieri C, Bianchi N, Landi C, Rottoli P. Analysis of serum amyloid A in sarcoidosis patients. *Respir Med* (2011) 105(5):775–80. doi: 10.1016/j.rmed.2010.12.010
70. Gungor S, Ozseker F, Yalcinsoy M, Akkaya E, Can G, Eroglu H, et al. Conventional markers in determination of activity of sarcoidosis. *Int Immunopharmacol* (2015) 25(1):174–9. doi: 10.1016/j.intimp.2015.01.015
71. Zhang Y, Chen X, Hu Y, Du S, Shen L, He Y, et al. Preliminary characterizations of a serum biomarker for sarcoidosis by comparative proteomic approach with tandem-mass spectrometry in ethnic Han Chinese patients. *Respir Res* (2013) 14(1):18. doi: 10.1186/1465-9921-14-18
72. Enyedi A, Csongrádi A, Altorjay IT, Beke GL, Váradi C, Enyedi EE, et al. Combined application of angiotensin converting enzyme and chitotriosidase analysis improves the laboratory diagnosis of sarcoidosis. *Clin Chim Acta* (2020) 500:155–62. doi: 10.1016/j.cca.2019.10.010
73. Brandwein SR, Medsger TAJr, Skinner M, Sipe JD, Rodnan GP, Cohen AS. Serum amyloid A protein concentration in progressive systemic sclerosis (scleroderma). *Ann Rheum Dis* (1984) 43(4):586–9. doi: 10.1136/ard.43.4.586
74. Lakota K, Carns M, Podlusky S, Mrak-Poljsak K, Hinchcliff M, Lee J, et al. Serum amyloid A is a marker for pulmonary involvement in systemic sclerosis. *PloS One* (2015) 10(1):e0110820. doi: 10.1371/journal.pone.0110820
75. Lis-Święty A, Widuchowska M, Brzezińska-Wcisło L, Kucharz E. High acute phase protein levels correlate with pulmonary and skin involvement in patients with diffuse systemic sclerosis. *J Int Med Res* (2018) 46:1634–9. doi: 10.1177/0300060518760955
76. Wang CM, Deng JH, Mao GF, He JL, Shi X. Serum Amyloid A: A Potential Biomarker Assessing Disease Activity in Systemic Lupus Erythematosus. *Med Sci Monit* (2020) 26:e923290. doi: 10.12659/MSM.923290
77. Boyd TA, Eastman PS, Huynh DH, Qureshi F, Sasso EH, Bolce R, et al. Correlation of serum protein biomarkers with disease activity in psoriatic arthritis. *Expert Rev Clin Immunol* (2020) 16(3):335–41. doi: 10.1080/1744666X.2020.1729129
78. Duzova A, Bakkaloglu A, Besbas N, Topaloglu R, Ozen S, Ozaltin F, et al. Role of A-SAA in monitoring subclinical inflammation and in colchicine dosage in familial Mediterranean fever. *Clin Exp Rheumatol* (2003) 21:509–14.
79. Lachmann HJ, Sengül B, Yavuzşen TU, Booth DR, Booth SE, Bybee A, et al. Clinical and subclinical inflammation in patients with familial Mediterranean fever and in heterozygous carriers of MEFV mutations. *Rheumatol (Oxford)* (2006) 45(6):746–50. doi: 10.1093/rheumatology/kei279
80. Berkun Y, Padeh S, Reichman B, Zaks N, Rabinovich E, Lidar M, et al. A Single Testing of Serum Amyloid A Levels as a Tool for Diagnosis and Treatment Dilemmas in Familial Mediterranean Fever. *Semin Arthritis Rheumatol* (2007) 37:182–8. doi: 10.1016/j.semarthrit.2007.03.005
81. Yalçinkaya F, Cakar N, Acar B, Tutar E, Güriz H, Elhan AH, et al. The value of the levels of acute phase reactants for the prediction of familial Mediterranean fever associated amyloidosis: a case control study. *Rheumatol Int* (2007) 27(6):517–22. doi: 10.1007/s00296-006-0265-6
82. Kallinich T, Wittkowski H, Keitzer R, Roth J, Foell D. Neutrophil-derived S100A12 as novel biomarker of inflammation in familial Mediterranean fever. *Ann Rheum Dis* (2010) 69(4):677–82. doi: 10.1136/ard.2009.114363
83. Lofty HM, Marzouk H, Farag Y, Nabih M, Khalifa IAS, Mostafa N, et al. Serum Amyloid A Level in Egyptian Children with Familial Mediterranean Fever. *Int J Rheumatol* (2016) 1:1–6. doi: 10.1155/2016/7354018
84. Cakan M, Karadag SG, Tanatar A, Sonmez HE, Ayaz NA. The Value of Serum Amyloid A Levels in Familial Mediterranean Fever to Identify Occult Inflammation During Asymptomatic Periods. *J Clin Rheumatol* (2021) 27 (1):1–4. doi: 10.1097/RHU.0000000000001134
85. Bilginer Y, Ozaltin F, Basaran C, Duzova A, Besbas N, Topaloglu R, et al. Evaluation of intima media thickness of the common and internal carotid arteries with inflammatory markers in familial Mediterranean fever as possible predictors for atherosclerosis. *Rheumatol Int* (2008) 28(12):1211–6. doi: 10.1007/s00296-008-0605-9
86. Mohamed R, El-Bassyouni HT, Elwan SH, Youness E, Soliman DR, Shehata GM, et al. Carotid intima-media thickness, lipid profile, serum amyloid A and vitamin D status in children with familial Mediterranean fever. *Egyptian Rheumatologist* (2020) 42(3):237–40. doi: 10.1016/j.ejr.2020.05.005
87. Sargsyan Y, Sargsyan A. Endothelial biomarkers in patients with familial Mediterranean fever associated vascular disease and vasculopathy. *Pediatr Rheumatol* (2015) 13(1):O16. doi: 10.1186/1546-0096-13-S1-O16
88. Aygündüz M, Bavbek N, Öztürk M, Kaftan O, Koşar A. Kirazli A.Serum beta 2-microglobulin reflects disease activity in Behçet's disease. *Rheumatol Int* (2002) 22(1):5–8. doi: 10.1007/s00296-002-0180-4
89. Cantarini L, Pucino V, Vitale A, Talarico R, Lucherini OM, Magnotti F. et al. Immunometabolic biomarkers of inflammation in Behçet's disease: relationship with epidemiological profile, disease activity and therapeutic regimens. *Clin Exp Immunol* (2016) 184(2):197–207. doi: 10.1111/cei.12768
90. Vitale A, Rigante D, Lupalco G, Brizi MG, Caso F, Franceschini R, et al. Serum amyloid A in Behcet's disease. *Clin Rheumatol* (2014) 33(8):1165–7. doi: 10.1007/s10067-014-2555-9
91. Sota J, Vitale A, Rigante D, Orlando I, Lucherini OM, Simpatico A, et al. Correlation of Serum Amyloid-A Levels, Clinical Manifestations, Treatment, and Disease Activity in Patients with Behçet's Disease. *Isr Med Assoc J* (2018) 20(8):517–21. doi: 10.1038/s41433-019-0740-4
92. Lee HJ, Kim JH, Kim SW, Joo HA, Lee HW, Kim YS, et al. Proteomic Analysis of Serum Amyloid A as a Potential Marker in Intestinal Behçet's Disease. *Digestive Dis Sci* (2017) 62(8):1953–62. doi: 10.1007/s10620-017-4606-y
93. Hawkins PN, Lachmann HJ, Aganna E, McDermott MF. Spectrum of Clinical Features in Muckle-Wells Syndrome and Response to Anakinra. *Arthritis Rheumatol* (2004) 50(2):607–12. doi: 10.1002/art.2003
94. Scarpioni R, Rigante D, Cantarini L, Ricardi M, Albertazzi V, Melfa L, et al. Renal involvement in secondary amyloidosis of Muckle-Wells syndrome: marked improvement of renal function and reduction of proteinuria after therapy with human anti-interleukin1β monoclonal antibody canakinumab. *Clin Rheumatol* (2015) 34:1311–6. doi: 10.1007/s10067-013-2481-2
95. Hoffman HM, Throne ML, Amar NJ, Cartwright RC, Kivitz AJ, Soo Y, et al. Long-term efficacy and safety profile of rilonacept in the treatment of cryopryin-associated periodic syndromes: results of a 72-week open-label extension study. *Clin Ther* (2012) 34(10):2091–103. doi: 10.1016/j.clinthera.2012.09.009
96. Goldbach-Mansky R, Shroff SD, Wilson M, Snyder C, Plehn S, Barham B. A pilot study to evaluate the safety and efficacy of the long-acting interleukin-1 inhibitor rilonacept (Interleukin-1 Trap) in patients with familial cold autoinflammatory syndrome. *Arthritis Rheumatol* (2008) 58(8):2432–42. doi: 10.1002/art.23620
97. Wikén M, Hallén B, Kullenberg T, Koskinen LO. Development and effect of antibodies to anakinra during treatment of severe CAPS: sub-analysis of a long-term safety and efficacy study. *Clin Rheumatol* (2018) 37(12):3381–6. doi: 10.1007/s10067-018-4196-x
98. Connolly M, Marrelli A, Blades M, McCormick J, Maderna P, Godson C, et al. Acute serum amyloid A induces migration, angiogenesis, and inflammation in synovial cells in vitro and in a human rheumatoid arthritis/SCID mouse chimera model. *J Immunol* (2010) 184(11):6427–37. doi: 10.4049/jimmunol.0902941
99. Ishii W, Matsuda M, Nakamura A, Nakamura N, Suzuki A, Ikeda S. Abdominal fat aspiration biopsy and genotyping of serum amyloid A contribute to early diagnosis of reactive AA amyloidosis secondary to rheumatoid arthritis. *Intern Med* (2003) 42(9):800–5. doi: 10.2169/internalmedicine
100. Migita K, Eguchi K, Tsukada T, Kawabe Y, Takashima H, Mine M, et al. Increased circulating serum amyloid A protein derivatives in rheumatoid arthritis patients with secondary amyloidosis. *Lab Invest* (1996) 75(3):371–5.
101. Gorlier C, Sellam J, Laurans L, Simon T, Giurgea I, Bastard JP, et al. In familial Mediterranean fever, soluble TREM-1 plasma level is higher in case of amyloidosis. *Innate Immun* (2019) 25(8):487–90. doi: 10.1177/1753425919870847
102. Lachmann HJ, Goodman HJB, Gilbertson JA, Gallimore JR, Sabin CA, Gillmore JD, et al. Natural history and outcome in systemic AA amyloidosis. *N Engl J Med* (2007) 356(23):2361–71. doi: 10.1056/NEJMoa070265

103. Gillmore JD, Lovat LB, Persey MR, Pepys MB, Hawkins PN. Amyloid load and clinical outcome in AA amyloidosis in relation to circulating concentration of serum amyloid A protein. *Lancet* (2001) 358(9275):24–9. doi: 10.1016/S0140-6736(00)05252-1
104. Perry ME, Stirling A, Hunter JA. Effect of etanercept on serum amyloid A protein (SAA) levels in patients with AA amyloidosis complicating inflammatory arthritis. *Clin Rheumatol* (2008) 27(7):923–5. doi: 10.1007/s10067-008-0875-3
105. Nakamura T, Higashi S, Tomoda K, Tsukano M, Shono M. Effectiveness of etanercept vs cyclophosphamide as treatment for patients with amyloid A amyloidosis secondary to rheumatoid arthritis. *Rheumatol (Oxford)* (2012) 51(11):2064–9. doi: 10.1093/rheumatology/kes190
106. Miyagawa I, Nakayamada S, Saito K, Hanami K, Nawata M, Sawamukai N, et al. Study on the safety and efficacy of tocilizumab, an anti-IL-6 receptor antibody, in patients with rheumatoid arthritis complicated with AA amyloidosis. *Mod Rheumatol* (2014) 24(3):405–9. doi: 10.3109/14397595.2013.844294
107. Lane T, Gillmore JD, Wechalekar AD, Hawkins PN, Lachmann HJ. Therapeutic blockade of interleukin-6 by tocilizumab in the management of AA amyloidosis and chronic inflammatory disorders: a case series and review of the literature. *Clin Exp Rheumatol* (2015) 33(6 Suppl 94):S46–53.
108. Okuda Y, Ohnishi M, Matoba K, Jouyama K, Yamada A, Sawada N, et al. Comparison of the clinical utility of tocilizumab and anti-TNF therapy in AA amyloidosis complicating rheumatic diseases. *Mod Rheumatol* (2014) 24 (1):137–43. doi: 10.3109/14397595.2013.854048
109. Xu B, Fan CY, Wang AL, Zou YL, Yu YH, He C, et al. Suppressed T cell-mediated immunity in patients with COVID-19: A clinical retrospective study in Wuhan, China. *J Infect* (2020) 81(1):e51–60. doi: 10.1016/j.jinf.2020.04.012
110. Shi F, Wu T, Zhu X, Ge Y, Zeng X, Chi Y, et al. Association of viral load with serum biomakers among COVID-19 cases. *Virology* (2020) 546:122–6. doi: 10.1016/j.virol.2020.04.011
111. Wang D, Li R, Wang J, Jiang Q, Gao C, Yang J, et al. Correlation analysis between disease severity and clinical and biochemical characteristics of 143 cases of COVID-19 in Wuhan, China: a descriptive study. *BMC Infect Dis* (2020) 20(1):519. doi: 10.1186/s12879-020-05242-w
112. Li H, Xiang X, Ren H, Xu L, Zhao L, Chen X, et al. Serum Amyloid A is a biomarker of severe Coronavirus Disease and poor prognosis. *J Infection* (2020) 80(6):646–55. doi: 10.1016/j.jinf.2020.03.035
113. Li X, Wang L, Yan S, Yang F, Xiang L, Zhu J, et al. Clinical characteristics of 25 death cases with COVID-19: A retrospective review of medical records in a single medical center, Wuhan, China. *Int J Infect Dis* (2020) 94:128–32. doi: 10.1016/j.ijid.2020.03.053
114. Mo XN, Su ZQ, Lei CL, Chen DF, Peng H, Chen RC, et al. Serum amyloid A is a predictor for prognosis of COVID-19. *Respirology* (2020) 25(7):764–5. doi: 10.1111/resp.13840
115. Watson G, See CG, Woo P. Use of somatic cell hybrids and fluorescence in situ hybridization to localize the functional serum amyloid A (SAA) genes to chromosome 11p15.4-p15.1 and the entire SAA superfamily to chromosome 11p15. *Genomics* (1994) 23(3):694–6. doi: 10.1006/geno.1994.1559
116. Jumeau C, Awad F, Assrawi E, Cobret L, Duquesnoy P, Giurgea I, et al. Expression of SAA1, SAA2 and SAA4 genes in human primary monocytes and monocyte-derived macrophages. *PloS One* (2019) 14(5):e0217005. doi: 10.1371/journal.pone.0217005
117. Kluve-Beckerman B, Drumm ML, Benson MD. Nonexpression of the human serum amyloid A three (SAA3) gene. *DNA Cell Biol* (1991) 10(9):651–61. doi: 10.1089/dna.1991.10.651
118. Steel DM, Sellar GC, Uhlar CM, Simon S, deBeer FC, Whitehead AS. A constitutively expressed serum amyloid A protein gene is closely linked to, and shares structural similarities with, an acute phase serum amyloid A protein gene. *Genomics* (1993) 16(2):447–54. doi: 10.1006/geno.1993.1209
119. Blank N, Hegenbart U, Lohse P, Beimler J, Röcken C, Ho AD, et al. Risk factors for AA amyloidosis in Germany. *Amyloid* (2015) 22:(1):1–7. doi: 10.3109/13506129.2014.980942
120. Booth DR, Booth SE, Gillmore JD, Hawkins PN, Pepys MB. SAA1 alleles as risk factors in reactive systemic AA amyloidosis. *Amyloid* (1998) 5(4):262–5. doi: 10.3109/13506129809007299
121. Utku U, Dilek M, Akpolat I, Bedir A, Akpolat T. SAA1 alpha/alpha alleles in Behcet's disease related amyloidosis. *Clin Rheumatol* (2007) 26:927–9. doi: 10.1007/s10067-006-0435-7
122. Moriguchi M, Terai C, Koseki Y, Uesato M, Nakajima A, Inada S, et al. Influence of genotypes at SAA1 and SAA2 loci on the development and the length of latent period of secondary AA-amyloidosis in patients with rheumatoid arthritis. *Hum Genet* (1999) 105(4):360–6. doi: 10.1007/s004399900150
123. Ajiro J, Narita I, Sato F, Saga D, Hasegawa H, Kuroda T, et al. SAA1 gene polymorphisms and the risk of AA amyloidosis in Japanese patients with rheumatoid arthritis. *Mod Rheumatol* (2006) 16(5):294–9. doi: 10.3109/s10165-006-0500-8
124. Nakamura T, Higashi S, Tomoda K, Tsukano M, Baba S, Shono M. Significance of SAA1.3 allele genotype in Japanese patients with amyloidosis secondary to rheumatoid arthritis. *Rheumatol (Oxford)* (2006) 45(1):43–9. doi: 10.1093/rheumatology/kei112
125. Moriguchi M, Terai C, Kaneko H, Koseki Y, Kajiyama H, Uesato M, et al. A novel single-nucleotide polymorphism at the 50-flanking region of SAA1 associated with risk of type AA amyloidosis secondary to rheumatoid arthritis. *Arthritis Rheumatol* (2001) 44(6):1266–72. doi: 10.1002/1529-0131(200106)44:6<1266::AID-ART218>3.0.CO;2-3
126. Yamada T, Okuda Y, Takasugi K, Wang L, Marks D, Benson MD, et al. An allele of serum amyloid A1 associated with amyloidosis in both Japanese and Caucasians. *Amyloid* (2003) 10(1):7–11. doi: 10.3109/13506120308995250
127. Moriguchi M, Kaneko H, Terai C, Koseki Y, Kajiyama H, Inada S, et al. Relative transcriptional activities of SAA1 promoters polymorphic at position -13(T/C): potential association between increased transcription and amyloidosis. *Amyloid* (2005) 12:26–32. doi: 10.1080/13506120500032394
128. Thorn CF, Lu ZY, Whitehead AS. Regulation of the human acute phase serum amyloid A genes by tumour necrosis factor-alpha, interleukin-6 and glucocorticoids in hepatic and epithelial cell lines. *Scand J Immunol* (2004) 59:152–8. doi: 10.1111/j.0300-9475.2004.01369.x
129. Hagihara K, Nishikawa T, Sugamata Y, Song J, Isobe T, Taga T, et al. Essential role of STAT3 in cytokine-driven NF-κB-mediated serum amyloid A gene expression. *Genes Cells* (2005) 10(11):1051–63. doi: 10.1111/j.1365-2443.2005.00900.x
130. Migita K, Koga T, Komori A, Torigoshi T, Maeda Y, Izumi Y, et al. Influence of Janus kinase inhibition on interleukin 6-mediated induction of acute-phase serum amyloid A in rheumatoid synovium. *J Rheumatol* (2011) 38 (11):2309–17. doi: 10.3899/jrheum.101362
131. Hagihara K, Nishikawa T, Isobe T, Song J, Sugamata Y, Yoshizaki K. IL-6 plays a critical role in the synergistic induction of human serum amyloid A (SAA) gene when stimulated with proinflammatory cytokines as analyzed with an SAA isoform real-time quantitative RT-PCR assay system. *Biochem Biophys Res Commun* (2004) 314(2):363–9. doi: 10.1016/j.bbrc.2003.12.096
132. Yoshizaki K. Pathogenic Role of IL-6 Combined with TNF-alfa or IL-1 in the Induction of Acute Phase Proteins SAA and CRP in Chronic Inflammatory Diseases. *Adv Exp Med Biol* (2011) 691:141–50. doi: 10.1007/978-1-4419-6612-4_15
133. Kushner I, Jiang SL, Zhang D, Lozanski G, Samols D. Do post-transcriptional mechanisms participate in induction of C-reactive protein and serum amyloid A by IL-6 and IL-1? *Ann NY Acad Sci* (1995) 762:102–7. doi: 10.1111/j.1749-6632.1995.tb32318.x
134. Steel DM, Roger JT, DeBeer MC, DeBeer FC, Whitehead AS. Biosynthesis of human acute-phase serum amyloid A protein (A-SAA) in vitro: the roles or mRNA accumulation, poly (A) tail shortening and translational efficiency. *Biochem J* (1993) 291(Pt 3):701–7. doi: 10.1042/bj2910701
135. Lozanski G, Jiang SL, Samols D. Kushner I. C-reactive protein and serum amyloid A mRNA stability following induction by cytokines. *Cytokine* (1996) 8(7):534–40. doi: 10.1006/cyto.1996.0072
136. Tanaka F, Migita K, Kawabe Y, Aoyagi T, Ida H, Kawakami A, et al. Interleukin-18 induces serum amyloid A (SAA) protein production from rheumatoid synovial fibroblasts. *Life Sci Feb* (2004) 13(74):1671–9. doi: 10.1016/j.lfs.2003.08.025
137. Thorn CF, Whitehead AS. Differential glucocorticoid enhancement of the cytokine-driven transcriptional activation of the human acute phase serum amyloid A genes, SAA1 and SAA2. *JImmunol* (2002) 1(169):399–406. doi: 10.4049/jimmunol.169.1.399
138. O'Hara R, Murphy EP, Whitehead AS, FitzGerald O, Bresnihan B. Acute-phase serum amyloid A production by rheumatoid arthritis synovial tissue. *Arthritis Res* (2000) 2(2):142–4. doi: 10.1186/ar78
139. Connolly M, Veale DJ, Fearon U. Acute serum amyloid A regulates cytoskeletal rearrangement, cell matrix interactions and promotes cell

migration in rheumatoid arthritis. *Ann Rheum Dis* (2011) 70(7):1296–303. doi: 10.1136/ard.2010.142240

140. Koga T, Torigoshi T, Motokawa S, Miyashita T, Maeda Y, Nakamura M, et al. Serum amyloid A-induced IL-6 production by rheumatoid synoviocytes. *FEBS Lett* (2008) 582(5):579–85. doi: 10.1016/j.febslet.2008.01.022
141. Furlaneto CJ, Campa A. A novel function of serum amyloid A: a potent stimulus for the release of tumor necrosis factor-alpha, interleukin-1beta, and interleukin-8 by human blood neutrophil. *Biochem Biophys Res Commun* (2000) 268(2):405–8. doi: 10.1006/bbrc.2000.2143
142. Lee MS, Yoo SA, Cho CS, Suh PG, Kim WU, Ryu SH. Serum amyloid A binding to formyl peptide receptor-like 1 induces synovial hyperplasia and angiogenesis. *J Immunol* (2006) 177(8):5585–94. doi: 10.4049/jimmunol.177.8.5585
143. He R, Sang H, Ye RD. Serum amyloid A induces IL-8 secretion through a G protein-coupled receptor, FPRL1/LXA4R. *Blood* (2003) 101(4):1572–81. doi: 10.1182/blood-2002-05-1431
144. Mullan RH, McCormick J, Connolly M, Bresnihan B, Veale DJ, Fearon U. A role for the high-density lipoprotein receptor SR-B1 in synovial inflammation via serum amyloid-A. *Am J Pathol* (2010) 176(4):1999–2008. doi: 10.2353/ajpath.2010.090014
145. Hong C, Shen C, Ding H, Huang S, Mu Y, Su H, et al. An involvement of SR-B1 mediated p38 MAPK signaling pathway in serum amyloid A-induced angiogenesis in rheumatoid arthritis. *Mol Immunol* (2015) 66(2):340–5. doi: 10.1016/j.molimm.2015.03.254
146. Sandri S, Rodriguez D, Gomes E, Monteiro HP, Russo M, Campa A. Is serum amyloid A an endogenous TLR4 agonist? *J Leukoc Biol* (2008) 83(5):1174–80. doi: 10.1189/jlb.0407203
147. Li W, Zhu S, Li J, D'Amore J, D'Angelo J, Yang H, et al. Serum amyloid A stimulates PKR expression and HMGB1 release possibly through TLR4/RAGE receptors. *Mol Med* (2015) 21:515–25. doi: 10.2119/molmed.2015.00109
148. He RL, Zhou J, Hanson CZ, Chen J, Cheng N, Ye RD. Serum amyloid A induces G-CSF expression and neutrophilia via Toll-like receptor 2. *Blood* (2009) 113(2):429–37. doi: 10.1182/blood-2008-03-139923
149. Cheng N, He R, Tian J, Ye PP, Ye RD. Cutting edge: TLR2 is a functional receptor for acute-phase serum amyloid A. *J Immunol* (2008) 181(1):22–6. doi: 10.4049/jimmunol.181.1.22
150. Connolly M, Rooney PR, McGarry T, Maratha AX, McCormick J, Miggin SM, et al. Acute serum amyloid A is an endogenous TLR2 ligand that mediates inflammatory and angiogenic mechanisms. *Ann Rheum Dis* (2016) 75(7):1392–8. doi: 10.1136/annrheumdis-2015-207655
151. O'Reilly S, Cant R, Ciechomska M, Finnigan J, Oakley F, Hambleton S, et al. Serum amyloid A induces interleukin-6 in dermal fibroblasts via Toll-like receptor 2, interleukin-1 receptor-associated kinase 4 and nuclear factor-κB. *Immunology* (2014) 143(3):331–40. doi: 10.1111/imm.12260
152. Okamoto H, Katagiri Y, Kiire A, Momohara S, Kamatani N. Serum amyloid A activates nuclear factor-kappaB in rheumatoid synovial fibroblasts through binding to receptor of advanced glycation end-products. *J Rheumatol* (2008) 35(5):752–6.
153. Mullan RH, Bresnihan B, Golden-Mason L, Markham T, O'Hara R, FitzGerald O, et al. Acute-phase serum amyloid A stimulation of angiogenesis, leukocyte recruitment, and matrix degradation in rheumatoid arthritis through an NF-kappaB-dependent signal transduction pathway. *Arthritis Rheumatol* (2006) 54 (1):105–14. doi: 10.1002/art.21518
154. Migita K, Kawabe Y, Tominaga M, Origuchi T, Aoyagi T, Eguchi K, et al. Serum amyloid A protein induces production of matrix metalloproteinases by human synovial fibroblasts. *Lab Invest* (1998) 78(5):535–9.
155. Vallon R, Freuler F, Desta-Tesdu N, Robeva A, Dawson J, Wenner P, et al. Serum amyloid A (apoSAA) expression is up-regulated in rheumatoid arthritis and induces transcription of matrix metalloproteinases. *J Immunol* (2001) 166(4):2801–7. doi: 10.4049/jimmunol.166.4.2801
156. O'Hara R, Murphy EP, Whitehead AS, FitzGerald O, Bresnihan B. Local expression of the serum amyloid A and formyl peptide receptor-like 1 genes in synovial tissue is associated with matrix metalloproteinase production in patients with inflammatory arthritis. *Arthritis Rheumatol* (2004) 50(6):1788–99. doi: 10.1002/art.20301
157. Kobayashi A, Naito S, Enomoto H, Shiomoi T, Kimura T, Obata K, et al. Serum levels of matrix metalloproteinase 3 (stromelysin 1) for monitoring synovitis in rheumatoid arthritis. *Arch Pathol Lab Med* (2007) 131(4):563–70. doi: 10.1043/1543-2165(2007)131[563:SLOMMS]2.0.CO;2
158. Satomura K, Torigoshi T, Koga T, Maeda Y, Izumi Y, Jiuchi Y, et al. (SAA) induces pentraxin 3 (PTX3) production in rheumatoid synoviocytes. *Mod Rheumatol* (2013) 23(1):28–35. doi: 10.3109/s10165-012-0630-0
159. Aggarwal S, Ghilardi N, Xie MH, de Sauvage FJ, Gurney AL. Interleukin-23 promotes a distinct CD4 T cell activation state characterized by the production of interleukin-17. *J Biol Chem* (2003) 278:1910–14. doi: 10.1074/jbc.M207577200
160. Hirota K, Yoshitomi H, Hashimoto M, Maeda S, Teradaira S, Sugimoto N, et al. Preferential recruitment of CCR6- expressing Th17 cells to inflamed joints via CCL20 in rheumatoid arthritis and its animal model. *J Exp Med* (2007) 204:2803–12. doi: 10.1084/jem.20071397
161. Migita K, Koga T, Torigoshi T, Maeda Y, Miyashita T, Izumi Y, et al. Serum amyloid A protein stimulates CCL20 production in rheumatoid synoviocytes. *Rheumatol (Oxford)* (2009) 48(7):741–7. doi: 10.1093/rheumatology/kep089
162. Lucherini M, Lopalco G, Cantarini L, Emmi G, Lopalco A, Venerito V, et al. Critical regulation of Th17 cell differentiation by serum amyloid-A signalling in Behcet's disease. *Immunol Lett* (2018) 201:38–44. doi: 10.1016/j.imlet.2018.10.013
163. Metawi SA, Abbas D, Kamal MM, Ibrahim MK. Serum and synovial fluid levels of interleukin-17 in correlation with disease activity in patients with RA. *Clin Rheumatol* (2011) 30(9):1201–7. doi: 10.1007/s10067-011-1737-y
164. Shen H, Goodall JC, Hill Gaston JS. Frequency and phenotype of peripheral blood Th17 cells in ankylosing spondylitis and rheumatoid arthritis. *Arthritis Rheumatol* (2009) 60(6):1647–56. doi: 10.1002/art.24568
165. Romero-Sanchez C, Jaimes DA, Londoño J, De Avila J, Castellanos JE, Bello JM. Association between Th-17 cytokine profile and clinical features in patients with spondyloarthritis. *Clin Exp Rheumatol* (2011) 29(5):828–34.
166. Bissonnette R, Nigen S, Langley RG, Lynde CW, Tan J, Fuentes-Duculan J, et al. Increased expression of IL-17A and limited involvement of IL-23 in patients with palmo-plantar (PP) pustular psoriasis or PP pustulosis; results from a randomised controlled trial. *J Eur Acad Dermatol Venereol* (2014) 28 (10):1298–305. doi: 10.1111/jdv.12272
167. Braun J, Baraliakos X, Deodhar A, Baeten D, Sieper J, Emery P, et al. Effect of secukinumab on clinical and radiographic outcomes in ankylosing spondylitis: 2-year results from the randomised phase III MEASURE 1 study. *Ann Rheum Dis* (2017) 76(6):1070–7. doi: 10.1136/annrheumdis-2016-209730
168. Migita K, Koga T, Satomura K, Izumi M, Torigodhi T, Maeda Y, et al. Serum amylodi A triggers the mosodium urate mediated mature interleukin 1ß production from human synovial fibroblasts. *Arthritis Res Ther* (2012) 14(3): R119. doi: 10.1186/ar3849
169. Migita K, Izumi Y, Fujikawa K, Agematsu K, Masumoto J, Jiuchi Y, et al. Dysregulated mature IL-1β production in familial Mediterranean fever. *Rheumatol (Oxford)* (2015) 54(4):660–5. doi: 10.1093/rheumatology/keu359
170. Niemi K, Teirilä L, Lappalainen J, Rajamäki K, Baumann MH, Öörni K, et al. Serum amyloid A activates the NLRP3 inflammasome via P2X7 receptor and a cathepsin B-sensitive pathway. *J Immunol* (2011) 186(11):6119–28. doi: 10.4049/jimmunol.1002843
171. Husby G, Natvig JB, Sletten K. New, third class of amyloid fibril protein. *J Exp Med* (1974) 139(3):773–8. doi: 10.1084/jem.139.3.773
172. Migita K, Yamasaki S, Shibatomi K, Ida H, Kawakami M,, Eguchi K. Impaired degradation of serum amyloid A (SAA) protein by cytokine-stimulated monocytes. *Clin Exp Immunol* (2001) 123(3):408–11. doi: 10.1046/j.1365-2249.2001.01472.x
173. Magy N, Benson MD, Liepnieks JL, Kluve-Beckerman B. Cellular events associated with the initial phase of AA amyloidogenesis: insights from a human monocyte model. *Amyloid* (2007) 14(1):51–63. doi: 10.1080/13506120601116575
174. Stix B, Kähne T, Sletten K, Raynes J, Roessner A, Röcken C. Proteolysis of AA amyloid fibril proteins by matrix metalloproteinases-1, -2, and -3. *Am J Pathol* (2001) 159(2):561–70. doi: 10.1016/s0002-9440(10)61727-0
175. Van der Hilst JCH, Yamada T, Op den Camp HJM, van der Meer JWM, Drenth JPH, Simon A. Increased susceptibility of serum amyloid A 1.1 to degradation by MMP-1: potential explanation for higher risk of type AA amyloidosis. *Rheumatol (Oxford)* (2008) 47(11):1651–4. doi: 10.1093/rheumatology/ken371
176. Tolle M, Huang T, Schuchardt M, Jankowski V, Prufer N, Jankowski J, et al. High-density lipoprotein loses its anti-inflammatory capacity by

accumulation of pro-inflammatory-serum amyloid A. *Cardiovasc Res* (2012) 94(1):154–62. doi: 10.1093/cvr/cvs089
177. Artl A, Marsche G, Lestavel S, Sattler W, Malle E. Role of serum amyloid A during metabolism of acute-phase HDL by macrophages. *Arterioscler Thromb Vasc Biol* (2000) 20(3):763–72. doi: 10.1161/01.atv.20.3.763
178. Gaal K, Tarr T, Lorincz H, Borbas V, Seres I, Harangi M, et al. High-density lipopoprotein antioxidant capacity, subpopulation distribution and paraoxonase-1 activity in patients with systemic lupus erythematosus. *Lipids Health Dis* (2016) 15:60. doi: 10.1186/s12944-016-0229-0
179. McMahon M, Grossman J, FitzGerald J, Dahlin-Lee E, Wallace DJ, Thong BY, et al. Proinflammatory high-density lipoprotein as a biomarker for atherosclerosis in patients with systemic lupus erythematosus and rheumatoid arthritis. *Arthritis Rheumatol* (2006) 54:2541–9. doi: 10.1002/art.21976
180. Meek RL, Urieli-Shoval, Benditt EP. Expression of apolipo-protein serum amyloid A mRNA in human atherosclerotic lesions and cultured vascular cells: implications for serum amyloid A function. *Proc Natl Acad Sci USA* (1994) 91(8):3186–90. doi: 10.1073/pnas.91.8.3186
181. Mechtcheriakova D, Schabbauer G, Lucerna M, Clauss M, de Martin R, Binder BR, et al. Specificity, diversity, and convergence in VEGF and TNF-alpha signaling events leading to tissue factor up-regulation via EGR-1 in endothelial cells. *FASEB J* (2001) 15:230–42. doi: 10.1096/fj.00-0247com
182. Zhao Y, Zhou S, Heng CK. Impact of serum amyloid A on tissue factor and tissue factor pathway inhibitor expression and activity in endothelial cells. *Arterioscler Thromb Vasc Biol* (2007) 27:1645–50. doi: 10.1161/ATVBAHA.106.137455
183. Chami B, Barrie N, Cai X, Wang X, Paul M, Morton-Chandra R, et al. Serum amyloid A receptor blockade and incorporation into high-density lipoprotein modulates its pro-inflammatory and pro-thrombotic activities on vascular endothelial cells. *Int J Mol Sci* (2015) 16(5):11101–24. doi: 10.3390/ijms160511101
184. Witting PK, Song C, Hsu K, Hua S, Parry SN, Aran R, et al. The acute-phase protein serum amyloid A induces endothelial dysfunction that is inhibited by high-density lipoprotein. *Free Radic Biol Med* (2011) 51:1390–8. doi: 10.1016/j.freeradbiomed.2011.06.031
185. Lingwood D, Binnington B, Rog T, Vattulainen I, Grzybek M, Coskun U, et al. Cholesterol modulates glycolipid conformation and receptor activity. *Nat Chem Biol* (2011) 7:260–2. doi: 10.1038/nchembio.551
186. Lakota K, Mrak-Poljsak K, Bozic B, Tomsic M, Sodin-Semrl S. Serum amyloid A activation of human coronary artery endothelial cells exhibits a neutrophil promoting molecular profile. *Microvasc Res* (2013) 90:55–63. doi: 10.1016/j.mvr.2013.07.011
187. Wang X, Chai H, Wang Z, Lin PH, Yao Q, Chen C. Serum amyloid A induces endothelial dysfunction in porcine coronary arteries and human coronary artery endothelial cells. *Am J Physiol Heart Circ Physiol* (2008) 295:2399–408. doi: 10.1152/ajpheart.00238.2008
188. Migita K, Miyashita T, Ishibashi H, Maeda Y, Nakamura M, Yatsuhashi H, et al. Suppressive effect of leflunomide metabolite (A77 1726) on metalloproteinase production in IL-1beta stimulated rheumatoid synovial fibroblasts. *Clin Exp Immunol* (2004) 137(3):612–6. doi: 10.1111/j.1365-2249.2004.02555.x
189. Rubin DT, Naik S, Kondragunta V, Rao T, Jain A. Detection of adalimumab and antibodies to adalimumab using a homogeneous mobility shift assay. *Curr Med Res Opin* (2017) 33(5):837–43. doi: 10.1080/03007995.2017.1289908
190. O'Neill L, Rooney P, Molloy D, Connolly M, McCormick J, McCarthy G, et al. Regulation of Inflammation and Angiogenesis in Giant Cell Arteritis by Acute-Phase Serum Amyloid A. *Arthritis Rheumatol* (2015) 67(9):2447–56. doi: 10.1002/art.39217
191. Chen ES, Song Z, Willett MH, Heine S, Yung RC, Liu MC, et al. Serum amyloid A regulates granulomatous inflammation in sarcoidosis through Toll-like receptor-2. *Am J Respir Crit Care Med* (2010) 181(4):360–73. doi: 10.1164/rccm.200905-0696OC
192. Bons JA, Drent M, Bouwman FG, Mariman EC, van Dieijen-Visser MP, Wodzig WK. Potential biomarkers for diagnosis of sarcoidosis using proteomics in serum. *Respir Med* (2007) 101(8):1687–95. doi: 10.1016/j.rmed.2007.03.002
193. Moore BJB, June CH. Cytokine release syndrome in severe COVID-19. *Science* (2020) 368(6490):473–4. doi: 10.1126/science.abb8925
194. Christenson K, Björkman L, Ahlin S, Olsson M, Sjöholm K, Karlsson A, et al. Endogenous Acute Phase Serum Amyloid A Lacks Pro-Inflammatory Activity, Contrasting the Two Recombinant Variants That Activate Human Neutrophils through Different Receptors. *Front Immunol* (2013) 22(4):92. doi: 10.3389/fimmu.2013.00092
195. Bjorkman L, Raynes JG, Shah C, Karlsson A, Dahlgren C, Bylund J. The proinflammatory activity of recombinant serum amyloid A is not shared by the endogenous protein in the circulation. *Arthritis Rheumatol* (2010) 62:1660–5. doi: 10.1002/art.27440
196. Yamada T, Okuda Y, Takasugi K, Itoh K, Igari J. Relative serum amyloid A (SAA) values: the influence of SAA1 genotypes and corticosteroid treatment in Japanese patients with rheumatoid arthritis. *Ann Rheum Dis* (2001) 60 (2):124–7. doi: 10.1136/ard.60.2.124
197. Griffiths K, Maxwell AP, McCarter RV, Nicol P, Hogg RE, Harbinson M, et al. Serum amyloid A levels are associated with polymorphic variants in the serum amyloid A 1 and 2 genes. *Ir J Med Sci* (2019) 188:1175–83. doi: 10.1007/s11845-019-01996-8
198. Zhang J, Guo W, Shi C, Zhang Y, Zhang C, Zhang L, et al. Copy number variations in serum amyloid A play a role in the determination of its individual baseline concentrations. *Clin Chem* (2018) 64:402–4. doi: 10.1373/clinchem.2017.279372
199. O'Brien KD, Brehm BJ, Seeley RJ, Bean J, Wener MH, Daniels S, et al. Diet-induced weight loss is associated with decreases in plasma serum amyloid A and C-reactive protein independent of dietary macronutrient composition in obese subjects. *J Clin Endocrinol Metab* (2005) 90:2244–9. doi: 10.1210/jc.2004-1011
200. Horiuchi Y, Hirayama S, Soda S, Seino U, Kon M, Ueno T, et al. Statin therapy reduces inflammatory markers in hypercholesterolemic patients with high baseline levels. *J Atheroscler Thromb* (2010) 17:722–9. doi: 10.5551/jat.3632
201. Giugliano D, Ceriello A, Esposito K. The effects of diet on inflammation: emphasis on the metabolic syndrome. *J Am Coll Cardiol* (2006) 48:677–85. doi: 10.1016/j.jacc.2006.03.052
202. Pruett BS, Pruett SB. An explanation for the paradoxical induction and suppression of an acute phase response by ethanol. *Alcohol* (2006) 39:105–10. doi: 10.1016/j.alcohol.2006.08.003
203. Al-Sieni AI, Al-Alawy AI, Al-Shehri ZS, Al-Abbasi FA. Serum amyloid-A protein and serum rheumatoid factor as serological surrogate markers for smoking risk factor in Saudi population. *Pak J Pharm Sci* (2013) 26:239–43.

8

The Immunoregulatory Role of Myeloid-Derived Suppressor Cells in the Pathogenesis of Rheumatoid Arthritis

Lan Yan [1†], Mingge Liang [1†], Tong Yang [1], Jinyu Ji [1], Goutham Sanker Jose Kumar Sreena [1], Xiaoqiang Hou [2], Meiqun Cao [3] and Zhitao Feng [1,2*]*

[1] *Medical College of China Three Gorges University, Yichang, China,* [2] *The Institute of Rheumatology, The First College of Clinical Medical Sciences, China Three Gorges University, Yichang, China,* [3] *Shenzhen Institute of Geriatrics, Shenzhen Second People's Hospital, The First Affiliated Hospital of Shenzhen University, Shenzhen, China*

***Correspondence:**
Meiqun Cao
mqcao111@163.com
Zhitao Feng
zhitao.feng@ctgu.edu.cn

†These authors have contributed equally to this work

Myeloid-derived suppressor cells (MDSCs) are a group of cells that regulate the immune response and exert immunosuppressive effects on various immune cells. Current studies indicate that MDSCs have both anti-inflammatory effects and proinflammatory effects on rheumatoid arthritis (RA) and RA animal models. MDSCs inhibit $CD4^+$ T cells, which secrete proinflammatory factors such as IFN-γ, IL-2, IL-6, IL-17, and TNF-α, by inhibiting iNOS, ROS, and IFN-γ and promoting the production of the anti-inflammatory factor IL-10. MDSCs can suppress dendritic cells by reducing MHC-II and CD86 expression, expand Treg cells *in vitro* through the action of IL-10, inhibit B cells through NO and PGE_2, and promote Th17 cell responses by secreting IL-1β. As a type of osteoclast precursor cell, MDSCs can differentiate into osteoclasts through activation of the NF-κB pathway via IL-1α. Overall, our study reviews the research progress related to MDSCs in RA, focusing on the effects of MDSCs on various types of cells and aiming to provide ideas to help reveal the important role of MDSCs in RA.

Keywords: myeloid-derived suppressor cell, rheumatoid arthritis, immune cell, immune regulation, cell therapy

Rheumatoid arthritis (RA) is a chronic inflammatory autoimmune disease mediated by a variety of immune cells that is mainly defined by the erosive destruction of the joints in the extremities. The basic pathological changes are the infiltration of inflammatory cells, the destruction of cartilage, and the erosion of bone (1). The pathogenesis involves the T cell activation pathway (2), B cells (3), macrophages, osteoclasts (OCs) (4), dendritic cells (DCs) (5), and so on. Since the body's immune system is a complex network-regulation system, it is composed of innate immunity and adaptive immunity and involves interactions and regulation among innate immune cells, antigen-presenting cells, adaptive immune cells, etc. Myeloid-derived suppressor cells (MDSCs), inhibitory cells expressing the markers CD11b and Gr-1, have been found to be abundant in infection (6), tumors (7), inflammation (8), and other diseases and negatively regulate the body's immune function. MDSCs are a special group of cells that regulate the immune response. They can exert their immunosuppressive effects on a variety of immune cells through different mechanisms, resulting in declines in the body's innate and adaptive immune functions and promoting the development and progression of diseases. There have been many reports showing that MDSCs have a strong immunosuppressive effect under abnormal conditions, but the roles of MDSCs and their subgroups in autoimmune arthritis are still controversial. Therefore, this article aims to review the role of MDSCs in the pathogenesis of RA and provide a theoretical basis for future research.

ORIGIN OF MDSCs

MDSCs, which are composed of bone marrow progenitor cells and immature myeloid cells (IMCs), are a heterogeneous cell group composed of morphologically, phenotypically, and functionally diverse but also highly immunosuppressive myeloid cells (8). Under normal conditions, IMCs develop into mature DCs, macrophages, and granulocytes after being generated in the bone marrow and then participate in immune responses in specific target organs. However, under the pathological conditions of a tumor, inflammation, infection, trauma, autoimmune disease, etc., various factors can contribute to the formation of MDSCs; vascular endothelial growth factor (VEGF), granulocyte-macrophage colony-stimulating factor (GM-CSF), interleukin (IL)-4, and other cytokines can block IMC differentiation (9). IMCs inhibit their own differentiation by releasing immunosuppressive factors, such as arginase-1 (Arg-1), inducible nitric oxide synthase (iNOS), nitric oxide (NO), and reactive oxygen species (ROS), ensuring that myeloid precursor cells cannot mature. IMCs expand *in vivo*, migrate out of the bone marrow, and accumulate in the peripheral blood and spleen or lesions, where they form MDSCs (10–12). Initially, in the field of tumor biology, MDSCs were considered to be immunosuppressive cells related to tumor expansion that accumulated near tumors and in the peripheral blood, promoted immune escape by tumor cells, and accelerated disease progression (13, 14). Recent research has found that MDSCs play an important immunosuppressive role in various immune diseases, so research on MDSCs in autoimmune diseases has expanded (15, 16). Under pathological conditions, dilated MDSCs can be identified in the blood, surrounding lymphoid tissues, the spleen, cancerous tissues, and inflamed sites in the corresponding target organs. They can inhibit other immune cells through direct contact or cytokine secretion, which usually inhibits the immune response (17).

PHENOTYPES OF MDSCs

The phenotypes of MDSCs are very different in mice and humans. MDSCs lack the most basic surface recognition features due to blocked differentiation, so MDSCs are morphologically indistinguishable from granulocytes and monocytes (18).

In mice, MDSCs have specific surface markers and are defined as cells that coexpress the myeloid antigens CD11b and Gr-1. According to the morphology of this cell population and the difference in the expression levels of the two Gr-1 epitopes, Ly6G and Ly6C, they can be divided into two subsets: monocytic MDSCs (M-MDSCs) and granulocytic MDSCs (G-MDSCs), which have the phenotypes $CD11b^{+}Ly6G^{-}Ly6C^{high}$ and $CD11b^{+}Ly6G^{+}Ly6C^{low}$, respectively (19, 20). The subgroups of M-MDSCs and G-MDSCs can also be divided by CD49d and CD11b expression patterns, and their phenotypes are $CD11b^{+}Ly6G^{+/-}Ly6C^{high}CD49d^{+}$ and $CD11b^{+}Ly6G^{+}Ly6C^{low/-}CD49d^{-}$. Additionally, some surface molecules, such as IL-4Rα, F4/80, CD80, CD31, and CD115, can be used to recognize the inhibitory functions of MDSC subgroups (21).

In patients, MDSCs can also be divided into M-MDSCs and G-MDSCs. Because CD33 and CD11b are coexpressed in human subsets, which also express CD14 and CD15, respectively, the phenotypes of human M-MDSCs and G-MDSCs can be expressed as $CD33^{+}CD11b^{+}CD14^{+}$ and $CD33^{+}CD11b^{+}CD15^{+}CD14^{-}$, respectively (22, 23). In addition, because MDSCs lack surface markers expressed by mature myeloid cells or lymphoid cells and express the MHC-II molecule HLA-DR, they can also be defined as $CD33^{+}CD11b^{+}HLA\text{-}DR^{-/low}$. Due to their lack of lineage-specific antigens (Lin), such as CD3, CD19, and CD56, MDSCs are often described as $Lin^{-}CD11b^{+}CD33^{+}HLA\text{-}DR^{-}$ (24, 25). MDSCs express various surface markers and are divided into different subsets, probably because of different transcription factors and immunomodulatory molecules, such as cytokines, growth factors, and inflammatory mediators, which are presented in different disease microenvironments, blocking the normal differentiation of IMCs and thereby causing these cells to arrest in various stages of development. Therefore, MDSCs have different surface marker expression patterns at different stages. The complexity of these surface marker patterns leads to the heterogeneity of MDSCs. Thus, according to the actual pathological condition, MDSCs show different inhibitory capabilities and functional mechanisms (**Tables 1, 2**).

REGULATION BETWEEN MDSCs AND IMMUNE CELLS

MDSCs and $CD4^{+}$ T Cells, Including Their Subpopulations

$CD4^{+}$ T cells are a subset of lymphocytes that play an important role in specific immune responses. Antigen-presenting cells can activate self-reactive $CD4^{+}$ T cells by presenting cognate antigens, which results in the T cells differentiating into various types of $CD4^{+}$ helper T cells subpopulations, including Th1 cells, Th2 cells, and Th17 cells; these T cells can also differentiate into regulatory T cells (Treg cells) (36). T cells play an important role in the immune response involved in RA.

Regulatory Effect of MDSCs on $CD4^{+}$ T Cells

Kurko et al. found that MDSCs exist in the synovial tissue of RA patients. Most of these MDSCs exhibit a neutrophil phenotype and morphology and can inhibit T cell infiltration in RA. This suggests that the increase in MDSC numbers observed in the synovial fluid (SF) of RA patients may be beneficial (26). Fujii et al. found that when the severity of arthritis in collagen-induced arthritis (CIA) mice peaked, MDSCs accumulated in the spleen; adoptive transfer of MDSCs into CIA mice could reduce the severity of disease and the numbers of $CD4^{+}$ T cells and Th17 cells in the lymph nodes. MDSCs could also inhibit the proliferation of $CD4^{+}$ T cells, their differentiation into Th17 cells *in vitro* and the production of proinflammatory factors secreted by $CD4^{+}$ T cells such as IFN-γ, IL-2, IL-6, and TNF-α and promote the production of the anti-inflammatory factor

TABLE 1 | Subpopulations and phenotypes of MDSCs in RA patients.

Source	Sample	Subset	Phenotypes	Function	Reference
RA patient	Synovial fluid	G-MDSCs	$CD11b^+CD33^+HLA\text{-}DR^{lo/-}CD14^-CD15^+$	Inhibit T cells proliferation	(26)
	Synovial fluid	M-MDSCs	$CD11b^+CD33^+HLA\text{-}DR^{lo/-}CD14^+CD15^-$	/	(26)
	Peripheral blood	G-MDSCs	$CD14^-HLA\text{-}DR^-CD33^+CD11b^+$	The proportion of MDSCs is negatively correlated with the proportion of Th1 cells	(27)
	Peripheral blood	G-MDSCs	$CD14^-HLA\text{-}DR^-CD33^+CD11b^+$	The proportion of MDSCs is negatively correlated with the proportion of Th1 cells	(28)
	Synovial fluid	/	$CD11b^+CD33^+$	Promote the differentiation of human Th17 cells *in vitro*	(29)
	Peripheral blood	MDSCs	$CD11b^+CD33^+$	Positive correlated with Th17 cells and RA activity	(30)
	Peripheral blood	MDSCs	$CD14^-HLA\text{-}DR^-CD33^+CD11b^+$	Th17 cells were negatively correlated with MDSCs	(31)
	Peripheral blood	/	$CD11b^+CD33^+$	MDSCs increased significantly in RA patients with high disease activity and promoted B cell proliferation *in vitro*	(32)

TABLE 2 | Subpopulations and phenotypes of MDSCs in animal models.

Source	Sample	Subset	Phenotypes	Function	Reference
DBA/1J mice	Spleen	G-MDSCs	$CD11b^+Gr\text{-}1^{high}$	Reduction at an early stage, related to the expansion of Th17 cells	(30)
CIA model	Spleen	M-MDSCs	$CD11b^+Gr\text{-}1^{medium}$	Increased at a late stage, promotes Th17 cells differentiation *in vivo*	(30)
	Spleen	G-MDSCs	$CD11b^+Ly6C^+Ly6G^+$	Inhibit T cells proliferation and Th1, Th17 cells differentiation	(25)
	Spleen	M-MDSCs	$CD11b^+Ly6C^+Ly6G^-$	Moderately inhibits T cells proliferation, but its adoptive transfer does not affect Th1 and Th17 responses *in vivo*	(25)
	Bone marrow	M-MDSCs	$CD11b^+Ly6C^{high}Ly6G^-$	Inhibit the proliferation of T cells, B cells	(33)
	Spleen	M-MDSCs	$CD11c^-CD11b^+Ly6G^-Ly6C^{high}$	IL-10-mediated reduction of joint inflammation after adoptive transfer	(34)
	Spleen	G-MDSCs	$CD11c^-CD11b^+Ly6G^+Ly6C^{low}$	Inhibit Th17 differentiation and promote Treg cells expansion	(34)
C57BL/6 mice	Spleen, Paw	M-MDSCs	$CD11b^+Ly6C^{high}Ly6G^-$	Inhibit T cells proliferation and IFN-γ secretion, promote Th17 cells differentiation *in vitro*	(29)
CIA model		G-MDSCs	$CD11b^+Ly6C^{low}Ly6G^+$	No effect of inhibiting T cells proliferation and IFN-γ secretion *in vitro*	(29)
BALB/c mice PGIA model	Synovial fluid	G-MDSCs	$Ly6G^{high}Ly6C^{int/low}$	Inhibits DC maturation and specific T cells proliferation	(35)

RA, Rheumatoid Arthritis; CIA, Collagen-induced arthritis; PGIA, Proteoglycan-induced mouse arthritis model; G-MDSCs, granulocytic myeloid-derived suppressor cells; M-MDSCs, monocytic myeloid-derived suppressor cells; DC, dendritic cells.

IL-10 secreted by $CD4^+$ T cells, which suggests that MDSCs play an important role in the regulation of CIA by inhibiting the proinflammatory response of $CD4^+$ T cells (37). Crook et al. (33) found that in autoimmune arthritis, M-MDSCs inhibit the proliferation of autologous $CD4^+$ T cells in the CIA model in a manner dependent on iNOS and IFN-γ. Egelston et al. (35) found that the synovial fluid of proteoglycan-induced arthritis (PGIA) mice contains a large number of MDSCs, which can inhibit T cell proliferation effectively through iNOS and ROS. Park et al. (34) found that MDSCs derived from CIA mice reduced IL-17 production and increased FOXP3 expression in $CD4^+$ T cells *in vitro*. In RA-associated interstitial lung disease (RA-ILD), Sendo et al. (38) found that $CD11b^+Ly6C^{high}$ cells (M-MDSCs) isolated from the lungs could develop the $CD11b^+Gr\text{-}1^{dim}$ phenotype when cultured with GM-CSF and IL-4-producing cells and the $CD11b^+Gr\text{-}1^{dim}$ cells could inhibit T cell proliferation. In addition, lung MDSCs inhibit the proliferation of $CD4^+$ T cells in an MDSC density-dependent manner and inhibit the differentiation of $CD4^+$ T cells into Th17 cells (39).

Obviously, in RA patients, MDSCs can inhibit infiltrating T cells in the joints. In autoimmune arthritis mice, MDSCs mainly inhibit $CD4^+$ T cells through iNOS, ROS, and IFN-γ. MDSCs can inhibit $CD4^+$ T cell proliferation, differentiation into Th17 cells, and secretion of proinflammatory factors such as IFN-γ, IL-2, IL-6, IL-17, and TNF-α and promote the production of the anti-inflammatory factor IL-10. The production of IL-10 increases

FOXP3 expression *in vitro*. These results suggest that MDSCs play a crucial role in the immune regulation occurring during RA.

Regulatory Effect of MDSCs on Th1 Cells

Th1 cells play an important role in the development of RA (40). Th1 cells and the signature cytokine IFN-γ play important roles in RA inflammation, and one of the methods to treat RA is to inhibit the Th1 response (41).

Studies have found that peripheral blood MDSCs in RA patients are positively correlated with disease activity and that the proportion of MDSCs is negatively correlated with the proportion of Th1 cells, which suggests that in the peripheral blood of RA patients, MDSCs and Th1 cells may be mutually antagonistic and participate in the development of RA together (27, 28). Park et al. (34) injected MDSCs into CIA mice *in vivo* and found that the number of Th1 cells in the spleen of the mice decreased, suggesting that MDSCs have an inhibitory effect on Th1 cells. Wang et al. (25) found that adoptive transfer of G-MDSCs into CIA mice reduces joint inflammation and the frequency of Th1 cells in the draining lymph node, suggesting that G-MDSCs have an inhibitory effect on Th1 cells in CIA that reduces joint inflammation.

All these studies have shown that MDSCs are negatively associated with Th1 cells in the peripheral blood of RA patients and the spleen of CIA mice. Further studies are required to fully understand the role of MDSCs in the regulation of Th1 cells during the pathological development of RA.

Regulatory Effect of MDSCs on Th17 Cells

Th17 cells are a subset of inflammatory CD4$^+$ T cells that mainly secrete IL-17. Studies have found that Th17 cells are associated with many autoimmune diseases, including RA, psoriasis, and multiple sclerosis (42). Studies have also found that blocking the function of Th17 cells may inhibit the development of RA. As a class of immunosuppressive cells, MDSCs play an essential role in the development of RA, and recent studies have found that in RA, MDSCs have a regulatory effect on Th17 cells.

Guo et al. found that the frequency of MDSCs in the synovial tissue of RA patients was positively associated with the level of IL-17A. Additionally, the MDSCs of RA patients and CIA mice could both promote the differentiation of human Th17 cells *in vitro*, and MDSCs could promote Th17/IL-17 responses. The increase in Th17 cells infiltration that occurs during the progression of CIA affected the accumulation of MDSCs, and the removal of MDSCs reduced the frequency of Th17 cells in the spleen of CIA mice, which suggests that MDSCs are positively correlated with Th17 cells and that MDSCs have certain proinflammatory effects. In addition, M-MDSCs were more effective than G-MDSCs in promoting Th17 cell differentiation (29). Zhang et al. found that the numbers of CD14$^+$HLA-DR$^{-/low}$ cells in the peripheral blood of RA patients were significantly higher than those in healthy controls and that the expansion of CD14$^+$HLA-DR$^{-/low}$ cells was closely associated with Th17 cells and Disease Activity Score-28 (DAS28) results. In CIA mice, the depletion of MDSCs *in vivo* led to the inhibition of T cell proliferation and reductions in IL-17A and IL-1β production, while adoptive transfer of MDSCs could lead to increased disease severity in mice, including joint swelling, cell infiltration, bone erosion, and cartilage destruction, and significantly increased serum IL-17A and IL-1β levels, which suggests that MDSCs play important roles in the development of RA and CIA (30). Studies have found that MDSCs are the main source of IL-1β, that MDSCs in CIA mice can express high levels of IL-1β and that MDSCs promote the differentiation of Th17 cells and CD4$^+$ T cells via the IL-1β signaling pathway, which suggests that MDSCs in CIA mice can promote the Th17 cell response through high expression of IL-1β (29, 30, 43). Cheng et al. found that the proportion of CD11b$^+$Gr1$^+$ MDSCs in their CIA group was positively correlated with the proportion of Th17 cells. After coculturing MDSCs and CD4$^+$ T cells, the proinflammatory factor IL-1β was highly expressed, while after blocking IL-1β, Th17 cell numbers, and IL-17A, STAT3, and RORγt mRNA expression levels were significantly reduced, which suggests that MDSCs, as a potential source of IL-1β, have a proinflammatory effect, mediating CD4$^+$ T cell differentiation into Th17 cells (44). Jiao et al. (31) found that in the peripheral blood of RA patients, Th17 cells were negatively correlated with MDSCs. Li et al. (45) noted that G-MDSCs could suppress the production of Th17 cells by secreting exosomes to ameliorate the pathology of CIA mice. Studies have found that adoptive transfer of MDSCs is beneficial in autoimmune arthritis and can reduce the number of Th17 cells in the draining lymph nodes and joint tissues, thereby reducing joint inflammation (25, 37, 46).

The above research shows that MDSC numbers are increased in the peripheral blood of RA patients, which promotes increases in the levels Th17 cells, IL-17A, and IL-1β. MDSCs can enhance the response of Th17 cells by secreting IL-1β, which suggests that MDSCs are mainly responsible for promoting the inflammatory effect. However, another study found that MDSCs were negatively correlated with Th17 cells in the peripheral blood of RA patients, suggesting that MDSCs can reduce the number of Th17 cells to relieve joint inflammation. MDSCs can promote Th17 cell responses in RA, mainly by secreting IL-1β, but MDSCs can also have an inhibitory effect on Th17 cells; the specific mechanism is not clear. Therefore, further research on the regulatory effect of MDSCs on Th17 cells in RA could clarify the role of MDSCs in RA.

Regulatory Effect of MDSCs on Treg Cells

In RA, Treg cells can be recruited to inflamed joints to exert a local inhibitory effect, which leads to increased levels of Treg cells in the joint synovial fluid and decreased levels in the peripheral blood (47). Some studies have found that MDSCs can participate in the development of RA by regulating Treg cells.

Park et al. showed that the number of Tregs in the spleen of mice treated with MDSCs increased and that the injection of G-MDSCs into CIA mice could promote Treg cell proliferation and weaken the joint inflammation in the mice. Treg cells were expanded *in vitro* in the presence of an anti-IL-10 antibody, and this antibody blocked the expansion effect of MDSCs on Treg cells, suggesting that without IL-10, MDSCs cannot inhibit joint inflammation. This may suggest that IL-10 plays an important role in the enhancement of Treg responses by MDSCs (34).

The above research suggests that G-MDSCs can promote the proliferation of Treg cells in CIA mice and that via IL-10, MDSCs can promote the proliferation of Treg cells *in vitro*. Further studies on the interaction among MDSCs, IL-10, and Treg cells in RA may help better clarify the role of MDSCs in RA.

Regulatory Effect of MDSCs on B Cells

B cells play a major role in the pathogenesis of RA, which not only promotes the production of autoantibodies but also regulates the function of T cells and DCs and promotes the development of ectopic lymphoid neoplasia and release of inflammatory mediators (48). At present, B cell-targeted therapy is effective in early and late established RA (49). Some studies have found that MDSCs have a regulatory effect on B cells in RA.

Crook et al. (33) showed that M-MDSCs in CIA mouse bone marrow could inhibit the proliferation and activation of B cells and produce specific antibodies through nitric oxide (NO) and prostaglandin E2 (PGE_2) to suppress the immune response. Another analysis of the peripheral blood of RA patients found that MDSC numbers were significantly increased in RA patients with high disease activity and these MDSCs promoted B cells proliferation *in vitro* (32).

MDSCs can inhibit B cells via NO and PGE_2 in the CIA model and promote B cell expansion in the peripheral blood of RA patients. The difference in effect may be due to the different sources of MDSCs, but further research is still needed. Overall, MDSCs may participate in the development of RA through B cell regulation, but the specific regulation of B cells by MDSCs still needs to be further explored.

Regulatory Effect of MDSCs on Macrophages

One of the typical symptoms of RA is inflammation caused by the accumulation of fibroblasts, lymphocytes, neutrophils, and monocytes/macrophages. Among these cells, activated macrophages are the main source of proinflammatory cytokines and chemokines, including TNF-α, IL-6, CXCL4, and CXCL7. Activated macrophages can activate endothelial cells and induce inflammation in the synovium and the production of OCs, eventually leading to joint damage (50, 51). In the pathogenesis of RA, macrophages play an important role. The increase in the number of macrophages in the synovium is considered an early biomarker of RA, and numerical changes can be used to distinguish effective treatment, ineffective treatment, and placebo treatment (52). Some studies have found that in the process of RA, MDSCs can regulate macrophages.

To evaluate the effect of MDSCs on macrophages *in vivo*, Zhang et al. (46) examined the frequency of macrophages in the draining lymph nodes and joint tissues of CIA mice treated with a phosphate-buffered saline (PBS) solution and MDSCs and found that the numbers of $CD11b^{+}CD68^{+}$ macrophages in the CIA mice treated with MDSCs were significantly reduced in the draining lymph nodes and joint tissues, suggesting that adoptive transfer of MDSCs can reduce the degrees of arthritis and histological damage in the CIA model by suppressing macrophages.

Macrophages play a key role in the pathological development of RA, and the regulatory mechanism by which MDSCs affect macrophages is currently uncertain. Therefore, further research on the MDSC-mediated regulatory mechanism modulating macrophages in RA may provide new ideas to clarify the specific roles of MDSCs in RA and the treatment of RA.

Regulatory Effect of MDSCs on DCs

DCs are important innate immune cells and professional antigen-presenting cells. They play a vital role in the initiation of immunity. Some studies have found that DCs play an important role in the pathological process of RA (53). Studies have found that MDSCs have a regulatory effect on DCs.

To study the possible effects of synovial fluid (SF) cells on DC maturation, Egelston et al. observed MHC-II and CD86 expression by DCs cultured alone or in the presence of SF cells (90% $Gr\text{-}1^{+}CD11b^{+}$ myeloid cells with a neutrophil morphology). The levels of MHC-II and CD86 in the DCs were significantly reduced by coculture with SF cells compared to culturing without SF cells after 24 h. This may suggest that $Gr\text{-}1^{+}CD11b^{+}$ SF cells significantly reduce the expression levels of MHC-II and CD86, both of which play key roles in antigen presentation by DCs, while the results for $Gr\text{-}1^{+}CD11b^{+}$ cells also indicate that the SF cells of PGIA mice have characteristics of MDSCs, suggesting that MDSCs inhibit the maturation and activation of DCs *in vitro* (35).

The SF cells of arthritic joints in PGIA mice appear to have characteristics of MDSCs and can inhibit DCs by reducing the expression of MHC-II and CD86. Further investigations on the immunomodulatory effects of MDSCs on DCs may provide new ideas related to the immunomodulatory functions of MDSCs in RA.

Regulatory Effect of MDSCs on OCs

Bone erosion is a sign of severe RA. Studies have found that OCs play a major role in bone resorption. Increased OC numbers or activity often leads to cartilage and bone destruction (54), and cytokines such as IL-1α, IL-1β, IL-6, IL-11, TNF-α, and M-CSF can provide signals for OC differentiation and bone resorption (55). Some studies have found that MDSCs are one of the types of OC precursor cells.

Sawant et al. cocultured MDSCs isolated from the bone marrow of breast cancer bone metastatic tumor-bearing mice with M-CSF and RANKL and stained the cells with TRAP to observe the expression of F4-80 during OC differentiation. They found that MDSCs are a new group of true OC progenitor cells and that MDSCs differentiate into OCs in a manner dependent on NO and have bone destruction function both *in vivo* and *in vitro*, suggesting that targeting MDSCs in breast cancer patients may reduce primary tumor growth and bone metastasis growth (56). Su et al. (57) found that in periodontitis, *Porphyromonas gingivalis* can induce the expansion of three subpopulations of MDSCs ($Ly6G^{++}Ly6C^{+}$, $Ly6G^{+}Ly6C^{++}$, and $Ly6G^{+}Ly6C^{+}$), and the $CD11b^{+}Ly6G^{+}Ly6C^{++}$ subpopulation can differentiate into OCs and exert inhibitory effects on T cells, which suggests that MDSCs not only have an immunosuppressive effect but also promote OC development.

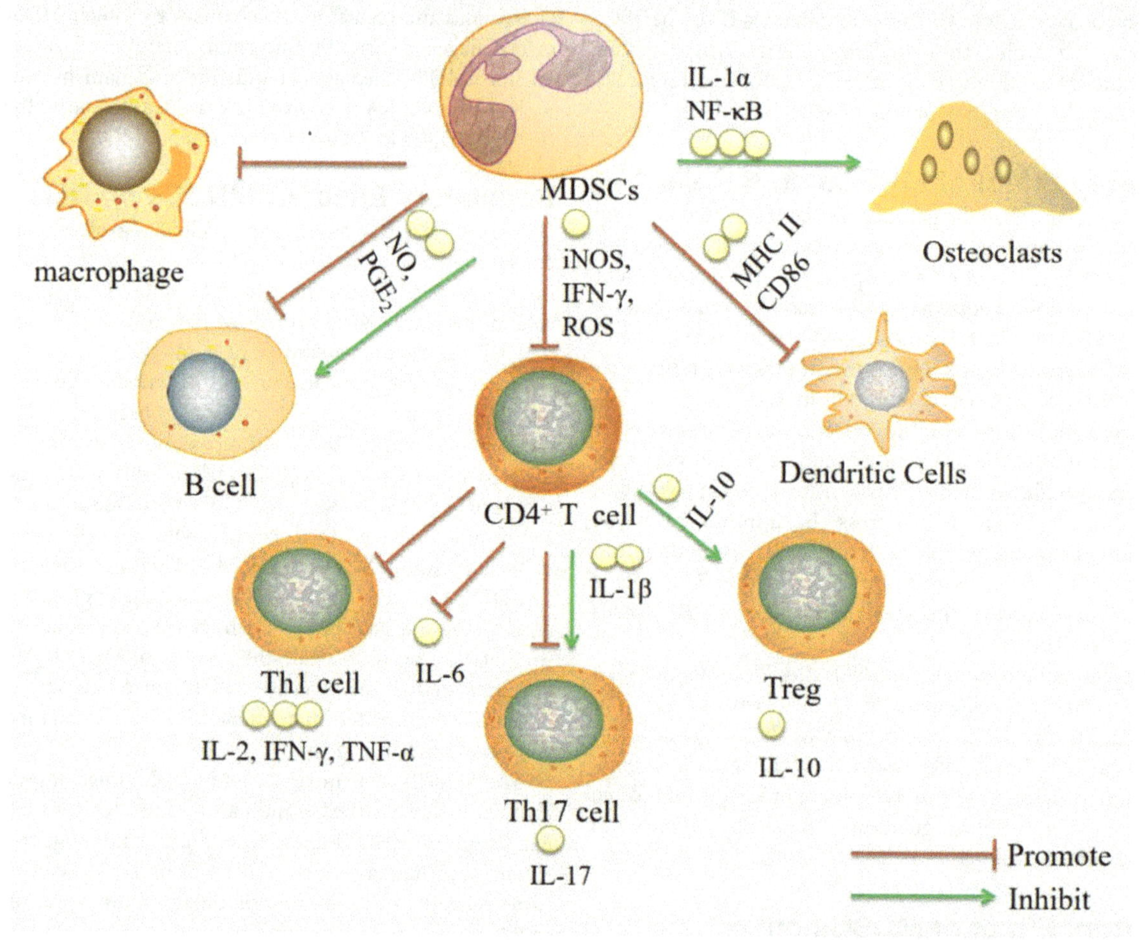

FIGURE 1 | Immuregulatory effect of MDSCs on immune cells. IL-1α, interleukin-1α; NF-κB, nuclear transcription factor kappa B; iNOS, inducible nitric oxide synthase; IFN-γ, interferon-γ; ROS, reactive oxygen species; NO, nitric oxide; PGE2, Prostaglandin E2; IL-1β, Interleukin-1β; IL-10, Interleukin-10; IL-2, Interleukin-2; IL-6, Interleukin-6; IL-17, Interleukin-17; TNF-α, Tumor Necrosis Factor-α.

Recent studies have found that MDSCs, as precursor cells of OCs, play an important role in the development of autoimmune arthritis. Zhang et al. found that compared with that in the bone marrow of normal mice, the number of MDSCs in the bone marrow of CIA mice was significantly increased and that the CIA MDSCs were more likely to differentiate into OCs and contribute to bone resorption, thereby causing bone destruction. When MDSCs were cocultured with M-CSF and RANKL, they differentiated into OCs, while differentiation was inhibited when they were cocultured with an inhibitor of NF-κB. These results suggest that NF-κB plays an important role in the differentiation of MDSCs into OCs and that IL-1α activates the NF-κB pathway. Furthermore, when OC differentiation medium is supplemented with IL-1α (10 ng/ml), the differentiation of MDSCs into OCs is enhanced, suggesting that IL-1α can activate the NF-κB pathway to promote OC differentiation (58).

It is clear that MDSCs can differentiate into OCs in tumors and inflammatory diseases and have bone destruction functions *in vivo*. In CIA mice, MDSCs are one of the types of OC precursor cells. In the context of culture with M-CSF and RANKL, IL-1α can activate the NF-κB pathway to promote MDSC differentiation into OCs, resulting in an increased degree of bone destruction. Whether bone destruction is related to the number of circulating MDSCs and whether MDSCs can be used as a biomarker to evaluate the aggressiveness of RA still need further study.

CONCLUSION

Similar reviews have also studied the roles of MDSCs in autoimmune arthritis. Li et al. (45) reviewed the effects and actions of MDSC subpopulations during the development of autoimmune arthritis and reported that both MDSC subpopulations play important roles in regulating the proliferation, response, and differentiation of $CD4^+$ T cells during the progression of autoimmune arthritis. Rajabinejad et al. (59) described the functions of MDSCs and the relationship between MDSCs and inflammation in RA, concluding that there are two different hypotheses related to MDSC function in RA: MDSCs can exert a proinflammatory effect by increasing the number of Th17 cells, but MDSCs can also increase the population of Tregs to produce an anti-inflammatory effect. In our review, we have integrated the literature on the regulatory effects of MDSCs on immune cells in the field of RA, describing the functions of MDSCs in arthritis model mice and RA patients and focusing on the effects of MDSCs on various types of cells. We report that the proinflammatory and anti-inflammatory functions of MDSCs are not only mediated by increasing the number of Th17 cells and the number of Tregs, respectively.

MDSCs have both proinflammatory and anti-inflammatory functions in RA and RA animal models. The proinflammatory function is mainly supported by the following observations: MDSCs can increase Th17 cell, B cell, and OC activity. MDSCs can promote Th17 cell responses by secreting IL-1β. As precursors of OCs, MDSCs can differentiate into OCs via NF-κB pathway signaling activated by IL-1α. The anti-inflammatory effect is mainly supported by the following observations: MDSCs can inhibit $CD4^+$ T cells, Th1 cells, Th17 cells, B cells, macrophages, and DCs and promote Treg cell expansion. MDSCs inhibit $CD4^+$ T cells, which secrete proinflammatory factors such as IFN-γ, IL-2, IL-6, IL-17, and TNF-α, by inhibiting iNOS, ROS, and IFN-γ and promote the production of the anti-inflammatory factor IL-10. MDSCs can suppress DCs by reducing MHC-II and CD86 expression. MDSCs can expand Treg cells *in vitro* through the action of IL-10. MDSCs can inhibit B cells through NO and PGE_2 (**Figure 1**).

However, there are no reports on the relationship between MDSCs and NK cells in RA, and Nausch et al. (60) found that in RMA-S tumor mice, M-MDSCs could express retinoic acid early inducible-1 (RAE-1) ligand to interact with NKG2D ligands on NK cells and activate NK cells to produce large amounts of IFN-γ. This suggests that MDSCs have a regulatory effect on NK cells and that studying the interaction between MDSCs and NK cells may provide new ideas related to the mechanism involving MDSCs in the pathological process of RA.

MDSCs are IMCs and have an inhibitory effect on the antitumor immune response. MDSCs play a key role in maintaining immunosuppression under chronic inflammatory conditions, so inhibition of MDSC expansion and activation by MDSC-targeted agents may increase the efficiency of the immune system. At present, many drugs targeting MDSCs have been applied for tumor treatment, and the immunosuppressive effects of these drugs have also been shown to affect autoimmune diseases (61). Nishimura et al. (62) found that the JAK inhibitor tofacitinib could significantly promote the proliferation of MDSCs in the bone marrow of SKG mice and improve the arthritic process. In other autoimmune diseases, MDSCs have been found to have a regulatory effect on immune cells. Iwata et al. (63) found that in the MRL-Faslpr lupus mouse model, $CD11b^+Gr\text{-}1^{low}$ cells inhibited the proliferation of $CD4^+$ T cells through Arg-1, and the percentage of $CD11b^+Gr\text{-}1^{low}$ cells was increased in the spleen, kidneys, and blood of 10-week-old lupus mice, suggesting that these cells contribute to immune regulation. Knier et al. (64) found that in experimental autoimmune encephalomyelitis, $Ly6G^+$ neutrophils differentiated into MDSCs in the central nervous system of wild-type mice in a STAT3-dependent manner, controlling the accumulation and activation of B cells in this compartment, and therapeutic interventions that modulate the interaction of MDSCs with B cells might prevent the continuation of the inflammatory response in the central nervous system compartment in chronic autoimmune diseases (where local aggregates of B cells are drivers of immunopathology) (64).

In conclusion, existing studies have suggested that MDSCs play an important role in RA. The heterogeneity, plasticity, and multiple phenotypes of MDSCs regulate T cells, B cells, DCs, OCs, macrophages, and other cells through various mechanisms to influence the immune response. However, given the existing mechanisms, it is difficult to provide a comprehensive hypothesis to explain the specific role of MDSCs. The differentiation, expansion, and migration of MDSCs are also constrained by many factors, so cell therapy also faces many obstacles (17). Understanding the inherent multifunctional nature of MDSCs and the ability to influence organ-specific targets will help elucidate the mechanisms of autoimmune diseases and possible new treatments (65). Therefore, further study of the mechanism of action of MDSCs in RA may provide new ideas for the diagnosis, treatment, and prognosis of RA.

AUTHOR CONTRIBUTIONS

ZF and MC conceived the review. LY, ML, TY, JJ, and XH searched databases and drafted the manuscript. ZF, GJ, and MC amended the final manuscript. All authors contributed to the article and approved the submitted version.

ACKNOWLEDGMENTS

Special thanks to GJ for English language editing.

REFERENCES

1. Aletaha D, Smolen JS. Diagnosis and management of rheumatoid arthritis: a review. *JAMA*. (2018) 320:1360–72. doi: 10.1001/jama.2018.13103
2. Smolen JS, Aletaha D, Barton A, Burmester GR, Emery P, Firestein GS, et al. Rheumatoid arthritis. *Nat Rev Dis Primers*. (2018) 4:18001. doi: 10.1038/nrdp.2018.1
3. Alivernini S, Tolusso B, Fedele AL, Clara DM, Gianfranco F, Elisa G. The B side of rheumatoid arthritis pathogenesis.

Pharmacol Res. (2019) 149:104465. doi: 10.1016/j.phrs.2019.104465
4. Liu H, Zhu Y, Gao Y, Qi D, Zhao L, Zhao L. Nr1d1 modulates synovial inflammation and bone destruction in rheumatoid arthritis. *Cell Death Dis.* (2020) 11:129. doi: 10.1038/s41419-020-2314-6
5. Leal Rojas IM, Mok WH, Pearson FE, Minoda Y, Kenna TJ, Barnardet RT, et al. Human blood Cd1c dendritic cells promote Th1 and Th17 effector function in memory Cd4 T cells. *Front Immunol.* (2017) 8:971. doi: 10.3389/fimmu.2017.00971
6. Tandeka M, Anca D, Plessiset ND. Corrigendum: the emerging role of myeloid-derived suppressor cells in tuberculosis. *Front Immunol.* (2019) 10:1528. doi: 10.3389/fimmu.2019.01528
7. Tian X, Shen H, Li Z, Wang T, Wang S. Tumor-derived exosomes, myeloid-derived suppressor cells, and tumor microenvironment. *J Hematol Oncol.* (2019) 12:84. doi: 10.1186/s13045-019-0772-z
8. Leija MG, Gonzalez RJ, Sandoval BJ, Higuera SI, Espinoza IM, González GR, et al. Long non-coding RNAs: regulators of the activity of myeloid-derived suppressor cells. *Front Immunol.* (2019) 10:1734. doi: 10.3389/fimmu.2019.01734
9. Wu H, Yi HF, Yang YG. The role of MDSC in autoimmune diseases. *Chin J Immunol.* (2017) 33:321–7. doi: 10.3969/j.issn.1000-484X.2017.03.001
10. Ugel S, Delpozzo F, Desantis G. Therapeutic targeting of myeloid-derived suppressor cells. *Curr Opin Pharmacol.* (2009) 9:470–81. doi: 10.1016/j.coph.2009.06.014
11. Gabrilovich DI, Nagaraj S. Myeloid-derived suppressor cells as regulators of the immune system. *Nat Rev Immunol.* (2009) 9:162–74. doi: 10.1038/nri2506
12. Wynn TA. Myeloid-cell differentiation redefined in cancer. *Nat Immunol.* (2013) 14:197–9. doi: 10.1038/ni.2539
13. Parker KH, Beury DW, Ostrand-Rosenberg S. Myeloid-derived suppressor cells: critical cells driving immune suppression in the tumor microenvironment. *Adv Cancer Res.* (2015) 128:95–139. doi: 10.1016/bs.acr.2015.04.002
14. Gabrilovich DI, Ostrand-Rosenberg S, Bronte V. Coordinated regulation of myeloid cells by tumors. *Nat Rev Immunol.* (2012) 12:253–68. doi: 10.1038/nri3175
15. Sica A, Massarotti M. Myeloid suppressor cells in cancer and autoimmunity. *J Autoimmun.* (2017) 85:117–25. doi: 10.1016/j.jaut.2017.07.010
16. Barnie PA, Zhang P, Lv H, Wang D, Su X, Su Z, et al. Myeloid-derived suppressor cells and myeloid regulatory cells in cancer and autoimmune disorders. *Exp Ther Med.* (2017) 13:378–88. doi: 10.3892/etm.2016.4018
17. Boros P, Ochando J, Zeher M. Myeloid-derived suppressor cells and autoimmunity. *Hum Immunol.* (2016) 77:631–6. doi: 10.1016/j.humimm.2016.05.024
18. Zhao C, Guo J, Li HZ. The function of myeloid-derived suppressor cells and its relationship with autoimmune diseases. *J Cell Mol Immunol.* (2015) 31:1433–36. doi: 10.13423/j.cnki.cjcmi.007533
19. Peranzoni E, Zilio S, Marigo I, Dolcetti L, Zanovello P, Mandruzzato S, et al. Myeloid-derived suppressor cell heterogeneity and subset definition. *Curr Opin Immunol.* (2010) 22:238–44. doi: 10.1016/j.coi.2010.01.021
20. Ribechini E, Greifenberg V, Sandwick S, Lutz MB. Subsets, expansion, and activation of myeloid-derived suppressor cells. *Med Microbiol Immunol.* (2010) 199:273–81. doi: 10.1007/s00430-010-0151-4
21. Forghani P, Khorramizadeh MR, Waller EK. Natural suppressor cells; past, present, and future. *Front Biosci (Elite Ed).* (2012) 4:1237–45. doi: 10.2741/e454
22. Greten TF, Manns MP, Korangy F. Myeloid-derived suppressor cells in human disease. *Int Immunopharmacol.* (2011) 11:802–7. doi: 10.1016/j.intimp.2011.01.003
23. Ko JS, Bukowski RM, Fincke JH. Myeloid-derived suppressor cells: a novel therapeutic target. *Curr Oncol Rep.* (2009) 11:87–93. doi: 10.1007/s11912-009-0014-6
24. Wesolowski R, Markowitz J, Iii WEC. Myeloid-derived suppressor cells - a new therapeutic target in the treatment of cancer. *J Immunother Cancer.* (2013) 1:10. doi: 10.1186/2051-1426-1-10
25. Wang WH, Jiao ZJ, Duan TH, Liu MH, Lu LW. Functional characterization of myeloid-derived suppressor cell subpopulations during the development of experimental arthritis. *Eur J Immunol.* (2015) 45:464–73. doi: 10.1002/eji.201444799
26. Kurko J, Vida A, Glant TT, Scanzello CR, Katz SR, Nair A, et al. Identification of myeloid-derived suppressor cells in the synovial fluid of patients with rheumatoid arthritis: a pilot study. *BMC Musculoskelet Disord.* (2014) 15:281. doi: 10.1186/1471-2474-15-281
27. Xu WM, Gong AH, Wang H, Hua SH, Wang XH, Chen Y, et al. Detection of peripheral blood myeloid-derived suppressor cells in patients with rheumatoid arthritis and its correlation analysis with Thl/Th2 cells. *J Jiangsu Univ.* (2013) 23:140–3.
28. Liu HX, Zheng Y, Luo XJ, Wang P, Peng P, Jiang ZJ. Detection of peripheral blood myeloid-derived inhibitory cells in patients with rheumatoid arthritis and their correlation with Th1/Th2 cells. *Lab Med Clin Med.* (2014) 11:3134–6. doi: 10.3969/j.issn.1672-9455.2014.22.019
29. Guo C, Hu F, Yi H, Feng ZT, Li CZ, Shi LJ, et al. Myeloid-derived suppressor cells have a proinflammatory role in the pathogenesis of autoimmune arthritis. *Ann Rheum Dis.* (2015) 75:278–85. doi: 10.1136/annrheumdis-2014-205508
30. Zhang H, Wang S, Huang Y, Wang H, Zhao J, Gaskin F, et al. Myeloid-derived suppressor cells are proinflammatory and regulate collagen-induced arthritis through manipulating Th17 cell differentiation. *Clin Immunol.* (2015) 157:175–86. doi: 10.1016/j.clim.2015.02.001
31. Jiao Z, Hua S, Wang W, Wang H, Gao J, Wang X. Increased circulating myeloid-derived suppressor cells correlated negatively with Th17 cells in patients with rheumatoid arthritis. *Scand J Rheumatol.* (2013) 42:85–90. doi: 10.3109/03009742.2012.716450
32. Chen W, Hu FL, Liu HJ, Xu LL, Li YN, Li ZG. Myeloid-derived suppressor cells from rheumatoid arthritis promote their own B cell proliferation. *J Peking Univ.* (2017) 49:819–23. doi: 10.3969/j.issn.1671-167X.2017.05.013
33. Crook KR, Jin M, Weeks MF, Rampersad RR, Baldi RM, Glekas AS, et al. Myeloid-derived suppressor cells regulate T cell and B cell responses during autoimmune disease. *J Leukoc Biol.* (2015) 97:573–82. doi: 10.1189/jlb.4A0314-139R
34. Park MJ, Lee SH, Kim EK, Lee EJ, Baek JA, Park SH, et al. Interleukin-10 produced by myeloid-derived suppressor cells is critical for the induction of tregs and attenuation of rheumatoid inflammation in mice. *Sci Rep.* (2018) 8:3753. doi: 10.1038/s41598-018-21856-2
35. Egelston C, Kurkó J, Besenyei T, Tryniszewska B, Rauch TA, Glant TT, et al. Suppression of dendritic cell maturation and T cell proliferation by synovial fluid myeloid cells from mice with autoimmune arthritis. *Arthritis Rheum.* (2012) 64:3179–88. doi: 10.1002/art.34494
36. Zazueta-Favela D, Donis-Maturano L, Licea-Navarro AF, Bernáldez-Sarabia J, Dan KWL, Cota-Arceet JM. Marine peptides as immunomodulators: derived synthetic conotoxins induce Il-10 production by regulatory T cells (Cd4foxp3). *Immunopharmacol Immunotoxicol.* (2019) 41:463–8. doi: 10.1080/08923973.2019.1641114
37. Fujii W, Ashihara E, Hirai H, Nagahara H, Kajitani N, Fujioka K, et al. Myeloid-derived suppressor cells play crucial roles in the regulation of mouse collagen-induced arthritis. *J Immunol.* (2013) 191:1073–81. doi: 10.4049/jimmunol.1203535
38. Sendo S, Saegusa J, Okano T, Takahashi S, Akashi K, Morinobu A, et al. Cd11b+Gr-1 tolerogenic dendritic cell-like cells are expanded in interstitial lung disease in SKG mice. *Arthritis Rheumatol.* (2017) 69:2314–27. doi: 10.1002/art.40231
39. Sendo S, Saegusa J, Yamada H, Nishimura K, Morinobu A, et al. Tofacitinib facilitates the expansion of myeloid-derived suppressor cells and ameliorates interstitial lung disease in SKG mice. *Arthritis Res Ther.* (2019) 21:184. doi: 10.1186/s13075-019-1963-2
40. Wang Z, Zhuo F, Chu P, Yang XL, Zhao G. Germacrone alleviates collagen-induced arthritis via regulating Th1/Th2 balance and Nf-κb activation. *Biochem Biophys Res Commun.* (2019) 518:560–4. doi: 10.1016/j.bbrc.2019.08.084
41. Guggino G, Giardina AR, Raimondo S, Giardina G, Sireci G, Dieli F, Peralta M, et al. Targeting Il-6 signaling in early rheumatoid arthritis is followed by Th1 and Th17 suppression and Th2 expansion. *Clin Exp Rheumatol.* (2014) 32:77–81. Available online at: https://europepmc.org/article/med/24429356
42. Tesmer LA, Lundy SK, Sarkar S, Fox D. A Th17 cells in human disease. *Immunol Rev.* (2008) 223:87–113. doi: 10.1111/j.1600-065X.2008.00628.x
43. Yi H, Guo C, Yu X, Zuo D, Wang XY. Mouse Cd11b+Gr-1+ myeloid cells can promote Th17 cell differentiation and experimental

autoimmune encephalomyelitis. *J Immunol.* (2012) 189:4295–304. doi: 10.4049/jimmunol.1200086

44. Cheng SY, Chen XY, Li HW, Xie Y, Li F, Zeng HS. Myeloid-derived inhibitory cells in the collagen-induced arthritis model promote the differentiation of Th17 cells through interleukin-1β. *Chin J Clin Immun Allergy.* (2018) 12:11–20.
45. Li M, Zhu D, Wang TT, Xia XL, Tian J, Wang SJ. Roles of myeloid-derived suppressor cell subpopulations in autoimmune arthritis. *Front Immunol.* (2018) 9:2849. doi: 10.3389/fimmu.2018.02849
46. Zhang L, Zhang ZM, Zhang HL, Wu M, Wang YX. Myeloid-derived suppressor cells protect mouse models from autoimmune arthritis via controlling inflammatory response. *Inflammation.* (2014) 37:670–7. doi: 10.1007/s10753-013-9783-z
47. Wang Y, Tian J, Wang S. The potential therapeutic role of myeloid-derived suppressor cells in autoimmune arthritis. *Semin Arthritis Rheum.* (2016) 45:490–5. doi: 10.1016/j.semarthrit.2015.07.003
48. Martin F, Chan AC. B cell immunobiology in disease: evolving concepts from the clinic. *Ann Rev Immunol.* (2006) 24:467–96. doi: 10.1146/annurev.immunol.24.021605.090517
49. Gerlag DM, Safy M, Maijer KI, Tang MW, Tas SW, Starmans-Kool MJF, et al. Effects of B-cell directed therapy on the preclinical stage of rheumatoid arthritis: the PRAIRI study. *Ann Rheum Dis.* (2019) 149:104465. doi: 10.1136/annrheumdis-2017-212763
50. Dimitroulas T, Nikas SN, Trontzas P, Kitas GD. Biologic therapies and systemic bone loss in rheumatoid arthritis. *Autoimmun Rev.* (2013) 12:958–66. doi: 10.1016/j.autrev.2013.03.015
51. Yeo L, Adlard N, Biehl M, Juarez M, Smallie T, Snow M, et al. Expression Of chemokines Cxcl4 and Cxcl7 by synovial macrophages defines an early stage of rheumatoid arthritis. *Ann Rheum Dis.* (2016) 75:763–71. doi: 10.1136/annrheumdis-2014-206921
52. Wijbrandts CA, Vergunst CE, Haringman JJ, Gerlag DM, Smeets TJM, Paul PT. Absence of changes in the number of synovial sublining macrophages after ineffective treatment for rheumatoid arthritis: implications for use of synovial sublining macrophages as a biomarker. *Arthritis Rheum.* (2007) 56:3869–71. doi: 10.1002/art.22964
53. Liu D, Li T, Luo H, Zuo XX, Liu SJ, Wu SY. The effect of the cholinergic anti-inflammatory pathway on collagen-induced arthritis involves the modulation of dendritic cell differentiation. *Arthritis Res Therapy.* (2018) 20:263. doi: 10.1186/s13075-018-1759-9
54. Rodan GA, Martin TJ. Therapeutic approaches to bone diseases. *Science.* (2000) 289:1508–14. doi: 10.1126/science.289.5484.1508
55. Gravallese EM, Manning C, Tsay A, Naito A, Pan C, Amento E, et al. Synovial tissue in rheumatoid arthritis is a source of osteoclast differentiation factor. *Arthritis Rheum.* (2000) 43:250–8. doi: 10.1002/1529-0131(200002)43:2<250::AID-ANR3>3.0.CO;2-P
56. Sawant A, Deshane J, Jules J, Lee CM, Harris AB, Feng X, et al. Myeloid-derived suppressor cells function as novel osteoclast progenitors enhancing bone loss in breast cancer. *Cancer Res.* (2013) 73:672–82. doi: 10.1158/0008-5472.CAN-12-2202
57. Su LK, Xu QG, Zhang P, Michalek SM, Katz J. Phenotype and function of myeloid-derived suppressor cells induced by *Porphyromonas gingivalis* infection. *Infect Immun.* (2017) 85:E00213–17. doi: 10.1128/IAI.00213-17
58. Zhang H, Huang Y, Wang S, Fu R, Guo CH, Wang HY, et al. Myeloid-derived suppressor cells contribute to bone erosion in collagen-induced arthritis by differentiating to osteoclasts. *J Autoimmun.* (2015) 65:82–9. doi: 10.1016/j.jaut.2015.08.010
59. Rajabinejad M, Salari F, Gorgin KA, Rezaiemanesh A. The role of myeloid-derived suppressor cells in the pathogenesis of rheumatoid arthritis; anti- or Pro-inflammatory cells? *Artif Cells Nanomed Biotechnol.* (2019) 47:4149–58. doi: 10.1080/21691401.2019.1687504
60. Nausch N, Galani IE, Schlecker E, Cerwenka A. Mononuclear myeloid-derived "suppressor" cells express RAE-1 and activate natural killer cells. *Blood.* (2008) 112:4080–9. doi: 10.1182/blood-2008-03-143776
61. Lecot P, Sarabi M, Abrantes MP, Mussard J, Koenderman L, Caux C, et al. Neutrophil heterogeneity in cancer: from biology to therapies. *Front Immunol.* (2019) 10:2155. doi: 10.3389/fimmu.2019.02155
62. Nishimura K, Saegusa J, Matsuki F, Akashi K, Kageyama G, Morinobu A. Tofacitinib facilitates the expansion of myeloid-derived suppressor cells and ameliorates arthritis in SKG mice. *Arthritis Rheumatol.* (2015) 67:893–902. doi: 10.1002/art.39007
63. Iwata Y, Furuichi K, Kitagawa K, Hara A, Okumura T, Kokubo S, et al. Involvement of Cd11b+ Gr-1 low cells in autoimmune disorder in MRL-FAS LPR mouse. *Clin Exp Nephrol.* (2010) 14:411–7. doi: 10.1007/s10157-010-0309-9
64. Knier B, Hiltensperger M, Sie C, Aly L, Lepennetier G, Engleitneret T, et al. Myeloid-derived suppressor cells control B cell accumulation in the central nervous system during autoimmunity. *Nat Immunol.* (2018) 19:1341–51. doi: 10.1038/s41590-018-0237-5
65. Glenn JD, Liu C, Whartenby KA. Frontline science: induction of experimental autoimmune encephalomyelitis mobilizes Th17-promoting myeloid-derived suppressor cells to the lung. *J Leukoc Biol.* (2019) 105:829–41. doi: 10.1002/JLB.4HI0818-335R

9

IL-33 Gene Polymorphisms as Potential Biomarkers of Disease Susceptibility and Response to TNF Inhibitors in Rheumatoid Arthritis, Ankylosing Spondylitis and Psoriatic Arthritis Patients

Milena Iwaszko[1], Joanna Wielińska[1], Jerzy Świerkot[2], Katarzyna Kolossa[3], Renata Sokolik[2], Bartosz Bugaj[2], Monika Chaszczewska-Markowska[1], Sławomir Jeka[3,4] and Katarzyna Bogunia-Kubik[1]*

[1] Laboratory of Clinical Immunogenetics and Pharmacogenetics, Hirszfeld Institute of Immunology and Experimental Therapy, Polish Academy of Sciences, Wrocław, Poland, [2] Department of Rheumatology and Internal Medicine, Wroclaw Medical University, Wrocław, Poland, [3] Department of Rheumatology and Connective Tissue Diseases, Jan Biziel University Hospital No. 2, Bydgoszcz, Poland, [4] Ludwik Rydygier Collegium Medicum in Bydgoszcz, Nicolaus Copernicus University, Toruń, Poland

***Correspondence:**
Milena Iwaszko
milena.iwaszko@hirszfeld.pl

Objective: Rheumatoid arthritis (RA), ankylosing spondylitis (AS), and psoriatic arthritis (PsA) belong to inflammatory rheumatic diseases, the group of conditions of unknown etiology. However, a strong genetic component in their pathogenesis has been well established. A dysregulation of cytokine networks plays an important role in the development of inflammatory arthritis. Interleukin 33 (IL-33) is a recently identified member of the IL-1 family. To date, the significance of IL-33 in inflammatory arthritis has been poorly studied. This research aimed to investigate the potential of *IL-33* gene polymorphisms to serve as biomarkers for disease susceptibility and TNF inhibitor response in RA, AS, and PsA patients.

Materials and Methods: In total, 735 patients diagnosed with RA, AS, and PsA and 229 healthy individuals were enrolled in the study. Genotyping for three single nucleotide polymorphisms (SNPs) within the *IL-33* gene, namely, rs16924159 (A/G), rs10975519 (T/C), and rs7044343 (C/T), was performed using polymerase chain reaction amplification employing LightSNiP assays.

Results: In the present study, the *IL-33* rs10975519 CC genotype was associated with a decreased risk of developing RA in females, while the *IL-33* rs16924159 polymorphism was associated with the efficacy of anti-TNF therapy and clinical parameters for RA and AS patients. The *IL-33* rs16924159 AA genotype correlated with higher disease activity and worse clinical outcomes in RA patients treated with TNF inhibitors, and AS patients carrying the *IL-33* rs16924159 AA genotype had higher disease activity and a worse response to anti-TNF therapy. That indicates a deleterious role of the *IL-33* rs16924159 AA genotype in the context of RA, as well as AS.

Conclusions: The obtained results suggest that *IL-33* gene polymorphisms might be potential candidate biomarkers of disease susceptibility and anti-TNF treatment response in patients with inflammatory rheumatic diseases.

Keywords: rheumatoid arthritis, psoriatic arthritis, ankylosing spondylitis, spondyloarthritis, *IL-33* gene polymorphism, anti-TNF therapy, TNF inhibitors

INTRODUCTION

Inflammatory arthritis comprises a diverse group of rheumatic diseases characterized by inflammation of synovial joints and systemic manifestations. Rheumatoid arthritis (RA), psoriatic arthritis (PsA), and ankylosing spondylitis (AS) constitute the most common subtypes of inflammatory arthritis. The worldwide prevalence of inflammatory arthritis amounts to approximately 3%. The exact etiology of RA, PsA, and AS has not been elucidated; however, there is evidence that genetic factors may contribute to their development.

An imbalanced cytokine network plays a crucial role in the pathogenesis of inflammatory arthritis (1, 2). Interleukin-33 (IL-33) constitutes a recently identified member of the IL-1 family that includes IL-1α, IL-1β, IL-1Ra, and IL-18. IL-33 is a dual-function protein, acting both as an endogenous danger signal and a nuclear factor (3, 4). This cytokine is constitutively expressed in the nuclei of endothelial and epithelial cells, acts as a nuclear repressor factor, and is involved in gene transcription regulation (5–7). In response to cellular damage, full-length IL-33 is rapidly released into the extracellular matrix, initiating an inflammatory response (8, 9). This cytokine functions as an alarmin, alerting the immune system and triggering the inflammatory process (8, 10).

IL-33 is predominantly expressed in epithelial, endothelial, and immune cells, including dendritic cells, macrophages, mast cells, and activated Th2 cells. IL-33 interacts with a receptor complex formed by orphan receptor ST2 (also known as IL-1RL1) and IL-1 receptor (IL-1RAcP) (11, 12). Two major ST2 isoforms result from the alternative splicing of gene transcripts: a full-length transmembrane form (ST2L) and a soluble form (sST2) (9). sST2 does not possess transmembrane and cytoplasmic domains and functions as a decoy receptor. IL-33 binding by sST2 inhibits the IL-33/ST2L interaction and, subsequently, IL-33–mediated signaling (13). ST2L expression has been detected for various types of immune cells: natural killer (NK) and NKT cells, innate lymphoid cell type II (ILC2), Th2 lymphocytes, dendritic cells, macrophages, regulatory T cells (Treg), B cells, eosinophils, basophils, and mast cells.

Following IL-33/ST2L binding, co-receptor recruitment of IL-1R accessory protein (IL-1RAP) is indispensable for signal transduction (14). The IL-33/ST2/IL-1RAcP complex induces recruitment of an adaptor protein, myeloid differentiation factor 88 (MyD88), that results in the activation of interleukin-1 receptor-associated kinases 1 and 4 (IRAK1/4) and tumor necrosis factor (TNF) receptor-associated factor 6 (TRAF6). These proteins trigger a downstream activation of the nuclear factor-κB (NF-κB) and the mitogen-activated protein kinase (MAPK) pathways (involving p38, JNKs c-Jun N-terminal kinases, and ERK extracellular signal-regulated kinase), leading to a proliferation of pro-inflammatory cytokine synthesis (9, 15).

IL-33 is predominantly involved in the Th2-mediated immune response by inducing IL-4, IL-5, and IL-13 cytokine production (16) and is crucial for the activation of Th2 cells, mast cells, eosinophils, basophils, dendritic cells (DC), and ILC2 cells (17). IL-33 was initially regarded as a mediator of the Th2-mediated immune response; however, it has also been implicated in Th1-associated immunity (3, 18). IL-33–mediated signaling is involved in the activation of Th1 cells, CD8+ T cells, NK and NKT cells, neutrophils, macrophages, and B cells (19–23). Moreover, IL-33 enhances the Th17 immune response, promotes an expansion of regulatory T (Treg) cells and DCs differentiation (24–27). The IL-33/ST2L axis is also involved in the generation of cytokines with pro-inflammatory potential, including IL–1β, IL-6, and tumor necrosis factor-α (TNF-α) (24, 28, 29).

IL-33 constitutes an essential component of both innate and adaptive immunity (6). This pleiotropic cytokine can target a broad range of immune cells and exerts multiple effects on immune system functions. The pleiotropic character of IL-33 indicates its potential as an essential player in the pathogenesis of autoimmune diseases. It has been revealed that dysregulation within the IL-33/ST2L axis contributes to the development of various diseases, including cardiovascular disorders, cancer, and infectious diseases (9, 15, 19). An increasing body of evidence also implies a crucial role of IL-33 in the pathogenesis of autoimmune disorders, such as inflammatory bowel disease, multiple sclerosis, psoriasis, and diabetes (9, 15).

This research aimed to investigate the potential of *IL-33* gene polymorphisms as predictors of disease susceptibility and biomarkers of anti-TNF therapy response in major autoimmune rheumatic diseases, including RA, AS, and PsA.

MATERIALS AND METHODS

Study Group

In total, 964 cases and controls were enrolled, including 466 RA, 143 AS, and 126 PsA patients. The control group consisted of 229 healthy individuals. The patients were recruited from the Department of Rheumatology and Internal Medicine at Wrocław Medical University, Poland, and the Department of

Rheumatology and Connective Tissue Diseases at Collegium Medicum, Bydgoszcz, Poland. RA was diagnosed according to the 2010 American College of Rheumatology/European League Against Rheumatism (ACR/EULAR) Classification Criteria for Rheumatoid Arthritis; all patients diagnosed with AS fulfilled the 1984 modified New York Criteria; PsA diagnoses were established according to the Classification Criteria for Psoriatic Arthritis (CASPAR).

The following demographic and clinical data were collected from all studied patients: gender, body mass index (BMI), disease onset, disease duration, medications received, C-reactive protein (CRP) levels, erythrocyte sedimentation rate (ESR), tender joint count (TJC), swollen joint count (STC), rheumatoid factor (RF) levels, anti-cyclic citrullinated peptide antibody (anti-CCP) levels (for RA patients), HLA-B27 status (for AS patients), Disease Activity Score-28 (DAS28), the Bath Ankylosing Spondylitis Disease Activity Index (BASDAI) (for AS and PsA patients), and the visual analog scale (VAS, ranging from 0 to 100 mm) of pain, and health assessment questionnaires (HAQs) and global health assessments (self-reported and from a physician) were used. The detailed demographic and clinical characteristics of the RA, AS, and PsA patients are depicted in **Table 1**.

The eligibility criteria were: age over 18 years; Caucasian ethnicity; confirmed diagnosis of RA, AS, or PsA; resistance to treatment with at least two disease-modifying anti-rheumatic drugs (DMARDs) for RA and PsA patients; resistance to treatment with at least two non-steroidal anti-rheumatic drugs for AS and PsA patients; the presence of active disease before the initiation of anti-TNF therapy; and the commencement of treatment with one of the four anti-TNF biological agents (adalimumab, etanercept, infliximab, certolizumab, or golimumab) at the time of the study. A complete medical history and a physical examination were also required.

The exclusion criteria adopted in the research were as follows: age below 18 years, the coexistence of other autoimmune disorders, infections with hepatotropic viruses or human immunodeficiency virus, infections resistant to therapy, a history of malignancy, the coexistence of other severe acute or chronic medical condition, pregnancy or breastfeeding, alcohol or drug abuse, poor clinical records, and an unwillingness or inability to cooperate.

Patients were examined before commencing the TNF blocking therapy and after 12 and 24 weeks of the treatment. Age- and sex-matched controls (without any family history of rheumatic diseases) from the Blood Bank of Wroclaw served as the control group. All participants were of Caucasian ancestry, and written informed consent was obtained. The study protocol was approved by the Wroclaw Medical University Ethics Committee.

Anti-TNF Treatment Regimen

The patients were administered the following anti-TNF agents: infliximab, adalimumab, etanercept, and certolizumab pegol. The patients received recommended doses of TNF blockers: 3 mg/kg body weight of infliximab given as intravenous infusions at weeks 0, 2, and 6 and every 8 weeks thereafter, subcutaneous injections of 40 mg adalimumab every other week, 50 mg etanercept every week, and 400 mg certolizumab pegol at weeks 0, 2, and 4 and 200 mg every 2 weeks thereafter, and 50 mg of golimumab once a month. Stable doses of methotrexate (MTX), glucocorticoids, and non-steroidal anti-inflammatory drugs were allowed. Therapeutic responses were assessed at weeks 12 and 24 after anti-TNF therapy initiation.

TABLE 1 | Patients' and controls' characteristics.

	RA patients N = 466	AS patients N = 143	PsA patients N = 126	Controls N = 229
Demographics				
Sex [females/males (% of females)]	368/98 (79.0)	36/107 (25.2)	62/64 (49.2)	98/131 (42.8)
Age (years) [mean (± SD)]	51.6 (± 12.3)	44.4 (± 13.0)	47.9 (± 12.1)	45.5 (± 11.9)
Clinical data				
Disease duration (years) [mean (± SD)]	12.7 (± 8.1)	12.0 (± 9.8)	10.7 (± 10.3)	
Disease onset (years) [mean (± SD)]	39.1 (± 12.6)	31.9 (± 9.6)	38.3 (± 12.6)	
DAS28 at baseline [mean (± SD)]	6.4 (± 0.7)		5.5 (± 1.3)	
CRP at baseline [mean (± SD)]	23.4 (± 34.0)	30.0 (± 56.7)	12.6 (± 17.3)	
BASDAI at baseline [mean (± SD)]		7.5 (± 1.4)	7.7 (± 1.0)	
VAS at baseline [mean (± SD)]	77.6 (± 11.9)	80.5 (± 10.8)	72.2 (± 16.0)	
HLA-B27 positive [%]		87.2		
RF positive [%]	68.3			
Anti-CCP positive [%]	90.0			
Anti-TNF drugs				
Etanercept [%]	26.6	30.8	32.5	
Adalimumab [%]	18.9	43.4	33.3	
Infliximab [%]	1.7	1.4	1.6	
Certolizumab pegol [%]	3.2	11.9	1.6	
Golimumab [%]		8.4	10.3	
Concomitant treatment				
Glucocorticosteroids [%]	91.0	20.5	21.4	
Methotrexate [%]	92.0	31.1	61.1	

RA, rheumatoid arthritis; AS, ankylosing spondylitis; PsA, psoriatic arthritis; DAS28, disease activity score 28; CRP, C-reactive protein; BASDAI, Bath Ankylosing Spondylitis Disease Activity Index; VAS, visual analog scale; HLA-B27, human leukocyte antigen B27; RF, rheumatoid factor; anti-CCP, anti cyclic citrullinated peptide antibodies; SD, standard deviation.

Assessment of the Disease Activity and Therapeutic Response

Disease activity in the RA patients was calculated with DAS28. DAS28 is a composite index incorporating four variables: Number of swollen and tender joints, CRP level, and a self-reported global health assessment (VAS, mm). High disease activity was defined by DAS28 > 5.1, moderate by 3.2 < DAS28 ≤ 5.1, and DAS28 ≤ 3.2 referred to low disease activity. EULAR response criteria were used to measure anti-TNF treatment efficacy, which combines the improvement in DAS28 scores between the initial and final score with the DAS28 score at the time of evaluation (30).

Bath Ankylosing Spondylitis Disease Activity Index (BASDAI) was employed to assess AS patient disease activity. BASDAI is a composite index comprising an evaluation using a VAS scale (range, 0–10 cm, where 0 = none and 100 = very severe) of the following components: Fatigue, spinal pain, enthesitis, peripheral joint pain/swelling, morning stiffness duration, and morning stiffness severity. A BASDAI of 50 (at least 50% improvement from baseline BASDAI or absolute score change of 2; scale 0–10) indicates a good response to therapy (31).

In the PsA cohort, DAS28 and BASDAI were used to assess disease activity status. As the anti-TNF therapy outcome measure, the psoriatic arthritis response criteria (PsARC) were employed. These criteria included TJC, SJC (assessing 68 and 66 joints, respectively, including the distal interphalangeal joints in the hands and feet), patient (PtGA) and provider (PrGA) global assessment of disease activity. An improvement of at least 30% in at least one joint count and one other measure and no decrease in the other measurements was defined as a positive therapeutic outcome (32, 33).

SNP Selection and Genotyping

The selection of genetic variants within the *IL-33* gene was based on an analysis of the available literature and search results from the HapMap and NCBI dbSNP databases. Information of the predicted functional consequences of SNPs was obtained using the SNPinfo Web Server (34). The studied SNPs were characterized with minor allele frequencies above 10% (1000 Genomes Project) (35).

Peripheral venous blood from each subject was collected in ethylenediaminetetraacetic acid (EDTA) anticoagulant tubes. DNA isolation was carried out using a Maxwell 16 Blood DNA Purification Kit (Promega Corp., Madison, WI, USA). The *IL-33* SNPs were detected by real-time PCR using LightCycler Technology with SimpleProbe probes (LightSNiP assays) designed by TIB MolBiol (Berlin, Germany). Genotyping was performed on a LightCycler 480 Real-Time PCR system (Roche Diagnostics, Rotkreuz, Switzerland) according to the manufacturer's instructions.

Statistical Analysis

The Population Genetics R package (cran:genetics, version 1.3.8.1) was used for testing the Hardy–Weinberg equilibrium (HWE) of the genotype distributions of the examined *IL-33* polymorphisms. For the presentation of categorical variables, frequencies and percentages were used, while means and standard deviations were calculated for continuous variables. A Fisher's exact test was used to detect differences in the genotype and allele frequencies between patients and controls. Fisher's exact or Wilcoxon's tests were applied to assess the relationships between the *IL–33* genetic variants and clinical parameters. RA patients' relative changes of DAS28 scores between baseline and weeks 12 as well as 24 were calculated for each patient by dividing a latter value by a baseline one. Analyses of the distributions of the *IL-33* genotypes and alleles within patient groups for their associations with therapeutic effect were performed using Fisher's exact test. RA patients with a good and moderate EULAR response were grouped together and compared to patients with no response. Stratification analyses employed the Cochran–Mantel–Haenszel χ^2 test for count data, followed by a post-hoc groupwise association test of genotypes (cran:rcompanion, version 2.3.26). Bonferroni corrected p_c values were calculated by multiplying the observed p value by 27 (3 diseases × 3 outcomes × 3 models). Level of statistical significance was set at 5 % ($p_c < 0.05$), uncorrected $p < 0.05$ was considered suggestive. Assuming the aforementioned significance level, the additive model, the minor allele frequency of 0.2, and effect size of 1.50, our study had 55 % power in the AS patients, 53% in the PsA patients, and 82 % in case of the RA patients. All statistical calculations, except power, were performed using R software environment (version 3.6.3; x86_64-pc-linux-gnu) (36). Statistical power calculations were performed with the Genetic Association Study Power Calculator (https://csg.sph.umich.edu/abecasis/cats/gas_power_calculator).

RESULTS

Genotype and Allele Distributions of IL-33 Polymorphisms in the RA, AS, PsA Patients and Healthy Controls

The genotype distributions of the examined *IL-33* polymorphisms in control group were in Hardy–Weinberg equilibrium ($p = 0.88$ for rs10975519, $p = 0.57$ for rs16924159, and $p = 0.67$ for rs7044343). The frequency of the genotypes and alleles of the *IL-33* rs10975519, rs16924159, or rs7044343 did not differ between the RA patients and controls, and no significant differences were found between the controls and AS or PsA patients (**Table 2**).

However, gender-stratified analysis of the genotype and allele distributions revealed differences between female RA patients and female controls regarding the *IL-33* rs10975519 polymorphism (**Figure 1**). The *IL-33* rs10975519 CC genotype was less frequent among female patients than female controls ($p = 0.008$, p_c = NS, OR = 0.54, $CI_{95\%}$ = 0.33–0.86). On the contrary, female patients more frequently possessed the *IL-33* rs10975519 CG genotype than female controls ($p = 0.004$, p_c = NS, OR = 1.97, $CI_{95\%}$ = 1.22–3.25). No association remained significant after Bonferroni correction, however. No gender-

TABLE 2 | Gender-stratified analysis of the *IL-33* genotypes frequencies in rheumatoid arthritis, ankylosing spondylitis, and psoriatic arthritis patients.

	rs10975519			rs16924159			rs7044343		
	CC	**CT**	**TT**	**AA**	**AG**	**GG**	**CC**	**CT**	**TT**
RA									
Female patients	142 (38.7%)	188 (51.2%)	37 (10.1%)	52 (14.2%)	182 (49.6%)	133 (36.2%)	48 (33.2%)	197 (53.7%)	122 (33.2%)
Male patients	43 (43.9%)	51 (52.0%)	4 (4.1%)	13 (13.3%)	46 (46.9%)	39 (39.8%)	7 (7.1%)	55 (56.1%)	36 (36.7%)
Female controls	53 (54.1%)	34 (34.7%)	11 (11.2%)	16 (16.3%)	45 (45.9%)	13 (13.3%)	13 (13.3%)	44 (44.9%)	41 (41.8%)
Male controls	51 (38.9%)	66 (50.4%)	14 (10.7%)	13 (9.9%)	66 (50.4%)	52 (39.7%)	18 (13.7%)	68 (51.9%)	45 (34.4%)
AS									
Female patients	**7 (19.4%)**[a]	23 (63.9%)	6 (16.7%)	10 (27.8%)	16 (44.4%)	10 (27.8%)	**8 (22.2%)**[b]	22 (61.1%)	6 (16.7%)
Male patients	47 (44.3%)	48 (45.3%)	11 (10.4%)	11 (10.4%)	57 (53.8%)	38 (35.8%)	18 (17.0%)	46 (43.4%)	42 (39.6%)
Female controls	53 (54.1%)	34 (34.7%)	11 (11.2%)	16 (16.3%)	45 (45.9%)	37 (37.8%)	13 (13.3%)	44 (44.9%)	41 (41.8%)
Male controls	51 (38.9%)	66 (50.4%)	14 (10.7%)	13 (9.9%)	66 (50.4%)	52 (39.7%)	18 (13.7%)	68 (51.9%)	45 (34.4%)
PsA									
Female patients	26 (41.9%)	27 (43.5%)	9 (14.5%)	8 (12.9%)	29 (46.8%)	25 (40.3%)	10 (16.4%)	30 (49.2%)	21 (34.4%)
Male patients	29 (45.3%)	26 (40.6%)	9 (14.1%)	12 (18.8%)	27 (42.2%)	25 (39.1%)	11 (17.2%)	29 (45.3%)	24 (37.5%)
Female controls	53 (54.1%)	34 (34.7%)	11 (11.2%)	16 (16.3%)	45 (45.9%)	37 (37.8%)	13 (13.3%)	44 (44.9%)	41 (41.8%)
Male controls	51 (38.9%)	66 (50.4%)	14 (10.7%)	12 (18.8%)	66 (50.4%)	52 (39.7%)	18 (13.7%)	68 (51.9%)	45 (34.4%)

[a]CMH: p=0.001, p_c=0.032, OR=0.47, $CI_{95\%}$=(0.30–0.74); groupwise (females): p_c=0.002; [b]CMH: p = 0.001, p_c = 0.027, OR = 0.46, $CI_{95\%}$ = (0.29–0.72); groupwise (females): p_c=0.038. RA, rheumatoid arthritis; AS, ankylosing spondylitis; PsA, psoriatic arthritis; CMH, Cochran-Mantel-Haenszel χ^2 test; p_c, value with Bonferroni correction.

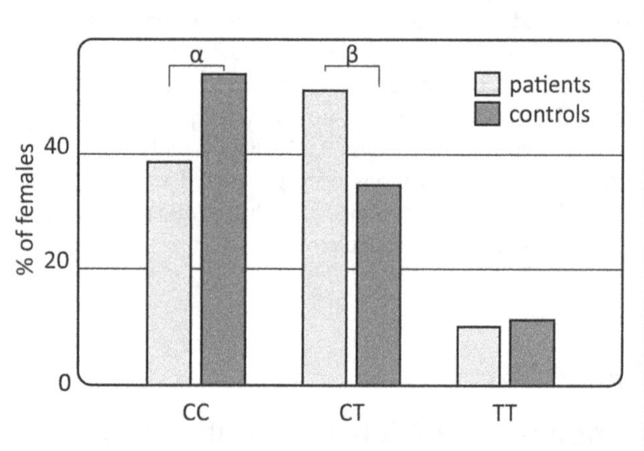

FIGURE 1 | Association of the *IL-33* rs10975519 polymorphism with rheumatoid arthritis susceptibility in females. Differences are indicated as "[α]CC *vs* CT+TT, p=0.008, p_c=NS, OR=0.54, $CI_{95\%}$=(0.33; 0.86); [β]CT *vs* CC+TT, p=0.004, p_c=NS, OR=1.97, $CI_{95\%}$=(1.22; 3.25); NS, non-significant; p_c, value with Bonferroni correction.

dependent associations were detected between *IL-33* rs16924159 or rs7044343 and disease risk in the RA cohort.

Gender-Stratified Analysis of the *IL-33* Genotype and Allele Frequencies in the RA, AS, and PsA Patients

A significant difference in the genotype and allele distribution was found for the *IL-33* rs10975519 genetic variant in the AS patients (**Table 2**). The frequency of the *IL-33* rs10975519 CC genotype was increased in male AS patients compared to females (p=0.001, p_c=0.032, OR = 0.47, $CI_{95\%}$ = 0.30–0.74). The comparison between females and males diagnosed with AS in accordance with the *IL-33* rs7044343 polymorphism also revealed significant relationships. A frequency of the *IL-33* rs7044343 CC genotype was increased in the females with AS, as compared to the males (p=0.001, p_c = 0.027, OR = 0.46, $CI_{95\%}$ = 0.29–0.72). The analysis involving the *IL-33* rs16924159 SNP polymorphism in relation to the patients' gender showed no significant associations.

The gender stratification analysis did not show any associations with any of the studied *IL-33* genetic variants in the RA and PsA patients (**Table 3**).

Effect of *IL-33* Polymorphisms on the Effectiveness of Anti-TNF Therapy in Patients Diagnosed With RA, AS, and PsA

The anti-TNF therapy clinical outcome was associated with the *IL-33* rs16924159 variant in the RA patients (**Table 4**). The *IL-33* rs16924159 AA genotype was more frequently observed among

TABLE 3 | Comparison of the *IL-33* genotypes and alleles frequencies between patients diagnosed with rheumatoid arthritis, ankylosing spondylitis, psoriatic arthritis, and healthy subjects.

	Controls	RA	AS	PsA
rs10975519				
C	308 (67.2%)	611 (65.5%)	179 (62.6%)	163 (64.7%)
T	150 (32.8%)	321 (34.4%)	54 (37.4%)	89 (35.3%)
CC	104 (45.4%)	186 (39.9%)	54 (37.8%)	55 (43.7%)
CT	100 (43.7%)	239 (51.3%)	71 (49.7%)	53 (42.1%)
TT	25 (10.9%)	41 (8.8%)	18 (12.6%)	18 (14.3%)
rs16924159				
A	169 (36.9%)	358 (38.4%)	116 (40.6%)	96 (38.1%)
G	289 (63.1%)	574 (61.6%)	170 (59.4%)	156 (61.9%)
AA	29 (12.7%)	65 (13.9%)	21 (14.7%)	20 (15.9%)
AG	111 (48.5%)	228 (48.9%)	74 (51.7%)	56 (44.4%)
GG	89 (38.9%)	173 (37.1%)	48 (33.6%)	50 (39.7%)
rs7044343				
C	174 (38.0%)	362 (38.8%)	122 (42.7%)	101 (40.4%)
T	284 (62.0%)	570 (61.2%)	164 (57.3%)	149 (59.6%)
CC	31 (13.5%)	55 (11.8%)	27 (18.9%)	21 (16.8%)
CT	112 (48.9%)	252 (54.1%)	68 (47.6%)	59 (47.2%)
TT	86 (37.6%)	159 (34.1%)	48 (33.6%)	45 (36.0%)

RA, rheumatoid arthritis; AS, ankylosing spondylitis; PsA, psoriatic arthritis.

TABLE 4 | Analysis of the *IL-33* genotypes distributions with regard to therapeutic response to anti-TNF agents in rheumatoid arthritis, ankylosing spondylitis and psoriatic arthritis patients.

	rs10975519			rs16924159			rs7044343		
	CC	**CT**	**TT**	**AA**	**AG**	**GG**	**CC**	**CT**	**TT**
RA									
12th week									
Responders	26 (37.1%)	39 (55.7%)	5 (7.1%)	10 (14.3%)	33 (47.1%)	27 (38.6%)	7 (10.0%)	39 (55.7%)	24 (34.3%)
Non-responders	145 (40.7%)	181 (50.8%)	30 (8.4%)	46 (12.9%)	178 (50.0%)	132 (37.1%)	42 (11.8%)	193 (54.2%)	121 (34.0%)
24th week									
Responders	98 (40.7%)	125 (51.9%)	18 (7.5%)	**25 (10.4%)**[a]	124 (51.5%)	**92 (38.2%)**[b]	27 (11.2%)	129 (53.5%)	85 (35.3%)
Non-responders	56 (38.6%)	76 (52.4%)	13 (9.0%)	27 (18.6%)	68 (46.9%)	50 (34.5%)	16 (11.0%)	81 (55.9%)	48 (33.1%)
AS									
12th week									
Responders	34 (32.4%)	56 (53.3%)	15 (14.3%)	18 (17.1%)	50 (47.6%)	37 (35.2%)	23 (21.9%)	51 (48.6%)	31 (29.5%)
Non-responders	18 (52.9%)	15 (44.1%)	1 (2.9%)	3 (8.8%)	22 (64.7%)	9 (26.5%)	2 (5.9%)	17 (50.0%)	15 (44.1%)
24th week									
Responders	46 (36.8%)	64 (51.2%)	15 (12.0%)	**15 (12.0%)**[c]	66 (52.8%)	**44 (35.2%)**[d]	24 (19.2%)	60 (48.0%)	41 (32.8%)
Non-responders	3 (37.5%)	4 (50.0%)	1 (12.5%)	4 (36.4%)	3 (27.3%)	4 (36.4%)	1 (12.5%)	5 (62.5%)	2 (25.0%)
PsA									
12th week									
Responders	32 (41.6%)	35 (45.5%)	10 (13.0%)	13 (16.9%)	35 (45.5%)	29 (37.7%)	15 (19.5%)	37 (48.1%)	25 (32.5%)
Non-responders	12 (40.0%)	14 (46.7%)	4 (13.3%)	5 (16.7%)	14 (46.7%)	11 (36.7%)	6 (20.0%)	14 (46.7%)	10 (33.3%)
24th week									
Responders	38 (47.5%)	33 (41.3%)	9 (11.3%)	13 (16.3%)	36 (45.0%)	31 (38.8%)	13 (16.5%)	37 (46.8%)	29 (36.7%)
Non-responders	12 (46.2%)	11 (42.3%)	3 (11.5%)	4 (15.4%)	12 (46.2%)	10 (38.5%)	4 (15.4%)	12 (46.2%)	10 (38.5%)

[a]*AA vs AG+GG, $p = 0.030$, p_c = NS, OR = 0.51, $CI_{95\%}$ = 0.27–0.95;* [b]*GG vs AA, $p = 0.046$, p_c = NS, OR = 1.98, $CI_{95\%}$=(0.99–3.98);* [c]*AA vs AG+GG, $p = 0.015$, p_c = NS, OR = 0.14, $CI_{95\%}$ = (0.02–0.83);* [d]*GG vs AA, p=0.024, p_c=NS, OR=11.22, $CI_{95\%}$ = 1.01–588.34.*

RA, rheumatoid arthritis; EULAR, European League Against Rheumatism; AS, ankylosing spondylitis; BASDAI, Bath Ankylosing Spondylitis Disease Activity Index; PsA, psoriatic arthritis; PsARC, Psoriatic Arthritis Response Criteria; NS, non-significant; p_c, value with Bonferroni correction.

the RA patients with worse response to anti-TNF agents after 24 weeks than the other genotypes ($p = 0.030$, p_c = NS, OR = 1.97, $CI_{95\%}$ = 1.05–3.72). Moreover, the presence of the *IL-33* rs16924159 GG genotype was associated with a good response to anti-TNF treatment at the 24th week ($p = 0.046$, p_c = NS, OR = 1.98, $CI_{95\%}$ = 0.99–3.98). However, with Bonferroni adjustment no effect reached significance. There were no differences between the other two studied *IL-33* polymorphisms and the clinical outcomes of the anti-TNF treatment among the RA patients.

Differences were also detected between the *IL-33* rs16924159 polymorphism and anti-TNF therapy efficacy in the AS patients (**Table 4**). After 24 weeks of treatment, a lack of response was more frequently observed in patients carrying the AA genotype than the other genotypes ($p = 0.015$, p_c = NS, OR = 7.15, $CI_{95\%}$ = 1.20–42.87). Additionally, an elevated frequency of the *IL-33* rs16924159 A allele was detected among patients with no response to anti-TNF agents after 24 weeks ($p = 0.032$, p_c = NS, OR = 3.51, $CI_{95\%}$ = 1.08–13.31). On the contrary, *IL-33* rs16924159 GG genotype frequencies were increased in patients who responded to anti-TNF treatment after 24 weeks compared to the AA genotype ($p = 0.024$, p_c = NS, OR = 11.22, $CI_{95\%}$ = 1.01–588.34).

There were no differences between the other two studied *IL-33* polymorphisms and the anti-TNF therapy outcomes among the RA and AS patients. No significant relationships in the genotype or allele distribution of the studied *IL-33* polymorphism and anti-TNF agent efficacy were found for the PsA patients (**Table 4**).

Clinical Parameters of the RA, AS, and PsA Patients and *IL-33* Genotype and Allele Distributions

Comparisons of the *IL-33* genotypes and alleles among the RA, AS, and PsA patients were performed using clinical laboratory parameters. Association between DAS28 and the distribution of the *IL-33* rs16924159 genotype was observed in the RA patients at week 24 of treatment (**Figure 2**). The *IL-33* rs16924159 AA genotype was more common among RA patients with higher DAS28 after 24 weeks of therapy than the other genotypes ($p = 0.023$, p_c = NS, OR = 1.97, $CI_{95\%}$ = 1.06–3.67). On the contrary, RA patients bearing the *IL-33* rs16924159 GG genotype had lower values of DAS28 at week 24 of anti-TNF treatment than patients carrying the other genotypes ($p = 0.049$, p_c = NS, OR = 1.97, $CI_{95\%}$ = 1.00–3.93). After Bonferroni correction, the associations were no longer significant.

Differences were detected in the RA patients between the *IL-33* rs16924159 genotype and relative changes in DAS28 values during treatment (**Figure 2**). Patients bearing the *IL-33* rs16924159 GG genotype had larger DAS28 reductions at week 12 of anti-TNF treatment than carriers of the AA genotype ($p = 0.036$, p_c = NS, W = 2396.5). This trend was also observed after 24 weeks of treatment. Lesser relative changes in DAS28 values were observed in patients with the *IL-33* rs16924159 AA genotype than the other genotypes (p=0.030, p_c=NS, W=5265.5). Patients homozygous for the *IL-33* rs16924159 GG genotype demonstrated a greater decrease in DAS28 values between baseline and week 24 than patients possessing the AA

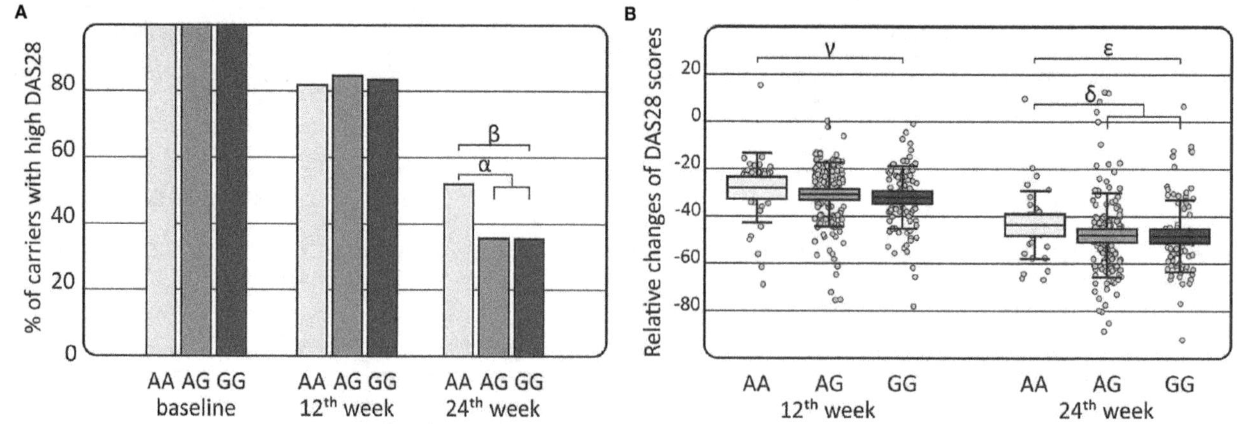

FIGURE 2 | Association of the *IL-33* rs16924159 polymorphism with disease activity in rheumatoid arthritis patients. **(A)** Comparison of *IL-33* rs16924159 genotype frequencies with DAS28 score at baseline as well as at 12th and 24th weeks after commencing of anti-TNF therapy; **(B)** Comparison of *IL-33* rs16924159 genotype frequencies with relative change in DAS28 between baseline and 12th week, as well as 24th week after commencing of anti-TNF therapy; Differences are indicated as; $^{\alpha}$AA *vs* AG+GG, p=0.023, p_c=NS, OR= 1.97, $CI_{95\%}$=(1.06; 3.67); $^{\beta}$GG *vs* AA, p=0.049, p_c=NS, OR=0.51, $CI_{95\%}$=(0.25; 1.00); $^{\gamma}$AA *vs* GG, p=0.036, p_c=NS, W=2396.5; $^{\delta}$AA *vs* AG+GG, p=0.030, p_c=NS, W=5265.5; $^{\varepsilon}$GG vs AA, p=0.016, p_c=NS, W=2301.0; DAS28, disease activity score 28; NS, non-significant; p_c, value with Bonferroni correction.

genotype (p = 0.016, p_c = NS, W = 2301.0). No other studied *IL-33* polymorphism was associated with any clinical parameters in the gender-stratified or whole RA cohort.

A significant association in the *IL-33* rs16924159 genotype distribution with regard to disease activity was found in the AS patients (**Table 5**). AS patients carrying the *IL-33* rs16924159 AA genotype displayed higher baseline BASDAI scores than patients possessing the other genotypes (p = 0.001, p_c = 0.027, W = 1821.0). On the contrary, lower baseline BASDAI scores were observed in AS patients bearing the *IL-33* rs16924159 GG genotype than AA homozygous patients (p = 0.003, p_c = 0.081, W = 718.0).

A comparison of clinical parameters with genotype frequencies and alleles of the *IL-33* variants did not show any associations in the PsA patients (**Table 5**).

DISCUSSION

A growing body of evidence highlights the role of the IL-33 signaling pathway in inflammatory arthritis. Significantly increased IL-33 levels have been detected in RA patients' serum and synovial fluid, and IL-33 levels have been shown to

TABLE 5 | Analysis of the *IL-33* genotypes distributions with regard to baseline clinical parameters of rheumatoid arthritis, ankylosing spondylitis and psoriatic arthritis patients.

	rs10975519			rs16924159			rs7044343		
	CC	CT	TT	AA	AG	GG	CC	CT	TT
RA									
RF+	85 (65.4%)	126 (71.2%)	20 (64.5%)	33 (70.2%)	107 (65.2%)	91 (71.7%)	25 (62.5%)	136 (73.1%)	70 (62.5%)
anti-CCP+	104 (89.7%)	148 (89.7%)	28 (93.3%)	43 (93.5%)	139 (91.4%)	98 (86.7%)	36 (94.7%)	156 (90.2%)	88 (88.0%)
CRP	24.4 (± 34.5)	22.1 (± 30.5)	26.7 (± 47.5)	22.7 (± 27.5)	22.6 (± 33.4)	24.8 (± 36.8)	25.5 (± 43.5)	23.0 (± 31.0)	23.4 (± 34.9)
VAS	79.4 (± 10.3)	76.1 (± 12.5)	77.6 (± 13.4)	74.8 (± 12.3)	77.4 (± 12.1)	78.8 (± 11.0)	76.4 (± 12.9)	77.0 (± 12.6)	78.8 (± 10.0)
DAS28	6.4 (± 0.7)	6.4 (± 0.7)	6.5 (± 0.7)	6.4 (± 0.7)	6.4 (± 0.7)	6.5 (± 0.7)	6.4 (± 0.7)	6.4 (± 0.7)	6.4 (± 0.6)
AS									
CRP	27.6 (± 28.5)	34.8 (± 77.0)	22.4 (± 28.7)	20.3 (± 17.7)	33.5 (± 75.2)	30.5 (± 28.3)	23.5 (± 27.6)	32.6 (± 75.1)	29.9 (± 29.8)
VAS	80.7 (± 9.8)	81.0 (± 11.5)	78.5 (± 10.9)	84.1 (± 7.1)	80.3 (± 10.3)	79.5 (± 11.1)	80.2 (± 10.6)	80.6 (± 10.0)	80.8 (± 11.4)
BASDAI	7.6 (± 1.4)	7.8 (± 1.3)	7.2 (± 1.2)	**8.2 (± 1.2)[a]**	7.5 (± 1.4)	**7.5 (± 1.4)[b]**	7.5 (± 1.1)	7.7 (± 1.2)	7.7 (± 1.3)
PsA									
CRP	12.0 (± 17.6)	13.1 (± 17.1)	10.4 (± 16.2)	10.2 (± 12.5)	11.4 (± 17.3)	14.0 (± 18.6)	9.9 (± 15.2)	14.1 (± 17.7)	11.1 (± 17.2)
VAS	72.6 (± 14.8)	72.9 (± 15.9)	68.9 (± 19.0)	65.5 (± 18.6)	72.2 (± 14.4)	75.1 (± 15.6)	71.2 (± 18.3)	72.6 (± 15.4)	71.8 (± 15.4)
BASDAI	7.2 (± 1.4)	7.7 (± 1.4)	7.2 (± 1.2)	8.4 (± 1.1)	7.3 (± 1.4)	7.3 (± 1.4)	7.5 (± 1.1)	7.6 (± 1.6)	7.3 (± 1.3)

[a]*AA vs AG+GG, p=0.001, p_c=0.027, W=1821.0;* [b]*GG vs AA, p = 0.003, p_c = NS, W = 718.0.*

RA, rheumatoid arthritis; SJC, swollen joints count; TJC, tender joints count; RF, rheumatoid factor; anti-CCP, anti cyclic citrullinated peptide antibody; CRP, C-reactive protein; VAS, visual analog scale; DAS28, disease activity score 28; AS, ankylosing spondylitis; BASDAI, Bath Ankylosing Spondylitis Disease Activity Index; PsA, psoriatic arthritis; NS, non-significant; p_c, value with Bonferroni correction.

positively correlate with disease severity, rheumatoid factor, and anticitrullinated protein antibodies (37–39). Furthermore, a reduction in serum IL-33 concentration in RA patients after anti-TNF therapy has been reported (38, 40). In addition, decreased levels of IL-33 have not been observed in patients unresponsive to TNF inhibitors (37). It has also been reported that TNF stimulates the IL-33 expression on both mRNA and protein levels in cultured synovial fibroblasts derived from RA patients (41–43). On the contrary, it has been shown that IL-33 affects TNF-dependent effects, enhancing the production of pro-inflammatory mediators, including IL-6, IL-8, and monocyte chemotactic protein-1 (MCP-1) and the pro-destructive molecules matrix metalloproteinase-1 (MMP–1), MMP-3, and TIMP-1 (41).

In the present study, the *IL-33* rs16924159 polymorphism was associated with anti-TNF therapy efficacy and clinical parameters in RA and AS patients. The *IL-33* rs16924159 AA genotype was correlated with higher disease activity and worse clinical outcomes in RA patients treated with TNF inhibitors. AS patients carrying the *IL-33* rs16924159 AA genotype had higher disease activity and a worse response to anti-TNF therapy; these results indicate a deleterious role of the *IL-33* rs16924159 AA genotype in RA and AS. A significant association was also found for the *IL-33* rs10975519 genetic variant. The *IL-33* rs10975519 CC genotype was associated with a decreased risk of developing RA among females. We did not find in the literature any gene candidate study investigating these SNPs in RA or PsA patients. One other study by Fan et al. addressed the relationships between the *IL-33* rs16924159 and rs10975519 polymorphisms and AS development; however, all subjects in this study were of Chinese ethnicity (44). The study reported a correlation between the rs10975519 CC genotype and a diminished predisposition to AS, but no association between *IL-33* rs16924159 and AS susceptibility was found (44). The *IL-33* rs10975519 C allele was previously associated with higher susceptibility to ischemic stroke in a Chinese cohort by Guo et al. (45). The *IL-33* rs10975519 variant was also studied in Chinese patients diagnosed with autoimmune thyroid diseases, systemic lupus, and coronary artery disease, although no significant relationships were revealed (46–48). The *IL-33* rs16924159 AA polymorphism was found to be associated with an increased risk of recurrent miscarriage (49). On the other hand, the rs16924159 A allele has been identified as a protective allele in asthma development (50). No association has been found between the *IL-33* rs16924159 and coronary artery disease or coronary heart disease in Mexican or Chinese populations, respectively (51, 52). There is also no significant relationship between this polymorphism and the risk of ischemic stroke (45). *IL-33* loci did not reach genome-wide level of statistical significance in previous GWAS studies in RA patients (53). No associations were also found with respect to disease susceptibility in previous GWAS studies involving AS and PsA patients (54–56). These results are in line with the results from the present study. None of the studied *IL-33* genetic variants was associated with RA, AS, or PsA risk in the whole cohort of patients. However, in the present study, significant association was observed between the *IL-33* rs10975519 genetic variant and predisposition to RA in females. Alas, in the aforementioned GWAS studies sex-stratified analyses were not applied, so no conclusions can be drawn. In the present study, significant relationships were also observed between the *IL-33* genetic variants and anti-TNF efficacy in RA as well as AS patients. However, GWAS studies investigating outcome of anti-TNF therapy in RA patients didn't identify genome-wide significant association for *IL-33* loci (57, 58). Interestingly, in a study investigating transcriptomic profile, *IL-33* genome-level expression was found significantly upregulated in RA patients that responded to anti-TNF therapy (59). The inconsistency between the studies might be attributed to differences in inclusion and outcome criteria between studies or false-positive associations obtained. Also, anti-TNF response is considered to be polygenic with many small-effect variants, which might be missed in GWAS analysis. Therefore, results derived from this study require validation in larger patient cohorts from Caucasian population.

Herein, no association was found between the *IL-33* rs7044343 polymorphism and RA susceptibility or anti-TNF treatment efficacy. Interestingly, a previous study using a Chinese cohort reported a significant association of the *IL-33* rs7044343 CC genotype with a decreased predisposition to RA (60). The *IL-33* rs7044343 C allele has also been shown to be strongly associated with a diminished risk of Alzheimer's disease in a study encompassing various populations (61). A meta-analysis performed by Zhong et al. also noted the *IL-33* rs7044343 C allele as a protective factor for Alzheimer disease (AD) development (62). However, no significant association was found in another study regarding Chinese patients diagnosed with AD (63). On the contrary, the rs7044343 C allele was identified as a risk factor for susceptibility to Behçet's disease and systemic sclerosis (64, 65). In line with these findings, the *IL-33* rs7044343 T allele has been associated with a decreased risk of coronary artery disease (51). The *IL-33* rs7044343 genetic variant was also examined for associations with asthma development in a Tunisian cohort; however, no significant relationships were found (66). Although, several other polymorphisms within the *IL-33* gene have been shown to be significantly associated with asthma susceptibility in various populations (50). A significant relationship was also found between the *IL-33* rs7044343 polymorphism and ischemic stroke in a Chinese cohort (67). On the contrary, there were no associations between the *IL-33* rs7044343 polymorphism and inflammatory bowel disease or idiopathic achalasia in an Italian cohort (68, 69). The *IL-33* rs7044343 polymorphism was also investigated in patients diagnosed with giant cell arteritis and chronic obstructive pulmonary disease; however, no significant correlations were detected (70, 71).

The discord between our studies' results and the aforementioned studies using Chinese cohorts most likely comes from genetic differences between the studied populations or inadequate sample sizes, particularly for AS and PsA cohorts. Indeed, the present study's main limitation was the limited sample size, possibly resulting in insufficient power for detecting associations.

Among the AS patient cohort, gender-specific associations in genotype distributions were found for all two studied genetic variants of *IL-33*. The *IL-33* rs1097559 CC genotype was less frequently observed among female AS patients than males, and the frequency of the *IL-33* rs7044343 TT genotype was significantly decreased in female patients. AS affects men more frequently than women, with male to female ratio of 3:1 (72, 73). Gender-related differences have been also detected with regard to clinical manifestation, radiographic damage and efficacy of biologic treatment. Female patients have higher disease activity defined as BASDAI and worse response to biologic treatment as compared to males (73–76). On the other hand, men are more likely to experience severe radiographic damage (77, 78). However, molecular mechanisms underlying these differences are currently unknown. No GWAS study performed to date on AS patients included sex-specific analyses. Some gene candidate studies reported gender-specific associations between studied genetic variants and AS. Polymorphisms within *ANKH* gene were found to be associated with AS susceptibility in a gender-dependent manner (79). Also, sex-related differences were observed in a haplotype distribution of specific tissue non-specific alkaline phosphatase (*TNAP*) gene (80). In addition, in the study conducted by Gracey et al., authors observed that gene expression profiles in AS patients differed between males and females (81).

The current study constitutes the first report of associations between *IL-33* gene polymorphisms and rheumatic diseases in a Caucasian population. The results indicated that *IL-33* polymorphisms might be associated with rheumatic disease risk and anti-TNF treatment outcomes in Caucasians. Nevertheless, additional studies with larger sample sizes and different populations are needed to validate these findings and to establish the exact role of *IL-33* polymorphisms in rheumatic diseases.

ETHICS STATEMENT

The studies involving human participants were reviewed and approved by the Wroclaw Medical University Ethics Committee. The patients/participants provided their written informed consent to participate in this study.

AUTHOR CONTRIBUTIONS

MI contributed to the conception and design of the study, genotyping, and statistical analyses and drafted and finalized the manuscript. JW performed most of the genotyping of patient and control samples, participated in the collection of literature data. JS, KK, RS, BB, and SJ provided clinical data and patient samples. MC-M prepared the control samples and their description. KB-K contributed to the conception and design of the study, drafted and finalized the manuscript, and secured funding All authors contributed to the article and approved the submitted version.

ACKNOWLEDGMENTS

The authors thank the Regional Centre of Transfusion Medicine and Blood Bank in Wroclaw for providing control samples.

REFERENCES

1. Noack M, Miossec P. Selected Cytokine Pathways in Rheumatoid Arthritis. *Semin Immunopathol* (2017) 39:365.e83. doi: 10.1007/s00281-017-0619-z
2. Livshits G, Kalinkovich A. Hierarchical, Imbalanced Pro-Inflammatory Cytokine Networks Govern the Pathogenesis of Chronic Arthropathies. *Osteoarthritis Cartilage* (2018) 26:7–17. doi: 10.1016/j.joca.2017.10.013
3. Cayrol C, Girard J-P. Interleukin-33 (IL-33): A Nuclear Cytokine From the IL-1 Family. *Immunol Rev* (2018) 281:154–68. doi: 10.1111/imr.12619
4. Gajardo Carrasco T, Morales RA, Perez F, Terraza C, Yanez L, Campos-Mora M, et al. Alarmin' Immunologists: IL-33 as a Putative Target for Modulating T Cell-Dependent Responses. *Front Immunol* (2015) 6:232. doi: 10.3389/fimmu.2015.00232
5. Carriere V, Roussel L, Ortega N, Lacorre DA, Americh L, Aguilar L, et al. IL-33, the IL-1-like Cytokine Ligand for ST2 Receptor, is a Chromatin-Associated Nuclear Factor In Vivo. *Proc Natl Acad Sci USA* (2007) 104:282–7. doi: 10.1073/pnas.0606854104
6. Drake LY, Kita H. IL-33: Biological Properties, Functions, and Roles in Airway Disease. *Immunol Rev* (2017) 278:173–84. doi: 10.1111/imr.12552
7. Moussion C, Ortega N, Girard JP. The IL-1-like Cytokine IL-33 is Constitutively Expressed in the Nucleus of Endothelial Cells and Epithelial Cells In Vivo: A Novel 'Alarmin'? *PloS One* (2008) 3(10):e3331. doi: 10.1371/journal.pone.0003331
8. Cayrol C, Girard JP. The IL-1-Like Cytokine IL-33 is Inactivated After Maturation by Caspase-1. *Proc Natl Acad Sci USA* (2009) 106:9021–26. doi: 10.1073/pnas.0812690106
9. Griesenauer B, Paczesny S. The ST2/IL-33 Axis in Immune Cells During Inflammatory Diseases. *Front Immunol* (2017) 8:475. doi: 10.3389/fimmu.2017.00475 eCollection 2017.
10. Nefla M, Holzinger D, Berenbaum F, Jacques C. The Danger From Within: Alarmins in Arthritis. *Nat Rev Rheumatol* (2016) 12:669–83. doi: 10.1038/nrrheum.2016.162
11. Chackerian AA, Oldham ER, Murphy EE, Schmitz J, Pflanz S, Kastelein RA. IL-1 Receptor Accessory Protein and ST2 Comprise the IL-33 Receptor Complex. *J Immunol* (2007) 179:2551–5. doi: 10.4049/jimmunol.179.4.2551
12. Liu X, Hammel M, He Y, Tainer JA, Jeng US, Zhang L, et al. Structural Insights Into the Interaction of IL-33 With its Receptors. *Proc Natl Acad Sci USA* (2013) 110:14918–23. doi: 10.1073/pnas.1308651110
13. Hayakawa H, Hayakawa M, Kume A, Tominaga S. Soluble ST2 Blocks interleukin-33 Signaling in Allergic Airway Inflammation. *J Biol Chem* (2007) 282:26369–80. doi: 10.1074/jbc.M704916200

14. Martin MU. Special Aspects of interleukin-33 and the IL-33 Receptor Complex. *Semin Immunol* (2013) 25:449–57. doi: 10.1016/j.smim.2013.10.006
15. Liew FY, Girard J-P, Turnquist HR. Interleukin-33 in Health and Disease. *Nat Rev Immunol* (2016) 16:676–89. doi: 10.1038/nri.2016.95
16. Schmitz J, Owyang A, Oldham E, Song Y, Murphy E, McClanahan TK, et al. Il-33, an Interleukin-1-Like Cytokine That Signals Via the IL-1 Receptor-Related Protein ST2 and Induces T Helper Type 2- Associated Cytokines. *Immunity* (2005) 23:479–90. doi: 10.1016/j.immuni.2005.09.015
17. Cayrol C, Girard J-P. IL-33: An Alarmin Cytokine With Crucial Roles in Innate Immunity, Inflammation and Allergy. *Curr Opin Immunol* (2014) 31:31–7. doi: 10.1016/j.coi.2014.09.004
18. Smithgall MD, Comeau MR, Park Yoon B-R, Kaufman D, Armitage R, Smith DE. IL-33 Amplifies Both Th1- and Th2-type Responses Through its Activity on Human Basophils, Allergen-Reactive Th2 Cells, iNKT and NK Cells. *Int Immunol* (2008) 20:1019–30. doi: 10.1093/intimm/dxn060
19. Afferni C, Buccione C, Andreone S, Galdiero MR, Varricchi G, Marone G, et al. The Pleiotropic Immunomodulatory Functions of IL-33 and its Implications in Tumor Immunity. *Front Immunol* (2018) 9:2601. doi: 10.3389/fimmu.2018.02601
20. Bonilla WV, Frohlich A, Senn K, Kallert S, Fernandez M, Johnson S, et al. The Alarmin Interleukin-33 Drives Protective Antiviral CD8(+) T Cell Responses. *Science* (2012) 335:984–89. doi: 10.1126/science.1215418
21. Bourgeois E, Van LP, Samson M, Diem S, Barra A, Roga S, et al. The pro-Th2 Cytokine IL-33 Directly Interacts With Invariant NKT and NK Cells to Induce IFN-Gamma Production. *Eur J Immunol* (2009) 39:1046–55. doi: 10.1002/eji.200838575
22. Gao K, Li X, Zhang L, Bai L, Dong W, Shi G, et al. Transgenic Expression of IL-33 Activates CD8(+) T Cells and NK Cells and Inhibits Tumor Growth and Metastasis in Mice. *Cancer Lett* (2013) 335:463–71. doi: 10.1016/j.canlet.2013.03.002
23. Sattler S, Ling GS, Xu D, Hussaarts L, Romaine A, Zhao H, et al. IL- 10-Producing Regulatory B Cells Induced by IL-33 (Breg(Il-33)) Effectively Attenuate Mucosal Inflammatory Responses in the Gut. *J Autoimmun* (2014) 50:107–22. doi: 10.1016/j.jaut.2014.01.032
24. Besnard A-G, Togbe D, Guillou N, Erard F, Quesniaux V, Ryffel B. IL-33-Activated Dendritic Cells are Critical for Allergic Airway Inflammation. *Eur J Immunol* (2011) 41:1675–86. doi: 10.1002/eji.201041033
25. Matta BM, Lott JM, Mathews LR, Liu Q, Rosborough BR, Blazar BR, et al. IL-33 is an Unconventional Alarmin That Stimulates IL-2 Secretion by Dendritic Cells to Selectively Expand IL-33R/ST2(+) Regulatory T Cells. *J Immunol* (2014) 193:4010–20. doi: 10.4049/jimmunol.1400481
26. Mayuzumi N, Matsushima H, Takashima A. IL-33 Promotes DC Development in BM Culture by Triggering GM-CSF Production. *Eur J Immunol* (2009) 39:3331–42. doi: 10.1002/eji.200939472
27. Schiering C, Krausgruber T, Chomka A, Frohlich A, Adelmann K, Wohlfert EA, et al. The Alarmin IL-33 Promotes Regulatory T-cell Function in the Intestine. *Nature* (2014) 513:564–8. doi: 10.1038/nature13577
28. Li P, Ma H, Han D, Mou K. Interleukin-33 Affects Cytokine Production by Keratinocytes in Vitiligo. *Clin Exp Dermatol* (2014) 40:163–70. doi: 10.1111/ced.12464
29. Rank MA, Kobayashi T, Kozaki H, Bartemes KR, Squillace DL, Kita H. IL-33-activated Dendritic Cells Induce an Atypical TH2-Type Response. *J Allergy Clin Immunol* (2009) 123:1047–54. doi: 10.1016/j.jaci.2009.02.026
30. Fransen J, van Riel PLCM. The Disease Activity Score and the EULAR Response Criteria. *Clin Exp Rheumatol* (2005) 23:S93–99. doi: 10.1016/j.rdc.2009.10.001
31. Zochling J, Braun J. Assessment of Ankylosing Spondylitis. *Clin Exp Rheumatol* (2005) 23(5Suppl 39):S133–41. doi: 10.1016/j.berh.2006.03.011
32. Fransen J, Antoni C, Mease PJ, Uter W, Kavanaugh A, Kalden JR, et al. Performance of Response Criteria for Assessing Peripheral Arthritis in Patients With Psoriatic Arthritis: Analysis of Data From Randomised Controlled Trials of Two Tumour Necrosis Factor Inhibitors. *Ann Rheum Dis* (2006) 65:1373–8. doi: 10.1136/ard.2006.051706
33. Mease PJ, Antoni CE, Gladman DD, Taylor W. Psoriatic Arthritis Assessment Tools in Clinical Trials. *Ann Rheum Dis* (2005) 64 Suppl 2:ii49–54. doi: 10.1136/ard.2004.034165
34. Xu Z, Taylor JA. SNP info: Integrating GWAS and Candidate Gene Information Into Functional SNP Selection for Genetic Association Studies. *Nucleic Acids Res* (2009) 37:W600–5. doi: 10.1093/nar/gkp290
35. Auton A, Brooks LD, Durbin RM, Garrison EP, Kang HM, Korbel JO, et al. A Global Reference for Human Genetic Variation. *Nature* (2015) 526:68–74. doi: 10.1038/nature15393
36. Core Team R. *R: A Language and Environment for Statistical Computing.* Vienna, Austria: R Foundation for Statistical Computing (2016). Available at: http://www.Rproject.org/.
37. Matsuyama Y, Okazaki H, Tamemoto H, Kimura H, Kamata Y, Nagatani K, et al. Increased Levels of Interleukin 33 in Sera and Synovial Fluid From Patients With Active Rheumatoid Arthritis. *J Rheumatol* (2010) 37:18–25. doi: 10.3899/jrheum.090492
38. Mu R, Huang HQ, Li YH, Li C, Ye H, Li ZG. Elevated Serum Interleukin 33 is Associated With Autoantibody Production in Patients With Rheumatoid Arthritis. *J Rheumatol* (2010) 37:2006–13. doi: 10.3899/jrheum.100184
39. Xiangyang Z, Lutian Y, Lin Z, Liping X, Hui S, Jing L. Increased Levels of interleukin-33 Associated With Bone Erosion and Interstitial Lung Diseases in Patients With Rheumatoid Arthritis. *Cytokine* (2012) 58:6–9. doi: 10.1016/j.cyto.2011.12.010
40. Kageyama Y, Torikai E, Tsujimura K, Kobayashi M. Involvement of IL-33 in the Pathogenesis of Rheumatoid Arthritis: The Effect of Etanercept on the Serum Levels of IL-33. *Mod Rheumatol* (2012) 22:89–93. doi: 10.1007/s10165-011-0480-1
41. Kunisch E, Chakilam S, Gandesiri M, Kinne RW. IL-33 Regulates TNF- a Dependent Effects in Synovial Fibroblasts. *Int J Mol Med* (2012) 29:530–40. doi: 10.3892/ijmm.2012.883
42. Palmer G, Talabot-Ayer D, Lamacchia C, Toy D, Seemayer CA, Viatte S, et al. Inhibition of Interleukin-33 Signaling Attenuates the Severity of Experimental Arthritis. *Arthritis Rheum* (2009) 60:738–49. doi: 10.1002/art.24305
43. Xu D, Jiang HR, Li Y, Pushparaj PN, Kurowska-Stolarska M, Leung BP, et al. IL-33 Exacerbates Autoantibody-Induced Arthritis. *J Immunol* (2010) 184:2620–26. doi: 10.4049/jimmunol.0902685
44. Fan D, Ding N, Yang T, Wu S, Liu S, Liu L, et al. Single Nucleotide Polymorphisms of the Interleukin-33 (Il-33) Gene are Associated With Ankylosing Spondylitis in Chinese Individuals: A Case-Control Pilot Study. *Scand J Rheumatol* (2014) 43:374. doi: 10.3109/03009742.2014.882408
45. Guo L, Zhou X, Guo X, Zhang X, Sun Y. Association of interleukin-33 Gene Single Nucleotide Polymorphisms With Ischemic Stroke in North Chinese Population. *BMC Med Genet* (2013) 14:109. doi: 10.1186/1471-2350-14-109
46. Guo J, Xiang Y, Peng YF, Huang HT, Lan Y, Wei YS. The Association of Novel IL-33 Polymorphisms With sIL-33 and Risk of Systemic Lupus Erythematosus. *Mol Immunol* (2016) 77:1–7. doi: 10.1016/j.molimm.2016.07.001
47. Tu X, Nie S, Liao Y, Zhang H, Fan Q, Xu C, et al. The IL-33-ST2L Pathway is Associated With Coronary Artery Disease in a Chinese Han Population. *Am J Hum Genet* (2013) 93:65. doi: 10.1016/j.ajhg.2013.08.009
48. Wang X, Zhu YF, Li DM, Qin Q, Wang Q, Muhali FS, et al. Polymorphisms of ST2-IL18R1-IL18RAP Gene Cluster: A New Risk for Autoimmune Thyroid Diseases. *Int J Immunogenet* (2016) 43:18–24. doi: 10.1111/iji.12240
49. Yue J, Tong Y, Xie L, Ma T, Yang J. Genetic Variant in IL-33 is Associated With Idiopathic Recurrent Miscarriage in Chinese Han Population. *Sci Rep* (2016) 6:23806. doi: 10.1038/srep23806
50. Grotenboer NS, Ketelaar ME, Koppelman GH, Nawijn MC. Decoding Asthma: Translating Genetic Variation in IL33 and IL1RL1 Into Disease Pathophysiology. *J Allergy Clin Immunol* (2013) 131:856–65. doi: 10.1016/j.jaci.2012.11.028
51. Angeles-Martinez J, Posadas-Sanchez R, Llorente L, Alvarez-Leon E, Ramirez-Bello J, Villarreal-Molina T, et al. The rs7044343 Polymorphism of the Interleukin 33 Gene Is Associated With Decreased Risk of Developing Premature Coronary Artery Disease and Central Obesity, and Could be Involved in Regulating the Production of IL-33. *PloS One* (2017) 12: e0168828. doi: 10.1371/journal.pone.0168828
52. Wu F, He M, Wen Q, Zhang W, Yang J, Zhang X, et al. Associations Between Variants in IL-33/ST2 Signaling Pathway Genes and Coronary Heart Disease Risk. *Int J Mol Sci* (2014) 15:23227–39. doi: 10.3390/ijms151223227
53. Okada Y, Wu D, Trynka G, Raj T, Terao C, Ikari K, et al. Genetics of Rheumatoid Arthritis Contributes to Biology and Drug Discovery. *Nature* (2014) 506:376–81. doi: 10.1038/nature12873
54. Australo-Anglo-American Spondyloarthritis C, Reveille JD, Sims AM, Danoy P, Evans DM, Leo P, et al. Genome-Wide Association Study of Ankylosing Spondylitis Identifies Non-MHC Susceptibility Loci. *Nat Genet* (2010) 42:123–7. doi: 10.1038/ng.513

55. Ellinghaus D, Jostins L, Spain SL, Cortes A, Bethune J, Han B, et al. Analysis of Five Chronic Inflammatory Diseases Identifies 27 New Associations and Highlights Disease-Specific Patterns at Shared Loci. *Nat Genet* (2016) 48:510–8. doi: 10.1038/ng.3528
56. International Genetics of Ankylosing Spondylitis Consortium (IGAS), Cortes A, Hadler J, Pointon JP, Robinson PC, Karaderi T, et al. Identification of Multiple Risk Variants for Ankylosing Spondylitis Through High-Density Genotyping of Immune-Related Loci. *Nat Genet* (2013) 45:730–8. doi: 10.1038/ng.2667
57. Massey J, Plant D, Hyrich K, Morgan AW, Wilson AG, Spiliopoulou A, et al. Genome-Wide Association Study of Response to Tumour Necrosis Factor Inhibitor Therapy in Rheumatoid Arthritis. *Pharmacogenomics J* (2018) 18:657–64. doi: 10.1038/s41397-018-0040-6
58. Umi·evi· Mirkov M, Cui J, Vermeulen SH, Stahl EA, Toonen EJM, Makkinje RR, et al. Genome-Wide Association Analysis of Anti-TNF Drug Response in Patients With Rheumatoid Arthritis. *Ann Rheum Dis* (2013) 72:1375–81. doi: 10.1136/annrheumdis-2012-202405
59. Sellam J, Marion-Thore S, Dumont F, Jacques S, Garchon H-J, Rouanet S, et al. Use of Whole-Blood Transcriptomic Profiling to Highlight Several Pathophysiologic Pathways Associated With Response to Rituximab in Patients With Rheumatoid Arthritis: Data From a Randomized, Controlled, Open-Label Trial. *Arthritis Rheumatol* (2014) 66:2015–25. doi: 10.1002/art.38671
60. Li C, Mu R, Guo J, Wu X, Tu X, Liu X, et al. Genetic Variant in IL33 is Associated With Susceptibility to Rheumatoid Arthritis. *Arthritis Res Ther* (2014) 16:R105. doi: 10.1186/ar4554
61. Chapuis J, Hot D, Hansmannel F, Kerdraon O, Ferreira S, Hubans C, et al. Transcriptomic and Genetic Studies Identify IL-33 as a Candidate Gene for Alzheimer's Disease. *Mol Psychiatry* (2009) 14:1004–16. doi: 10.1038/mp.2009.10
62. Zhong X, Liu MY, He M, Du K, Wei MJ. Association of Interleukin-33 Gene Polymorphisms With Susceptibility to Late Onset Alzheimer's Disease: A Meta-Analysis. *Neuropsychiatr Dis Treat* (2017) 13:2275–84. doi: 10.2147/NDT.S138073
63. Yu JT, Song JH, Wang ND, Wu ZC, Zhang Q, Zhang N, et al. Implication of IL-33 Gene Polymorphism in Chinese Patients With Alzheimer's Disease. *Neurobiol Aging* (2012) 33:1014.e11–1014.e14. doi: 10.1016/j.neurobiolaging.2010.07.003
64. Koca SS, Pehlivan, Kara M, Alibaz-Oner F, Oztuzcu S, Yilmaz N, et al. The IL-33 Gene is Related to Increased Susceptibility to Systemic Sclerosis. *Rheumatol Int* (2016) 36:579–84. doi: 10.1007/s00296-015-3417-8
65. Koca SS, Kara M, Deniz F, Ozgen M, Demir CF, Ilhane N, et al. Serum IL-33 Level and IL-33 Gene Polymorphisms in Behçet's Disease. *Rheumatol Int* (2015) 35:471–7. doi: 10.1007/s00296-014-3111-2
66. Charrad R, Kaabachi W, Berraies A, Hamzaoui K, Hamzaoui A. IL-33 Gene Variants and Protein Expression in Pediatric Tunisian Asthmatic Patients. *Cytokine* (2017) 104:85–91. doi: 10.1016/j.cyto.2017.09.028
67. Li S, Wang Z, Liu X, Li Y, Shi C, Wu J, et al. Association of Common Variants in the IL-33/ST2 Axis With Ischemic Stroke. *Curr Neurovasc Res* (2019) 16:494–501. doi: 10.2174/1567202616666191029112334
68. Latiano A, Palmieri O, Pastorelli L, Vecchi M, Pizarro TT, Bossa F, et al. Associations Between Genetic Polymorphisms in IL-33, IL1R1 and Risk for Inflammatory Bowel Disease. *PloS One* (2013) 8:e62144. doi: 10.1371/journal.pone.0062144
69. Latiano A, Palmieri O, Bossa F, Latiano T, Corritore G, de Santo E, et al. Impact of Genetic Polymorphisms on the Pathogenesis of Idiopathic Achalasia: Association With IL33 Gene Variant. *Hum Immunol* (2014) 75:364–9. doi: 10.1016/j.humimm.2014.01.004
70. Márquez A, Solans R, Hernández-Rodríguez J, Cid MC, Castañeda S, Ramentol M, et al. A Candidate Gene Approach Identifies an IL33 Genetic Variant as a Novel Genetic Risk Factor for GCA. *PloS One* (2014) 9:e113476. doi: 10.1371/journal.pone.0113476
71. Xu X, Li H, Liu Q, Zhang H. Interleukin-33 Gene Polymorphisms and Chronic Obstructive Pulmonary Disease in the Chinese Han Population. *J Int Med Res* (2020) 48:300060520962340. doi: 10.1177/0300060520962340
72. Gran JT, Husby G. Ankylosing Spondylitis in Women. *Semin Arthritis Rheum* (1990) 19:303–12. doi: 10.1016/0049-0172(90)90053-i
73. Van der Horst-Bruinsma IE, Zack DJ, Szumski A, Koenig AS. Female Patients With Ankylosing Spondylitis: Analysis of the Impact of Gender Across Treatment Studies. *Ann Rheum Dis* (2013) 72:1221–4. doi: 10.1136/annrheumdis-2012-202431
74. Glintborg B, Ostergaard M, Krogh NS, Dreyer L, Kristensen HL, Hetland ML. Predictors of Treatment Response and Drug Continuation in 842 Patients With Ankylosing Spondylitis Treated With Anti- Tumour Necrosis Factor: Results From 8 Years' Surveillance in the Danish Nationwide DANBIO Registry. *Ann Rheum Dis* (2010) 69:2002–8. doi: 10.1136/ard.2009.124446
75. Roussou E, Sultana S. Spondyloarthritis in Women: Differences in Disease Onset, Clinical Presentation, and Bath Ankylosing Spondylitis Disease Activity and Functional Indices (BASDAI and BASFI) Between Men and Women With Spondyloarthritides. *Clin Rheumatol* (2011) 30:121–7. doi: 10.1007/s10067-010-1581-5
76. Webers C, Essers I, Ramiro S, Stolwijk C, Landewé R, van der Heijde D, et al. Gender-Attributable Differences in Outcome of Ankylosing Spondylitis: Long-Term Results From the Outcome in Ankylosing Spondylitis International Study. *Rheumatology* (2016) 55:419–28. doi: 10.1093/rheumatology/kev340
77. Lee W, Reveille JD, Davis JCJr, Learch TJ, Ward MM, Weisman MH. Are There Gender Differences in Severity of Ankylosing Spondylitis? *Results PSOAS cohort Ann Rheum Dis* (2007) 66:633–8. doi: 10.1136/ard.2006.060293
78. Ward MM, Hendrey MR, Malley JD, Learch TJ, Davis JCJr, Reveille JD, et al. Clinical and Immunogenetic Prognostic Factors for Radiographic Severity in Ankylosing Spondylitis. *Arthritis Rheum* (2009) 61:859–66. doi: 10.1002/art.24585
79. Tsui HW, Inman RD, Reveille JD, Tsui FW. Association of a TNAP Haplotype With Ankylosing Spondylitis. *Arthritis Rheum* (2007) 56:234–43. doi: 10.1002/art.22307
80. Tsui HW, Inman RD, Paterson AD, Reveille JD, Tsui FW. ANKH Variants Associated With Ankylosing Spondylitis: Gender Differences. *Arthritis Res Ther* (2005) 7:R513–25. doi: 10.1186/ar1701
81. Gracey E, Yao Y, Green B, Qaiyum Z, Baglaenko Y, Lin A, et al. Sexual Dimorphism in the Th17 Signature of Ankylosing Spondylitis. *Arthritis Rheumatol* (2016) 68:679–89. doi: 10.1002/art.39464

10

Recent Developments in Clinical Applications of Mesenchymal Stem Cells in the Treatment of Rheumatoid Arthritis and Osteoarthritis

Joel Jihwan Hwang [1†], *Yeri Alice Rim* [2†], *Yoojun Nam* [2] *and Ji Hyeon Ju* [2,3*]

[1] *College of Public Health and Social Justice, Saint Louis University, St. Louis, MO, United States,* [2] *Catholic Induced Pluripotent Stem Cell Research Center, College of Medicine, The Catholic University of Korea, Seoul, South Korea,* [3] *Division of Rheumatology, Department of Internal Medicine, Seoul St. Mary's Hospital, Institute of Medical Science, College of Medicine, The Catholic University of Korea, Seoul, South Korea*

***Correspondence:**
Ji Hyeon Ju
juji@catholic.ac.kr

†These authors have contributed equally to this work

Mesenchymal stem cell (MSC) therapies have been used as cell-based treatments for decades, owing to their anti-inflammatory, immunomodulatory, and regenerative properties. With high expectations, many ongoing clinical trials are investigating the safety and efficacy of MSC therapies to treat arthritic diseases. Studies on osteoarthritis (OA) have shown positive clinical outcomes, with improved joint function, pain level, and quality of life. In addition, few clinical MSC trials conducted on rheumatoid arthritis (RA) patients have also displayed some optimistic outlook. The largely positive outcomes in clinical trials without severe side effects establish MSCs as promising tools for arthritis treatment. However, further research is required to investigate its applicability in clinical settings. This review discusses the most recent advances in clinical studies on MSC therapies for OA and RA.

Keywords: mesenchymal stem cell, rheumatoid arthritis, osteoarthritis, cartilage, cell therapy

INTRODUCTION

The first study on mesenchymal stem cells (MSCs) was published in 1966 by Fridenshtein et al., who cultured bone-forming cells from guinea-pig bone marrow and spleen cells (1, 2). Subsequent studies have characterized MSCs as clonogenic progenitor cells capable of differentiating into mesoderm-derived cells such as osteoblasts, chondrocytes, and adipocytes (1, 3–5). The term "mesenchymal stem cell" was first used in 1991 to represent cells originating from embryonic mesodermal tissues (5, 6). While, MSCs imply mesenchymal "stem" or "stromal" cells at the same time, it is suggested only to refer progenitor cells with self-renewal and differentiation ability as "mesenchymal stem cells." Mesenchymal stromal cells, on the other hand, refer to a bulk population of cells with immunomodulatory and homing properties. Some researchers, however, have recently argued that MSCs should be renamed "medicinal signaling cells" because these cells secrete therapeutic regenerative bioactive factors to stimulate the site- and tissue-specific resident stem cells of patients rather than differentiating into tissue-producing cells (7). Nevertheless, the wide clinical potential of MSCs, which ranges from repairing simple tissue tears to regulating immunological diseases, remains to be fully elucidated (2). Hence, researchers worldwide continue to explore the applications of MSCs. Notably, there were 1,043 trials involving 47,548 patients conducted between 2011 and 2018 (2).

Although the criteria for defining human MSCs are not concrete and subject to changes, most researchers agree on the three defining characteristics of human MSCs established by the International Society of Cellular Therapy (ISCT) (8, 9). The first general characteristic of MSCs is plastic adherence where cells with clonal expansion ability can be maintained for several passages in plastic culture dishes while excluding the subpopulation of cells with hematopoietic functions (9, 10). This characteristic is generally believed to encompass all types of MSCs without any exceptions. The second feature of human MSCs is the unique set of positive and negative surface markers expressed on these cells; the ICST has proposed CD105 (endoglin), CD73 (ecto-5′-nucleotidase), and CD90 (Thy-1) as the surface markers of MSCs. In contrast, MSCs lack the expression of hematopoietic and endothelial markers, such as CD45, CD34, CD14, CD11b, CD79α, CD19, and human leukocyte antigen (HLA)-DR (8, 9). Although the list proposed by the ICST is generally agreed upon by researchers, this criterion is the most disputed; some researchers regard CD34, CD45, and CD14 as negative markers, while STRO-1, CD29, CD73, CD90, CD105, CD106, CD166, CD146, and CD44 are considered positive markers (11). Multiple studies have also discovered variations from this criterion. For instance, fractions of adipose tissue derived-MSCs (AT-MSCs) were observed to express CD34 when insulin-like growth factor 1 (IGF-1) was added to the culture media (12). Moreover, the expression of the negative marker HLA-DR was upregulated in murine and human MSCs after exposure to interferon-γ (IFN-γ) (13, 14). Hence, positive and negative surface markers are not widely used to classify *in vitro*-expanded MSCs, and further research is needed to clarify this criterion. The final and most defining characteristic of MSCs is the ability to differentiate into osteoblasts, adipocytes, and chondroblasts *in vitro* (8). As mentioned earlier, the differentiation potential of MSCs into various cell lineages was a factor in their early classification as a type of stem cell and remains one of their key traits (6).

Abbreviations: ACPA, anti-citrullinated protein antibodies; AI, arthritis index; AIA, antigen-induced arthritis; ALK, activin receptor-like kinase; AT-MSC, adipose tissue-derived mesenchymal stem cell; BMAC, bone marrow aspirate concentration; BM-MSC, bone marrow-derived mesenchymal stem cell; CD, cluster of differentiation; DAS28, disease activity score; DMARD, disease-modifying anti-rheumatic drug; ECM, extracellular matrix; FLS, fibroblast-like synoviocytes; GFP-MSC, green fluorescent protein-positive mesenchymal stem cells; HA, hyaluronic acid; HAQ, health assessment questionnaire; HKA angle, hip-knee-ankle angle; HLA, human leukocyte antigen; ICOAP pain questionnaire, measure of Intermittent and Constant Osteoarthritis Pain questionnaire; ICST, International Society of Cellular Therapy; IFN- γ, interferon gamma; IGF-1, insulin-like growth factor 1; IKDC, International Knee Documentation Committee; IL, interleukin; K-L grade, Kellgren-Lawrence grade; KOOS, Knee Injury and Osteoarthritis Outcome Score; MMP, matrix metalloproteinases; MRI, magnetic resonance imaging; MSC, mesenchymal stem cell; NPRS, Numeric Pain Rating Scale; NF-κB, nuclear factor-kappa B; OA, osteoarthritis; OP-1, osteogenic protein 1; PGA, patient global assessment; RA, rheumatoid arthritis; ROS, reactive oxygen species; GWAS, genome-wide association studies; SF-36 Questionnaire, 36-Item Short Form Survey; SM-MSC, synovium-derived mesenchymal stem cell; SNP, single nucleotide polymorphism; TNF, tumor necrosis factor; UCB-MSC, umbilical cord blood-derived mesenchymal stem cell; VAS, visual analog scale; WOMAC index, Western Ontario and McMaster Universities Osteoarthritis index; WORMS, whole-organ MRI scoring.

The first clinical studies involving MSCs assessed their therapeutic potential in hematopoiesis, osteogenesis imperfecta, Hurler syndrome, and metachromatic leukodystrophy (15–19). These studies provided initial safety assessments for MSCs and encouraged further research to thoroughly examine their clinical efficacy (15). Recent decades have seen clinical trials conducted on these cells, especially for autoimmune, neurodegenerative, cardiovascular, and bone and cartilage diseases (20). However, the number of approved MSC treatments worldwide remains limited. Asian countries have approved more MSC treatments than other countries; South Korea has approved four MSC therapies, whereas Japan and India have each approved one (**Table 1**).

HUMAN TISSUES CONTAINING MSCs AND THE VARIOUS POTENTIALS OF THESE CELLS

The ISCT MSC committee recommends not to use the term mesenchymal "stem" cells unless there is rigorous *in vitro* and *in vivo* functional evidence that can provide the self-renewal and differentiation ability (9). While MSCs are found in various parts of the human body, MSCs isolated from the bone marrow (BM), umbilical cord blood, periosteum, dental pulp, adipose tissue, and growth plate were confirmed to have stem cell-like properties [**Figure 1**; (21–23)]. In this section, we will discuss four sites where MSCs are frequently found and used for treatment of arthritic diseases: the bone marrow, umbilical cord, adipose tissue, and synovial membrane (24). To select a suitable MSC source for treatment, both advantages and disadvantages of MSC acquisition including the potential side effects and limitations (e.g., cell quality, number, and the difficulty and invasiveness of the isolation process) must be considered (25).

Bone marrow was the initial extraction site used by Fridenshtein et al. (1). After years of animal studies, the isolation and expansion of human bone marrow-derived MSCs (BM-MSCs) in culture were first conducted in 1992 (2, 26). With the safety and effectiveness of BM-MSCs confirmed through multiple clinical trials, they have become the most widely-used source of MSCs characterized by remarkable differentiation potential (27). However, there are several limitations of BM-MSCs. Most importantly, the yields, along with the differentiation and repair potential, are heavily dependent on the donor characteristics, such as disease condition and age (25). Furthermore, BM-MSC harvesting is challenging and inefficient, as only 0.001–0.01% of bone marrow cells are MSCs (27, 28). The risk of infection during the isolation of cells from the bone marrow also cannot be ignored. Consequently, a more effective and less invasive procedure is required, and scientists have attempted to identify new extraction sites (27, 28).

In 2000, human umbilical cord blood was recognized as an alternative source of MSCs (29). Umbilical cord blood-derived MSCs (UCB-MSCs) show rapid self-renewal and differentiation capabilities, thereby promoting tissue repair and modulation of immune responses; moreover, these cells are

TABLE 1 | A list of approved cell therapy products around the world and a graphical image of countries where MSC therapies are approved and clinically used.

Name	Country	Product description	Date of market approval	Current status
Prochymal (MESOBLAST INTERNATIONAL SARL)	Canada	Allogeneic *ex vivo*-cultured adult human mesenchymal stromal cells for the management of acute graft-vs.-host disease (aGVHD) in pediatric patients	May 2, 2015	The product was never marketed in Canada
Stempeucel® (Stempeutics Research)	India	*Ex vivo*-cultured adult allogeneic mesenchymal stromal cells for the treatment of critical limb ischemia due to thromboangiitis obliterans (Buerger disease)	May 2016	On the market, limited release (200 patients on a cost recovery basis), post-market surveillance study required
Temcell HS (JCR Pharmaceuticals Co. Ltd.)	Japan	Allogeneic mesenchymal stromal cells for the treatment of aGVHD	September 2015	On the market
Prochymal (Osiris Therapeutics Incorporated)	New Zealand	Allogeneic *ex vivo*-cultured adult human mesenchymal stromal cells indicated for the rescue of patients with NLT 6 month to 17 year of age with aGVHD, refractory to treatment with systemic corticosteroid therapy or other immunosuppressive agents	June 14, 2012	Approval lapsed
NEURONATA-R® (Corestem, Inc.)	South Korea	Autologous bone marrow mesenchymal stromal cell therapy for amyotrophic lateral sclerosis	July 30, 2014	Orphan product
Cupistem® (Anterogen)	South Korea	Autologous adipose tissue-derived mesenchymal stromal cell therapy for Crohn's fistula	January 18, 2012	Covered by insurance as of 2014, orphan product
CARTISTEM® (Medipost Co., Ltd.)	South Korea	Human umbilical cord blood-derived mesenchymal stromal cells for the treatment of knee articular cartilage defects in patients with osteoarthritis (ICRS grade IV)	January 18, 2012	On the Market
Cellgram®-AMI (Pharmicell Co., Ltd.)	South Korea	Autologous bone barrow-derived mesenchymal stromal cells for patients with acute myocardial infarction (left ventricular ejection fraction improvement)	July 1, 2011	Name at time of approval was Hearticellgram®-AMI, on the market
Ixmyelocel-T (Vericel)	USA	Autologous expanded multicellular (mesenchymal cells, monocytes, and alternatively activated macrophages) product for patients with advanced heart failure due to ischemic dilated cardiomyopathy	May 10, 2017	Orphan product
Alofisel® (Takeda Pharma A/S)	European Union	Allogenic adipose tissue-derived mesenchymal cells used for complex anal fistulas in adults with Crohn's disease	March 23, 2018	Orphan product

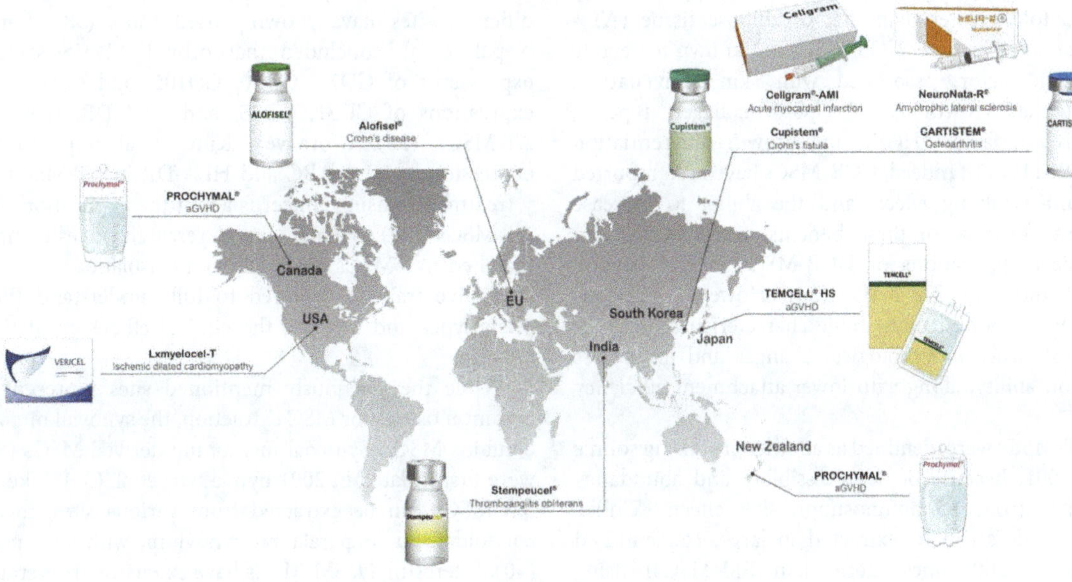

Asian countries have approved more MSC treatments than other countries. South Korea has approved four MSC therapies, while Japan and India have each approved one.

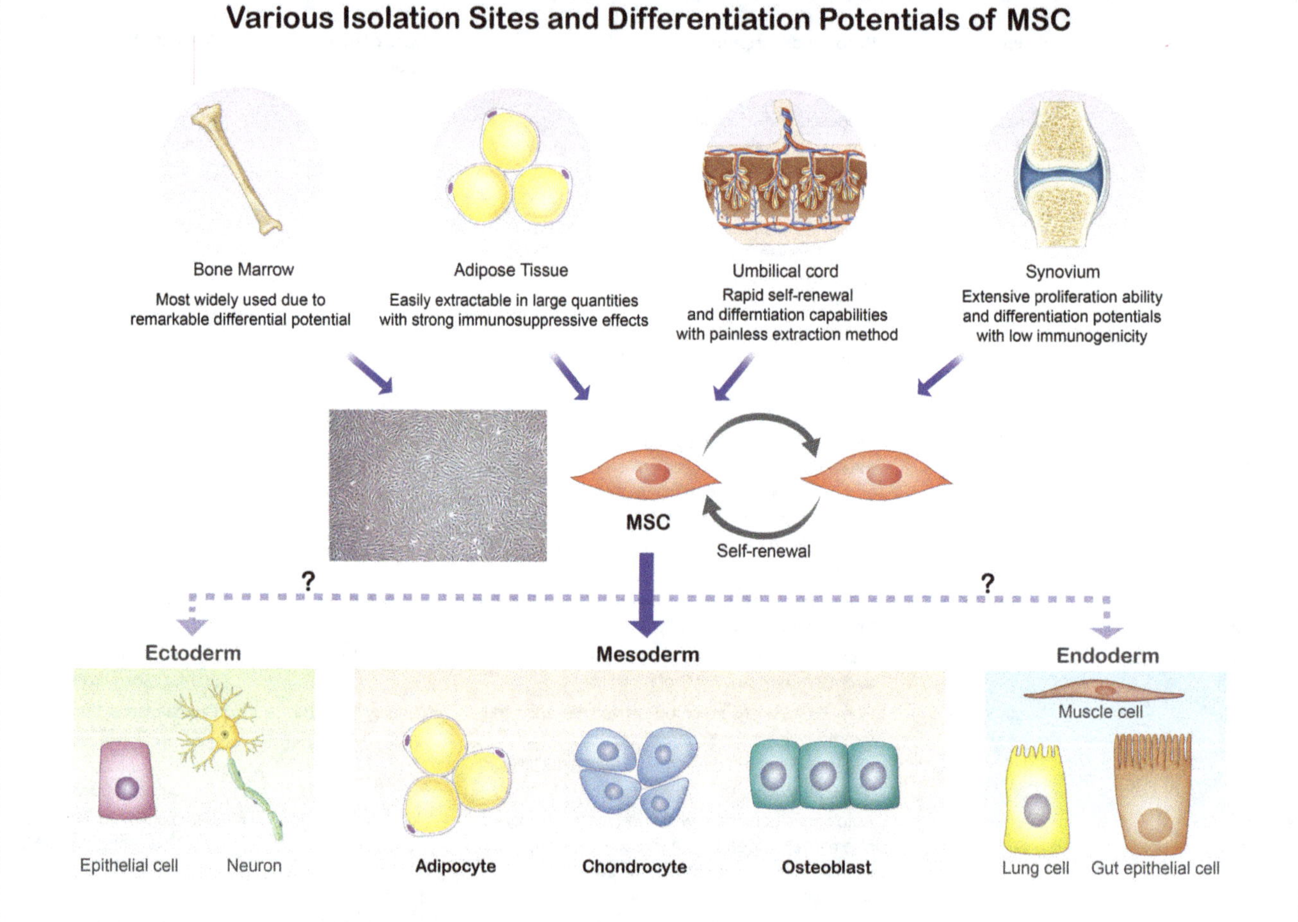

FIGURE 1 | Various isolation sites and differentiation potentials of MSCs. Bone marrow, adipose tissue, umbilical cord, and synovium are common sites for MSC extraction. The isolated MSCs can be differentiated into adipocytes, chondrocytes, myocytes, and osteoblasts.

easy to access with painless extraction procedures (30). UCB-MSCs have rapid proliferation rates that are approximately three- to four-fold greater than that of adipose tissue (AT)-MSCs (31, 32). Furthermore, UCB-MSCs are known to secrete multiple growth factors associated with skin rejuvenation, such as epithelial growth factor (EGF), collagen type 1, hepatocyte growth factor (HGF), and growth differentiation factor-11 (GDF-11) (33). Indeed, UCB-MSCs have been reported to possess anti-wrinkling effects and the ability to increase dermal density. Because of these benefits, researchers claim that the clinical applications of UCB-MSCs extend beyond the limits of those of BM-MSCs (34). However, previous studies have also reported undesirable characteristics of UCB-MSCs, such as earlier morphological changes and faster loss of amplification ability, along with lower attachment efficiency (31, 35, 36).

Human AT-MSCs were identified as another promising source of MSCs in 2001, because of its accessibility and abundancy as well as its stronger immunosuppressive effects. Unlike BM-MSCs, AT-MSCs can be extracted in large, concentrated quantities (about 500 times more than BM-MSCs) using relatively simple procedures and local anesthesia (37). Another benefit of AT-MSCs is that they can be extracted from various human body sites; however, AT-MSCs extracted from different sites have shown varied traits (38). For instance, Nepali et al. concluded that orbital AT-MSCs have higher expressions of CD73, CD90, CD105, and CD146, but lower expressions of CD31, CD45, and HLA-DR, than abdominal AT-MSCs (38). Moreover, Kim et al. reported increased expression of HLA-ABC and HLA-DR in AT-MSCs after IFN-γ treatment, raising concerns about the application of allogenic AT-MSCs (32). Hence, more research investigating donor-matched AT-MSCs from different isolation sites and their respective traits is required to fully understand the defining phenotypes and increase the clinical efficiency of these MSCs (28, 38).

While the previously mentioned sites represent the most common tissues for MSC extraction, the synovial membrane also contains MSCs. Synovial membrane-derived MSCs (SM-MSCs) were first isolated in 2001 by De Bari et al. (39). Like AT-MSCs, SM-MSCs can be extracted from various sites, including the cotyloid fossa or paralabral synovium, with site-specific traits (40). Interestingly, SM-MSCs have extensive proliferative ability, multilineage differentiation potential, and low immunogenicity relative to other MSCs (39, 41). Due to higher expression of type II collagen, aggrecan, and SRY-box transcription factor 9 in SM-MSCs, they have demonstrated higher chondrogenic potential than MSCs from other sources and are expected to be more widely used for cartilage repair and joint homeostasis treatments (42–44). Moreover, a study by Sakaguchi et al. concluded that SM-MSCs and BM-MSCs have greater osteogenic and adipogenic potentials than other MSCs; however, SM-MSCs foster relatively low-density expansions *in vitro* compared to BM-MSCs (41, 45).

APPLICATIONS OF MSC THERAPIES FOR CARTILAGE INJURIES

The safety and efficacy of MSCs in the treatment of joint-related diseases and cartilage injuries have been continuously examined over the recent decades. Concurrently, the prevalence of cartilage lesions have also significantly increased during this period, as the early incidence rates of this condition have roughly tripled from 1996 to 2011 (46, 47). Despite the high prevalence rate, a universally efficient method for articular cartilage repair is yet to be developed (48). Current surgical options include arthroplasty, microfracture, and autologous chondrocyte implantation (49). The promising qualities of MSC-based therapies could potentially provide effective, less invasive procedures to repair articular cartilage defects. In an experimental trial, BM-MSCs were transplanted into the patellae of two patients with full-thickness articular cartilage defects (50). Two years after transplantation, the arthroscopic results showed significant improvements in the walking abilities of both patients (50). Similarly, another case study involving a judo athlete diagnosed with a full-thickness cartilage defect in the medial femoral condyle exhibited recovery within months after the implantation of MSC-embedded collagen gel with reduced pain (51). Furthermore, a 2010 study compared the clinical outcomes of cartilage lesion repair between implantations of first-generation autologous chondrocytes and BM-MSCs in groups of 36 patients each; all patients showed improvements in quality of life with no significant differences between the groups (52). Therefore, it was concluded that BM-MSC treatment is a cost-efficient option for cartilage lesion repair with minimal donor-site morbidity and fewer surgical procedures than autologous chondrocyte implantation (52). Thus, multiple clinical trials have revealed the promising potential of MSC therapy in cartilage repair.

Variations in the general characteristics of rheumatoid arthritis (RA) and osteoarthritis (OA) largely depend on their etiologies and initial symptoms. RA is a chronic systemic autoimmune disease characterized by joint inflammation and bone erosion (53, 54), whereas OA is a degenerative joint disease that triggers the gradual loss of articular cartilage (55, 56). While increased bone spur growth is observed in osteoarthritic joints during the early stages, RA joints initially experience synovial inflammation (**Figure 2**). Ultimately, patients diagnosed with either joint condition suffer from severe cartilage inflammation and loss of mobility (56, 57). In this review, we will further discuss the use of MSCs in these two respective joint diseases.

APPLICATIONS OF MSC THERAPIES IN OA

General Characteristics of OA

OA is the most common degenerative joint disease (55). Its initial symptoms include loss of articular cartilage followed by progressive to joint stiffness, swelling, pain, and loss of mobility (56). The prevalence rate of OA is extremely high, affecting more than 250 million people worldwide (58–60). With increases in the aging and obese populations, the prevalence of OA is predicted to increase to 67 million by 2030 (61). Hence, an effective and safe OA treatment is urgently required.

Like RA, OA is also divided into two groups based on its etiology: primary and secondary (59). Primary OA is idiopathic and gene-dependent, whereas secondary OA mainly originates from traumatic events (58, 62, 63). Despite different etiologies, the two types of OA progress in similar directions, ultimately resulting in the loss and destruction of articular cartilage (55).

Although aging is one of the biggest risk factors for OA, the underlying mechanisms and related factors are yet to be definitively established (55, 56, 64). An imbalance in the production and activities of catabolic mediators in aging cells is a cause of the destruction and loss of articular cartilage (65). A disturbed ratio of the transforming growth factor β (TGF-β) receptors activin receptor-like kinase 1 (ALK1) and ALK5 triggers the downregulation of the TGF-β pathway and induces matrix metalloproteinase (MMP) expression, which degrades structural proteins in the cartilage (55, 66). The exact reason for this imbalance in signaling is assumed to be the senescent phenotype of OA chondrocytes, but a clear explanation is still required (65). Age-related mitochondrial dysfunction has also been suggested to promote the development of OA (66, 67). Aged articular chondrocytes and other cells display increased secretion of reactive oxygen species (ROS), and thereby elevated oxidative stress (67–69). The production of ROS ultimately alters mitochondrial function, leaving them unable to synthesize proteoglycans, the primary building blocks of the cartilage extracellular matrix (ECM) (70).

Genetic predisposition is another major risk factor of primary OA, with almost 30–65% of OA risk being genetically determined (56, 64, 71, 72). Recent genome-wide association studies (GWAS) have drastically expanded our understanding of the genetic risk factors of OA (71, 73). Currently, 90 loci are known to pose significant OA genetic risks, and 80 possible gene mutations or single nucleotide polymorphisms (SNPs) have been identified to be involved in OA pathogenesis (74). These include genes encoding other structural factors (*Col2a1*, *Col9a1*, and *Col11a1*) and bone morphogenetic proteins (*Gdf5*) (75–81). There are various ongoing studies focused on fully uncovering the genetic risk factors of OA. Most notably, a 2019 study analyzed ~77,000 patients with OA and 378,000 undiagnosed individuals from the UK Biobank cohort to identify 52 novel OA-associated signals (74). While most studies have specifically investigated OA susceptibility loci in Europeans or those of

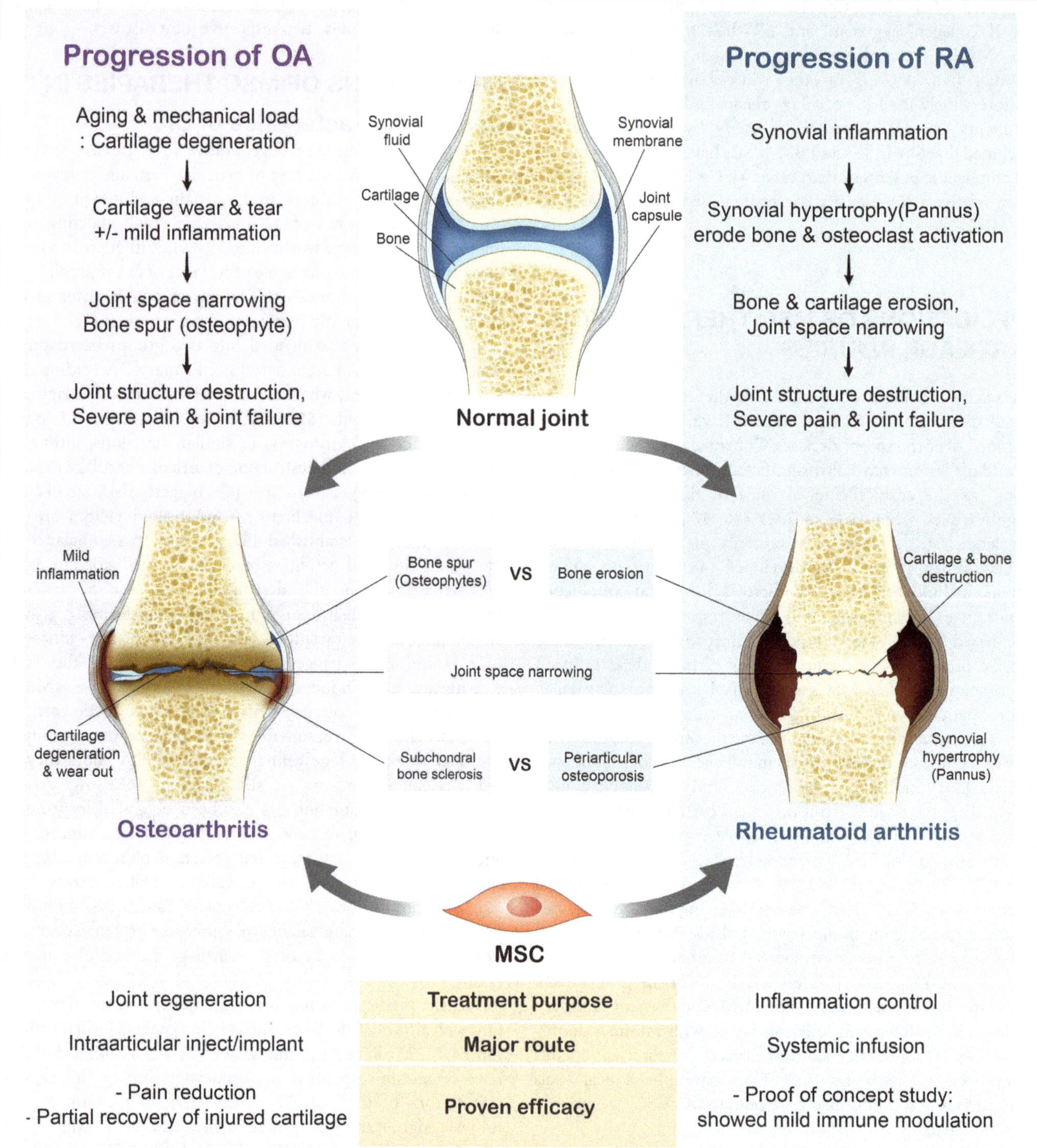

FIGURE 2 | Progression of rheumatoid arthritis (RA) and osteoarthritis (OA). In contrast to the healthy joint, the osteoarthritic joint has thinned cartilage and the bone ends rub together. Joints diagnosed with RA have swollen, inflamed synovial membranes and undergo bone erosion. The cartilage erosion seen in the later stages of arthritis ultimately leads to the loss of mobility.

European descent, there have also been studies targeting other populations (82–85). A 2020 study by Zhao et al. showed a significant correlation between the SNP rs10896015 in the *LTBP3* gene and hip OA among the Chinese population (86). Furthermore, another study revealed that the SNP rs4238326 in the *ALDH1A2* gene, which was previously reported to trigger hand OA in European populations, is also linked to knee OA risk (86, 87).

Obesity has become a highly prevalent disease in contemporary society and it is estimated to spread to almost 20% of the global population by 2030 (88). Obese patients with unhealthy diets are exposed to multiple risk factors of OA, as one study reports a 24% increase in the likelihood of developing OA in obese individuals compared to those of healthy weight (89). First and foremost, mechanical overload in joints promotes ROS production by OA chondrocytes, which further aggravates cartilage degradation (90). A recent study concluded that there is a 2.5-times higher likelihood of patients with diabetic knee OA experiencing knee pain compared to patients with non-diabetic knee OA due to accelerated cartilage damage (91). Furthermore, obesity has also been associated with the secretion of adipokines, thus contributing to low-grade systemic inflammation (92–95). The expression levels of pro-inflammatory cytokines, such as interleukin (IL)-1β, IL-6, IL-8, and tumor necrosis factor-α (TNF-α), are increased in obese individuals (96–101). Inflammatory factors activate the nuclear factor-κB (NF-κB) signaling pathway and ultimately result in the upregulation of MMPs, subsequently targeting the ECM (102–104). Lastly, meta-analysis studies have shown a significant relationship between obesity and dose-response. Patients with higher body mass indices are less likely to be dose-responsive and show continual clinical consequences (89, 105, 106).

Although moderate physical activity is encouraged to improve one's general health, repetition or incorrect execution of movements is the prevailing cause of OA in both young and older adults (56, 64, 107). From a comprehensive review of recent studies, common occupational activities such as sitting (hip and knee OA), lifting (knee OA), driving (knee OA), and squat (lower limb OA) have been associated with increased risk of OA (108, 109). These activities, if repeated, could be detrimental to the joint, as a study calculated the risk of developing localized OA to be twice as likely in individuals with occupations demanding repetitive physical activities compared to the average population (110). Moreover, although recreational sports activities are known to lower the occurrence of OA, elite athletes participating in competitive sports are extremely prone to OA, as incorrect execution of movements may disturb joint stabilization (111–114). In a systematic review including over 8,400 subjects, it was concluded that soccer, weightlifting, and wrestling were the sports with the highest prevalence of knee OA (112). Furthermore, it has been reported that OA prevalence rates in contact sports, such as rugby, are twice as high as those in non-contact sports (113).

Clinical Trials Using MSCs in OA

We also reviewed recent clinical trials that used MSC-based treatments in patients with OA (**Table 2**). A clinical trial by Kim et al. involved 49 patients (55 knees) with isolated full-thickness cartilage lesions and Kellgren-Lawrence (K-L) grade 1 or 2 OA with symptoms of knee joint pain and/or functional limitations despite non-surgical treatments for a minimum of 3 months (115). AT-MSCs were harvested from each patient's buttocks via tumescent liposuction. Upon isolation, AT-MSCs were loaded into a fibrin glue product and surgically implanted into the lesion site. Implanted knees were immobilized with a knee brace for 2 weeks post-surgery, followed by passive joint exercises. During the follow-ups, it was reported that the mean International Knee Documentation Committee (IKDC) score increased from 37.7 to 67.3, and the Tegner Activity Scale from 2.2 to 3.8. Both scores showed significant improvements in patients, with 74.5% of them expressing better satisfaction. In addition, age and lesion size were identified as independent factors affecting clinical outcomes. Patients over 60 years of age with lesion sizes >6.0 cm^2 showed less favorable results. Although there were some variations in the results due to these factors, the overall clinical outcomes of MSC implantation in OA patients were encouraging, with successful results.

In 2016, Shapiro et al. conducted a randomized, single-blinded, placebo-controlled trial in 25 patients with mild to moderate bilateral knee OA who had previously received conventional treatments, such as activity modification or physical therapy (116). Each patient had ~52 mL of bone marrow harvested from their respective superior iliac crests. The marrow cells were then analyzed for the positive and negative co-expression of surface markers to fulfill the minimal criteria for defining MSCs. Upon confirmation, 5 mL of cells were mixed with 10 mL of previously separated platelet-poor bone marrow plasma to be injected into a randomly assigned knee of each patient (13 patients received MSCs in their right knee, and 12 patients in their left knee). The contralateral knees subsequently underwent an intra-articular injection of 15 mL of sterile saline, and served as controls. After 1 week, 3 months, and 6 months, the Measure of Intermittent and Constant Osteoarthritis Pain (ICOAP) questionnaire and visual analog scale (VAS) pain scores of the two groups were recorded. The VAS pain scores and answers to the ICOAP questionnaires indicated significant improvements throughout the follow-up periods in both the bone marrow aspirate concentration group and the placebo group. Furthermore, both groups showed increased activity levels and decreases in self-reported pain medication usage, with no difference in the degree of improvement from baseline. The efficacy of MSC injection was questioned, as there was no difference in pain-mediating capabilities between the knees treated with the BM-MSC injection vs. saline.

In 2016, Pers et al. published a phase I, prospective, bicentric, single-arm, open-label, dose-escalating clinical trial report of AT-MSC injection in patients with knee OA (117). The 18 patients selected for the trial were 50–75 years of age with K-L grade 3–4 knee OA. The subjects were first divided into three consecutive cohorts with increasing dosages: 2×10^6 (low dose), 10×10^6 (medium dose), and 50×10^6 (high dose) cells. The primary outcome assessed the safety of the trial, while the secondary outcome measured clinical efficacy. The AT-MSCs were extracted from the respective patients through liposuction and the prepared AT-MSC dosages were administered via intra-articular injections to the knee joints. In the primary outcome assessment, no adverse events from either liposuction or intra-articular injection were observed. However, one patient who had hypertension and hyperlipidemia suffered from unstable angina pectoris without increased levels

TABLE 2 | Clinical trials using MSCs in OA.

Year	References	Sample	Source of MSC	Injection method	Treatment group	Result
2015	Kim et al. (115)	49 patients	AT-MSCs	Loaded into fibrin glue product to be surgically implanted into lesion site	Patients received approximately same amount of MSC (4.3×10^6) via arthroscopic procedure	Patients showed overall satisfaction with improved mean IKDC and Tegner activity scores. Regarding the efficacy of MSC implantation, it was concluded that there was a cutoff for both age (>60 years old) and cartilage lesion size (>6.0 cm^2)
2016	Shapiro et al. (116)	25 patients	BM-MSCs	Combined with platelet-poor plasma for injection	25 patients were randomly divided into two groups. 12 patients had BMAC injected in their left knee and placebo in their right, while 13 patients were injected BMAC on their right knee and placebo in their left. The BMAC product had a median of 34,400 MSCs	Significant improvements in ICOAP scores, VAS pain scores, activity level, and pain medication usage were observed from both placebo and treated knees. No adverse events were reported which ensured the safety of MSC treatment
2016	Pers et al. (117)	18 patients	AT-MSCs	Intra-articular injection in the knee joint	18 patients were divided into 3 cohorts with increasing dosage: 2×10^6 (low dose), 10×10^6 (medium dose), and 50×10^6 (high dose)	Only the low dosage group showed statistically significant improvements in all categories of WOMAC index, VAS pain score, and KOOS index. The medium dose group showed improvements in some categories. The high dose group did not have any statistically significant results. Thus, there was an inverse dose effect
2018	Matas et al. (118)	26 patients (with 8 serving as controls)	UCB-MSCs	Intra-articular injection	Patients in the control group received hyaluronic acid treatment and MSC-treated patients were divided into two groups ($n = 9$). The first group received single dose of UCB-MSC (20×10^6), while the second group received two dosages (20×10^6) 6 months apart	Some patients in MSC treated groups showed acute synovitis after injection. No serious adverse events were reported. Improvements in pain and function with lower WOMAC and VAS pain scores was observed compared to the control group without any differences in MRI scores
2019	Freitag et al. (119)	30 patients (with 10 serving as controls)	AT-MSCs	Intra-articular injection	Patients were separated equally into three groups ($n = 10$). The control group continued to receive conventional conservative management. The first treatment group received one MSC injection (1×10^8 AT-MSCs). The second treatment groups received two injections 6 months apart (1×10^8 AT-MSCs)	The two treated groups saw significant reduction in pain measured by NPRS and WOMAC scores. MSC injection was also concluded to reduce the rate of cartilage loss upon MRI analysis. Although minor discomfort and bruising was common for treated groups, no serious adverse events were reported
2019	Chahal et al. (120)	12 patients	BM-MSCs	Intra-articular injection	Patients were divided into four cohorts ($n = 3$). Each group received a single intra-articular injection of BM-MSCs. The first three cohorts received (1×10^6, 10×10^6, and 50×10^6 of BM-MSCs) The fourth cohort had each patient receive the different dosages of MSC listed above	Although four patients reported pain and swelling after injection, no other serious adverse events were reported. Patients who received higher dosages of MSCs saw more significant improvements in KOOS, WOMAC stiffness, quality of life, and symptoms
2019	Lee et al. (121)	24 patients (with 12 serving as control)	AT-MSCs	Intra-articular injection	Patients in the treated group received inter-articular injection of AT-MSC (1×10^8) in 3 mL of saline	The MSC treated group showed significant improvements in WOMAC and VAS scores. Furthermore, the size of the cartilage defect was increased in the control group, while no significant change was observed in the MSC group. No serious adverse events were reported

of cardiac markers 3 months after treatment. In addition, four other patients reported minor knee pain/joint effusion that resolved spontaneously or after treatment with non-steroidal anti-inflammatory drugs. Thus, the safety of AT-MSC treatment was further demonstrated. The secondary outcome was initially assessed using magnetic resonance imaging (MRI), which showed no correlation between MRI and clinical results, in addition to histologic analysis that showed no indication of tumor proliferation. In contrast to other studies, only the low dosage group presented statistically significant results in all categories of the Western Ontario and McMaster Universities Osteoarthritis (WOMAC) index, VAS pain score, and Knee Injury and Osteoarthritis Outcome Score (KOOS). This inverse dose effect could possibly be due to increased inflammation in the low-dose group. Despite limited resources and unclear explanations, Pers et al. further demonstrated the safety and promising potential of MSC treatment.

Matas et al. led a randomized, double-blinded, controlled clinical trial including 29 patients aged 40–65 years with K-L grade 1–3 knee OA (118). Patients were divided into three groups and received two injections 6-months apart. The hyaluronic acid (HA) group (control) received two HA injections (3 mL of Durolane). The MSC-1 group received UCB-MSC (2×10^7 UCB-MSCs and 5% AB plasma in 3 mL of saline) at baseline and was later injection with placebo (5% of AB plasma in 3 mL of saline), while the MSC-2 group received two UCB-MSC injections (2×10^7 UCB-MSCs and 5% AB plasma in 3 mL of saline). Although acute synovitis was common after UCB-MSC injections, no serious adverse events were observed during the trial. Clinical assessment revealed that the MSC-2 group had significantly lower total WOMAC indices than the HA control group at 12 months (4.2 vs. 15.2). In parallel with this result, the VAS score of the MSC-2 group was 2.4, while the VAS score of the HA group was 22.1. In contrast to the MSC-2 group, the MSC-1 group did show improvements through the first 9 months, but later became ineffective after receiving an HA injection. Overall, no patients in any group showed evidence of chondral damage or intra-articular calcifications upon MRI follow-up. The clinically significant results indicated that repeated administration of UC-MSCs dosage is a favorable and safe means of improving the clinical outcomes of patients with knee OA.

Freitag et al. conducted a randomized trial involving 30 patients aged 18 years or older with K-L grade 2–3 knee OA who had previously undergone primary conservative management of OA, such as weight management programs and bracing (119). The participants were first randomly divided into three groups: two treatment groups and one control group. The first group was injected once with 1×10^8 MSCs, while the second group received two injections of 1×10^8 MSCs 6 months apart. The third group served as the control with continued conservative treatments. MSCs were harvested from the adipose tissues of the patients and cultured until passage 2 prior to injection. AT-MSCs were then injected under ultrasound guidance into the intra-articular knee space. The primary outcomes measured the pain and functional changes after the procedure; the secondary outcome involved an MRI analysis after 12 months. Relative to the control, the two treated groups showed significant improvements in pain according to the numeric pain rating scale (NPRS) (6.7 and 6.5 to 2.6 and 2.3) and WOMAC scores (59.6 and 54.4 to 84 and 87.3). MRI analysis showed that 37% of the participants in the first treatment group exhibited further cartilage loss compared to the control. However, ~89% of the patients in the second treatment group showed marked improvement or no progression in cartilage loss. Furthermore, no serious adverse events were observed in the two treated groups during follow-up. Thus, it was concluded that AT-MSC therapy is a safe and effective treatment for knee OA and that frequent injections are preferable.

In 2019, Chahal et al. published a non-randomized, open-label, dose-escalation clinical study (120). This study included patients aged 40–65 years, who were diagnosed with K-L grade 3–4 knee OA and had failed to derive benefits from non-operative treatment regimens for at least 6 months. A total of 12 patients were divided into four cohorts. The first three cohorts were injected with 1×10^6, 2×10^7, and 5×10^7 BM-MSCs (extracted from the posterior superior spine, respectively). In the fourth cohort, three patients each received different BM-MSCs dosages consistent with the increasing dosage levels injected into the three previous cohorts. The primary outcome ensured the safety of the trial, and the secondary outcomes involved clinical, radiological, and biomarker assessments. Without any adverse events, patients saw significant improvements in KOOS and WOMAC stiffness scores, quality of life, and symptoms 12 months post-BM-MSC treatment. Moreover, patients treated with higher dosages demonstrated better chances of significant improvements compared to those treated with lower dosages. Hence, it was concluded from this study that BM-MSC treatment is safe with positive clinical outcomes, specifically at higher dosages.

In 2019, Lee et al. conducted a randomized, double-blinded, placebo-controlled study in 24 patients with knee OA aged 18–75 years, who had a mean pain intensity (VAS score) of 4 or higher for a minimum of 12 weeks with at least one grade 3–4 lesion (121). Patients were randomly divided into MSC and control groups. MSCs were then isolated from the abdominal subcutaneous adipose tissue via lipoaspiration. After the isolated AT-MSCs were cultured to passage 3, the MSC group was treated with an intra-articular injection of 1×10^6 AT-MSCs in 3 mL of saline, while the control group was injected with 3 mL of saline alone. The primary clinical outcome was evaluated 6 months after injection using the WOMAC index. In addition, the secondary outcomes comprised clinical scores, physical examination, radiological evaluation, and safety assessment. In the follow-up, the control group showed no drastic changes in any of the outcomes. On the contrary, the MSC group showed significant reductions in WOMAC and VAS scores for knee pain, from 60.0 to 26.7 and 6.8 to 3.4, respectively. Moreover, the physical and radiological examination data showed that the MSC-injected patients demonstrated a wider range of knee motion (127.9°-134.6°) and unchanged cartilage defects, in contrast to the enlargement seen in the control group. Finally, with all adverse events below grade 3 of the National Cancer Institute-Common Terminology Criteria for Adverse Events scale, the use of intermittent acetaminophen could remediate all treatment-related adverse events without any treatment discontinuations. Although some evaluations (K-L grade, HKA angle, quadriceps power, and the presence of joint effusion) did not show any difference or improvement between the MSC and control groups, it was concluded that the intra-articular injection of AT-MSCs resulted in satisfactory clinical and functional outcomes without serious short-term safety concerns.

APPLICATIONS OF MSC THERAPY IN RA

General Characteristics of RA

RA is a chronic systemic autoimmune disease that causes progressive disability and premature death (53). This disease initially affects the synovial joints and later progresses to the skin, eyes, heart, kidneys, and lungs (53, 57). Ultimately, the patient suffers from joint failure characterized by cartilage damage and severely weakened tendons and ligaments (57, 122). The prevalence rate of RA was reported to be ~0.5–1.0% across the global population in 2002, with females being twice as more likely to be affected due to unknown factors (123, 124).

Based on the presence or absence of anti-citrullinated protein antibodies, RA is divided into two major subtypes (53), which show significant differences in their respective genomes and have completely different pathophysiologies (125). The primary genetic risk factors of RA include alleles encoding the HLA-DR region (53, 126–130). Other critical components are environmental risk factors, such as exposure to tobacco smoke, and lifestyle factors, such as dietary habits (53, 128). As the mechanisms of RA development and its specific targeting of the joints remain unclear, further research is required to fully understand this process (53). The fulminant stage of RA involves hyperplastic synovium, cartilage damage, and bone erosion (53). Along with bone loss, both inflammation and autoimmune responses are potential causes of RA progression (53). This cascade of reactions is activated when fibroblast-like synoviocytes (FLSs) interact with immune cells of the innate and adaptive immune systems (53). Some of the immune cells responsible for inflammation are monocytes, macrophages, T lymphocytes, and B cells (53, 131, 132). The synovial membrane and cartilage undergo significant inflammation, causing hyperplastic synovium and cartilage destruction that eventually lead to bone erosion (54). Hyperplastic synovium is a critical characteristic of RA, and there are two hypotheses regarding its cause. The first is that the abnormal proliferation of FLSs ultimately leads to the production of inflammatory cytokines and mediators that continue joint destruction (53, 133). The second is that the resistance to apoptosis due to defects in tumor protein p53 triggers the hyperplastic synovium (53, 134). Here, the shortage of chondrocytes caused by apoptosis would result in cartilage degeneration and joint-space narrowing via directed adhesion and invasion (53, 135, 136).

Clinical Trials Using MSCs in RA

Compared to OA, relatively few trials have been performed in RA with MSCs. In some cases, it is said that MSC therapy is not suitable for RA given the growing armamentarium of other efficient therapeutic agents available in contrast to OA. Systemic administration of autologous MSCs seemed to cause an exacerbation of RA in a collagen-induced arthritis (CIA) RA animal model, whereas the results of administration of allogeneic MSCs were more successful. These results suggest that allogeneic MSCs are more effective in treatment for autoimmune disorders (137, 138). Although there have been a limited number of clinical trials of MSC treatment in RA patients, the safety and efficacy of therapy have been confirmed in several studies (139). Here, we have briefly reviewed recent clinical trials that used MSC-based treatments in patients with RA (**Table 3**).

Wang et al. conducted a randomized controlled clinical trial with 172 patients with RA who previously underwent unsuccessful chemotherapy treatments and were currently prescribed disease-modifying anti-rheumatic drugs (DMARDs) (140). The MSC-treated group ($n = 136$) received 4.0×10^7 UC-MSCs in 40 mL of stem cell solvent, while the control group ($n = 36$) received only 40 mL of stem cell solvent via intravenous infusion. The MSC-treated group was then further divided into three groups based on the intervals after the first treatment: Group 1 had a 3-month interval, Group 2 had a 6-month interval, and Group 3 had an 8-month interval between injections. The safety of the trial was assessed through radiographic and physical examinations, while disease activity was monitored via disease activity score 28 (DAS28) and the Health Assessment Questionnaire (HAQ). This study did not find serious side effects other than minor fevers and chills. Two weeks after the intravenous injection, the MSC-treated groups showed higher quality of life with reduced joint pain/swelling compared to that of the control group. Moreover, decreased DAS28 and HAQ scores were recorded in the MSC-treated group with repeated treatments, indicating a steady reduction in disease activity. Thus, treatment with a combination of DMARDs and UCB-MSC via injection was concluded to be safe and effective in reducing the long-term disease activity of refractory RA compared to that of conventional DMARDs treatment alone.

Park et al. conducted a clinical trial to test the safety of short-term application of UCB-MSCs in patients with RA (141). The nine participating patients, all aged 18 years or older, had baseline DAS28 assessments and were on a stable dose of methotrexate for a minimum of 12 weeks. Patients received different concentrations of UCB-MSCs via intravenous infusion. Follow-ups for the assessment of clinical and safety parameters were conducted 24 h, 3 days, 1 week, and 4 weeks after infusion. At 4 weeks post-infusion, no abnormalities were detected in the hematologic and chemical profiles; only minor elevations in serum uric acid levels were observed among patients. Hence, it was reported that there were no serious adverse events or dose-limiting toxicities due to the application of UCB-MSCs. UCB-MSC treatment reduced the disease activity of RA and dose-dependently reduced the DAS28 score and VAS pain scale.

Ghoryani et al. conducted a clinical trial to test the immunoregulatory effects of MSCs on 13 female patients with refractory RA, who had previously received maximum dosages of DMARDs (142). The patients had their respective BM-MSCs transplanted via a single dose (1×10^6 per kg of body weight) and were followed up at 1, 6, and 12 months post-transplantation. Patients showed a significant reduction in DAS28 score (from

TABLE 3 | Clinical trials using MSCs in RA.

Year	References	Sample	Source of MSC	Injection method	Treatment group	Result
2013	Wang et al. (140)	172 patients (with 36 patients serving as control)	UCB-MSCs	Intravenous injection	136 patients were divided into three groups based on the interval after the first injection Group 1 ($n = 76$): 3 month-interval Group 2 ($n = 45$): 6 month-interval Group 3 ($n = 15$): 8-month interval (4×10^4 cells per injection)	MSC injections with DMARDs treatment lowered the HAQ and DAS28 scores in 3–6 months follow-up compared to the control group who had only received DMARDs
2018	Park et al. (141)	9 patients	UCB-MSCs	Single intravenous infusion	Nine patients were divided into three groups depending on their injection dosage: 2.5×10^7, 5×10^7, or 1×10^8	No adverse events were recorded. Lower VAS and DAS28 scores were reported in patients who received higher dosages
2020	Ghoryani et al. (142)	13 patients	BM-MSCs	Single intravenous injection	13 patients each received a single intravenous injection of autologous BM-MSCs (1×10^6 per kg)	During the 12-month follow-up period, increased FOXP3, IL-10, and TGF-β1 expression were observed leading to a conclusion that BM-MSC treatment has immunoregulatory effects on regulatory T cells of RA patients

5.56 to 4.72) after 12 months of MSC treatment. Increased forkhead box P3 (FOXP3), IL-10, and TGF-β1 gene expressions were observed in patients treated with MSCs. Based on the increases in IL-10 and TGF-β, MSC therapy was concluded to have significant immunomodulatory effects in patients with refractory RA. Nevertheless, further research is required to investigate the possible effects of increasing/replicating the MSC dosages in patients for improved results.

STRATEGIES FOR FUTURE USE OF MSCs

The terminology debate over "stem" versus "stromal" has been argued in the past and is still ongoing (9). In 2005, the ISCT committee issued a paper that clarifies that the term MSC is not equivalent (or interchangeable) with mesenchymal stromal cell (143). While the MSCs previously discussed in our study refers to cells with self-renewal and differentiation, mesenchymal stromal cells refers to a bulk population of cells with secretory, immunomodulatory effects with additional homing ability (144–146). This is a critical point in studies using MSCs, as the ISCT MSC committee recommends to clarify whether MSC stands for "mesenchymal stromal cells" or "mesenchymal stem cells." However, currently, there is no surface marker that can be used to distinguish these two cell types. The ISCT MSC committee endorses the functional distinction between stromal and stem cells and suggests further analysis focused on their functionalities along with their secretomes. With advanced analysis at the single cells levels and mass cytometry using next-generation sequencing tools, it is important to distinguish the epigenomic, transcriptomic, and proteomic differences between the mesenchymal stromal cells and stem cells. Future studies that target treatment and regeneration of the defected joint tissue should consider thoroughly characterizing the attributes along with the stemness of the MSCs that are used in each study. Such detailed characterization of the investigated MSCs may suggest a unique subtype of MSCs for more direct targeting for the treatment of arthritic diseases.

CONCLUSION

In this review, we have summarized the current status of MSC therapies for OA and RA. While, OA had more promising studies and results compared to that of RA, MSC therapy has shown potential in both OA and RA treatments with reduced pain, improved joint function, and enhanced overall life satisfaction in patients. Clinical trials on OA and RA discussed in this review demonstrate that MSCs are a safe treatment option without serious adverse events. However, more studies are required to examine the long-term safety of MSC injections and their respective clinical applications. Future research studies employing the latest in technology can be the key to increasing scientific evidence concerning their efficacy and safety of MSC therapies. In addition, thorough examination and characterization of the studies already using MSCs are critical for the better understanding of MSCs and will allow them to become a leading candidate for the treatment of various diseases, including arthritic diseases.

AUTHOR CONTRIBUTIONS

JH and JJ concepted the topic, collected data, and wrote the manuscript. YR and YN reviewed and revised the work. JJ supervised this project. All authors contributed to the article and approved the submitted version.

REFERENCES

1. Fridenshtein A, Piatetskii S II, Petrakova KV. [Osteogenesis in transplants of bone marrow cells]. *Arkh Anat Gistol Embriol.* (1969) 56:3–11.
2. Pittenger MF, Discher DE, Peault BM, Phinney DG, Hare JM, Caplan AI. Mesenchymal stem cell perspective: cell biology to clinical progress. *NPJ Regen Med.* (2019) 4:22. doi: 10.1038/s41536-019-0083-6
3. Friedenstein AJ, Chailakhyan RK, Gerasimov UV. Bone marrow osteogenic stem cells: in vitro cultivation and transplantation in diffusion chambers. *Cell Tissue Kinet.* (1987) 20:263–72. doi: 10.1111/j.1365-2184.1987.tb01309.x
4. Friedenstein AJ, Chailakhjan RK, Lalykina KS. The development of fibroblast colonies in monolayer cultures of guinea-pig bone marrow and spleen cells. *Cell Tissue Kinet.* (1970) 3:393–403. doi: 10.1111/j.1365-2184.1970.tb00347.x
5. Gomez-Salazar M, Gonzalez-Galofre ZN, Casamitjana J, Crisan M, James W, Peault B. Five decades later, are mesenchymal stem cells still relevant? *Front Bioeng Biotechnol.* (2020) 8:148. doi: 10.3389/fbioe.2020.00148
6. Caplan AI. Mesenchymal stem cells. *J Orthop Res.* (1991) 9:641–50. doi: 10.1002/jor.1100090504
7. Caplan AI. Mesenchymal stem cells: time to change the name! *Stem Cells Transl Med.* (2017). 6:1445–51. doi: 10.1002/sctm.17-0051
8. Dominici M, Le Blanc K, Mueller I, Slaper-Cortenbach I, Marini F, Krause D, et al. Minimal criteria for defining multipotent mesenchymal stromal cells. The International Society for Cellular Therapy position statement. *Cytotherapy.* (2006) 8:315–7. doi: 10.1080/14653240600855905
9. Viswanathan S, Shi Y, Galipeau J, Krampera M, Leblanc K, Martin I, et al. Mesenchymal stem versus stromal cells: International Society for Cell & Gene Therapy [ISCT(R)] mesenchymal stromal cell committee position statement on nomenclature. *Cytotherapy.* (2019) 21:1019–24. doi: 10.1016/j.jcyt.2019.08.002
10. Via AG, Frizziero A, Oliva F. Biological properties of mesenchymal Stem Cells from different sources. *Muscles Ligaments Tendons J.* (2012) 2:154–62.
11. Saeed H, Ahsan M, Saleem Z, Iqtedar M, Islam M, Danish Z et al. Mesenchymal stem cells (MSCs) as skeletal therapeutics - an update. *J Biomed Sci.* (2016) 23:41. doi: 10.1186/s12929-016-0254-3
12. Bellagamba BC, Grudzinski PB, Ely PB, Nader PJH, Nardi NB, da Silva Meirelles L. Induction of expression of CD271 and CD34 in mesenchymal stromal cells cultured as spheroids. *Stem Cells Int.* (2018) 2018:7357213. doi: 10.1155/2018/7357213
13. Stagg J, Pommey S, Eliopoulos N, Galipeau, J. Interferon-gamma-stimulated marrow stromal cells: a new type of nonhematopoietic antigen-presenting cell. *Blood.* (2006) 107:2570–7. doi: 10.1182/blood-2005-07-2793
14. Romieu-Mourez R, Francois M, Boivin MN, Stagg J, Galipeau J. Regulation of MHC class II expression and antigen processing in murine and human mesenchymal stromal cells by IFN-gamma, TGF-beta, and cell density. *J Immunol.* (2007) 179:1549–8. doi: 10.4049/jimmunol.179.3.1549
15. Parekkadan B, Milwid JM. Mesenchymal stem cells as therapeutics. *Annu Rev Biomed Eng.* (2010) 12:87–117. doi: 10.1146/annurev-bioeng-070909-105309
16. Lazarus HM, Haynesworth, SE, Gerson SL, Rosenthal NS, CaplanAI. *Ex vivo* expansion and subsequent infusion of human bone marrow-derived stromal progenitor cells (mesenchymal progenitor cells): implications for therapeutic use. *Bone Marrow Transplant.* (1995) 16:557–64.
17. Koc ON, Gerson SL, Cooper BW, Dyhouse SM, Haynesworth SE, Caplan AI, et al. Rapid hematopoietic recovery after coinfusion of autologous-blood stem cells and culture-expanded marrow mesenchymal stem cells in advanced breast cancer patients receiving high-dose chemotherapy. *J Clin Oncol.* (2000) 18:307–16. doi: 10.1200/JCO.2000.18.2.307
18. Horwitz EM, Gordon PL, Koo WK, Marx JC, Neel MD, McNall RY, et al. Isolated allogeneic bone marrow-derived mesenchymal cells engraft and stimulate growth in children with osteogenesis imperfecta: implications for cell therapy of bone. *Proc Natl Acad Sci USA.* (2002) 99:8932–7. doi: 10.1073/pnas.132252399
19. Koc ON, Day J, Nieder M, Gerson SL, Lazarus HM, Krivit W. Allogeneic mesenchymal stem cell infusion for treatment of metachromatic leukodystrophy (MLD) and Hurler syndrome (MPS-IH). *Bone Marrow Transplant.* (2002) 30:215–22. doi: 10.1038/sj.bmt.1703650
20. Saeedi P, Halabian R, Imani Fooladi AA. A revealing review of mesenchymal stem cells therapy, clinical perspectives and modification strategies. *Stem Cell Investig.* (2019) 6:34. doi: 10.21037/sci.2019.08.11
21. Sacchetti, B, Funari, A, Remoli, C, Giannicola, G, Kogler, G, Liedtke, S, et al. No identical "mesenchymal stem cells" at different times and sites: human committed progenitors of distinct origin and differentiation potential are incorporated as adventitial cells in microvessels. *Stem Cell Rep.* (2016) 6:897–913. doi: 10.1016/j.stemcr.2016.05.011
22. Gronthos, S, Brahim, J, Li, W, Fisher LW, Cherman, N, Boyde, A et al. Stem cell properties of human dental pulp stem cells. *J Dent Res.* (2002) 81:531–5. doi: 10.1177/154405910208100806
23. Zannettino AC, Paton S, Arthur A, Khor F, Itescu S, Gimble JM, et al. Multipotential human adipose-derived stromal stem cells exhibit a perivascular phenotype in vitro and in vivo. *J Cell Physiol.* (2008) 214:413–21. doi: 10.1002/jcp.21210
24. Han, Y, Li, X, Zhang, Y, Han, Y, Chang, F, Ding, J. Mesenchymal stem cells for regenerative medicine. *Cells.* (2019) 8:886. doi: 10.3390/cells8080886
25. Fan XL, Zhang Y, Li X, Fu QL. Mechanisms underlying the protective effects of mesenchymal stem cell-based therapy. *Cell Mol Life Sci.* (2020) 77:2771–94. doi: 10.1007/s00018-020-03454-6
26. Haynesworth SE, Goshima J, Goldberg VM, Caplan AI. Characterization of cells with osteogenic potential from human marrow. *Bone.* (1992) 13:81–8. doi: 10.1016/8756-3282(92)90364-3
27. Pittenger MF, Mackay AM, Beck SC, Jaiswal RK, Douglas R, Mosca JD, et al. Multilineage potential of adult human mesenchymal stem cells. *Science.* (1999) 284:143–7. doi: 10.1126/science.284.5411.143
28. Mohamed-Ahmed S, Fristad I, Lie SA, Suliman S, Mustafa K, Vindenes H, et al. Adipose-derived and bone marrow mesenchymal stem cells: a donor-matched comparison. *Stem Cell Res Ther.* (2018) 9:168. doi: 10.1186/s13287-018-0914-1
29. Erices A, Conget P, Minguell JJ. Mesenchymal progenitor cells in human umbilical cord blood. *Br J Haematol.* (2000) 109:235–42. doi: 10.1046/j.1365-2141.2000.01986.x
30. Nagamura-Inoue T, He H. Umbilical cord-derived mesenchymal stem cells: their advantages and potential clinical utility. *World J Stem Cells.* (2014) 6:195–202. doi: 10.4252/wjsc.v6.i2.195
31. Chen JY, Mou XZ, Du XC, Xiang C. Comparative analysis of biological characteristics of adult mesenchymal stem cells with different tissue origins. *Asian Pac J Trop Med.* (2015) 8:739–46. doi: 10.1016/j.apjtm.2015.07.022
32. Kim JH, Jo CH, Kim HR, Hwang YI. Comparison of immunological characteristics of mesenchymal stem cells from the periodontal ligament, umbilical cord, and adipose tissue. *Stem Cells Int.* (2018) 2018:8429042. doi: 10.1155/2018/8429042
33. Kim YJ, Seo DH, Lee SH, Lee SH, An GH, Ahn HJ, et al. Conditioned media from human umbilical cord blood-derived mesenchymal stem cells stimulate rejuvenation function in human skin. *Biochem Biophys Rep.* (2018) 16:96–102. doi: 10.1016/j.bbrep.2018.10.007
34. Lu LL, Liu YJ, Yang SG, Zhao QJ, Wang X, Gong W, et al. Isolation and characterization of human umbilical cord mesenchymal stem cells with hematopoiesis-supportive function and other potentials. *Haematologica.* (2006) 91:1017–26.
35. Stanko P, Kaiserova K, Altanerova V, Altaner, C. Comparison of human mesenchymal stem cells derived from dental pulp, bone marrow, adipose tissue, and umbilical cord tissue by gene expression. *Biomed Pap Med Fac Univ Palacky Olomouc Czech Repub.* (2014) 158:373–7. doi: 10.5507/bp.2013.078
36. Schmelzer E, McKeel DT, Gerlach JC. Characterization of human mesenchymal stem cells from different tissues and their membrane encasement for prospective transplantation therapies. *Biomed Res Int.* (2019) 2019:6376271. doi: 10.1155/2019/6376271

37. Zuk PA, Zhu M, Mizuno H, Huang J, Futrell JW, Katz AJ, et al. Multilineage cells from human adipose tissue: implications for cell-based therapies. *Tissue Eng.* (2001) 7:211–28. doi: 10.1089/107632701300062859
38. Nepali S, Park M, Lew H, Kim O. Comparative analysis of human adipose-derived mesenchymal stem cells from orbital and abdominal fat. *Stem Cells Int.* (2018) 2018:3932615. doi: 10.1155/2018/3932615
39. De Bari C, Dell'Accio F, Tylzanowski P, Luyten FP. Multipotent mesenchymal stem cells from adult human synovial membrane. *Arthritis Rheum.* (2001) 44:1928–42. doi: 10.1002/1529-0131(200108)44:8<1928::AID-ART331>3.0.CO;2-P
40. Murata Y, Uchida S, Utsunomiya H, Hatakeyama A, Nakashima H, Chang A, et al. Synovial mesenchymal stem cells derived from the cotyloid fossa synovium have higher self-renewal and differentiation potential than those from the paralabral synovium in the hip joint. *Am J Sports Med.* (2018) 46:2942–53. doi: 10.1177/0363546518794664
41. Li N, Gao J, Mi L, Zhang G, Zhang L, Zhang N, et al. Synovial membrane mesenchymal stem cells: past life, current situation, and application in bone and joint diseases. *Stem Cell Res Ther.* (2020) 11:381. doi: 10.1186/s13287-020-01885-3
42. Kubosch EJ, Lang G, Furst D, Kubosch D, Izadpanah K, Rolauffs B, et al. The potential for synovium-derived stem cells in cartilage repair. *Curr Stem Cell Res Ther.* (2018) 13:174–84. doi: 10.2174/1574888X12666171002111026
43. Mochizuki T, Muneta T, Sakaguchi Y, Nimura A, Yokoyama A, Koga H, et al. Higher chondrogenic potential of fibrous synovium- and adipose synovium-derived cells compared with subcutaneous fat-derived cells: distinguishing properties of mesenchymal stem cells in humans. *Arthritis Rheum.* (2006) 54:843–53. doi: 10.1002/art.21651
44. Ogata Y, Mabuchi Y, Yoshida M, Suto EG, Suzuki N, Muneta, T, et al. Purified human synovium mesenchymal stem cells as a good resource for cartilage regeneration. *PLoS ONE.* (2015) 10:e0129096. doi: 10.1371/journal.pone.0129096
45. Sakaguchi Y, Sekiya I, Yagishita K, Muneta, T. Comparison of human stem cells derived from various mesenchymal tissues: superiority of synovium as a cell source. *Arthritis Rheum.* (2005) 52:2521–29. doi: 10.1002/art.21212
46. Mor A, Grijota M, Norgaard M, Munthe J, Lind M, Deruaz A, et al. Trends in arthroscopy-documented cartilage injuries of the knee and repair procedures among 15-60-year-old patients. *Scand J Med Sci Sports.* (2015) 25:e400–7. doi: 10.1111/sms.12330
47. Martin AR, Patel JM, Zlotnick HM, Carey JL, Mauck RL. Emerging therapies for cartilage regeneration in currently excluded 'red knee' populations. *NPJ Regen Med.* (2019) 4:12. doi: 10.1038/s41536-019-0074-7
48. Zylinska B, Silmanowicz P, Sobczynska-Rak A, Jarosz L, Szponder T. Treatment of articular cartilage defects: focus on tissue engineering. *In Vivo.* (2018) 32:1289–300. doi: 10.21873/invivo.11379
49. Du D, Hsu P, Zhu Z, Zhang, C. Current surgical options and innovation for repairing articular cartilage defects in the femoral head. *J Orthop Translat.* (2020) 21:122–8. doi: 10.1016/j.jot.2019.06.002
50. Wakitani S, Mitsuoka T, Nakamura N, Toritsuka Y, Nakamura Y, Horibe S, et al. Autologous bone marrow stromal cell transplantation for repair of full-thickness articular cartilage defects in human patellae: two case reports. *Cell Transplant.* (2004) 13:595–600. doi: 10.3727/000000004783983747
51. Kuroda R, Ishida K, Matsumoto T, Akisue T, Fujioka H, Mizuno K, et al. Treatment of a full-thickness articular cartilage defect in the femoral condyle of an athlete with autologous bone-marrow stromal cells. *Osteoarthritis Cartilage.* (2007) 15:226–31. doi: 10.1016/j.joca.2006.08.008
52. Nejadnik H, Hui JH, Feng Choong EP, Tai BC, Lee EH. Autologous bone marrow-derived mesenchymal stem cells versus autologous chondrocyte implantation: an observational cohort study. *Am J Sports Med.* (2010) 38:1110–6. doi: 10.1177/0363546509359067
53. Guo Q, Wang Y, Xu D, Nossent J, Pavlos NJ, Xu J, et al. Rheumatoid arthritis: pathological mechanisms and modern pharmacologic therapies. *Bone Res.* (2018) 6:15. doi: 10.1038/s41413-018-0016-9
54. Ouboussad L, Burska AN, Melville A, Buch MH. Synovial tissue heterogeneity in rheumatoid arthritis and changes with biologic and targeted synthetic therapies to inform stratified therapy. *Front Med.* (2019) 6:45. doi: 10.3389/fmed.2019.00045
55. Chen D, Shen J, Zhao W, Wang T, Han L, Hamilton JL, et al. Osteoarthritis: toward a comprehensive understanding of pathological mechanism. *Bone Res.* (2017) 5:16044. doi: 10.1038/boneres.2016.44
56. Musumeci G, Aiello FC, Szychlinska MA, Di Rosa M, Castrogiovanni P, Mobasheri A, et al. Osteoarthritis in the XXIst century: risk factors and behaviours that influence disease onset and progression. *Int J Mol Sci.* (2015) 16:6093–112. doi: 10.3390/ijms16036093
57. Bullock J, Rizvi SAA, Saleh AM, Ahmed SS, Do DP, Ansari RA, et al. Rheumatoid arthritis: a brief overview of the treatment. *Med Princ Pract.* (2018) 27:501–7. doi: 10.1159/000493390
58. Mora JC, Przkora R, Cruz-Almeida Y. Knee osteoarthritis: pathophysiology and current treatment modalities. *J Pain Res.* (2018) 11:2189–96. doi: 10.2147/JPR.S154002
59. Bannuru RR, Schmid CH, Kent DM, Vaysbrot EE, Wong JB, McAlindon TE. Comparative effectiveness of pharmacologic interventions for knee osteoarthritis: a systematic review and network meta-analysis. *Ann Intern Med.* (2015) 162:46–54. doi: 10.7326/M14-1231
60. Nelson AE, Allen KD, Golightly YM, Goode AP, Jordan JM. A systematic review of recommendations and guidelines for the management of osteoarthritis: the chronic osteoarthritis management initiative of the U.S. bone and joint initiative. *Semin Arthritis Rheum.* (2014) 43:701–12. doi: 10.1016/j.semarthrit.2013.11.012
61. Hootman JM, Helmick CG. Projections of US prevalence of arthritis and associated activity limitations. *Arthritis Rheum.* (2006) 54:226–9. doi: 10.1002/art.21562
62. Ryder JJ, Garrison K, Song F, Hooper L, Skinner J, Loke Y, et al. Genetic associations in peripheral joint osteoarthritis and spinal degenerative disease: a systematic review. *Ann Rheum Dis.* (2008) 67:584–91. doi: 10.1136/ard.2007.073874
63. Nordenvall R, Bahmanyar S, Adami J, Stenros C, Wredmark T, Fellander-Tsai, et al. A population-based nationwide study of cruciate ligament injury in Sweden, 2001-2009: incidence, treatment, and sex differences. *Am J Sports Med.* (2012) 40:1808–13. doi: 10.1177/0363546512449306
64. Vina ER, Kwoh CK. Epidemiology of osteoarthritis: literature update. *Curr Opin Rheumatol.* (2018) 30:160–7. doi: 10.1097/BOR.0000000000000479
65. Loeser RF. Aging processes and the development of osteoarthritis. *Curr Opin Rheumatol.* (2013) 25:108–13. doi: 10.1097/BOR.0b013e32835a9428
66. Loeser RF. The role of aging in the development of osteoarthritis. *Trans Am Clin Climatol Assoc.* (2017) 128:44–54.
67. Loeser RF. Aging and osteoarthritis. *Curr Opin Rheumatol.* (2011) 23:492–6. doi: 10.1097/BOR.0b013e3283494005
68. Naik E, Dixit VM. Mitochondrial reactive oxygen species drive proinflammatory cytokine production. *J Exp Med.* (2011) 208:417–20. doi: 10.1084/jem.20110367
69. Goodwin W, McCabe D, Sauter E, Reese E, Walter M, Buckwalter JA, et al. Rotenone prevents impact-induced chondrocyte death. *J Orthop Res.* (2010) 28:1057–63. doi: 10.1002/jor.21091
70. Zahan OM, Serban O, Gherman C, Fodor, D. The evaluation of oxidative stress in osteoarthritis. *Med Pharm Rep.* (2020) 93:12–22. doi: 10.15386/mpr-1422
71. Johnson VL, Hunter DJ. The epidemiology of osteoarthritis. *Best Pract Res Clin Rheumatol.* (2014) 28:5–15. doi: 10.1016/j.berh.2014.01.004
72. Deshpande BR, Katz JN, Solomon DH, Yelin EH, Hunter DJ, Messier SP, et al. Number of persons with symptomatic knee osteoarthritis in the us: impact of race and ethnicity, age, sex, and obesity. *Arthritis Care Res.* (2016) 68:1743–50. doi: 10.1002/acr.22897
73. Reynard LN, Barter MJ. Osteoarthritis year in review 2019: genetics, genomics and epigenetics. *Osteoarthritis Cartilage.* (2020) 28:275–84. doi: 10.1016/j.joca.2019.11.010
74. Tachmazidou I, Hatzikotoulas K, Southam L, Esparza-Gordillo J, Haberland V, Zheng J, et al. Identification of new therapeutic targets for osteoarthritis through genome-wide analyses of UK Biobank data. *Nat Genet.* (2019) 51:230–6. doi: 10.1038/s41588-018-0327-1
75. Loughlin J, Dowling B, Chapman K, Marcelline L, Mustafa Z, Southam L, et al. Functional variants within the secreted frizzled-related protein 3 gene are associated with hip osteoarthritis in females. *Proc Natl Acad Sci USA.* (2004) 101:9757–62. doi: 10.1073/pnas.0403456101
76. Bijsterbosch J, Kloppenburg M, Reijnierse M, Rosendaal FR, Huizinga TW, Slagboom PE, et al. Association study of candidate genes for the progression of hand osteoarthritis. *Osteoarthritis Cartilage.* (2013) 21:565–9. doi: 10.1016/j.joca.2013.01.011

77. Valdes AM, Spector TD, Tamm A, Kisand K, Doherty SA, Dennison EM, et al. Genetic variation in the SMAD3 gene is associated with hip and knee osteoarthritis. *Arthritis Rheum.* (2010) 62:2347–52. doi: 10.1002/art.27530
78. Rodriguez RR, Seegmiller RE, Stark MR, Bridgewater LC. A type XI collagen mutation leads to increased degradation of type II collagen in articular cartilage. *Osteoarthritis Cartilage.* (2004) 12:314–20. doi: 10.1016/j.joca.2003.12.002
79. Jeong C, Lee J.Y, Kim J, Chae H, Park HI, Kim M, et al. Novel COL9A3 mutation in a family diagnosed with multiple epiphyseal dysplasia: a case report. *BMC Musculoskelet Disord.* (2014) 15:371. doi: 10.1186/1471-2474-15-371
80. Carlson KM, Yamaga KM, Reinker KA, Hsia YE, Carpenter C, Abe LM, et al. Precocious osteoarthritis in a family with recurrent COL2A1 mutation. *J Rheumatol.* (2006) 33:1133–6.
81. Zhang R, Yao J, Xu P, Ji B, Luck JV, Chin B, et al. A comprehensive meta-analysis of association between genetic variants of GDF5 and osteoarthritis of the knee, hip and hand. *Inflamm Res.* (2015) 64:405–14. doi: 10.1007/s00011-015-0818-9
82. Styrkarsdottir U, Helgason H, Sigurdsson A, Norddahl GL, Agustsdottir AB, Reynard LN, et al. Whole-genome sequencing identifies rare genotypes in COMP and CHADL associated with high risk of hip osteoarthritis. *Nat Genet.* (2017) 49:801–5. doi: 10.1038/ng.3816
83. Zengini E, Hatzikotoulas K, Tachmazidou I, Steinberg J, Hartwig FP, Southam L, et al. Genome-wide analyses using UK Biobank data provide insights into the genetic architecture of osteoarthritis. *Nat Genet.* (2018) 50:549–58. doi: 10.1038/s41588-018-0079-y
84. Styrkarsdottir U, Lund SH, Thorleifsson G, Zink F, Stefansson OA, Sigurdsson JK, et al. Meta-analysis of Icelandic and UK data sets identifies missense variants in SMO, IL11, COL11A1 and 13 more new loci associated with osteoarthritis. *Nat Genet.* (2018) 50:1681–7. doi: 10.1038/s41588-018-0247-0
85. Styrkarsdottir U, Stefansson OA, Gunnarsdottir K, Thorleifsson G, Lund SH, Stefansdottir L, et al. Publisher Correction: GWAS of bone size yields twelve loci that also affect height, BMD, osteoarthritis or fractures. *Nat Commun.* (2019) 10:2358. doi: 10.1038/s41467-019-10425-4
86. Zhao T, Zhao J, Ma C, Wei J, Wei B, Liu J. Common variants in LTBP3 gene contributed to the risk of hip osteoarthritis in Han Chinese population. *Biosci Rep.* (2020) 40:BSR20192999. doi: 10.1042/BSR20192999
87. Chu M, Zhu X, Wang C, Rong J, Wang Y, Wang S, et al. The rs4238326 polymorphism in ALDH1A2 gene potentially associated with non-post traumatic knee osteoarthritis susceptibility: a two-stage population-based study. *Osteoarthritis Cartilage.* (2017) 25:1062–7. doi: 10.1016/j.joca.2017.01.003
88. Kelly T, Yang W, Chen CS, Reynolds K, He J. Global burden of obesity in 2005 and projections to 2030. *Int J Obes.* (2008) 32:1431–7. doi: 10.1038/ijo.2008.102
89. Qin B, Yang M, Fu H, Ma N, Wei T, Tang Q, et al. Body mass index and the risk of rheumatoid arthritis: a systematic review and dose-response meta-analysis. *Arthritis Res Ther.* (2015) 17:86. doi: 10.1186/s13075-015-0601-x
90. Eymard F, Parsons C, Edwards MH, Petit-Dop F, Reginster JY, Bruyere O, et al. Diabetes is a risk factor for knee osteoarthritis progression. *Osteoarthritis Cartilage.* (2015) 23:851–9. doi: 10.1016/j.joca.2015.01.013
91. Alenazi AM, Alshehri MM, Alothman S, Alqahtani BA, Rucker J, Sharma N, et al. The association of diabetes with knee pain severity and distribution in people with knee osteoarthritis using data from the osteoarthritis initiative. *Sci Rep.* (2020) 10:3985. doi: 10.1038/s41598-020-60989-1
92. Xie C, Chen Q. Adipokines: new therapeutic target for osteoarthritis? *Curr Rheumatol Rep.* (2019) 21:71. doi: 10.1007/s11926-019-0868-z
93. Berenbaum F. Osteoarthritis as an inflammatory disease (osteoarthritis is not osteoarthrosis!). *Osteoarthritis Cartilage.* (2013) 21:16–21. doi: 10.1016/j.joca.2012.11.012
94. Conde J, Scotece M, Gomez R, Lopez V, Gomez-Reino JJ, Gualillo O. Adipokines and osteoarthritis: novel molecules involved in the pathogenesis and progression of disease. *Arthritis.* (2011) 2011:203901. doi: 10.1155/2011/203901
95. Fain JN. Release of inflammatory mediators by human adipose tissue is enhanced in obesity and primarily by the nonfat cells: a review. *Mediators Inflamm.* (2010) 2010:513948. doi: 10.1155/2010/513948
96. Visser M. Higher levels of inflammation in obese children. *Nutrition.* (2001) 17:480–1. doi: 10.1016/s0899-9007(01)00509-3
97. Aygun AD, Gungor S, Ustundag B, Gurgoze MK, Sen Y. Proinflammatory cytokines and leptin are increased in serum of prepubertal obese children. *Mediators Inflamm.* (2005) 2005:180–3. doi: 10.1155/MI.2005.180
98. Pou KM, Massaro JM, Hoffmann U, Vasan RS, Maurovich-Horvat P, Larson MG, et al., Meigs JB, Lipinska I, Kathiresan S, et al. Visceral and subcutaneous adipose tissue volumes are cross-sectionally related to markers of inflammation and oxidative stress: the Framingham Heart Study. *Circulation.* (2007) 116:1234–41. doi: 10.1161/CIRCULATIONAHA.107.710509
99. Straczkowski M, Dzienis-Straczkowska S, Stepien A, Kowalska I, Szelachowska M, Kinalska I. Plasma interleukin-8 concentrations are increased in obese subjects and related to fat mass and tumor necrosis factor-alpha system. *J Clin Endocrinol Metab.* (2002) 87:4602–6. doi: 10.1210/jc.2002-020135
100. Shi C, Zhu L, Chen X, Gu N, Chen L, Zhu L, et al. IL-6 and TNF-alpha induced obesity-related inflammatory response through transcriptional regulation of miR-146b. *J Interferon Cytokine Res.* (2014) 34:342–8. doi: 10.1089/jir.2013.0078
101. Makki K, Froguel P, Wolowczuk I. Adipose tissue in obesity-related inflammation and insulin resistance: cells, cytokines, and chemokines. *ISRN Inflamm.* (2013) 2013:139239. doi: 10.1155/2013/139239
102. Xu L, Sun C, Zhang S, Xu X, Zhai L, Wang Y, et al. Sam68 promotes NF-kappaB activation and apoptosis signaling in articular chondrocytes during osteoarthritis. *Inflamm Res.* (2015) 64:895–902. doi: 10.1007/s00011-015-0872-3
103. Chow YY, Chin KY. The role of inflammation in the pathogenesis of osteoarthritis. *Mediators Inflamm.* (2020) 2020:8293921. doi: 10.1155/2020/8293921
104. Kapoor M, Martel-Pelletier J, Lajeunesse D, Pelletier JP, Fahmi H. Role of proinflammatory cytokines in the pathophysiology of osteoarthritis. *Nat Rev Rheumatol.* (2011) 7:33–42. doi: 10.1038/nrrheum.2010.196
105. Jiang L, Tian W, Wang Y, Rong J, Bao C, Liu Y, et al. Body mass index and susceptibility to knee osteoarthritis: a systematic review and meta-analysis. *Joint Bone Spine.* (2012) 79:291–7. doi: 10.1016/j.jbspin.2011.05.015
106. Raud B, Gay C, Guiguet-Auclair C, Bonnin A, Gerbaud L, Pereira B, et al. Level of obesity is directly associated with the clinical and functional consequences of knee osteoarthritis. *Sci Rep.* (2020) 10:3601. doi: 10.1038/s41598-020-60587-1
107. Chang AH, Lee JJ, Chmiel JS, Almagor O, Song J, Sharma L. Association of long-term strenuous physical activity and extensive sitting with incident radiographic knee osteoarthritis. *JAMA Netw Open.* (2020) 3:e204049. doi: 10.1001/jamanetworkopen.2020.4049
108. Schram B, Orr R, Pope R, Canetti E, Knapik J. Risk factors for development of lower limb osteoarthritis in physically demanding occupations: a narrative umbrella review. *J Occup Health.* (2020) 62:e12103. doi: 10.1002/1348-9585.12103
109. Gignac MAM, Irvin E, Cullen K, Van Eerd D, Beaton DE, Mahood Q, et al. Men and women's occupational activities and the risk of developing osteoarthritis of the knee, hip, or hands: a systematic review and recommendations for future research. *Arthritis Care Res.* (2020) 72:378–96. doi: 10.1002/acr.23855
110. Messier SP, Legault C, Mihalko S, Miller GD, Loeser RF, DeVita P, et al. The Intensive Diet and Exercise for Arthritis (IDEA) trial: design and rationale. *BMC Musculoskelet Disord.* (2009). 10:93. doi: 10.1186/1471-2474-10-93
111. Alentorn-Geli E, Samuelsson K, Musahl V, Green CL, Bhandari M, Karlsson J. The association of recreational and competitive running with hip and knee osteoarthritis: a systematic review and meta-analysis. *J Orthop Sports Phys Ther.* (2017) 47:373–90. doi: 10.2519/jospt.2017.7137
112. Driban JB, Hootman JM, Sitler MR, Harris KP, Cattano NM. Is participation in certain sports associated with knee osteoarthritis? A systematic review. *J Athl Train.* (2017) 52:497–506. doi: 10.4085/1062-6050-50.2.08
113. Hind K, Konerth N, Entwistle I, Theadom A, Lewis G, King D, et al. Cumulative sport-related injuries and longer term impact in retired male elite- and amateur-level rugby code athletes and non-

contact athletes: a retrospective study. *Sports Med.* (2020) 50:2051–61. doi: 10.1007/s40279-020-01310-y

114. Bullock GS, Collins GS, Peirce N, Arden NK, Filbay SR. Playing sport injured is associated with osteoarthritis, joint pain and worse health-related quality of life: a cross-sectional study. *BMC Musculoskelet Disord.* (2020) 21:111. doi: 10.1186/s12891-020-3136-5
115. Kim YS, Choi YJ, Koh YG. Mesenchymal stem cell implantation in knee osteoarthritis: an assessment of the factors influencing clinical outcomes. *Am J Sports Med.* (2015) 43:2293–2301. doi: 10.1177/0363546515588317
116. Shapiro SA, Kazmerchak SE, Heckman MG, Zubair AC, O'Connor MI. A prospective, single-blind, placebo-controlled trial of bone marrow aspirate concentrate for knee osteoarthritis. *Am J Sports Med.* (2017) 45:82–90. doi: 10.1177/0363546516662455
117. Pers YM, Rackwitz L, Ferreira R, Pullig O, Delfour C, Barry F, et al. Adipose mesenchymal stromal cell-based therapy for severe osteoarthritis of the knee: a phase i dose-escalation trial. *Stem Cells Transl Med.* (2016) 5:847–56. doi: 10.5966/sctm.2015-0245
118. Matas J, Orrego M, Amenabar D, Infante C, Tapia-Limonchi R, Cadiz MI, et al. Umbilical cord-derived Mesenchymal Stromal Cells (MSCs) for knee osteoarthritis: repeated msc dosing is superior to a single MSC dose and to hyaluronic acid in a controlled randomized phase I/II trial. *Stem Cells Transl Med.* (2019) 8:215–24. doi: 10.1002/sctm.18-0053
119. Freitag J, Bates D, Wickham J, Shah K, Huguenin L, Tenen A, et al. Adipose-derived mesenchymal stem cell therapy in the treatment of knee osteoarthritis: a randomized controlled trial. *Regen Med.* (2019) 14:213–30. doi: 10.2217/rme-2018-0161
120. Chahal J, Gomez-Aristizabal A, Shestopaloff K, Bhatt S, Chaboureau A, Fazio A, et al. Bone marrow mesenchymal stromal cell treatment in patients with osteoarthritis results in overall improvement in pain and symptoms and reduces synovial inflammation. *Stem Cells Transl Med.* (2019) 8:746–57. doi: 10.1002/sctm.18-0183
121. Lee WS, Kim HJ, Kim KI, Kim GB, Jin W. Intra-articular injection of autologous adipose tissue-derived mesenchymal stem cells for the treatment of knee osteoarthritis: a phase IIb, randomized, placebo-controlled clinical trial. *Stem Cells Transl Med.* (2019) 8:504–11. doi: 10.1002/sctm.18-0122
122. Lee JE, Kim IJ, Cho MS, Lee J. A case of rheumatoid vasculitis involving hepatic artery in early rheumatoid arthritis. *J Korean Med Sci.* (2017) 32:1207–10. doi: 10.3346/jkms.2017.32.7.1207
123. Silman AJ, Pearson JE. Epidemiology and genetics of rheumatoid arthritis. *Arthritis Res.* (2002) 4(Suppl. 3):S265–72. doi: 10.1186/ar578
124. Myasoedova E, Crowson CS, Turesson C, Gabriel SE, Matteson EL. Incidence of extraarticular rheumatoid arthritis in Olmsted County, Minnesota, in 1995-2007 versus 1985-1994: a population-based study. *J Rheumatol.* (2011) 38:983–9. doi: 10.3899/jrheum.101133
125. Daha NA, Toes RE. Rheumatoid arthritis: are ACPA-positive and ACPA-negative RA the same disease? *Nat Rev Rheumatol.* (2011) 7:202–3. doi: 10.1038/nrrheum.2011.28
126. Okada Y, Kim K, Han B, Pillai NE, Ong RT, Saw WY, et al. Risk for ACPA-positive rheumatoid arthritis is driven by shared HLA amino acid polymorphisms in Asian and European populations. *Hum Mol Genet.* (2014) 23:6916–26. doi: 10.1093/hmg/ddu387
127. Raychaudhuri S, Sandor C, Stahl EA, Freudenberg J, Lee HS, Jia X, et al. Five amino acids in three HLA proteins explain most of the association between MHC and seropositive rheumatoid arthritis. *Nat Genet.* (2012) 44:291–6. doi: 10.1038/ng.1076
128. Deane KD, Demoruelle MK, Kelmenson LB, Kuhn KA, Norris JM, Holers VM. Genetic and environmental risk factors for rheumatoid arthritis. *Best Pract Res Clin Rheumatol.* (2017) 31:3–18. doi: 10.1016/j.berh.2017.08.003
129. Michou L, Croiseau P, Petit-Teixeira E, du Montcel ST, Lemaire I, Pierlot C, et al. Validation of the reshaped shared epitope HLA-DRB1 classification in rheumatoid arthritis. *Arthritis Res Ther.* (2006) 8:R79. doi: 10.1186/ar1949
130. du Montcel ST, Michou L, Petit-Teixeira E, Osorio J, Lemaire I, Lasbleiz S, et al. New classification of HLA-DRB1 alleles supports the shared epitope hypothesis of rheumatoid arthritis susceptibility. *Arthritis Rheum.* (2005) 52:1063–8. doi: 10.1002/art.20989
131. Mellado M, Martinez-Munoz L, Cascio G, Lucas P, Pablos JL, Rodriguez-Frade JM. T cell migration in rheumatoid arthritis. *Front Immunol.* (2015) 6:384. doi: 10.3389/fimmu.2015.00384
132. Volkov M, van Schie KA, van der Woude D. Autoantibodies and B Cells: the ABC of rheumatoid arthritis pathophysiology. *Immunol Rev.* (2020) 294:148–63. doi: 10.1111/imr.12829
133. Bottini N, Firestein GS. Duality of fibroblast-like synoviocytes in RA: passive responders and imprinted aggressors. *Nat Rev Rheumatol.* (2013) 9:24–33. doi: 10.1038/nrrheum.2012.190
134. Lee YH, Ji JD, Kim A, Kim CH, Song GG. Expression of p53 protein in rheumatoid arthritis synovium. An immunohistochemical analysis. *Korean J Intern Med.* (1999) 14:59–65. doi: 10.3904/kjim.1999.14.1.59
135. Pap T, Korb-Pap A. Cartilage damage in osteoarthritis and rheumatoid arthritis–two unequal siblings. *Nat Rev Rheumatol.* (2015) 11:606–15. doi: 10.1038/nrrheum.2015.95
136. Kato K, Yasojima N, Tamura K, Ichikawa S, Sutherland K, Kato M, et al. Detection of fine radiographic progression in finger joint space narrowing beyond human eyes: phantom experiment and clinical study with rheumatoid arthritis patients. *Sci Rep.* (2019) 9:8526. doi: 10.1038/s41598-019-44747-6
137. El-Jawhari JJ, El-Sherbiny YM, Jones EA, McGonagle D. Mesenchymal stem cells, autoimmunity and rheumatoid arthritis. *QJM.* (2014) 107:505–14. doi: 10.1093/qjmed/hcu033
138. Augello A, Tasso R, Negrini SM, Cancedda R, Pennesi G. Cell therapy using allogeneic bone marrow mesenchymal stem cells prevents tissue damage in collagen-induced arthritis. *Arthritis Rheum.* (2007) 56:1175–86. doi: 10.1002/art.22511
139. Zhang Q, Li Q, Zhu J, Guo H, Zhai Q, Li B, et al. Comparison of therapeutic effects of different mesenchymal stem cells on rheumatoid arthritis in mice. *PeerJ.* (2019) 7:e7023. doi: 10.7717/peerj.7023
140. Wang L, Wang L, Cong X, Liu G, Zhou J, Bai B, et al. Human umbilical cord mesenchymal stem cell therapy for patients with active rheumatoid arthritis: safety and efficacy. *Stem Cells Dev.* (2013) 22:3192–202. doi: 10.1089/scd.2013.0023
141. Park EH, Lim HS, Lee S, Roh K, Seo KW, Kang KS, et al. Intravenous infusion of umbilical cord blood-derived mesenchymal stem cells in rheumatoid arthritis: a phase ia clinical trial. *Stem Cells Transl Med.* (2018) 7:636–42. doi: 10.1002/sctm.18-0031
142. Ghoryani M, Shariati-Sarabi Z, Tavakkol-Afshari J, Mohammadi M. The sufficient immunoregulatory effect of autologous bone marrow-derived mesenchymal stem cell transplantation on regulatory T cells in patients with refractory rheumatoid arthritis. *J Immunol Res.* (2020) 2020:3562753. doi: 10.1155/2020/3562753
143. Horwitz EM, Le Blanc K, Dominici M, Mueller I, Slaper-Cortenbach I, Marini FC, et al. Clarification of the nomenclature for MSC: the international society for cellular therapy position statement. *Cytotherapy.* (2005) 7:393–5. doi: 10.1080/14653240500319234
144. Sacchetti B, Funari A, Michienzi S, Di Cesare S, Piersanti S, Saggio I, et al. Self-renewing osteoprogenitors in bone marrow sinusoids can organize a hematopoietic microenvironment. *Cell.* (2007) 131:324–36. doi: 10.1016/j.cell.2007.08.025
145. Chan CKF, Gulati GS, Sinha R, Tompkins JV, Lopez M, Carter AC, et al. Identification of the human skeletal stem cell. *Cell.* (2018) 175:43–56.e21. doi: 10.1016/j.cell.2018.07.029
146. Le Blanc K, Mougiakakos D. Multipotent mesenchymal stromal cells and the innate immune system. *Nat Rev Immunol.* (2012) 12:383–96. doi: 10.1038/nri3209

11

Multipotent Mesenchymal Stromal Cells in Rheumatoid Arthritis and Systemic Lupus Erythematosus: From a Leading Role in Pathogenesis to Potential Therapeutic Saviors?

Jehan J. El-Jawhari[1,2], *Yasser El-Sherbiny*[1,2], *Dennis McGonagle*[3,4] *and Elena Jones*[3,4*]

[1] *Department of Biosciences, School of Science and Technology, Nottingham Trent University, Nottingham, United Kingdom,* [2] *Department of Clinical Pathology, Faculty of Medicine, Mansoura University, Mansoura, Egypt,* [3] *Faculty of Medicine and Health, Leeds Institute of Rheumatic and Musculoskeletal Medicine, University of Leeds, Leeds, United Kingdom,* [4] *The National Institute for Health Research Leeds Biomedical Research Centre, Chapel Allerton Hospital, Leeds, United Kingdom*

Correspondence:
Elena Jones
e.jones@leeds.ac.uk

The pathogenesis of the autoimmune rheumatological diseases including rheumatoid arthritis (RA) and systemic lupus erythematosus (SLE) is complex with the involvement of several immune cell populations spanning both innate and adaptive immunity including different T-lymphocyte subsets and monocyte/macrophage lineage cells. Despite therapeutic advances in RA and SLE, some patients have persistent and stubbornly refractory disease. Herein, we discuss stromal cells' dual role, including multipotent mesenchymal stromal cells (MSCs) also used to be known as mesenchymal stem cells as potential protagonists in RA and SLE pathology and as potential therapeutic vehicles. Joint MSCs from different niches may exhibit prominent pro-inflammatory effects in experimental RA models directly contributing to cartilage damage. These stromal cells may also be key regulators of the immune system in SLE. Despite these pro-inflammatory roles, MSCs may be immunomodulatory and have potential therapeutic value to modulate immune responses favorably in these autoimmune conditions. In this review, the complex role and interactions between MSCs and the haematopoietically derived immune cells in RA and SLE are discussed. The harnessing of MSC immunomodulatory effects by contact-dependent and independent mechanisms, including MSC secretome and extracellular vesicles, is discussed in relation to RA and SLE considering the stromal immune microenvironment in the diseased joints. Data from translational studies employing MSC infusion therapy against inflammation in other settings are contextualized relative to the rheumatological setting. Although safety and proof of concept studies exist in RA and SLE supporting experimental and laboratory data, robust phase 3 clinical trial data in therapy-resistant RA and SLE is still lacking.

Keywords: Multipotent Mesenchymal Stromal Cells, rheumatoid arthritis, systemic lupus erythematosus, autoimmunity, immune therapy, immunomodulaion

INTRODUCTION

The original description of multipotent mesenchymal stromal cells, previously known as mesenchymal stem cells (MSCs) that represented tissue-resident clonogenic stromal cells with multilineage osteogenic, chondrogenic, adipogenic and potentially other stromal lineage differentiation capacities emphasized their role in skeletal structure and integrity (1, 2). However, MSCs were later found to be capable of crosstalk with the immune system and have multifaceted additional immunomodulatory functions (3). Strong evidence of research over several years have shown that there are two-way interactions between MSCs and immune cells/factors (4, 5). The best characterized and popular MSCs for immunomodulatory therapies include bone marrow (BM)-MSCs, umbilical cord (UC)-MSCs and adipose-derived (AD)-MSCs. Whilst there is great interest in the use of MSCs for tissue regeneration and repair, the focus herein is in their less well-understood role in tissue homeostasis and immune regulation and on the attempts to translate this into novel immunomodulatory therapy strategies.

Major two-way communication exists between MSCs and immune cells. Cytokines exclusively derived from immune cells such as IL-22 can affect the survival, proliferation, and differentiation function of MSCs (6). Conversely, MSCs can initiate powerful contact-dependent and independent anti-inflammatory cascades that terminate immune responses in healthy condition (5). In contrast to this, MSCs can produce pro-inflammatory effects in pathological tissue environments and drive pathology (4, 7). In the context of RA, the cross-talk between MSCs and immune cells resident in the synovium presents a particular interest.

While MSCs were defined in 2006 as tripotential, plastic adherent cells with a characteristic surface phenotype according to International Society for Cell & Gene Therapy (ISCT) position statement (1), synovium-derived MSCs were first described in 2001 as clonogenic cells with the same ability to proliferate in culture and to have trilineage differentiation potential at the single-cell level (8). Subsequently, the typical surface phenotype of synovium-derived MSCs has been confirmed by flow cytometry (9). In contrast to synovium-derived MSCs, fibroblast-like synoviocytes terminology refers to a culture-expanded fibroblast population from synovium that has not been confirmed to have all MSC characteristics according to the strict ISCT criteria (9). A recent analysis of the literature revealed that both synovium-derived MSCs and fibroblast-like synoviocytes have similar fibroblastic morphology and no distinctive features clearly discriminating between both populations in terms of cell surface markers, differentiation potential or immunomodulatory functions (10, 11). Using the terminology of synovium-derived MSCs and fibroblast-like synoviocytes is likely to refer to the same cell population however, there is no complete agreement (12, 13) and further investigation is needed to clarify the relationship between these cells. Here, we refer to synovial multipotent mesenchymal stromal cells as "MSCs," but we use "fibroblast-like synoviocytes" for describing specific studies that used this terminology.

This review will focus on the interesting crosstalk between MSCs and immune cells and how this crosstalk impacts inflammatory mediators in two autoimmune/inflammatory joint diseases that both exhibit joint predilections; rheumatoid arthritis (RA) and systemic lupus erythematosus (SLE). We focus on these diseases in the experimental model settings and on preliminary clinical trials data emerging in humans where proof of concept preclinical studies showing systemic MSC infusion may be associated with beneficial impacts. Consolidating this knowledge is essential to understand further the emerging field of MSC use for immune homeostasis restoration and to facilitate the development and optimization of therapeutic methods, particularly for resistant rheumatologic autoimmune disease that is refractory to all existing therapies.

PATHOGENESIS OF RA AND SLE

The autoimmune diseases are self-directed inflammatory disorders characterized by progressive tissue destruction and a loss of tissue function if not adequately treated (14). Both RA and SLE are more common in females than males, but the ratio is exaggerated in SLE, where it is up to 10-fold more common in females (15). Autoantibody positive RA is typically progressive whereas SLE course is usually characterized by remission and relapse phases (16). SLE and RA have several shared genetic associations such as MHC-Class II genes and numerous genetic polymorphisms in genes linked to innate and adaptive immune cell function (17, 18).

Both RA and SLE are characterized by the presence of autoantibodies that predate clinical disease. The pathogenesis of SLE is particularly highlighted by over-activation of B-lymphocytes with excess production of autoantibodies and typically leads to multi-organ inflammation including skin, joint causing lupus arthritis (LA) and internal organs including the kidneys (18). In RA, the production of autoantibodies against citrullinated proteins in the joints and elsewhere is associated with the immune complex formation and pro-inflammatory cytokine production including TNF-α and IL-6 and this orchestrates extensive tissue damage. Although RA is much more joint centric than SLE, it is also viewed as a systemic disease and heterogeneous innate and adaptive mechanism may contribute to resistant disease where therapy remains suboptimal (19).

Despite differences in some molecular mechanisms, both RA and SLE are commonly characterized by the loss of peripheral immune tolerance that encompasses reduced T-reg cells in both settings (20, 21). Additionally, increased immune cell numbers and activation, especially in target end organs and excess production of cytokines and other immune mediators that culminates in chronic inflammation are common for both diseases (18). Given that a subgroup of RA and SLE cases are both refractory to all available conventional therapies, a need for experimental new therapy exists. Application of MSCs is one putative cell therapy strategy and has clinical data in the public domain for both the therapy of resistant RA and resistant SLE.

MSC FUNCTION IN HEALTHY JOINTS

When initially studied in the laboratory, MSCs were described as colony-forming fibroblasts with the capability to undergo massive clonal expansion (22). As mentioned, *in vitro* expanded MSCs have been characterized according to the ISCT criteria. These criteria include plastic adherence, lack of expression of hematopoietic lineage markers CD45, CD34, CD14 or CD11b, CD79 alpha, CD19, and HLA-DR, but the expression of surface molecules CD90, CD73, CD105 (1). The surface molecule CD271 is also considered as a distinctive marker for uncultured bone marrow (BM) and bone MSCs (23), which are most common and best-characterized MSCs within musculoskeletal tissues (24). Although not the focus of this article, MSCs are a reservoir of cells for the maintenance of subchondral bone, adipose tissue, ligaments, menisci, the synovial membrane and the synovial fluid homeostasis (4, 25). Interestingly, these MSCs are capable of migration toward the damaged areas e.g., MSCs can migrate from subchondral BM into the joint cavity as detected in underlining layers of proliferating synovial tissue (26), also MSCs were shown to be involved in the synovial hyperplasia in a mouse model of joint surface injury (27). Migratory chondroprogenitors have been found in damaged osteoarthritic cartilage (28), which could, in principle, originate from MSCs migrating upwards from the subchondral bone (29). At the synovio-entheseal complexes, populations of BM cells may theoretically have access to joint cavity via channels wide enough to facilitate MSCs passage from the subchondral bone plate (30). So, under normal condition, there may be potential for loco-regional migration of MSCs from different joint and bone MSC niches toward repair responses and possibly for immunomodulatory responses, but the latter is not well-studied.

A lesser appreciated role for MSCs comes from their immunomodulatory capabilities which have been well-reviewed elsewhere (5, 31, 32). Of note, most of the work pertaining to MSC immunomodulation in RA and SLE was conducted using culture expanded MSCs, but we have recently shown a potential immunosuppression capacity of uncultured MSCs in cancellous bones (33). Pro-inflammatory cytokines, IFN-γ TNF-α and IL-1 can induce or enhance the immunosuppressive capabilities by MSCs, a process that is termed "licensing" whereby pro-inflammatory cytokine treatment of MSCs increases their immunomodulatory capacity (4). Licensed MSCs can inhibit immune cells via soluble mediators; TGF-β, indoleamine 2,3-dioxygenase (IDO), inducible Nitric oxide synthases (iNOS), prostaglandin E2 (PGE2), IL-1 receptor antagonist (IL-1Ra) and tumor necrosis factor-inducible gene 6 (TSG6) (34–36). It must be pointed out that although the immunomodulatory function of MSCs was first reported in relationship to bone marrow MSCs (37), this property likely extends to other fibroblastic cells including synovial fibroblasts (38). It has also been reported that both synovium-derived MSCs and fibroblast-like synoviocytes possess similar immunomodulatory capacity by suppressing T cell proliferation via IDO and TGF-β -dependent mechanisms (39). Therefore, considering the immunomodulatory function of fibroblast-like synoviocytes alongside that of synovium-derived MSCs appears relevant, particularly as more data have emerged in this field recently (40).

Cell to cell contact is another important mechanism of MSC-mediated immunosuppression. Co-culture experiments between MSCs and NK cell lines have shown a change in the NK granule polarization (41). Additionally, MSCs can support neutrophil survival via a surface intercellular adhesion molecule 1 (ICAM-1)-dependent mechanism (42). Cellular interactions between MSCs and adaptive immune cells have also been reported. MSCs can suppress naïve T cell and memory T cell via ICAM-1 and vascular cell adhesion molecule 1 (VCAM-1) interactions (43). Similarly, MSCs can induce the Notch1/Forkhead box P3 (FOXP3) pathway in CD4+T cells and increase the percentage of CD4+CD25 FOXP3+cells (44). One of the surface proteins expressed on MSCs galectin-1 was linked to MSC-mediated immunosuppression of T lymphocytes (45). In addition to T cells, MSCs have been shown to increase the survival of quiescent B cells in cell-cell contact context (46) by activating p38 mitogen-activated protein kinase (MAPK) pathways (47). Therefore, it seems likely that the synovial MSCs not only contribute to normal joint tissue integrity and structure, but also have immunomodulatory characteristics qualifying their potential role in healthy joint homeostasis as well as RA or LA pathogenesis.

Outside the joint, MSCs and non-MSC stromal cells also exhibit similar immunomodulatory capabilities. For example, skin fibroblasts exert virtually the same immunomodulatory effects as BM-MSCs (48). An interesting aspect of the use of culture-expanded MSCs as effector cells for immunomodulation in RA is that these cells are given intravenously. However, there is little evidence for the physiological circulation of MSCs in humans, including patients with RA (49), which will be discussed further in this review.

ALTERED MSC FUNCTIONS IN RA AND SLE JOINTS

The intrinsic immunosuppressive role of MSCs within the joint may contribute to maintaining immune homeostasis within a healthy joint, while the opposite scenario could happen in the pathological microenvironment. As mentioned above, various stromal cell populations derived from synovial tissues have been assigned different terminologies. Fibroblast-like synoviocytes and Type B synoviocytes represent essentially the same cell type with the ability to produce proteoglycans, cytokines, arachidonic acid metabolites, and metalloproteinases (10). However, the term "fibroblast-like synoviocytes" is more commonly used to describe the pathogenic role of RA intimal fibroblasts in destructive joint inflammation unlike "synovial fibroblasts" that broadly defines all synovial-derived cells (50). All synovial fibroblasts and synovium-derived MSCs have similar morphology of spindle-shaped cells (51), but it has been proposed that these fibroblasts can be the aged form of MSCs probably with altered immune and repair related functions (12). Another suggestion was that MSCs and synovial fibroblasts could represent dissimilar functional stages of the same stromal cell lineage (13). Importantly, a recent study has identified and described two anatomically different subsets of fibroblasts accountable for mediating either inflammation or tissue damage in arthritis murine models (40). The synovial sub-lining cells, FAPα^{+} THY1^{+} fibroblasts were found to mediate inflammation in murine arthritis. In contrast, FAPα^{+} THY1^{-} located in synovial lining layer were linked to destructive bone changes and cartilage damage (40).

Although immune cells are key orchestrators of RA and SLE, there is evidence that fibroblast-like synoviocytes are also contributing to joint disease pathogenesis (50). When MSCs were harvested from RA patients, *in vitro* immunosuppression was evident, however, it seems that the microenvironment of RA joint reduced efficacy of MSCs to control the exaggerated immune response in this disease (4, 52). Citrullinated fibrinogen (a prominent auto-antigen in RA) can affect BM-MSC function by promoting IL-6, IL-8, CCL2 expression and reducing IDO via the involvement of toll-like receptor 4 (TLR-4) and NFκB pathway (53). Interestingly, while stimulation of TLR4 expressed on MSCs causes the production of pro-inflammatory cytokines IL-6 and IL-8, TLR3 engagement induced immunosuppressive MSCs to produce IDO (54, 55). Another defect reported in RA BM-MSCs is A20 downregulation leading to higher IL-6 expression levels, further contributing to RA progression (56). A20 is an anti-inflammatory protein that prevents NF-kB hyperactivation following excess exposure of cells to TNF-α (57). In summary, variable mechanisms could induce pro-inflammatory function of MSCs contributing to RA pathogenesis.

There are reports of MSC immunosuppressive functions alterations in SLE. It has been reported that BM-MSCs from SLE patients had less IDO production than healthy MSCs when both MSCs were licensed by IFN-γ (58). Thus, the modulation of IDO activity could be potentially useful to reinstate the functions of SLE BM-MSCs. Other studies showed lower expression of immunosuppressive cytokines such as TGF-β and IL-10 by SLE BM-MSCs because of abnormal activation of several JAK-STAT, p53/p21, PTEN/Akt, PI3K/Akt, and Wnt/beta-catenin signaling pathways (59–61). Despite evidence of less immunosuppression, the pro-inflammatory effect of SLE MSCs and mechanisms causing these changes are not fully clear.

Besides immunomodulatory alterations, several *in vitro* studies showed that SLE MSCs have a tendency toward senescence. Increased ROS indicating endoplasmic reticulum stress was linked to the senescence of SLE MSCs as detected by electron microscopy (62). Also, induced levels of senescence-related genes that block the cell cycle in MSCs from SLE patients were associated with limited proliferation and cell morphology showing deeply stained nucleus, and disordered cytoskeletal organization (63). These biological characters seemed to be linked to mitochondrial antiviral signaling protein (MAVS) that induces an IFN-β and ROS expression in SLE MSCs (64, 65). IFN-β is involved in cell senescence via p53 transcriptional and functional alterations of P53 (66). Senescence-associated cytokines, including IL-6, IL-8, and granulocyte–macrophage colony-stimulating factor (GM-CSF), significantly increased at the gene expression levels in SLE MSCs (64). Furthermore, increased susceptibility to death was suggested for SLE MSCs due to significantly low levels of an anti-apoptotic marker, Bcl-2 (67) and where SLE BM-MSCs were reported to have a normal karyotype (68).

In summary, the functions and proliferative capacity of MSCs are changed in RA and SLE either due to intrinsic or extrinsic reasons but all associated with chronic inflammation. Multiple subsets of immune cells are present in the autoimmune arthritis milieu, and their interactions with MSCs are discussed below.

MSCs INTERACTION WITH KEY IMMUNE CELL PLAYERS IN RA AND SLE

DCs and MSCs

In normal condition, MSCs have inhibitory effects on dendritic cells (DCs). MSCs can suppress the monocyte differentiation into DCs or switch monocyte differentiation into macrophages rather than antigen-presenting DCs via several mechanisms including IL-6, TSG-6, and COX-2/PGE2 (69–71). Furthermore, MSCs can inhibit the maturation, migration and antigen presentation of DCs as murine DCs co-cultured with murine MSCs also found to induce more T-reg cells (72). Additionally, the production of IL-1Ra via MSCs can inhibit the production of IL-1β, IL-6, and IL-23 by DCs in co-cultures (73).

Monocyte-derived DCs can acquire the phenotype of myeloid-derived suppressor cells (MDSC) via the growth-regulated oncogene (GRO) chemokines produced by human MSCs. These DCs were found to have high secretion of IL-10 and IL-4 but low expression of IL-12 and IFN-γ (74). Additionally, human MSCs were reported to promote the expansion of MDSCs expressing arginase-1 (ARG-1) and iNOS through hepatocyte growth factor bractice HGF-related mechanism (75). Another mechanism by which MSCs can support the survival of MDSCs is exosomes produced by MSCs that induce the anti-apoptotic proteins Bcl-xL and Mcl-1 as seen in tumor cells (76). The variety of mechanisms by which MSCs inhibit DC function indicate that MSCs might have an underestimated role of keeping immune hemostasis (mainly suppression). Interestingly, RA DCs highly express pro-inflammatory transcription factor NF-κB in correlation with the disease activity, and in response to local inflammatory mediators such as damage-associated molecular patterns (DAMPs) and TNF-α (77). The abnormally active DCs suggest the failure of immune control mechanisms, possibly including joint MSCs.

In RA, fibroblast-like synoviocytes or MSCs have been shown to function as antigen-presenting cells leading to T-lymphocyte activation and proliferation (78) when thrombospondin-1 expressed by these synoviocytes are engaged with CD47 on T-lymphocyte surface (79). Another mechanism that could explain how MSCs could act as DC-like cells is TLR activation directly involved in RA pathogenesis (80). TLR2 and 4 are highly expressed in the synovium (81) with the most abundant types of ligands for TLR2 and TLR4 including HSP22 and Biglycan (82, 83). A study has shown that RA-induced cytokines IL-12 and IL-18 together with IFN-γ cause an upregulation of TLR4 on synovial MSCs and consequently trigger the expression of pro-inflammatory cytokines IL-6 and TNF-α (81). The TLR-related pro-inflammatory functions of MSCs demonstrate MSC changes in RA, but it would be still valuable to investigate how DCs display their functions when co-cultured with synovial MSCs in RA milieu.

Plasmacytoid dendritic cells (pDCs) are the primary producers of IFN-α (84). In SLE, pDCs induce the differentiation of immature B-lymphocytes to plasma cells but not B-reg cells with induction of IFN-α secretion (85). In parallel, high IFN-α in SLE marked by increased plasmablasts and CD314 (86, 87) has been linked to defective T-reg cell function that promotes differentiation of CD4+ T effector cells (88). In contrast to hematopoietic cells, IFN-α seems to have less effect on MSCs. The gene expression levels of differentiation markers of native MSCs were found unaffected by IFN-α (89). However, when MSCs were treated with IFN-α within an *in vitro* culture condition, inhibition of cell proliferation was reported (89, 90). Additionally, the osteogenic differentiation potential of culture expanded MSCs was found to be suppressed by exposure to IFN-α (91). Considering IFN-α is one of the major players in SLE milieu, it remains to be established if this cytokine could affect immunomodulatory functions of MSCs at a functional level. Altogether, MSCs and DCs can behave differentially in normal condition, however these cells share some mechanisms related to pro-inflammatory cytokine release and TLR activation in autoimmune diseases such as RA and SLE.

Macrophages and MSCs

Macrophages are a source of bone morphogenetic proteins (BMPs) and Oncostatin M, which induce the proliferation and osteogenic differentiation of MSCs (92) and conversely, MSCs regulate macrophage function. Bone marrow MSCs can suppress monocyte differentiation into osteoclast via osteoprotegerin production (OPG) (93). Also, MSCs can drive macrophage polarization from their pro-inflammatory to anti-inflammatory types through the production of IDO, COX-2/PGE2, and TSG-6 (94). By a PGE2-dependent mechanism and IDO involvement, human MSCs attenuate pro-inflammatory function and enhance the anti-inflammatory role of macrophages that have increased phagocytic capacity and high production of IL-10 and TGF-β (95). Human MSCs also affect macrophages' functions to overproduce IL-10 and reduce IL-12 and TNF-α expression levels (96). Collectively, MSCs can induce the anti-inflammatory effect of macrophages.

Inflammatory joint resident macrophages in RA are stimulated by Th1 cells via IFN-γ to produce IL-1β and TNF-α acquiring pro-inflammatory phenotype and inducing a hyperimmune response in RA inflamed joint synovium (97). In parallel, MSCs within such an inflammatory microenvironment could also induce macrophage pro-inflammatory phenotype via TLR2 and TLR4 induction (4). Furthermore, RA-MSCs could have innate immune abilities with a production of GM-CSF that is a major macrophage activating factor (98). These data indicate the cumulative effect of MSCs and macrophages in the progression of arthritis.

In addition to their role in chronic inflammation, macrophages are involved in bone and cartilage repair. Macrophages can induce the expression of RANKL by MSCs promoting the osteoclast formation (99). Similarly, MSCs were shown to induce the osteoclastogenesis from BM hematopoietic stem cells although in a different mechanism via involvement of IL-6 (100). Furthermore, macrophages produce matrix metalloproteinases (MMPs) that aid to degrade the cartilage matrix (101). Additionally, macrophages produce TNF-α within inflammatory milieu reduce osteoblasts and promote osteoclasts (102, 103). TNF-α stimulates the production of M-CSF by MSCs, which, in turn, induces the differentiation of osteoclast progenitors (104). With regards to cartilage, TNF-α induces the death of mature chondrocytes and the growth of bone cells assisting the conversion from cartilage into bone (105). TNF-α also increases MMPs that could mediate cartilage degradation and angiopoietin production helping osteochondral angiogenesis (106). The bone and cartilage changes mediated by inflammatory cytokines could explain how MSCs within the inflammatory arthritis milieu cannot repair or overcome joint tissue damage. All these data demonstrate how chronic inflammation can affect immune cells and MSCs leading to joint tissue damage. While macrophages have a pro-inflammation effect and destructive role in RA joints' bone and cartilage, MSCs may be promoting these altered functions.

T-Lymphocytes and MSCs

T-lymphocytes are central players in orchestrating inflammation in RA and SLE. Joint resident lymphocytes in health or disease are in contact with joint resident MSCs and thus exhibit complex interactions. The effect of T-lymphocytes on MSCs pervasively impacts on all MSC functions. In addition to licensing effect, T-lymphocyte-derived cytokines IFN-γ and TNF-α can upregulate MSC migration (107), but block the MSC differentiation capacity (108).

Compared to Th1 cytokines, Th17 cells were reported as an osteoclastogenic helper T-lymphocyte subset also contributing to bone damage in arthritis (109). Furthermore, IL-17 can suppress the chondrogenic differentiation of MSCs via suppression of a key chondrogenesis transcriptional factor, SRY-box 9 (SOX9) and its activator cAMP-dependent protein kinase (PKA) (110). Innate lymphocytes cells (ILC3s) and Th17 cells commonly produce IL-17, but ILC3s also produce IL-22 and M-CSF cytokines (111). We have demonstrated that IL-22 could stimulate the proliferation and osteogenic differentiation of IFN-γ/TNF-α-licensed MSCs (6) indicating the complexity of how inflammatory milieu can affect the regenerative capacity of MSCs.

While T-lymphocytes affect MSC function, MSCs can in turn, affect T lymphocytes. The culture expanded synovial MSCs extracted from healthy subjects can inhibit T lymphocyte proliferation (112). Also, these MSCs can maintain the percentage of T-reg cells when in co-culture with T-reg enriched lymphocytes (113) further supporting the role of MSCs in maintaining immune tolerance. Some studies indicated that MSCs from RA patients could preserve T lymphocytes immunosuppression capacity *in vitro*. The co-culture of PBMCs with BM-MSCs, both from RA patients or healthy controls, resulted in decrease the production of TNF-α, IL-17, IL-6, IL-2, IFN-γ, and IL-9 by all T-lymphocyte subsets (naive, effector, and memory T-lymphocytes). Also, these MSCs induced the gene expression levels of anti-inflammatory cytokines IL-10 and

TGF-β by $CD4^+$ and $CD8^+$ T-lymphocytes (114). Another *in vitro* study showed that human RA synovial MSCs, in a fashion comparable with donor-matched BM-MSCs, suppressed T-cell response in a mixed lymphocyte reaction with a similar expression level of IDO (112). In contrast, another study showed that RA MSCs had an impaired function in inhibiting Th17 cells (115). Instead, RA fibroblast-like synoviocytes stimulated T-cells following interaction between CXCR4 on T-lymphocytes and SDF-1 on synoviocytes (116). The variability in the capacity of RA MSCs to suppress T-lymphocytes suggests that the altered immunosuppressive mechanism of these MSCs could probably be correlated to disease severity or donor variability.

Human MSCs produce HLA-G5 a non-classical MHC class I molecule, which has been linked to inhibition of the reactivity and cytolytic function of alloreactive T-lymphocytes (117). HLA-G5 was also found to be involved in the suppression of T-lymphocyte proliferation as well as promoting the differentiation shift toward T-reg cells (117). In SLE, the link between high levels of IL-10 and HLA-G and chronic pro-inflammatory status is not clear. The overall MSC and T-lymphocyte interactions seem to be complicated to explain how both cell types collaboratively promote chronic inflammation in autoimmune joint diseases. However, these interactions explain clearly how the regenerative capacity of MSCs could be limited in this inflammatory milieu.

B-Lymphocytes and MSCs

A supportive role for joint stromal and B-cell function in RA is a long-recognized phenomenon (86). Normal human MSCs can inhibit the proliferation and functions of B-lymphocytes (4). In contrast, RA fibroblast-like synoviocytes could promote B-lymphocyte migration, via SDF-1 and vascular cell adhesion molecule-1 (VCAM-1) dependent mechanisms (118, 119). Additionally, RA synovial stromal cell line could promote the survival and functions of B-lymphocytes via an increase in the expression of BCL-XL via a CD49/CD29-CD106-dependent mechanism (120). Also, RA synovial fibroblasts could promote B-lymphocyte survival by upregulation of IL-15 receptor on the surface of B-lymphocytes (121). Furthermore, RA fibroblast-like synoviocytes induced immunoglobulin class switching in B-lymphocytes (122). These data together indicate the changed function of MSCs toward B-lymphocytes in RA favoring inflammation.

BM-MSCs from SLE patients showed less immunosuppressive effects on B-lymphocytes compared to control MSCs. The effect of these SLE-MSCs on the proliferation and production of autoimmune antibodies was mediated via CCL2 (123). While BM-MSCs in SLE have defective immunosuppressive potential, these MSCs stimulated the growth and maturation of B lymphocytes (124). Furthermore, high expression of olfactory 1/early B-lymphocyte factor-associated zinc-finger (OAZ) gene that is linked to cell cycle control was detected for BM-MSCs from SLE patients. Interestingly, the down expression of this gene was associated with increased ability of MSCs to inhibit B-lymphocyte functions of autoantibody production (125). Although less characterized, MSCs seem to promote B-lymphocyte response in SLE in common with RA.

Collectively, MSCs seemed to be reprogrammed to support the pro-inflammatory functions of B-lymphocytes rather than immune response regulation in both RA and SLE. At the present, we would summarize the literature as suggesting that the multiple impacts of MSCs on the immune system outweigh any potential detrimental impacts on autoantibody production. Further investigations into the mechanisms underlying these changes would help to understand autoimmune pathogenicity and to optimize MSC-based therapies as discussed in the next sections.

THERAPEUTIC USE OF MSCs IN RA AND SLE

Animal Models of Using MSCs for Experimental RA and SLE

Several experimental models confirmed the potential effectiveness of MSCs for RA and SLE treatment via multiple anti-inflammatory mechanisms. Murine bone marrow MSCs have been shown to impair TLR-4 induced activation of DCs, thus reducing the DC migration to lymph nodes and excretion of antigen presentation (74). Additionally, UC-MSCs were effective for the treatment of RA, as shown in collagen-induced arthritis (CIA) mouse model. These MSCs reduced synovitis and articular destruction with declined levels of TNF-α and IL-1β in the serum and joints (126). Human AD-MSCs have been also effective in increasing T-reg cells and IL-10 levels and reducing the serum levels of TNF-α and anti-collagen type II in CIA model (127).

Similar to RA, murine SLE studies showed that the application of therapeutic human BM-MSCs showed a decrease in serum levels of anti-dsDNA antibodies and renal complement C3 expression (128, 129). Furthermore, allogeneic murine MSCs were effective in SLE mice compared with cyclophosphamide treatment (130). In another SLE experimental model, allogeneic MSCs enhanced the anti-inflammatory effects of immunosuppressant drugs with less adverse effects of these medications (131). In another study, allogeneic MSCs have reduced renal immunoglobulin G (IgG) deposition in SLE mice (132). Recently, a novel mechanism of how therapeutic MSCs can suppress chronic inflammation in SLE was described whereby transplantation of allogeneic UC-MSCs has been shown to increase the expression of $CD1c^+$DCs by promoting their proliferation and anti-apoptosis effect (133). Although, MSCs were found effective in controlling immune responses in RA and SLE experimental models by effects on DCs and both T and B lymphocytes, the outcomes on disease severity and markers were variable, and the potential reasons are discussed below.

The source of MSCs is one of the common variables used in preclinical RA and SLE studies. *In vitro* studies showed that UC-MSCs, AD-MSCs and BM-MSCs similarly inhibit the maturation of DCs, T cell proliferation and activate T-reg cell induction (134–138). In contrast, the superiority of UC-MSCs was reported in hampering the cytokine release from LPS-stimulated macrophages and in the induction of T-reg cells compared to BM-MSCs (139, 140). Other studies showed that AD-MSCs are more potent in inhibiting T cell activation and proliferation than UC-MSCs and BM-MSCs (141, 142). In contrast to *in vitro* studies, fewer studies directly compared the efficacy of different MSC sources in RA models. Synovial fluid-MSCs effectively improved the severity of collagen-induced arthritis more than BM-MSCs (143). In the second study, BM-MSCs, AD-MSCs, and UC-MSCs treated arthritis with no significant difference between the three groups (144). The meta analysis data of RA experimental models showed that AD-MSCs and UC-MSCs had better therapeutic effects on experimental RA than BM-MSCs. Interestingly, clinical scores were similar between UC-MSCs and AD-MSCs, but UC-MSCs demonstrated better outcomes using histological tissue scores (bone erosion, cartilage damage, and inflammation) (145). Reviewing SLE experimental models, different BM, AD or UC-MSCs were comparably effective as shown by the reduction of T effector cell number, increased T-reg cell number in the spleen and decreased antibody production and inflammatory cytokines in kidneys (146). Overall, the *in vitro* and preclinical data suggested a similarity of AD-MSC and UC-MSC potency probably followed by BM-MSCs to induce immunosuppression for RA and SLE experimental models.

While some studies showed no difference in immune compatibility of MSCs (147–149), other groups reported that allogeneic and syngeneic transplantation had no different effect on arthritis (150, 151). In contrast, using xenogeneic MSCs e.g., human-derived MSCs in RA experimental studies was more effective than the use of allogeneic or syngeneic murine MSCs (145). These data suggest that an appropriate level of immune incompatibility between donor MSCs and the host may benefit cell therapy.

The quantity of MSCs is another factor that could affect the therapeutic outcome. UC-MSCs was effective in improving mouse CIA in a dose-dependent manner in another study (152). Other two studies showed that the higher doses (2.5, 5 × 10^6) of either BM-, UC-, or AD-MSCs were more effective than a lower dose (1 × 10^6) for treating arthritis mice models (144, 153) indicating that adequate quantities of MSCs are essential for satisfactory therapeutic effect. In terms of the frequency of the doses, two doses were shown to be more effective than a single dose, and the therapy timing was more important than the number of BM-MSC doses (149). Other two studies reported that there was no difference between single or double doses of 1 × 10^6 BM-MSCs (150), or between two and five injections of AD- or BM-MSCs (144).

Interestingly, the administration time of the required quantity of therapeutic MSCs was investigated. Injection of MSCs during the early phase of disease was associated with favorable outcomes in RA animal models, and the earlier the MSC treatment, the more efficient treatment (153–155). However, in severe arthritis model, early MSC dose was not adequate to reduce the disease severity over the long term (149, 156). Overall, it is possible that variability in disease severity or the inherent immunomodulatory ability of injected MSCs could influence the outcomes using adequate doses of MSCs.

Route of administration was another factor to be assessed in preclinical models, and the data showed that injection of MSCs prior to the onset of arthritis via either IV or intra-peritoneal (IP) routes was similarly effective and better than administration after the onset of the disease (153). Furthermore, local implantation of MSCs, particularly when loaded on scaffolds were more effective in improvement of arthritis scores compared to intra-articular (IA) or IP (157). Finally, the passage number of culture-expanded MSCs and culture conditions are other factors that might impact the immunomodulatory potential of MSCs and necessitate further investigation.

Clinical Studies of Using MSCs for RA

The value of MSCs in autoimmune diseases or transplantation is mainly related to their basic immunosuppressive capacity and the bonus of a good safety profile (158). As mentioned, the immune system may activate inflammatory responses in MSCs; therefore, MSCs from non-inflamed environments may conversely modulate aberrant immune responses. Thus, the use of healthy MSCs is a promising tool for RA therapy particularly in the therapy of refractory disease (159).

There is a relative paucity of randomized controlled trials (RCT) of MSCs in RA and SLE and beyond that also a general lack of trials in other immune diseases settings (37, 160). Nevertheless, RCTs in the transplantation setting have suggested efficacy and safety of MSCs (158, 161). A systematic literature review and meta-analysis of MSC trials showed that only a minority were undertaken for an inflammatory disease where numbers were generally small, but safety was good (158, 161). It can be surmised that the promising laboratory mechanistic data on MSC immunomodulation and the supportive preclinical data, but there is a paucity of high-quality RCTs in RA and SLE.

The MSC-based therapy usually involves culture expansion of either autologous or allogeneic MSCs, and these cells are infused intravenously at an average of 1–2 million MSCs per kg of body weight (162). Several studies have investigated the use of (UC-MSCs in RA clinical trials (**Table 1**). Clinical studies using MSCs for treating refractory RA have considerably increased since 2011 with UC-MSCs used in nearly half of these studies. Therefore, it is not surprising that the therapeutic MSCs are 78% allogenic and 22% autologous. Additionally, both one dose and multiple doses are popular. Two early pilot studies have proved safety for MSCs in RA therapy. Ra et al. used autologous AD-MSC therapy for four RA patients, among other autoimmune diseases. These MSCs were infused intravenously in a single, double, or quadruple dose. The patients were monitored for 13 months, with all of them showing no adverse effect and improvement of Visual Analog Scale (VAS) and Korean Western Ontario McMaster (KWOMAC) scores (176). In another small pilot study, four refractory RA patients were treated with allogeneic BM-MSCs or UC-MSCs. These patients were given a single IV infusion of one million MSCs/kg of body weight. MSC-based therapy proved no adverse effects, and the therapy seemed less effective. After 24 months, three out of four patients had a moderate response measured using European league against rheumatism (EULAR) parameters, erythrocyte sedimentation rate (ESR), C reactive protein (CRP), disease activity score (DAS) 28, and VAS score (165).

TABLE 1 | Clinical trials for RA therapy using MSCs.

Phase	MSC source	Patients	Outcome	References
Phase I/II	UC allogeneic	64 patients	Three years follow-up: no serious adverse effects. Remission measured by ACR, DAS-28, ESR, and HAQ. Low levels of CRP, RF, anti-CCP antibodies, TNF-α and IL-6. Increase of blood T-reg cells.	(163)
Phase I/II	UC allogeneic	172 patients	The 8-month follow-up; no serious adverse effects Low levels of CRP, RF, anti-CCP antibodies, TNF-α and IL-6. Increase of blood T-reg cells.	(164)
Phase I	UC allogeneic	4 patients	3 patients had lower ESR, DAS-28, pain VAS score at 1 and 6 months. 2 patients had a EULAR moderate response at 6 months but a relapse at 7 and 23 months, respectively. No one had achieved the DAS-28-defined remission. No serious adverse events were reported.	(165)
Phase I/II randomized	UC allogeneic	105 patients refractory	Safety and good response indicated by initial IFN-γ induction then increase of IL-10 and T-reg cells/TH17 ratio.	(166)
Phase I	UC allogeneic	9 patients refractory	No major toxicity up to 4 weeks after the infusion. Reduction in serum erythrocyte sedimentation rate and DAS28 score. Reduced levels of IL-1β, IL-6, IL-8, and TNF-α.	(167)
Phase I/II	UC allogeneic	63 patients refractory	Efficacy and ACR20 response rates in 53.3% patients with MSC and in 93.3% patients with MSC combined with IFN-γ at 3-month follow-up. No new or unexpected safety issues were encountered in 1-year follow-up.	(168)
Phase 1	UC allogeneic	9 patients refractory	Safety, a decline in the DAS28-ESR, HAQ, and VAS scores as well as blood levels of ESR and CRP, IL-1β, IL-6, IL-8, and TNF-α.	(167)
Phase I/II non-randomized	UC allogeneic	64 patients refractory	Safe after 1 and 3 years. The ESR, CRP, RF were lower than that of pre-treatment. Decrease in HAQ and DAS28 scores.	(163)
Phase I	BM autologous	9 patients refractory	Increase T-reg cells. Decreasing trend in Th17. Decrease DAS28 and VAS scores.	(169)
Phase I	BM autologous	13 patients refractory	Increase gene expression of FOXP3 at month 12. Increasing in PBMC culture supernatant levels of IL-10 and TGF-β1.	(170)
Phase I/II randomized	BM autologous	30 patients	No adverse effects. Improvement in WOMAC, VAS score, but not beyond 12 months.	(171)
Phase I/II	BM autologous	20 patients Early RA	Ongoing NCT03186417[a]	
Phase I/II randomized	Adipose allogenic	53 patients	Well-tolerated therapy. ACR20 was 20–45% at 1-month and 0–25% at 3-month follow-up.	(172)
Phase II	BM-MSCs autologous	48 patients	There were positive clinical outcomes as observed using ACR, PGA, and HAQ.	(173)
Phase I	BM-MSCs autologous	13 refractory patients	A decrease in the blood levels of CD19+ B cells with a decreased expression of BR3, TACI, and BCMA receptors and blood BAFF and APRIL levels 12 months after the MSC infusion.	(174)
Phase I	BM-MSCs autologous	13 refractory patients	The blood levels of CXCL8, CXCL12, and CXCL13 were significantly decreased 6 months after MSCs transplantation but returned to pre-treatment levels after 12 months.	(175)

[a] *ClinicalTrials.gov. Available online at: http://clinicaltrials.gov/.*

BM, Bone marrow; UC, Umbilical; DAS28, 28-joint disease activity score; HAQ, Health index; EULAR, European League Against Rheumatism; FOXP3, forkhead box P3; WOMAC, Western Ontario and McMaster Universities Arthritis Index; VAS, visual analog scale; ACR20, American College of Rheumatology 20 responses; PGA, Patient global assessment.

Wang et al. have conducted two studies; one phase I/II clinical trial treating 172 RA patients with up to 8-month follow-up (164) and another study with 64 patients were followed up to 3 years for long term results (163). In both studies, patients were treated with a single dose of systematically injected allogeneic UC-MSCs (4×10^7 cells/patient) combined with low-dose DMARD treatments (leflunomide, hydroxychloroquine sulfate, or methotrexate). The outcomes were no serious adverse effects and a remission measured by the American College of Rheumatology improvement criteria (ACR), the DAS-28, ESR, and the Health Assessment Questionnaire (HAQ). Additionally, low levels of CRP, rheumatoid factor (RF), and anti-cyclic citrullinated peptide (anti-CCP) antibodies, TNF-α and IL-6 cytokines were reported. These clinical results, in addition to the increase in the percentage of blood T-reg cells were reported in both studies (163, 164).

A small study was conducted on nine RA patients who were not treated with any biologic compound but received IV allogeneic UC-MSCs. In this phase I clinical trial, the MSC doses were 2.5×10^7, 5×10^7, or 1×10^8 UC-MSCs per subject (167). The safety, the decline in the DAS28, HAQ, and VAS scores, as well as blood levels of ESR, CRP, IL-1β, IL-6, IL-8, and TNF-α, particularly with the higher dose of MSCs were noted.

Despite the promising effects of UC-MSCs in the above clinical studies, other reports indicated less effectiveness of using allogenic UC-MSCs even with a higher dose. A phase I clinical study treated 53 refractory RA patients with a single IV dose of 1×10^6 allogeneic UC-MSCs/kg of body weight. The results of up to 12 months follow-up confirmed the clinical safety of this MSC therapy (166). However, the clinical outcomes were variable with 54% of the patients achieved a good or moderate response, but 46% of the patients had no clinical response as measured by CRP, ESR, HAQ and DAS28 scores. Also, 8% of responders experienced a relapse by 24 weeks. With regards to laboratory findings, responders had increased blood levels of albumin, hemoglobin, T-reg cells and IL-10, but a decrease in anti-inflammatory mediators anti-CCP, IL-6, TNF-α, and Th17 cells. Interestingly, there was a positive association between high serum IFN-γ levels and reduced DAS28 score. In agreement, a recently published clinical study for 63 refractory RA patients showed that 1×10^6 IU of recombinant IFN-γ that injected intramuscularly increased the effectiveness of simultaneous delivered UC-MSCs (intravenous 1×10^6 MSCs/kg of body weight) by nearly 2-fold (168). Together these data further confirmed the perception that MSC immunosuppressive capacity is not constitutive, but dependent on a process of cytokine-related licensing that is acquired within inflammatory milieu and could be different between patients.

Another source of therapeutic MSCs is bone marrow with several studies that have been completed or ongoing (**Table 1**). In a multicenter randomized double-blind placebo-controlled sequential dose-escalation phase II study, allogeneic BM MSCs with high differentiation capacity expressing STRO-1 or STRO-3 markers were used (173). An infusion of 1×10^6 or 2×10^6 MPCs/kg of body weight were used in 48 patients in combination with DMARDs. There were positive clinical outcomes as observed using ACR, patient global assessment (PGA), and HAQ particularly with the higher dose. Furthermore, a pilot study involved nine refractory RA patients who were IV-infused with one dose of autologous BM-MSCs (1 to 2×10^6 cells/kg of body weight) combined with conventional therapy. Twelve-month follow-up showed no adverse effect, a significant decrease in DAS28-ESR, VAS scores and ESR, but no changes in blood inflammatory markers (169). Systemic injection of autologous BM-MSCs into refractory RA patients with 12 month-follow up demonstrated that the gene expression of forkhead box P3 (FOXP3) in peripheral blood mononuclear cells (PBMCs) was significantly induced (170). Furthermore, high levels of IL-10 and transforming growth factor-beta 1 (TGF-β1) were noted in the culture supernatant of PBMCs over the time course of treatment (170). Autologous BM-MSCs were also used in another study with promising effects, but up to 12 months follow up (171).

The first randomized multicenter clinical study using allogeneic AD-MSCs for RA was a double-blind placebo-controlled dose-escalation phase Ib/IIa trial (172). Fifty-three refractory RA patients were divided into three groups, having intravenous infused MSC doses of 1, 2, or 4×10^6 cells/kg of body weight. After a 6-month follow-up, a transient fever was noted, but a satisfactory response was observed using the EULAR criteria, DAS28-ESR, and CRP. No MSC dose-response was noted, probably because of the small number of RA patients in each group. With regards to inflammation markers, no significant changes in circulating T cell populations were observed. Interestingly, there was an indication of MSC immunogenicity in 19% of RA patients, but without apparent clinical significance (172).

A recent clinical study for 13 RA patients suggested that multiple doses of BM-MSCs or a higher dose of MSCs may be required to maintain immunosuppressive status (174). Also, this study has reported for the first time a decrease in the blood levels of CD19+ B cells with a decreased expression of BLyS receptor 3 (BR3), transmembrane activator and CAML interactor (TACI), and B-cell maturation antigen (BCMA) receptors and blood BAFF and APRIL levels 12 months after the MSC infusion. These results indicate that MSC therapy may decrease B cell proliferation. The same research group showed that blood levels of CXCL8, CXCL12, and CXCL13 were significantly decreased 6 months after BM-MSCs transplantation but returned to pre-treatment levels after 12 months (175).

Altogether, several clinical trials have offered support for the safety of MSCs particularly for resistant RA (165, 166, 168, 170–172). The variable outcomes regarding remission could be due to MSC type, dose, and frequency as well as donor factors such as age, health condition and immune status. Higher and multiples doses and availability of inflammatory licensing milieu for MSCs seem to favor better outcomes. Nevertheless, more randomized controlled trials are needed to establish efficacy. The source of therapeutic MSCs is an important point to consider for treating autoimmune arthritis particularly with tissue damages/lesions. Considering research findings that are indicating that autologous RA MSCs might not act efficiently as immunosuppressive cells, it is not surprising that allogenic MSCs are frequently used in RA patient studies. Most of the clinical trials have involved the systematic infusion of allogeneic MSCs from BM, AD, and UC (177). Furthermore, the therapeutic effect of injected allogeneic MSCs could be diminished probably due to activated immune mechanisms (178). More research is needed to compare how activated immune response and inflammatory milieu can affect the activities of infused allogeneic and autologous MSCs.

Clinical Studies of Using MSCs for SLE

The therapeutic management of SLE has historically focused on the use of intensive immunosuppressive agents such as steroids, methylprednisolone, cyclophosphamide and mycophenolate mofetil and latterly drugs that target B-cell and autoantibody axis (179). However, potentially serious side effects related to immune suppression e.g., infection and myelosuppression, as well as organ toxicity can arise (180, 181). Furthermore, some patients are resistant to these standard therapies (182). Consequently, there is a need to develop new approaches for SLE treatment.

Several clinical trials of MSCs in SLE are either completed or ongoing (**Table 2**). Application of therapeutic MSCs is a fairly new tool for SLE patients, but reported as safe with claims of effectiveness in refractory disease patients (184–186, 188, 190). One study tested the effect of intravenous infusion of UC-MSCs at 1×10^6/kg body weight to treat nine refractory SLE patients. No adverse events such as headache, nausea or vomiting were observed. There was no change in the blood picture, organ functions or tumorigenic marker levels (188). In another study, UC-MSCs were used for several autoimmune diseases, including SLE. The data showed 5-year and 8-year survival rates were 90.4 and 88.9%, respectively. The incidence rate of infections was 29.5, and 1.2% of patients experienced malignancies. Deaths rate was 0.2% mainly due to disease relapse and complications associated with the underlying disease (185). In another study, three patients were given 90×10^6 allogenic BM-MSCs and were followed up for 9 months. The results showed improvement as monitored by the SLE disease activity index (SLEDAI) and other markers such as proteinuria, lymphocyte and monocyte antigens antibodies (184). In contrast, 13 SLE patients were also treated with allogenic BM-MSCs with no adverse effect, but 2 out of 13 patients had disease replace (186). In a randomized study, 2 out of 12 patients treated with UC-MSCs had pneumonia while one patient in the control group (6 patients) had a stroke, and another had ascites (190).

Several studies demonstrated laboratory signs of SLE disease activity improvements. Using MSC therapy in either case studies or RCTs showed a reduction in SLE laboratory disease activity markers such as proteinuria (187, 190, 193). With regards to clinical remission, the results were variable. When 2×10^8 UC-MSCs were infused intravenously in 12 SLE patients, remission occurred in 75% of these patients compared to 83% remission in who had placebo (190). In a multi-center clinical study, two doses of intravenously infused UC-MSCs were well-tolerated with no adverse effects (192). Additionally, SLEDAI and BILAG scores for renal, hematopoietic and cutaneous systems were significantly improved. Blood levels of antinuclear antibody and anti-double-stranded DNA antibodies also decreased significantly at 3-month follow-up. There was 12% disease relapse detected after 6 months of follow-up (192). A 4-year study showed that half of 87 treatment-resistant SLE patients entered clinical remission at 4-year follow-up after allogenic BM- or UC-MSCs were infused intravenously (189). In this study, the popular dose (1×10^6 MSCs/kg of body weight) was used, but the overall rate of relapse was relatively high (189). In another study, UC-MSC infusion induced 100% disease remission for 16 resistant SLE patients after 28 months (191). Significant remission was reported according to the SLEDAI score, blood levels of anti-dsDNA antibody, albumin, Complement-3, and renal function. Additionally, an increase in T-reg cells and normalized Th1- and Th2-related cytokines were observed (191).

In a case study, autologous BM-MSC transplantation had no effect on SLE disease activity in 14 weeks of follow-up despite increasing T-reg cell counts (183). The transplantation of autologous MSCs could probably fail to inhibit the pathogenic immune reactions in SLE patients due to defective immunomodulatory functions (194). Both intrinsic and microenvironmental mechanisms seemed to be related to the defective functions of SLE MSCs. Therefore, improving the functions of autologous MSCs can be an alternative therapeutic approach. Collectively, most clinical studies up to date showed that MSC therapy for SLE had good but variable efficacy with 50–100% remission rate. Like RA clinical trials, the variation in the effectiveness of these MSC therapies could be related to the dose and type of MSCs, the clinical status of patients prior to therapy and the concurrent use of other immunosuppressive regimes. Most of the SLE clinical studies included a single dose of MSCS and showing variable outcomes. Therefore, larger studies are needed to validate the efficient dose and need for biological/inflammatory mediators.

Non-cellular and Apoptotic MSC-Based Therapy for RA and SLE

Extracellular vesicles (EVs), a part of MSC secretome, have recently attracted considerable attention as new therapeutic vehicles for treating RA and other immune-related diseases (195). The EVs are small vesicles excreted by parent cells, which carry nucleic acids, mitochondria and proteins within a lipid-bilayer membrane, and they can fuse with recipient cells, thus enabling direct cell-to-cell communication. MSC-derived EVs contain a large repertoire of miRNAs that can effectively regulate recipient's cell transcription toward inflammation reduction; furthermore, this MSC-EV cargo can be modified by MSC pre-conditioning. For example, the anti-inflammatory properties of MSC-EVs can be enhanced by MSC stimulation with TNF-α combined with IFN-γ (196). EVs derived from human MSCs containing miRNA-124a could help to reduce RA synovial hyperplasia as shown to inhibit the proliferation and migration of fibroblast-like synoviocyte cell line (197). In a porcine model of synovitis, BM MSC-EVs delivered intra-articularly, significantly reduced leukocyte counts and TNF levels in the synovial fluid (198). Thus, MSC-derived exosomes could be a new strategy for the treatment of RA.

The potential use of MSC-EVs for the treatment of SLE is also being explored. In contrast to MSCs themselves, EVs are easier to characterize and store, and being acellular entities, they carry

TABLE 2 | Clinical trials for SLE therapy using MSCs.

Phase	MSC source	Patients	Outcomes	References
Case study	BM autologous	2 patients	MSCs induced T-reg cells. No effect on disease at 14-week follow-up. One patient had a renal flare.	(183)
Phase II	BM allogenic	3 patients, high activity	SLEDAI scores: substantial remissions for 2 patients and partial for the third.	(184)
Phase I/II	BM allogenic	15 refractory patients	Decrease in Anti-dsDNA levels & the SLEDAI score at 12-month follow-up. 2 patients had a renal relapse. No serious adverse events were reported.	(185)
Phase I/II	BM/UC allogeneic	404 SLE and other autoimmune patients	The 5- and 8-year survival; 90.4 and 88.9%, respectively. Rate of infections was 29.5% and serious infections was 12.9% 1.2% patients experienced malignancies. MSC transplantation-related mortality was 0.2%.	(186)
Phase II	BM/UC allogeneic	81 refractory patients	60.5% remission rate. Improvement of GFR, BILAG and SLEDAI scores during 12-month visit by MSCT. 22.4% had experienced renal flare by 12-month follow-up Total disease activity evaluated by Systemic Lupus	(187)
Phase II	UC allogeneic	81 refractory patients	Good safety profile of MSCs in SLE patients. Normal Liver and heart function. No change in peripheral blood cell counts. No rise of serum tumor markers.	(188)
Phase II	UC or BM allogenic	87 refractory patients	Half of the patients entered clinical remission at 4 years. No adverse event was observed.	(189)
Phase II	UC allogeneic	18 patients	MSCs had no apparent additional effect. One patient had leukopenia, pneumonia and another died of severe pneumonia.	(190)
Phase II	UC allogenic	16 patients, refractory or had life-threatening visceral involvement	Increase in peripheral T-reg cells, balance between Th1 and Th2 cytokines. Significant reduction in disease activity in all patients (SLEDAI score, levels of serum ANA, anti-dsDNA antibody, serum albumin, and complement C3, and renal function. No recurrence, no treatment-related deaths	(191)
Phase I/II	UC allogenic	40 patients, active SLE	SLEDAI and BILAG scores were significantly improved. Decrease of serum antinuclear and anti-double-stranded DNA antibodies 0.12% disease relapse after 6 months.	(192)
Phase II	UC allogenic	81 patients	Ongoing, NCT02633163[a]	
Phase I	UC allogenic	7 patients	Not reported yet, NCT03174587[a]	
Phase I	UC allogenic	6 patients	Not reported yet, NCT03171194[a]	
Phase I/II	Olfactory mucosa	10 patients	Ongoing, NCT04184258[a]	
Phase I	UC allogenic	10 patients	Ongoing, NCT03219801[a]	
Phase I	Amniotic fluid	16 patients	Not reported yet, NCT04318600[a]	

[a]*ClinicalTrials.gov. Available online at: http://clinicaltrials.gov/.*
BM, Bone marrow; UC, Umbilical; BILAG, British Isles Lupus Assessment Group; SLEDAI, The Systemic Lupus Erythematosus Disease Activity Index 2000.

no concerns associated with MSC tumorigenicity or the risks of immune responses (in case of allogeneic cells). The success of preclinical testing of MSC-EVs for graft-vs.-host-disease or a mouse model of acute kidney injury indicates that the use of MSC-EVs for SLE treatment may hold future promise. However, there are currently only a few preclinical studies describing the use of MSC-EVs in SLE animal models (199, 200) and none so far in human patients.

Altogether it is safe to use MSCs or their EVs in RA treatment with some encouraging response noted, more work is needed to determine optimal MSC sources, concentrations and routes of administration. Future work should also consider the choice of the intervention therapy time in relation to inflammation status and it is a challenge that needs to be addressed by having more molecular biology studies. Similarly, there is a perception that allogeneic MSCs are a potential therapeutic tool for SLE unlike autologous MSCs, which have a defective immunomodulatory function and poorly proliferative. Even with possible immunological rejection, allogeneic MSCs are the usual vehicle for putative MSC based immunomodulatory therapies. Targeting autologous MSCs for improving their function could be another option. Future studies should aim to investigate the mechanism of the functional defect of SLE MSCs. Such data will improve our understanding of the pathogenesis of SLE and could introduce new methods modifying cell therapy using autologous MSCs for SLE and other autoimmune diseases.

In addition to secretory products from viable MSCs, the apoptotic MSCs have been shown to induce immunosuppression effects. Galleu et al. showed that MSCs used to treat graft-vs.-host disease (GvHD) undergo apoptosis in a perforin-dependent mechanism by recipient cytotoxic cells, and this process is required for MSC-mediated immunosuppression (201). Interestingly, the group reported that the response of patients with GvHD to therapeutic MSCs is positively correlated with high cytotoxic activity against infused MSCs. Furthermore, it has been shown that apoptotic MSCs, which are engulfed by recipient macrophages could induce the production of IDO, thus mediating immunosuppression (201). Therefore, the infusion of apoptotic MSCs generated *ex vivo* could be an alternative concept for new MSC-based therapies of autoimmune diseases such as RA and SLE.

DISCUSSION

The use of MSCs as cell therapy for an autoimmune disorder such as RA or SLE is promising, still some aspects of treatment need consideration and further clinical testing and optimization is required (**Figure 1**). Typically, the immunosuppressive effect of licensed-MSCs is the rationale behind using them as a potential tool for treating autoimmune diseases. Uniquely, several mechanisms have been proposed for how MSCs can display immunosuppression (**Figure 2**). These mechanisms include the production of soluble factors, cell-cell interactions, extracellular vesicles, and recently described apoptosis-mediated immunosuppression. The best characteristic mechanism is secretory products followed by cell to cell mechanisms. Newly emerged EV and apoptotic MSCs are more recent though interesting mode of MSC immunosuppressive functions (36, 202). Nevertheless, combined actions of MSCs is likely but need further verification. Furthermore, the simultaneous effect of MSCs on multiple immune cells makes them suitable for use in refractory autoimmune arthritis. The safety of MSCs in human therapies has been well-demonstrated with no major toxicity. The possibility of excess immunosuppression and tumor transformation was noted in experimental models of arthritis treated with MSCs, although none was recorded in human studies (203). A milieu of chronic inflammation is associated with autoimmune diseases, and such a milieu could affect the functions of MSCs (7). Synovial MSCs in RA and SLE might directly participate in the disease progression. In active disease, these MSCs seem to have pro-inflammatory phenotype and they are not effective in controlling the exaggerated immune response. The functions of MSCs in SLE and RA could be changed due to multiple mechanisms that are known, however more studies are also needed to investigate the causes. It is important to assess the immunomodulatory functions of native MSCs to verify if the alterations of these functions are related to cellular changes, microenvironment or both. Interestingly, we have assessed by *in vitro* assay of T-cell proliferation how uncultured non-hematopoietic cells of cancellous bone can display immunosuppressive effects (33).

Different factors could affect the outcomes of MSC-based clinical trials for RA and SLE. As discussed above, the high doses, early timing and more frequency of MSCs seem to correlate positively with the therapeutic outcomes. Additionally, licensing by inflammatory milieu, particularly IFN-γ, is an important factor to consider, but this may increase regulatory issues substantially and delay or deter translational research in this area. The extraction method, accessibility and processing could be other factors affecting the choice of one type of MSCs rather than others (204). While several sources for MSCs have been utilized for clinical trials, UC-MSCs are the most frequent, followed by BM-MSCs and AD-MSCs. BM-MSCs are the best characterized MSCs and proven safe for use in the different regenerative and inflammatory application. With regards to accessibility, UC is a non-invasive source of MSCs, while harvesting BM-MSCs or AD-MSCs would require a surgical procedure, could sometimes be hard to access and cause complications (204). Additionally, MSC yield and functional potential are dependent on donor factors (e.g., age and co-morbidity) (89, 205). Several *in vitro*, preclinical and clinical studies remain inconclusive but suggest that the immunosuppressive function of UC-MSCs and AD-MSCs could be more potent than that of BM-MSCs (137, 139, 145, 206). However, the source/type of MSCs is not currently considered a factor affecting the clinical therapeutic outcomes, particularly with no clinical studies comparing the outcomes side-by-side between the different types of MSCs.

All clinical trials of using MSCs in RA or SLE employed culture-expanded MSCs as these expanded cells provide adequate quantity for multiple and high doses. However, these *ex vivo* manipulated cells would require the FDA's regulations for testing and approval of culture, expansion and treatment, which are essential to avoid any complication, e.g., infection (207). Although the processing of MSCs is a costly process with complicated steps for safety and quality control (208), this therapy still has great potential, particularly for patients with refractory diseases. The alternatives could be native or minimally manipulated MSCs. The main problem of these native uncultured MSCs is the limited numbers and variability due to donor age and health conditions (23, 209, 210). Therefore, some additional procedures were suggested to enrich the native sources of MSCs, such as BM concentration (187).

In addition to the quantity, several studies have aimed to improve the quality of therapeutic MSCs, particularly autologous cells using genetic modifications or biological stimulation. Genetically modified BM-MSCs to overexpress IL-37 showed *in vitro* suppression of splenocyte proliferation, decreasing cytokines IL-1β, TNF-α, IL-17, and IL-6 and autoantibodies leading to an improvement of SLE signs in a mouse model (211). BM-MSCs in SLE have higher expression of miR-663, which is correlated with SLE disease activity, and miR-663 inhibition was found to reduce the disease progression in SLE mouse model (194). Other examples include overexpression of miR-146a in

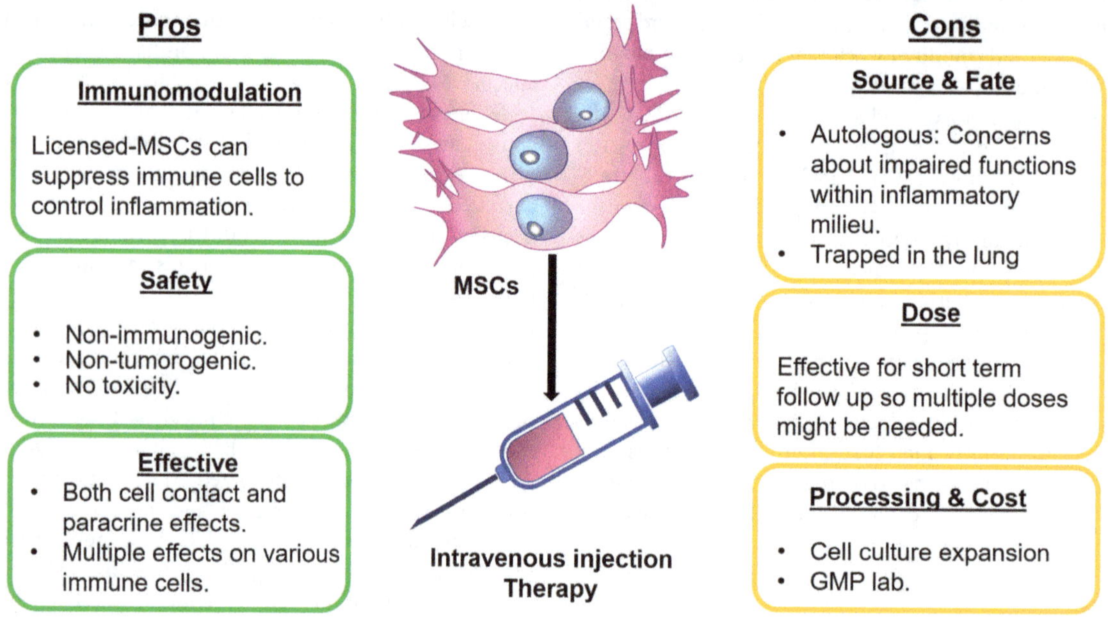

FIGURE 1 | Pros and Cons of using MSCs for RA and SLE therapies. Therapy of RA and SLE using MSCs have some advantages including the immunosuppression capacity. These cells are safe to use and having simultaneous effects on multiple immune cells and exhibition of both contact and non-contact activities. In contrast, autologous MSCs might not be effective or only effective for short term due to inflammatory milieu. Also, intravenously injected MSCs could be trapped in lungs. Additionally, this therapy usually necessitates GMP lab for expansion of MSCs in culture.

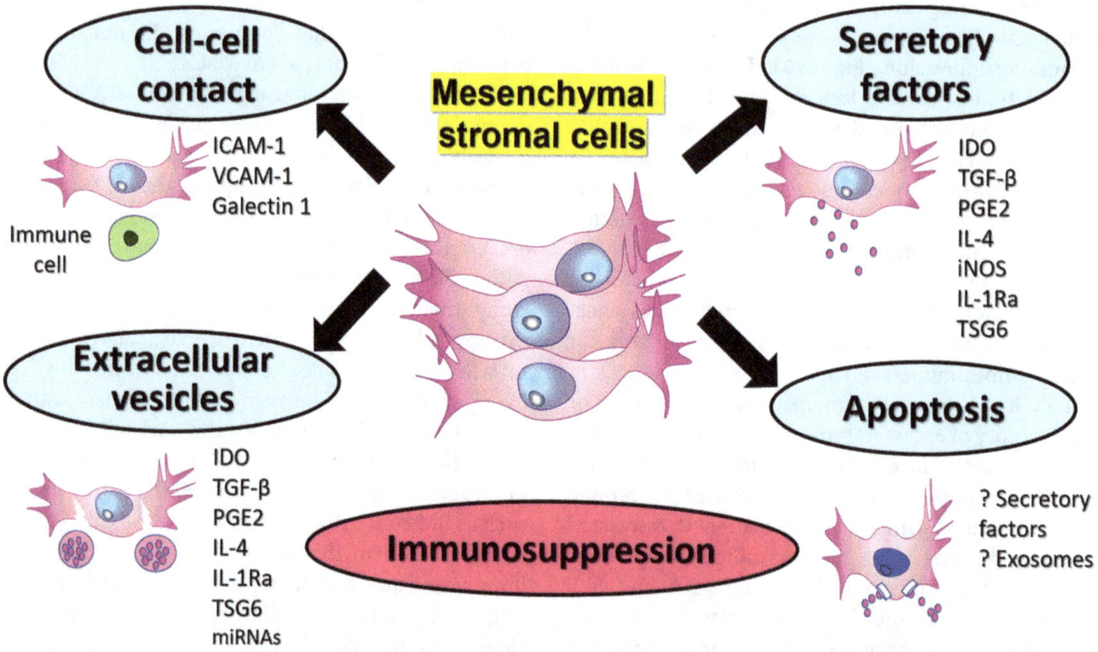

FIGURE 2 | Potential mechanisms of immunosuppression by therapeutic MSCs. Therapeutic MSCs could display immunosuppression via production of extracellular soluble factors. Cell to cell interactions between MSCs and immune cells can be mediated via surface molecules such as ICAM-1, VCAM-1, and Gelactin-1. Additionally, extracellular vesicles containing immunosuppressive factors and other proteins and miRNAs constitute another mechanism that could be used therapeutic for autoimmune diseases. Finally, apoptotic MSCs that can be engulfed by macrophages, and this could probably help to mediate immunosuppression via soluble factors or extracellular vesicles or exosomes.

MSCs that was associated with increased T-reg cells, FoxP3, TGFβ and IL-10 gene expression in CIA mice (212). Additionally, miR-320a inhibits the progression of RA and its induction in MSC exosomes or its target, CXCL9 helped to attenuate arthritis and bone destruction in CIA mouse model (213). It has also been shown that the transfection of IL-Ra gene in MSCs with long-term delivery via encapsulation in alginate-poly-L-lysine microcapsules can attenuate the inflammatory markers in CIA rat model (214). Other biological methods were proposed to augment autologous functions of MSCs. Endoplasmic Reticulum (ER)-stressed UC-MSCs further down-regulated peripheral CD4+CXCR5+ICOS+ T-lymphocytes associated with PGE2 and IL-6 increase in co-culture supernatant, suggesting that the immunosuppressive effect of MSCs could be enhanced by induction of ER stress (215). IL-4 has been shown as a potential therapeutic tool for autoimmune arthritis as its use in CIA mouse models was associated with an elevation of IL-13 levels and decreased IL-6 plasma concentrations (216). The mechanism of IL-4-linked immunosuppression is the ability to promote macrophage polarization into immunosuppressive cells via the suppression of Th1-mediated immune response as shown in proteoglycan-induced arthritis mice model (217). Similarly, IL-4 could increase MSC immunosuppressive effects by induction of T-reg cells as tested in a rat model of autoimmune colitis (218). While appear promising, genetic or other biological manipulations of RA and SLE MSCs can still carry considerable regulatory, ethical or safety concerns which may overweigh their therapeutic value.

The fate of infused MSCs is an interesting topic of cell-based therapeutic research. A model was proposed for a multistage process when MSCs enter the bloodstream as tethering and rolling, activation, arrest, diapedesis, and migration (219). Furthermore, preclinical studies demonstrated the presence of MSCs in inflamed tissues, and these MSCs able to induce different immunosuppressive, angiogenic, and anti-apoptotic effects (220, 221). Still, some challenges have been reported for intravenous infusion of MSCs. The systemic infusion of MSCs induces the expression of procoagulants like tissue factor (TF) on the surface of MSCs inducing instant blood-mediated inflammatory reaction (IBMIR) and complement activation. These reactions could induce cytotoxicity of infused MSCs (222, 223). Additionally, strong evidence showed that systematically injected MSCs are mostly trapped in the lungs, and few of these cells could circulate and reach the target site (224). Several methods have been suggested to overcome this issue by enhancing the migration of MSCs, modulating MSC surface markers or use of 3D cultures (225), but the secretory functions of MSCs might still be adequate. Interestingly, the death or trapping of therapeutic MSCs might still be advantageous as dead and apoptotic MSCs have been shown to have a potential immunomodulatory function (202). These apoptotic MSCs could induce IDO production by phagocytes helping immunosuppression (201), but it would be interesting to investigate further how apoptotic MSCs could control immune responses and how to exploit these cells for optimum therapies.

Overall, the legitimacy of MSC therapies for RA and SLE is currently increasing with various options for using different MSC types and administration approaches. However, future studies should focus on understanding why intrinsic/*in vivo* MSCs fail to function properly in autoimmune joint diseases, and how MSCs are being affected by chronic inflammatory milieu (226). These investigations would potentially help to introduce new therapeutic targets helping to correct the autoimmune reactions. MSC-based therapy in autoimmune joint disease could be further validated by having phase 3 clinical trials with large patient cohorts. More clinical studies are needed to directly compare the source and type of MSCs. While donor age appeared not affecting MSC functions (205), other factors such as the donor's disease, MSC culture conditions and mode of application should be also investigated for effect on autoimmune arthritis therapy.

AUTHOR CONTRIBUTIONS

JJE-J wrote the main parts of the first draft of the manuscript, prepared the figure, and updated all subsequent manuscript versions. YE-S helped with draft preparation and the tables. DM contributed to draft preparation and feedback on parts related to clinical aspects. EJ contributed into the draft preparation, provided the feedback on all sections, and wrote some parts related to exosome therapies. All authors contributed toward the design of the review, planning the sections, reviewed and made changes on the final draft, and agreed about the content.

REFERENCES

1. Dominici M, Le Blanc K, Mueller I, Slaper-Cortenbach I, Marini F, Krause D, et al. Minimal criteria for defining multipotent mesenchymal stromal cells. The International society for cellular therapy position statement. *Cytotherapy.* (2006) 8:315–7. doi: 10.1080/14653240600855905
2. Caplan AI. Mesenchymal stem cells: time to change the name! *Stem Cells Transl Med.* (2017) 6:1445–51. doi: 10.1002/sctm.17-0051
3. Wang Y, Chen X, Cao W, Shi Y. Plasticity of mesenchymal stem cells in immunomodulation: pathological and therapeutic implications. *Nat Immunol.* (2014) 15:1009–16. doi: 10.1038/ni.3002
4. El-Jawhari JJ, El-Sherbiny YM, Jones EA, McGonagle D. Mesenchymal stem cells, autoimmunity and rheumatoid arthritis. *QJM.* (2014) 107:505–14. doi: 10.1093/qjmed/hcu033
5. Gao F, Chiu SM, Motan DA, Zhang Z, Chen L, Ji HL, et al. Mesenchymal stem cells and immunomodulation: current status and future prospects. *Cell Death Dis.* (2016) 7:e2062. doi: 10.1038/cddis.2015.327
6. El-Zayadi AA, Jones EA, Churchman SM, Baboolal TG, Cuthbert RJ, El-Jawhari JJ, et al. IL-22 drives the proliferation, migration and osteogenic differentiation of human bone marrow mesenchymal stem cells (MSCs): A novel cytokine that may contribute to aberrant new bone formation in human SpA. *Rheumatology.* (2016) 56:488–93. doi: 10.1093/rheumatology/kew384
7. El-Jawhari JJ, Jones E, Giannoudis PV. The roles of immune cells in bone healing; what we know, do not know and future perspectives. *Injury.* (2016) 47:2399–406. doi: 10.1016/j.injury.2016.10.008
8. De Bari C, Dell'Accio F, Tylzanowski P, Luyten FP. Multipotent mesenchymal stem cells from adult human synovial membrane. *Arthritis Rheum.* (2001)

44:1928–42. doi: 10.1002/1529-0131(200108)44:8<1928::AID-ART331>3.0.CO;2-P

9. Karystinou A, Dell'Accio F, Kurth TB, Wackerhage H, Khan IM, Archer CW, et al. Distinct mesenchymal progenitor cell subsets in the adult human synovium. *Rheumatology.* (2009) 48:1057–64. doi: 10.1093/rheumatology/kep192
10. Li F, Tang Y, Song B, Yu M, Li Q, Zhang C, et al. Nomenclature clarification: synovial fibroblasts and synovial mesenchymal stem cells. *Stem Cell Res Ther.* (2019) 10:260. doi: 10.1186/s13287-019-1359-x
11. Sakaguchi Y, Sekiya I, Yagishita K, Muneta T. Comparison of human stem cells derived from various mesenchymal tissues: superiority of synovium as a cell source. *Arthritis Rheumatism.* (2005) 52:2521–9. doi: 10.1002/art.21212
12. Soundararajan M, Kannan S. Fibroblasts and mesenchymal stem cells: two sides of the same coin? *J Cell Physiol.* (2018) 233:9099–109. doi: 10.1002/jcp.26860
13. De Bari C. Are mesenchymal stem cells in rheumatoid arthritis the good or bad guys? *Arthritis Res Therapy.* (2015) 17:113. doi: 10.1186/s13075-015-0634-1
14. McGonagle D, McDermott MF. A proposed classification of the immunological diseases. *PLoS Med.* (2006) 3:e297. doi: 10.1371/journal.pmed.0030297
15. Hwang J, Lee J, Ahn JK, Park EJ, Cha HS, Koh EM. Clinical characteristics of male and female Korean patients with systemic lupus erythematosus: a comparative study. *Korean J Internal Med.* (2015) 30:242–9. doi: 10.3904/kjim.2015.30.2.242
16. Gyori N, Giannakou I, Chatzidionysiou K, Magder L, van Vollenhoven RF, Petri M. Disease activity patterns over time in patients with SLE: analysis of the Hopkins Lupus Cohort. *Lupus Sci Med.* (2017) 4:e000192. doi: 10.1136/lupus-2016-000192
17. Viatte S, Barton A. Genetics of rheumatoid arthritis susceptibility, severity, and treatment response. *Semin Immunopathol.* (2017) 39:395–408. doi: 10.1007/s00281-017-0630-4
18. Marion TN, Postlethwaite AE. Chance, genetics, and the heterogeneity of disease and pathogenesis in systemic lupus erythematosus. *Semin Immunopathol.* (2014) 36:495–517. doi: 10.1007/s00281-014-0440-x
19. McGonagle D, Watad A, Savic S. Mechanistic immunological based classification of rheumatoid arthritis. *Autoimmun Rev.* (2018) 17:1115–23. doi: 10.1016/j.autrev.2018.06.001
20. Tselios K, Sarantopoulos A, Gkougkourelas I, Boura P. CD4+CD25highFOXP3+ T regulatory cells as a biomarker of disease activity in systemic lupus erythematosus: a prospective study. *Clin Exp Rheumatol.* (2014) 32:630–9. doi: 10.1136/annrheumdis-2013-eular.1407
21. Zhang X, Zhang X, Zhuang L, Xu C, Li T, Zhang G, et al. Decreased regulatory T-cell frequency and interleukin-35 levels in patients with rheumatoid arthritis. *Experi Therap Med.* (2018) 16:5366–72. doi: 10.3892/etm.2018.6885
22. Friedenstein AJ, Chailakhjan RK, Lalykina KS. The development of fibroblast colonies in monolayer cultures of guinea-pig bone marrow and spleen cells. *Cell Tissue Kinet.* (1970) 3:393–403. doi: 10.1111/j.1365-2184.1970.tb00347.x
23. Cuthbert R, Boxall SA, Tan HB, Giannoudis PV, McGonagle D, Jones E. Single-platform quality control assay to quantify multipotential stromal cells in bone marrow aspirates prior to bulk manufacture or direct therapeutic use. *Cytotherapy.* (2012) 14:431–40. doi: 10.3109/14653249.2011.651533
24. Schett G, Gravallese E. Bone erosion in rheumatoid arthritis: mechanisms, diagnosis and treatment. *Nat Rev Rheumatol.* (2012) 8:656–64. doi: 10.1038/nrrheum.2012.153
25. Jones EA, English A, Henshaw K, Kinsey SE, Markham AF, Emery P, et al. Enumeration and phenotypic characterization of synovial fluid multipotential mesenchymal progenitor cells in inflammatory and degenerative arthritis. *Arthritis Rheumatism.* (2004) 50:817–27. doi: 10.1002/art.20203
26. Nakagawa S, Toritsuka Y, Wakitani S, Denno K, Tomita T, Owaki H, et al. Bone marrow stromal cells contribute to synovial cell proliferation in rats with collagen induced arthritis. *J Rheumatol.* (1996) 23:2098–103.
27. Sergijenko A, Roelofs AJ, Riemen AH, De Bari C. Bone marrow contribution to synovial hyperplasia following joint surface injury. *Arthritis Res Therapy.* (2016) 18:166. doi: 10.1186/s13075-016-1060-8
28. Koelling S, Kruegel J, Irmer M, Path JR, Sadowski B, Miro X, et al. Migratory chondrogenic progenitor cells from repair tissue during the later stages of human osteoarthritis. *Cell Stem Cell.* (2009) 4:324–35. doi: 10.1016/j.stem.2009.01.015
29. Sanjurjo-Rodriguez C, Baboolal TG, Burska AN, Ponchel F, El-Jawhari JJ, Pandit H, et al. Gene expression and functional comparison between multipotential stromal cells from lateral and medial condyles of knee osteoarthritis patients. *Sci Rep.* (2019) 9:9321. doi: 10.1038/s41598-019-45820-w
30. Benjamin M, Toumi H, Suzuki D, Redman S, Emery P, McGonagle D. Microdamage and altered vascularity at the enthesis-bone interface provides an anatomic explanation for bone involvement in the HLA-B27-associated spondylarthritides and allied disorders. *Arthritis Rheumatism.* (2007) 56:224–33. doi: 10.1002/art.22290
31. Wang M, Yuan Q, Xie L. Mesenchymal stem cell-based immunomodulation: properties and clinical application. *Stem Cells Int.* (2018) 2018:3057624. doi: 10.1155/2018/3057624
32. Wang LT, Ting CH, Yen ML, Liu KJ, Sytwu HK, Wu KK, et al. Human mesenchymal stem cells (MSCs) for treatment towards immune- and inflammation-mediated diseases: review of current clinical trials. *J Biomed Sci.* (2016) 23:76. doi: 10.1186/s12929-016-0289-5
33. El-Sherbiny YM, El-Jawhari JJ, Moseley TA, McGonagle D, Jones E. T cell immunomodulation by clinically used allogeneic human cancellous bone fragments: a potential novel immunotherapy tool. *Sci Rep.* (2018) 8:13535. doi: 10.1038/s41598-018-31979-1
34. Pohlers D, Beyer A, Koczan D, Wilhelm T, Thiesen HJ, Kinne RW. Constitutive upregulation of the transforming growth factor-beta pathway in rheumatoid arthritis synovial fibroblasts. *Arthritis Res Ther.* (2007) 9:R59. doi: 10.1186/ar2217
35. Marigo I, Dazzi F. The immunomodulatory properties of mesenchymal stem cells. *Semin Immunopathol.* (2011) 33:593–602. doi: 10.1007/s00281-011-0267-7
36. Siegel G, Schafer R, Dazzi F. The immunosuppressive properties of mesenchymal stem cells. *Transplantation.* (2009) 87(Suppl. 9):S45–9. doi: 10.1097/TP.0b013e3181a285b0
37. Le Blanc K, Ringden O. Immunomodulation by mesenchymal stem cells and clinical experience. *J Intern Med.* (2007) 262:509–25. doi: 10.1111/j.1365-2796.2007.01844.x
38. Khan IM, Bishop JC, Gilbert S, Archer CW. Clonal chondroprogenitors maintain telomerase activity and Sox9 expression during extended monolayer culture and retain chondrogenic potential. *Osteoarthritis Cartilage.* (2009) 17:518–28. doi: 10.1016/j.joca.2008.08.002
39. Haniffa MA, Wang XN, Holtick U, Rae M, Isaacs JD, Dickinson AM, et al. Adult human fibroblasts are potent immunoregulatory cells and functionally equivalent to mesenchymal stem cells. *J Immunol.* (2007) 179:1595–604. doi: 10.4049/jimmunol.179.3.1595
40. Croft AP, Campos J, Jansen K, Turner JD, Marshall J, Attar M, et al. Distinct fibroblast subsets drive inflammation and damage in arthritis. *Nature.* (2019) 570:246–51. doi: 10.1038/s41586-019-1263-7
41. Hu CD, Kosaka Y, Marcus P, Rashedi I, Keating A. Differential immunomodulatory effects of human bone marrow-derived mesenchymal stromal cells on natural killer cells. *Stem Cells Dev.* (2019) 28:933–43. doi: 10.1089/scd.2019.0059
42. Jiang D, Muschhammer J, Qi Y, Kugler A, de Vries JC, Saffarzadeh M, et al. Suppression of neutrophil-mediated tissue damage-a novel skill of mesenchymal stem cells. *Stem Cells.* (2016) 34:2393–406. doi: 10.1002/stem.2417
43. Ren G, Zhao X, Zhang L, Zhang J, L'Huillier A, Ling W, et al. Inflammatory cytokine-induced intercellular adhesion molecule-1 and vascular cell adhesion molecule-1 in mesenchymal stem cells are critical for immunosuppression. *J Immunol.* (2010) 184:2321–8. doi: 10.4049/jimmunol.0902023
44. Del Papa B, Sportoletti P, Cecchini D, Rosati E, Balucani C, Baldoni S, et al. Notch1 modulates mesenchymal stem cells mediated regulatory T-cell induction. *Eur J Immunol.* (2013) 43:182–7. doi: 10.1002/eji.201242643
45. Gieseke F, Bohringer J, Bussolari R, Dominici M, Handgretinger R, Muller I. Human multipotent mesenchymal stromal cells

use galectin-1 to inhibit immune effector cells. *Blood.* (2010) 116:3770–9. doi: 10.1182/blood-2010-02-270777

46. Franquesa M, Mensah FK, Huizinga R, Strini T, Boon L, Lombardo E, et al. Human adipose tissue-derived mesenchymal stem cells abrogate plasmablast formation and induce regulatory B cells independently of T helper cells. *Stem Cells.* (2015) 33:880–91. doi: 10.1002/stem.1881
47. Tabera S, Perez-Simon JA, Diez-Campelo M, Sanchez-Abarca LI, Blanco B, Lopez A, et al. The effect of mesenchymal stem cells on the viability, proliferation and differentiation of B-lymphocytes. *Haematologica.* (2008) 93:1301–9. doi: 10.3324/haematol.12857
48. Cappellesso-Fleury S, Puissant-Lubrano B, Apoil PA, Titeux M, Winterton P, Casteilla L, et al. Human fibroblasts share immunosuppressive properties with bone marrow mesenchymal stem cells. *J Clin Immunol.* (2010) 30:607–19. doi: 10.1007/s10875-010-9415-4
49. Churchman SM, Jones EA, Roshdy T, Cox G, Boxall SA, McGonagle D, et al. Transient existence of circulating mesenchymal stem cells in the deep veins in humans following long bone intramedullary reaming. *J Clin Med.* (2020) 9:968. doi: 10.3390/jcm9040968
50. Bottini N, Firestein GS. Duality of fibroblast-like synoviocytes in RA: passive responders and imprinted aggressors. *Nat Rev Rheumatol.* (2013) 9:24–33. doi: 10.1038/nrrheum.2012.190
51. Kim YS, Lee HJ, Yeo JE, Kim YI, Choi YJ, Koh YG. Isolation and characterization of human mesenchymal stem cells derived from synovial fluid in patients with osteochondral lesion of the talus. *Am J Sports Med.* (2015) 43:399–406. doi: 10.1177/0363546514559822
52. Djouad F, Fritz V, Apparailly F, Louis-Plence P, Bony C, Sany J, et al. Reversal of the immunosuppressive properties of mesenchymal stem cells by tumor necrosis factor alpha in collagen-induced arthritis. *Arthritis Rheumatism.* (2005) 52:1595–603. doi: 10.1002/art.21012
53. Sun Y, Deng W, Yao G, Chen W, Tang X, Feng X, et al. Citrullinated fibrinogen impairs immunomodulatory function of bone marrow mesenchymal stem cells by triggering toll-like receptor. *Clin Immunol.* (2018) 193:38–45. doi: 10.1016/j.clim.2018.01.008
54. Waterman RS, Tomchuck SL, Henkle SL, Betancourt AM. A new mesenchymal stem cell (MSC) paradigm: polarization into a pro-inflammatory MSC1 or an Immunosuppressive MSC2 phenotype. *PLoS ONE.* (2010) 5:e10088. doi: 10.1371/journal.pone.0010088
55. Opitz CA, Litzenburger UM, Lutz C, Lanz TV, Tritschler I, Koppel A, et al. Toll-like receptor engagement enhances the immunosuppressive properties of human bone marrow-derived mesenchymal stem cells by inducing indoleamine-2,3-dioxygenase-1 via interferon-beta and protein kinase R. *Stem Cells.* (2009) 27:909–19. doi: 10.1002/stem.7
56. Feng Z, Zhai Y, Zheng Z, Yang L, Luo X, Dong X, et al. Loss of A20 in BM-MSCs regulates the Th17/Treg balance in rheumatoid arthritis. *Sci Rep.* (2018) 8:427. doi: 10.1038/s41598-017-18693-0
57. Priem D, Devos M, Druwe S, Martens A, Slowicka K, Ting AT, et al. A20 protects cells from TNF-induced apoptosis through linear ubiquitin-dependent and -independent mechanisms. *Cell Death Dis.* (2019) 10:692. doi: 10.1038/s41419-019-1937-y
58. Wang D, Feng X, Lu L, Konkel JE, Zhang H, Chen Z, et al. A CD8 T cell/indoleamine 2,3-dioxygenase axis is required for mesenchymal stem cell suppression of human systemic lupus erythematosus. *Arthritis Rheumatol.* (2014) 66:2234–45. doi: 10.1002/art.38674
59. Gu Z, Tan W, Feng G, Meng Y, Shen B, Liu H, et al. Wnt/beta-catenin signaling mediates the senescence of bone marrow-mesenchymal stem cells from systemic lupus erythematosus patients through the p53/p21 pathway. *Mol Cell Biochem.* (2014) 387:27–37. doi: 10.1007/s11010-013-1866-5
60. Chen H, Shi B, Feng X, Kong W, Chen W, Geng L, et al. Leptin and neutrophil-activating peptide 2 promote mesenchymal stem cell senescence through activation of the phosphatidylinositol 3-Kinase/Akt pathway in patients with systemic lupus erythematosus. *Arthritis Rheumatol.* (2015) 67:2383–93. doi: 10.1002/art.39196
61. Tan W, Gu Z, Shen B, Jiang J, Meng Y, Da Z, et al. PTEN/Akt-p27(kip1) signaling promote the BM-MSCs senescence and apoptosis in SLE patients. *J Cell Biochem.* (2015) 116:1583–94. doi: 10.1002/jcb.25112
62. Gu Z, Meng Y, Tao T, Guo G, Tan W, Xia Y, et al. Endoplasmic reticulum stress participates in the progress of senescence of bone marrow-derived mesenchymal stem cells in patients with systemic lupus erythematosus. *Cell Tissue Res.* (2015) 361:497–508. doi: 10.1007/s00441-015-2131-x
63. Nie Y, Lau C, Lie A, Chan G, Mok M. Defective phenotype of mesenchymal stem cells in patients with systemic lupus erythematosus. *Lupus.* (2010) 19:850–9. doi: 10.1177/0961203310361482
64. Gao L, Bird AK, Meednu N, Dauenhauer K, Liesveld J, Anolik J, et al. Bone marrow-derived mesenchymal stem cells from patients with systemic lupus erythematosus have a senescence-associated secretory phenotype mediated by a mitochondrial antiviral signaling protein-interferon-beta feedback loop. *Arthritis Rheumatol.* (2017) 69:1623–35. doi: 10.1002/art.40142
65. Shi D, Li X, Chen H, Che N, Zhou S, Lu Z, et al. High level of reactive oxygen species impaired mesenchymal stem cell migration via overpolymerization of F-actin cytoskeleton in systemic lupus erythematosus. *Pathol Biol.* (2014) 62:382–90. doi: 10.1016/j.patbio.2014.07.009
66. Moiseeva O, Mallette FA, Mukhopadhyay UK, Moores A, Ferbeyre G. DNA damage signaling and p53-dependent senescence after prolonged beta-interferon stimulation. *Mol Biol Cell.* (2006) 17:1583–92. doi: 10.1091/mbc.e05-09-0858
67. Li X, Liu L, Meng D, Wang D, Zhang J, Shi D, et al. Enhanced apoptosis and senescence of bone-marrow-derived mesenchymal stem cells in patients with systemic lupus erythematosus. *Stem Cells Dev.* (2012) 21:2387–94. doi: 10.1089/scd.2011.0447
68. Sun LY, Zhang HY, Feng XB, Hou YY, Lu LW, Fan LM. Abnormality of bone marrow-derived mesenchymal stem cells in patients with systemic lupus erythematosus. *Lupus.* (2007) 16:121–8. doi: 10.1177/0961203306075793
69. Djouad F, Charbonnier LM, Bouffi C, Louis-Plence P, Bony C, Apparailly F, et al. Mesenchymal stem cells inhibit the differentiation of dendritic cells through an interleukin-6-dependent mechanism. *Stem Cells.* (2007) 25:2025–32. doi: 10.1634/stemcells.2006-0548
70. Liu Y, Yin Z, Zhang R, Yan K, Chen L, Chen F, et al. MSCs inhibit bone marrow-derived DC maturation and function through the release of TSG-6. *Biochem Biophys Res Commun.* (2014) 450:1409–15. doi: 10.1016/j.bbrc.2014.07.001
71. Spaggiari GM, Abdelrazik H, Becchetti F, Moretta L. MSCs inhibit monocyte-derived DC maturation and function by selectively interfering with the generation of immature DCs: central role of MSC-derived prostaglandin E2. *Blood.* (2009) 113:6576–83. doi: 10.1182/blood-2009-02-203943
72. Cahill EF, Tobin LM, Carty F, Mahon BP, English K. Jagged-1 is required for the expansion of CD4+ CD25+ FoxP3+ regulatory T cells and tolerogenic dendritic cells by murine mesenchymal stromal cells. *Stem Cell Res Ther.* (2015) 6:19. doi: 10.1186/s13287-015-0021-5
73. Kikodze N, Pantsulaia I, Chikovani T. The role of T regulatory and Th17 cells in the pathogenesis of rheumatoid arthritis (Review). *Georgian Med News.* (2016) 261:62–8.
74. Jiang XX, Zhang Y, Liu B, Zhang SX, Wu Y, Yu XD, et al. Human mesenchymal stem cells inhibit differentiation and function of monocyte-derived dendritic cells. *Blood.* (2005) 105:4120–6. doi: 10.1182/blood-2004-02-0586
75. Yen BL, Yen ML, Hsu PJ, Liu KJ, Wang CJ, Bai CH, et al. Multipotent human mesenchymal stromal cells mediate expansion of myeloid-derived suppressor cells via hepatocyte growth factor/c-met and STAT3. *Stem Cell Rep.* (2013) 1:139–51. doi: 10.1016/j.stemcr.2013.06.006
76. Wang J, De Veirman K, De Beule N, Maes K, De Bruyne E, Van Valckenborgh E, et al. The bone marrow microenvironment enhances multiple myeloma progression by exosome-mediated activation of myeloid-derived suppressor cells. *Oncotarget.* (2015) 6:43992–4004. doi: 10.18632/oncotarget.6083
77. Wehr P, Purvis H, Law SC, Thomas R. Dendritic cells, T cells and their interaction in rheumatoid arthritis. *Clin Experi Immunol.* (2019) 196:12–27. doi: 10.1111/cei.13256
78. Tran CN, Davis MJ, Tesmer LA, Endres JL, Motyl CD, Smuda C, et al. Presentation of arthritogenic peptide to antigen-specific T cells by fibroblast-like synoviocytes. *Arthritis Rheum.* (2007) 56:1497–506. doi: 10.1002/art.22573
79. Vallejo AN, Yang H, Klimiuk PA, Weyand CM, Goronzy JJ. Synoviocyte-mediated expansion of inflammatory T cells in rheumatoid synovitis is dependent on CD47-thrombospondin 1 interaction. *J Immunol.* (2003) 171:1732–40. doi: 10.4049/jimmunol.171.4.1732

80. Huang QQ, Pope RM. The role of toll-like receptors in rheumatoid arthritis. *Curr Rheumat Rep.* (2009) 11:357–64. doi: 10.1007/s11926-009-0051-z
81. Radstake TR, Roelofs MF, Jenniskens YM, Oppers-Walgreen B, van Riel PL, Barrera P, et al. Expression of toll-like receptors 2 and 4 in rheumatoid synovial tissue and regulation by proinflammatory cytokines interleukin-12 and interleukin-18 via interferon-gamma. *Arthritis Rheum.* (2004) 50:3856–65. doi: 10.1002/art.20678
82. Roelofs MF, Boelens WC, Joosten LA, Abdollahi-Roodsaz S, Geurts J, Wunderink LU, et al. Identification of small heat shock protein B8 (HSP22) as a novel TLR4 ligand and potential involvement in the pathogenesis of rheumatoid arthritis. *J Immunol.* (2006) 176:7021–7. doi: 10.4049/jimmunol.176.11.7021
83. Schaefer L, Babelova A, Kiss E, Hausser HJ, Baliova M, Krzyzankova M, et al. The matrix component biglycan is proinflammatory and signals through Toll-like receptors 4 and 2 in macrophages. *J Clin Invest.* (2005) 115:2223–33. doi: 10.1172/JCI23755
84. Swiecki M, Colonna M. The multifaceted biology of plasmacytoid dendritic cells. *Nat Rev Immunol.* (2015) 15:471–85. doi: 10.1038/nri3865
85. Menon M, Blair PA, Isenberg DA, Mauri C. A regulatory feedback between plasmacytoid dendritic cells and regulatory B cells is aberrant in systemic lupus erythematosus. *Immunity.* (2016) 44:683–97. doi: 10.1016/j.immuni.2016.02.012
86. Vital EM, Dass S, Buch MH, Henshaw K, Pease CT, Martin MF, et al. B cell biomarkers of rituximab responses in systemic lupus erythematosus. *Arthritis Rheumatism.* (2011) 63:3038–47. doi: 10.1002/art.30466
87. El-Sherbiny YM, Md Yusof MY, Psarras A, Hensor EMA, Kabba KZ, Dutton K, et al. B cell tetherin: a flow cytometric cell-specific assay for response to type I interferon predicts clinical features and flares in systemic lupus erythematosus. *Arthritis Rheumatol.* (2020) 72:769–79. doi: 10.1002/art.41187
88. Yan B, Ye S, Chen G, Kuang M, Shen N, Chen S. Dysfunctional CD4+,CD25+ regulatory T cells in untreated active systemic lupus erythematosus secondary to interferon-alpha-producing antigen-presenting cells. *Arthritis Rheumatism.* (2008) 58:801–12. doi: 10.1002/art.23268
89. Ganguly P, Burska AN, Davis CLM, El-Jawhari JJ, Giannoudis PV, Jones EA. Intrinsic Type 1 Interferon (IFN1) profile of uncultured human bone marrow CD45(low)CD271(+) multipotential stromal cells (BM-MSCs): the impact of donor age, culture expansion and IFNalpha and IFNbeta stimulation. *Biomedicines.* (2020) 8:214. doi: 10.3390/biomedicines8070214
90. Peiffer I, Eid P, Barbet R, Li ML, Oostendorp RA, Haydont V, et al. A sub-population of high proliferative potential-quiescent human mesenchymal stem cells is under the reversible control of interferon alpha/beta. *Leukemia.* (2007) 21:714–24. doi: 10.1038/sj.leu.2404765
91. Oreffo RO, Romberg S, Virdi AS, Joyner CJ, Berven S, Triffitt JT. Effects of interferon alpha on human osteoprogenitor cell growth and differentiation *in vitro. J Cell Biochem.* (1999) 74:372–85 doi: 10.1002/(SICI)1097-4644(19990901)74:3<372::AID-JCB6>3.0.CO;2-H
92. Guihard P, Danger Y, Brounais B, David E, Brion R, Delecrin J, et al. Induction of osteogenesis in mesenchymal stem cells by activated monocytes/macrophages depends on oncostatin M signaling. *Stem Cells.* (2012) 30:762–72. doi: 10.1002/stem.1040
93. Oshita K, Yamaoka K, Udagawa N, Fukuyo S, Sonomoto K, Maeshima K, et al. Human mesenchymal stem cells inhibit osteoclastogenesis through osteoprotegerin production. *Arthritis Rheumatism.* (2011) 63:1658–67. doi: 10.1002/art.30309
94. Pajarinen J, Lin T, Gibon E, Kohno Y, Maruyama M, Nathan K, et al. Mesenchymal stem cell-macrophage crosstalk and bone healing. *Biomaterials.* (2019) 196:80–9. doi: 10.1016/j.biomaterials.2017.12.025
95. Vasandan AB, Jahnavi S, Shashank C, Prasad P, Kumar A, Prasanna SJ. Human Mesenchymal stem cells program macrophage plasticity by altering their metabolic status via a PGE2-dependent mechanism. *Sci Rep.* (2016) 6:38308. doi: 10.1038/srep38308
96. Kim J, Hematti P. Mesenchymal stem cell-educated macrophages: a novel type of alternatively activated macrophages. *Experi Hematol.* (2009) 37:1445–53. doi: 10.1016/j.exphem.2009.09.004
97. Kinne RW, Brauer R, Stuhlmuller B, Palombo-Kinne E, Burmester GR. Macrophages in rheumatoid arthritis. *Arthritis Res.* (2000) 2:189–202. doi: 10.1186/ar86
98. Alvaro-Gracia JM, Zvaifler NJ, Firestein GS. Cytokines in chronic inflammatory arthritis. IV. Granulocyte/macrophage colony-stimulating factor-mediated induction of class II MHC antigen on human monocytes: a possible role in rheumatoid arthritis. *J Exp Med.* (1989) 170:865–75. doi: 10.1084/jem.170.3.865
99. Udagawa N, Takahashi N, Akatsu T, Tanaka H, Sasaki T, Nishihara T, et al. Origin of osteoclasts: mature monocytes and macrophages are capable of differentiating into osteoclasts under a suitable microenvironment prepared by bone marrow-derived stromal cells. *Proc Natl Acad Sci USA.* (1990) 87:7260–4. doi: 10.1073/pnas.87.18.7260
100. Mbalaviele G, Jaiswal N, Meng A, Cheng L, Van Den Bos C, Thiede M. Human mesenchymal stem cells promote human osteoclast differentiation from CD34+ bone marrow hematopoietic progenitors. *Endocrinology.* (1999) 140:3736–43. doi: 10.1210/endo.140.8.6880
101. Dreier R, Wallace S, Fuchs S, Bruckner P, Grassel S. Paracrine interactions of chondrocytes and macrophages in cartilage degradation: articular chondrocytes provide factors that activate macrophage-derived pro-gelatinase B (pro-MMP-9). *J Cell Sci.* (2001) 114:3813–22.
102. Lam J, Takeshita S, Barker JE, Kanagawa O, Ross FP, Teitelbaum SL. TNF-alpha induces osteoclastogenesis by direct stimulation of macrophages exposed to permissive levels of RANK ligand. *J Clin Investig.* (2000) 106:1481–8. doi: 10.1172/JCI11176
103. Gilbert L, He X, Farmer P, Boden S, Kozlowski M, Rubin J, et al. Inhibition of osteoblast differentiation by tumor necrosis factor-alpha. *Endocrinology.* (2000) 141:3956–64. doi: 10.1210/endo.141.11.7739
104. Kitaura H, Zhou P, Kim HJ, Novack DV, Ross FP, Teitelbaum SL. M-CSF mediates TNF-induced inflammatory osteolysis. *J Clin Investig.* (2005) 115:3418–27. doi: 10.1172/JCI26132
105. Aizawa T, Kon T, Einhorn TA, Gerstenfeld LC. Induction of apoptosis in chondrocytes by tumor necrosis factor-alpha. *J Orthopaedic Res.* (2001) 19:785–96. doi: 10.1016/S0736-0266(00)00078-4
106. Lehmann W, Edgar CM, Wang K, Cho TJ, Barnes GL, Kakar S, et al. Tumor necrosis factor alpha (TNF-alpha) coordinately regulates the expression of specific matrix metalloproteinases (MMPS) and angiogenic factors during fracture healing. *Bone.* (2005) 36:300–10. doi: 10.1016/j.bone.2004.10.010
107. Haasters F, Prall WC, Westphal I, Bocker W, Padula D, Mutschler W, et al. Overexpression of dnIKK in mesenchymal stem cells leads to increased migration and decreased invasion upon TNFalpha stimulation. *Biochem Biophys Res Commun.* (2013) 436:265–70. doi: 10.1016/j.bbrc.2013.05.091
108. Liu Y, Wang L, Kikuiri T, Akiyama K, Chen C, Xu X, et al. Mesenchymal stem cell-based tissue regeneration is governed by recipient T lymphocytes via IFN-gamma and TNF-alpha. *Nat Med.* (2011) 17:1594–601. doi: 10.1038/nm.2542
109. Sato K, Suematsu A, Okamoto K, Yamaguchi A, Morishita Y, Kadono Y, et al. Th17 functions as an osteoclastogenic helper T cell subset that links T cell activation and bone destruction. *J Experi Med.* (2006) 203:2673–82. doi: 10.1084/jem.20061775
110. Kondo M, Yamaoka K, Sonomoto K, Fukuyo S, Oshita K, Okada Y, et al. IL-17 inhibits chondrogenic differentiation of human mesenchymal stem cells. *PLoS ONE.* (2013) 8:e79463. doi: 10.1371/journal.pone.0079463
111. Cupedo T, Crellin NK, Papazian N, Rombouts EJ, Weijer K, Grogan JL, et al. Human fetal lymphoid tissue-inducer cells are interleukin 17-producing precursors to RORC+ CD127+ natural killer-like cells. *Nat Immunol.* (2009) 10:66–74. doi: 10.1038/ni.1668
112. Djouad F, Bony C, Haupl T, Uze G, Lahlou N, Louis-Plence P, et al. Transcriptional profiles discriminate bone marrow-derived and synovium-derived mesenchymal stem cells. *Arthritis Res Ther.* (2005) 7:R1304–15. doi: 10.1186/ar1827
113. Hagmann S, Gotterbarm T, Muller T, Baesig AM, Gantz S, Dreher T, et al. The influence of bone marrow and synovium derived mesenchymal stromal cells from osteoarthritis patients on regulatory T-cells in coculture. *Clin Exp Immunol.* (2013) 173:454–62. doi: 10.1111/cei.12122
114. Pedrosa M, Gomes J, Laranjeira P, Duarte C, Pedreiro S, Antunes B, et al. Immunomodulatory effect of human bone marrow-derived mesenchymal

stromal/stem cells on peripheral blood T cells from rheumatoid arthritis patients. *J Tissue Eng Regen Med.* (2020) 14:16–28. doi: 10.1002/term.2958
115. Sun Y, Deng W, Geng L, Zhang L, Liu R, Chen W, et al. Mesenchymal stem cells from patients with rheumatoid arthritis display impaired function in inhibiting Th17 cells. *J Immunol Res.* (2015) 2015:284215. doi: 10.1155/2015/284215
116. Bradfield PF, Amft N, Vernon-Wilson E, Exley AE, Parsonage G, Rainger GE, et al. Rheumatoid fibroblast-like synoviocytes overexpress the chemokine stromal cell-derived factor 1 (CXCL12), which supports distinct patterns and rates of CD4+ and CD8+ T cell migration within synovial tissue. *Arthritis Rheum.* (2003) 48:2472–82. doi: 10.1002/art.11219
117. Selmani Z, Naji A, Zidi I, Favier B, Gaiffe E, Obert L, et al. Human leukocyte antigen-G5 secretion by human mesenchymal stem cells is required to suppress T lymphocyte and natural killer function and to induce CD4+CD25highFOXP3+ regulatory T cells. *Stem Cells.* (2008) 26:212–22. doi: 10.1634/stemcells.2007-0554
118. Burger JA, Zvaifler NJ, Tsukada N, Firestein GS, Kipps TJ. Fibroblast-like synoviocytes support B-cell pseudoemperipolesis via a stromal cell-derived factor-1- and CD106 (VCAM-1)-dependent mechanism. *J Clin Invest.* (2001) 107:305–15. doi: 10.1172/JCI11092
119. Reparon-Schuijt CC, van Esch WJ, van Kooten C, Rozier BC, Levarht EW, Breedveld FC, et al. Regulation of synovial B cell survival in rheumatoid arthritis by vascular cell adhesion molecule 1 (CD106) expressed on fibroblast-like synoviocytes. *Arthritis Rheum.* (2000) 43:1115–21. doi: 10.1002/1529-0131(200005)43:5<1115::AID-ANR22>3.0.CO;2-A
120. Hayashida K, Shimaoka Y, Ochi T, Lipsky PE. Rheumatoid arthritis synovial stromal cells inhibit apoptosis and up-regulate Bcl-xL expression by B cells in a CD49/CD29-CD106-dependent mechanism. *J Immunol.* (2000) 164:1110–6. doi: 10.4049/jimmunol.164.2.1110
121. Benito-Miguel M, Garcia-Carmona Y, Balsa A, Bautista-Caro MB, Arroyo-Villa I, Cobo-Ibanez T, et al. IL-15 expression on RA synovial fibroblasts promotes B cell survival. *PLoS ONE.* (2012) 7:e40620. doi: 10.1371/journal.pone.0040620
122. Bombardieri M, Kam NW, Brentano F, Choi K, Filer A, Kyburz D, et al. A BAFF/APRIL-dependent TLR3-stimulated pathway enhances the capacity of rheumatoid synovial fibroblasts to induce AID expression and Ig class-switching in B cells. *Ann Rheum Dis.* (2011) 70:1857–65. doi: 10.1136/ard.2011.150219
123. Che N, Li X, Zhang L, Liu R, Chen H, Gao X, et al. Impaired B cell inhibition by lupus bone marrow mesenchymal stem cells is caused by reduced CCL2 expression. *J Immunol.* (2014) 193:5306–14. doi: 10.4049/jimmunol.1400036
124. Traggiai E, Volpi S, Schena F, Gattorno M, Ferlito F, Moretta L, et al. Bone marrow-derived mesenchymal stem cells induce both polyclonal expansion and differentiation of B cells isolated from healthy donors and systemic lupus erythematosus patients. *Stem Cells.* (2008) 26:562–9. doi: 10.1634/stemcells.2007-0528
125. Feng X, Che N, Liu Y, Chen H, Wang D, Li X, et al. Restored immunosuppressive effect of mesenchymal stem cells on B cells after olfactory 1/early B cell factor-associated zinc-finger protein down-regulation in patients with systemic lupus erythematosus. *Arthritis Rheumatol.* (2014) 66:3413–23. doi: 10.1002/art.38879
126. Zhang Q, Li Q, Zhu J, Guo H, Zhai Q, Li B, et al. Comparison of therapeutic effects of different mesenchymal stem cells on rheumatoid arthritis in mice. *PeerJ.* (2019) 7:e7023. doi: 10.7717/peerj.7023
127. El-Gendy H, Hawass SE, Awad M, Mohsen MA, Amin M, Abdalla HA, et al. Comparative study between human mesenchymal stem cells and etanercept as immunomodulatory agents in rat model of rheumatoid arthritis. *Immunol Res.* (2020) 68:255–68. doi: 10.1007/s12026-020-09132-w
128. Zhou K, Zhang H, Jin O, Feng X, Yao G, Hou Y, et al. Transplantation of human bone marrow mesenchymal stem cell ameliorates the autoimmune pathogenesis in MRL/lpr mice. *Cell Mol Immunol.* (2008) 5:417–24. doi: 10.1038/cmi.2008.52
129. Sun L, Akiyama K, Zhang H, Yamaza T, Hou Y, Zhao S, et al. Mesenchymal stem cell transplantation reverses multiorgan dysfunction in systemic lupus erythematosus mice and humans. *Stem Cells.* (2009) 27:1421–32. doi: 10.1002/stem.68
130. Choi EW, Lee M, Song JW, Shin IS, Kim SJ. Mesenchymal stem cell transplantation can restore lupus disease-associated miRNA expression and Th1/Th2 ratios in a murine model of SLE. *Sci Rep.* (2016) 6:38237. doi: 10.1038/srep38237
131. Hajkova M, Hermankova B, Javorkova E, Bohacova P, Zajicova A, Holan V, et al. Mesenchymal stem cells attenuate the adverse effects of immunosuppressive drugs on distinct T Cell subopulations. *Stem Cell Rev Rep.* (2017) 13:104–15. doi: 10.1007/s12015-016-9703-3
132. Gu F, Molano I, Ruiz P, Sun L, Gilkeson GS. Differential effect of allogeneic versus syngeneic mesenchymal stem cell transplantation in MRL/lpr and (NZB/NZW)F1 mice. *Clin Immunol.* (2012) 145:142–52. doi: 10.1016/j.clim.2012.08.012
133. Yuan X, Qin X, Wang D, Zhang Z, Tang X, Gao X, et al. Mesenchymal stem cell therapy induces FLT3L and CD1c(+) dendritic cells in systemic lupus erythematosus patients. *Nat Commun.* (2019) 10:2498. doi: 10.1038/s41467-019-10491-8
134. Xishan Z, Baoxin H, Xinna Z, Jun R. Comparison of the effects of human adipose and bone marrow mesenchymal stem cells on T lymphocytes. *Cell Biol Int.* (2013) 37:11–8. doi: 10.1002/cbin.10002
135. Castro-Manrreza ME, Mayani H, Monroy-Garcia A, Flores-Figueroa E, Chavez-Rueda K, Legorreta-Haquet V, et al. Human mesenchymal stromal cells from adult and neonatal sources: a comparative in vitro analysis of their immunosuppressive properties against T cells. *Stem Cells Dev.* (2014) 23:1217–32. doi: 10.1089/scd.2013.0363
136. Puissant B, Barreau C, Bourin P, Clavel C, Corre J, Bousquet C, et al. Immunomodulatory effect of human adipose tissue-derived adult stem cells: comparison with bone marrow mesenchymal stem cells. *Brit J Haematol.* (2005) 129:118–29. doi: 10.1111/j.1365-2141.2005.05409.x
137. Chao YH, Wu HP, Wu KH, Tsai YG, Peng CT, Lin KC, et al. An increase in CD3+CD4+CD25+ regulatory T cells after administration of umbilical cord-derived mesenchymal stem cells during sepsis. *PLoS ONE.* (2014) 9:e110338. doi: 10.1371/journal.pone.0110338
138. Saeidi M, Masoud A, Shakiba Y, Hadjati J, Mohyeddin Bonab M, Nicknam MH, et al. Immunomodulatory effects of human umbilical cord Wharton's jelly-derived mesenchymal stem cells on differentiation, maturation and endocytosis of monocyte-derived dendritic cells. *Iran J Allergy Asthma Immunol.* (2013) 12:37–49.
139. Barcia RN, Santos JM, Filipe M, Teixeira M, Martins JP, Almeida J, et al. What makes umbilical cord tissue-derived mesenchymal stromal cells superior immunomodulators when compared to bone marrow derived mesenchymal stromal cells? *Stem Cells Int.* (2015) 2015:583984. doi: 10.1155/2015/583984
140. Jin HJ, Bae YK, Kim M, Kwon SJ, Jeon HB, Choi SJ, et al. Comparative analysis of human mesenchymal stem cells from bone marrow, adipose tissue, and umbilical cord blood as sources of cell therapy. *Int J Mol Sci.* (2013) 14:17986–8001. doi: 10.3390/ijms140917986
141. Najar M, Raicevic G, Boufker HI, Fayyad Kazan H, De Bruyn C, Meuleman N, et al. Mesenchymal stromal cells use PGE2 to modulate activation and proliferation of lymphocyte subsets: Combined comparison of adipose tissue, Wharton's Jelly and bone marrow sources. *Cell Immunol.* (2010) 264:171–9. doi: 10.1016/j.cellimm.2010.06.006
142. Ribeiro A, Laranjeira P, Mendes S, Velada I, Leite C, Andrade P, et al. Mesenchymal stem cells from umbilical cord matrix, adipose tissue and bone marrow exhibit different capability to suppress peripheral blood B, natural killer and T cells. *Stem Cell Res Ther.* (2013) 4:125. doi: 10.1186/scrt336
143. Lee WJ, Hah YS, Ock SA, Lee JH, Jeon RH, Park JS, et al. Cell source-dependent in vivo immunosuppressive properties of mesenchymal stem cells derived from the bone marrow and synovial fluid of minipigs. *Experi Cell Res.* (2015) 333:273–88. doi: 10.1016/j.yexcr.2015.03.015
144. Park KH, Mun CH, Kang MI, Lee SW, Lee SK, Park YB. Treatment of collagen-induced arthritis using immune modulatory properties of human mesenchymal stem cells. *Cell Transplant.* (2016) 25:1057–72. doi: 10.3727/096368915X687949
145. Liu L, Wong CW, Han M, Farhoodi HP, Liu G, Liu Y, et al. Meta-analysis of preclinical studies of mesenchymal stromal cells to treat rheumatoid arthritis. *EBioMedicine.* (2019) 47:563–77. doi: 10.1016/j.ebiom.2019.08.073
146. Zhou T, Liao C, Li HY, Lin W, Lin S, Zhong H. Efficacy of mesenchymal stem cells in animal models of lupus nephritis: a meta-analysis. *Stem Cell Res Ther.* (2020) 11:48. doi: 10.1186/s13287-019-1538-9
147. Parolini O, Souza-Moreira L, O'Valle F, Magatti M, Hernandez-Cortes P, Gonzalez-Rey E, et al. Therapeutic effect of human amniotic

membrane-derived cells on experimental arthritis and other inflammatory disorders. *Arthritis Rheumatol.* (2014) 66:327–39. doi: 10.1002/art.38206

148. Yamout B, Hourani R, Salti H, Barada W, El-Hajj T, Al-Kutoubi A, et al. Bone marrow mesenchymal stem cell transplantation in patients with multiple sclerosis: a pilot study. *J Neuroimmunol.* (2010) 227:185–9. doi: 10.1016/j.jneuroim.2010.07.013
149. Bouffi C, Bony C, Courties G, Jorgensen C, Noel D. IL-6-dependent PGE2 secretion by mesenchymal stem cells inhibits local inflammation in experimental arthritis. *PLoS ONE.* (2010) 5:e14247. doi: 10.1371/journal.pone.0014247
150. Schurgers E, Kelchtermans H, Mitera T, Geboes L, Matthys P. Discrepancy between the in vitro and *in vivo* effects of murine mesenchymal stem cells on T-cell proliferation and collagen-induced arthritis. *Arthritis Res Therapy.* (2010) 12:R31. doi: 10.1186/ar2939
151. Sullivan C, Murphy JM, Griffin MD, Porter RM, Evans CH, O'Flatharta C, et al. Genetic mismatch affects the immunosuppressive properties of mesenchymal stem cells in vitro and their ability to influence the course of collagen-induced arthritis. *Arthritis Res Therapy.* (2012) 14:R167. doi: 10.1186/ar3916
152. Yu Y, Yoon KA, Kang TW, Jeon HJ, Sim YB, Choe SH, et al. Therapeutic effect of long-interval repeated intravenous administration of human umbilical cord blood-derived mesenchymal stem cells in DBA/1 mice with collagen-induced arthritis. *J Tissue Eng Regen Med.* (2019) 13:1134–42. doi: 10.1002/term.2861
153. Papadopoulou A, Yiangou M, Athanasiou E, Zogas N, Kaloyannidis P, Batsis I, et al. Mesenchymal stem cells are conditionally therapeutic in preclinical models of rheumatoid arthritis. *Ann Rheumatic Dis.* (2012) 71:1733–40. doi: 10.1136/annrheumdis-2011-200985
154. Augello A, Tasso R, Negrini SM, Cancedda R, Pennesi G. Cell therapy using allogeneic bone marrow mesenchymal stem cells prevents tissue damage in collagen-induced arthritis. *Arthritis Rheumatism.* (2007) 56:1175–86. doi: 10.1002/art.22511
155. Kim JH, Lee YT, Oh K, Cho J, Lee DS, Hwang YI. Paradoxical effects of human adipose tissue-derived mesenchymal stem cells on progression of experimental arthritis in SKG mice. *Cell Immunol.* (2014) 292:94–101. doi: 10.1016/j.cellimm.2014.10.005
156. Gonzalez MA, Gonzalez-Rey E, Rico L, Buscher D, Delgado M. Treatment of experimental arthritis by inducing immune tolerance with human adipose-derived mesenchymal stem cells. *Arthritis Rheumatism.* (2009) 60:1006–19. doi: 10.1002/art.24405
157. Liu H, Ding J, Wang J, Wang Y, Yang M, Zhang Y, et al. Remission of collagen-induced arthritis through combination therapy of microfracture and transplantation of thermogel-encapsulated bone marrow mesenchymal stem cells. *PLoS ONE.* (2015) 10:e0120596. doi: 10.1145/2818302
158. Thompson M, Mei SHJ, Wolfe D, Champagne J, Fergusson D, Stewart DJ, et al. Cell therapy with intravascular administration of mesenchymal stromal cells continues to appear safe: An updated systematic review and meta-analysis. *EClinicalMedicine.* (2020) 19:100249. doi: 10.1016/j.eclinm.2019.100249
159. Kearsley-Fleet L, Davies R, De Cock D, Watson KD, Lunt M, Buch MH, et al. Biologic refractory disease in rheumatoid arthritis: results from the British society for rheumatology biologics register for rheumatoid arthritis. *Ann Rheumatic Dis.* (2018) 77:1405–12. doi: 10.1136/annrheumdis-2018-213378
160. Martin I, Galipeau J, Kessler C, Le Blanc K, Dazzi F. Challenges for mesenchymal stromal cell therapies. *Sci Transl Med.* (2019) 11:480. doi: 10.1126/scitranslmed.aat2189
161. Tan J, Wu W, Xu X, Liao L, Zheng F, Messinger S, et al. Induction therapy with autologous mesenchymal stem cells in living-related kidney transplants: a randomized controlled trial. *JAMA.* (2012) 307:1169–77. doi: 10.1001/jama.2012.316
162. Wang D, Akiyama K, Zhang H, Yamaza T, Li X, Feng X, et al. Double allogenic mesenchymal stem cells transplantations could not enhance therapeutic effect compared with single transplantation in systemic lupus erythematosus. *Clin Dev Immunol.* (2012) 2012:273291. doi: 10.1155/2012/273291
163. Wang L, Huang S, Li S, Li M, Shi J, Bai W, et al. Efficacy and safety of umbilical cord mesenchymal stem cell therapy for rheumatoid arthritis patients: a prospective phase I/II study. *Drug Des Devel Ther.* (2019) 13:4331–40. doi: 10.2147/DDDT.S225613
164. Wang L, Wang L, Cong X, Liu G, Zhou J, Bai B, et al. Human umbilical cord mesenchymal stem cell therapy for patients with active rheumatoid arthritis: safety and efficacy. *Stem Cells Dev.* (2013) 22:3192–202. doi: 10.1089/scd.2013.0023
165. Liang J, Li X, Zhang H, Wang D, Feng X, Wang H, et al. Allogeneic mesenchymal stem cells transplantation in patients with refractory RA. *Clin rheumatol.* (2012) 31:157–61. doi: 10.1007/s10067-011-1816-0
166. Yang Y, He X, Zhao R, Guo W, Zhu M, Xing W, et al. Serum IFN-gamma levels predict the therapeutic effect of mesenchymal stem cell transplantation in active rheumatoid arthritis. *J Translat Med.* (2018) 16:165. doi: 10.1186/s12967-018-1541-4
167. Park EH, Lim HS, Lee S, Roh K, Seo KW, Kang KS, et al. Intravenous infusion of umbilical cord blood-derived mesenchymal stem cells in rheumatoid arthritis: a phase ia clinical trial. *Stem Cells Transl Med.* (2018) 7:636–42. doi: 10.1002/sctm.18-0031
168. He X, Yang Y, Yao M, Yang L, Ao L, Hu X, et al. Combination of human umbilical cord mesenchymal stem (stromal) cell transplantation with IFN-gamma treatment synergistically improves the clinical outcomes of patients with rheumatoid arthritis. *Ann Rheumatic Dis.* (2020) 79:1298–304. doi: 10.1136/annrheumdis-2020-217798
169. Ghoryani M, Shariati-Sarabi Z, Tavakkol-Afshari J, Ghasemi A, Poursamimi J, Mohammadi M. Amelioration of clinical symptoms of patients with refractory rheumatoid arthritis following treatment with autologous bone marrow-derived mesenchymal stem cells: A successful clinical trial in Iran. *Biomed Pharmacother.* (2019) 109:1834–40. doi: 10.1016/j.biopha.2018.11.056
170. Ghoryani M, Shariati-Sarabi Z, Tavakkol-Afshari J, Mohammadi M. The sufficient immunoregulatory effect of autologous bone marrow-derived mesenchymal stem cell transplantation on regulatory t cells in patients with refractory rheumatoid arthritis. *J Immunol Res.* (2020) 2020:3562753. doi: 10.1155/2020/3562753
171. Shadmanfar S, Labibzadeh N, Emadedin M, Jaroughi N, Azimian V, Mardpour S, et al. Intra-articular knee implantation of autologous bone marrow-derived mesenchymal stromal cells in rheumatoid arthritis patients with knee involvement: results of a randomized, triple-blind, placebo-controlled phase 1/2 clinical trial. *Cytotherapy.* (2018) 20:499–506. doi: 10.1016/j.jcyt.2017.12.009
172. Alvaro-Gracia JM, Jover JA, Garcia-Vicuna R, Carreno L, Alonso A, Marsal S, et al. Intravenous administration of expanded allogeneic adipose-derived mesenchymal stem cells in refractory rheumatoid arthritis (Cx611): results of a multicentre, dose escalation, randomised, single-blind, placebo-controlled phase Ib/IIa clinical trial. *Ann Rheumatic Dis.* (2017) 76:196–202. doi: 10.1136/annrheumdis-2015-208918
173. Gronthos S, Zannettino AC, Hay SJ, Shi S, Graves SE, Kortesidis A, et al. Molecular and cellular characterisation of highly purified stromal stem cells derived from human bone marrow. *J Cell Sci.* (2003) 116:1827–35. doi: 10.1242/jcs.00369
174. Gowhari Shabgah A, Shariati-Sarabi Z, Tavakkol-Afshari J, Ghasemi A, Ghoryani M, Mohammadi M. A significant decrease of BAFF, APRIL, and BAFF receptors following mesenchymal stem cell transplantation in patients with refractory rheumatoid arthritis. *Gene.* (2020) 732:144336. doi: 10.1016/j.gene.2020.144336
175. Gowhari Shabgah A, Shariati-Sarabi Z, Tavakkol-Afshari J, Ghoryani M, Mohammadi M. Possible anti-inflammatory effects of mesenchymal stem cells transplantation via changes in CXCL8 levels in patients with refractory rheumatoid arthritis. *Int J Mol Cell Med.* (2019) 8:191–9. doi: 10.22088/IJMCM.BUMS.8.3.191
176. Ra JC, Kang SK, Shin IS, Park HG, Joo SA, Kim JG, et al. Stem cell treatment for patients with autoimmune disease by systemic infusion of culture-expanded autologous adipose tissue derived mesenchymal stem cells. *J Translat Med.* (2011) 9:181. doi: 10.1186/1479-5876-9-181
177. Lopez-Santalla M, Fernandez-Perez R, Garin MI. Mesenchymal stem/stromal cells for rheumatoid arthritis treatment: an update on clinical applications. *Cells.* (2020) 91852. doi: 10.3390/cells90 81852

178. Prigozhina TB, Khitrin S, Elkin G, Eizik O, Morecki S, Slavin S. Mesenchymal stromal cells lose their immunosuppressive potential after allotransplantation. *Experi Hematol.* (2008) 36:1370–6. doi: 10.1016/j.exphem.2008.04.022
179. Grootscholten C, Ligtenberg G, Hagen EC, van den Wall Bake AW, de Glas-Vos JW, Bijl M, et al. Azathioprine/methylprednisolone versus cyclophosphamide in proliferative lupus nephritis. A randomized controlled trial. *Kidney Int.* (2006) 70:732–42. doi: 10.1038/sj.ki.5001630
180. Kamanamool N, McEvoy M, Attia J, Ingsathit A, Ngamjanyaporn P, Thakkinstian A. Efficacy and adverse events of mycophenolate mofetil versus cyclophosphamide for induction therapy of lupus nephritis: systematic review and meta-analysis. *Medicine.* (2010) 89:227–35. doi: 10.1097/MD.0b013e3181e93d00
181. Ishii S, Miwa Y, Otsuka K, Nishimi S, Nishimi A, Saito M, et al. Influence of renal complications on the efficacy and adverse events of tacrolimus combination therapy in patients with systemic lupus erythematosus (SLE) during a maintenance phase: a single-centre, prospective study. *Lupus Sci Med.* (2015) 2:e000091. doi: 10.1136/lupus-2015-000091
182. Nikpour M, Urowitz MB, Ibanez D, Gladman DD. Frequency and determinants of flare and persistently active disease in systemic lupus erythematosus. *Arthritis Rheumatism.* (2009) 61:1152–8. doi: 10.1002/art.24741
183. Carrion F, Nova E, Ruiz C, Diaz F, Inostroza C, Rojo D, et al. Autologous mesenchymal stem cell treatment increased T regulatory cells with no effect on disease activity in two systemic lupus erythematosus patients. *Lupus.* (2010) 19:317–22. doi: 10.1177/0961203309348983
184. Barbado J, Tabera S, Sanchez A, Garcia-Sancho J. Therapeutic potential of allogeneic mesenchymal stromal cells transplantation for lupus nephritis. *Lupus.* (2018) 27:2161–5. doi: 10.1177/0961203318804922
185. Liang J, Zhang H, Kong W, Deng W, Wang D, Feng X, et al. Safety analysis in patients with autoimmune disease receiving allogeneic mesenchymal stem cells infusion: a long-term retrospective study. *Stem Cell Res Ther.* (2018) 9:312. doi: 10.1186/s13287-018-1053-4
186. Liang J, Zhang H, Hua B, Wang H, Lu L, Shi S, et al. Allogenic mesenchymal stem cells transplantation in refractory systemic lupus erythematosus: a pilot clinical study. *Ann Rheumatic Dis.* (2010) 69:1423–9. doi: 10.1136/ard.2009.123463
187. Gu F, Wang D, Zhang H, Feng X, Gilkeson GS, Shi S, et al. Allogeneic mesenchymal stem cell transplantation for lupus nephritis patients refractory to conventional therapy. *Clin Rheumatol.* (2014) 33:1611–9. doi: 10.1007/s10067-014-2754-4
188. Wang D, Niu L, Feng X, Yuan X, Zhao S, Zhang H, et al. Long-term safety of umbilical cord mesenchymal stem cells transplantation for systemic lupus erythematosus: a 6-year follow-up study. *Clin Exp Med.* (2017) 17:333–40. doi: 10.1007/s10238-016-0427-0
189. Wang D, Zhang H, Liang J, Li X, Feng X, Wang H, et al. Allogeneic mesenchymal stem cell transplantation in severe and refractory systemic lupus erythematosus: 4 years of experience. *Cell Transplant.* (2013) 22:2267–77. doi: 10.3727/096368911X582769c
190. Deng D, Zhang P, Guo Y, Lim TO. A randomised double-blind, placebo-controlled trial of allogeneic umbilical cord-derived mesenchymal stem cell for lupus nephritis. *Ann Rheumatic Dis.* (2017) 76:1436–9. doi: 10.1136/annrheumdis-2017-211073
191. Sun L, Wang D, Liang J, Zhang H, Feng X, Wang H, et al. Umbilical cord mesenchymal stem cell transplantation in severe and refractory systemic lupus erythematosus. *Arthritis Rheumatism.* (2010) 62:2467–75. doi: 10.1002/art.27548
192. Wang D, Li J, Zhang Y, Zhang M, Chen J, Li X, et al. Umbilical cord mesenchymal stem cell transplantation in active and refractory systemic lupus erythematosus: a multicenter clinical study. *Arthritis Res Therapy.* (2014) 16:R79. doi: 10.1186/ar4520
193. Zhou T, Li HY, Liao C, Lin W, Lin S. Clinical efficacy and safety of mesenchymal stem cells for systemic lupus erythematosus. *Stem Cells Int.* (2020) 2020:6518508. doi: 10.1155/2020/6518508
194. Geng L, Tang X, Zhou K, Wang D, Wang S, Yao G, et al. MicroRNA-663 induces immune dysregulation by inhibiting TGF-beta1 production in bone marrow-derived mesenchymal stem cells in patients with systemic lupus erythematosus. *Cell Mol Immunol.* (2019) 16:260–74. doi: 10.1038/cmi.2018.1
195. Yang JH, Liu FX, Wang JH, Cheng M, Wang SF, Xu DH. Mesenchymal stem cells and mesenchymal stem cell-derived extracellular vesicles: potential roles in rheumatic diseases. *World J Stem Cells.* (2020) 12:688–705. doi: 10.4252/wjsc.v12.i7.688
196. Krampera M, Cosmi L, Angeli R, Pasini A, Liotta F, Andreini A, et al. Role for interferon-gamma in the immunomodulatory activity of human bone marrow mesenchymal stem cells. *Stem Cells.* (2006) 24:386–98. doi: 10.1634/stemcells.2005-0008
197. Meng HY, Chen LQ, Chen LH. The inhibition by human MSCs-derived miRNA-124a overexpression exosomes in the proliferation and migration of rheumatoid arthritis-related fibroblast-like synoviocyte cell. *BMC Musculoskeletal Disord.* (2020) 21:150. doi: 10.1186/s12891-020-3159-y
198. Casado JG, Blazquez R, Vela FJ, Alvarez V, Tarazona R, Sanchez-Margallo FM. Mesenchymal stem cell-derived exosomes: immunomodulatory evaluation in an antigen-induced synovitis porcine model. *Front Vet Sci.* (2017) 4:39. doi: 10.3389/fvets.2017.00039
199. Perez-Hernandez J, Redon J, Cortes R. Extracellular vesicles as therapeutic agents in systemic lupus erythematosus. *Int J Mol Sci.* (2017) 18:717. doi: 10.3390/ijms18040717
200. Sharma J, Hampton JM, Valiente GR, Wada T, Steigelman H, Young MC, et al. Therapeutic development of mesenchymal stem cells or their extracellular vesicles to inhibit autoimmune-mediated inflammatory processes in systemic lupus erythematosus. *Front Immunol.* (2017) 8:526. doi: 10.3389/fimmu.2017.00526
201. Galleu A, Riffo-Vasquez Y, Trento C, Lomas C, Dolcetti L, Cheung TS, et al. Apoptosis in mesenchymal stromal cells induces in vivo recipient-mediated immunomodulation. *Sci Transl Med.* (2017) 9:7828. doi: 10.1126/scitranslmed.aam7828
202. Weiss ARR, Dahlke MH. Immunomodulation by mesenchymal stem cells (MSCs): mechanisms of action of living, apoptotic, and dead MSCs. *Front Immunol.* (2019) 10:1191. doi: 10.3389/fimmu.2019.01191
203. Chapelin F, Khurana A, Moneeb M, Gray Hazard FK, Chan CFR, Nejadnik H, et al. Tumor formation of adult stem cell transplants in rodent arthritic joints. *Mol Imaging Biol.* (2019) 21:95–104. doi: 10.1007/s11307-018-1218-7
204. Berebichez-Fridman R, Montero-Olvera PR. Sources and clinical applications of mesenchymal stem cells: state-of-the-art review. *Sultan Qaboos Univ Med J.* (2018) 18:e264–e77. doi: 10.18295/squmj.2018.18.03.002
205. Ganguly P, El-Jawhari JJ, Burska AN, Ponchel F, Giannoudis PV, Jones EA. The analysis of *in vivo* aging in human bone marrow mesenchymal stromal cells using colony-forming unit-fibroblast assay and the CD45(low)CD271(+) phenotype. *Stem Cells Int.* (2019) 2019:5197983. doi: 10.1155/2019/5197983
206. Mattar P, Bieback K. Comparing the immunomodulatory properties of bone marrow, adipose tissue, and birth-associated tissue mesenchymal stromal cells. *Front Immunol.* (2015) 6:560. doi: 10.3389/fimmu.2015.00560
207. Mendicino M, Bailey AM, Wonnacott K, Puri RK, Bauer SR. MSC-based product characterization for clinical trials: an FDA perspective. *Cell Stem Cell.* (2014) 14:141–5. doi: 10.1016/j.stem.2014.01.013
208. Capelli C, Pedrini O, Valgardsdottir R, Da Roit F, Golay J, Introna M. Clinical grade expansion of MSCs. *Immunol Lett.* (2015) 168:222–7. doi: 10.1016/j.imlet.2015.06.006
209. El-Jawhari JJ, Cuthbert R, McGonagle D, Jones E, Giannoudis PV. The CD45lowCD271high cell prevalence in bone marrow samples may provide a useful measurement of the bone marrow quality for cartilage and bone regenerative therapy. *J Bone Joint Surg Am Vol.* (2017) 99:1305–13. doi: 10.2106/JBJS.16.01138
210. Siegel G, Kluba T, Hermanutz-Klein U, Bieback K, Northoff H, Schafer R. Phenotype, donor age and gender affect function of human bone marrow-derived mesenchymal stromal cells. *BMC Med.* (2013) 11:146. doi: 10.1186/1741-7015-11-146
211. Xu J, Chen J, Li W, Lian W, Huang J, Lai B, et al. Additive therapeutic effects of mesenchymal stem cells and IL-37 for systemic lupus erythematosus. *J Am Soc Nephrol.* (2020) 31:54–65. doi: 10.1681/ASN.2019050545
212. Tavasolian F, Hosseini AZ, Soudi S, Naderi M. miRNA-146a improves immunomodulatory effects of MSC-derived

exosomes in rheumatoid arthritis. *Curr Gene Ther.* (2020) 20:297–312. doi: 10.2174/1566523220666200916120708

213. Meng Q, Qiu B. Exosomal MicroRNA-320a derived from mesenchymal stem cells regulates rheumatoid arthritis fibroblast-like synoviocyte activation by suppressing CXCL9 expression. *Front Physiol.* (2020) 11:441. doi: 10.3389/fphys.2020.00441
214. Hu J, Li H, Chi G, Yang Z, Zhao Y, Liu W, et al. IL-1RA gene-transfected bone marrow-derived mesenchymal stem cells in APA microcapsules could alleviate rheumatoid arthritis. *Int J Clin Exp Med.* (2015) 8:706–13.
215. Wei J, Ouyang X, Tang Y, Li H, Wang B, Ye Y, et al. ER-stressed MSC displayed more effective immunomodulation in RA CD4(+)CXCR5(+)ICOS(+) follicular helper-like T cells through higher PGE2 binding with EP2/EP4. *Mod Rheumatol.* (2020) 30:509–16. doi: 10.1080/14397595.2019.1651446
216. Hemmerle T, Doll F, Neri D. Antibody-based delivery of IL4 to the neovasculature cures mice with arthritis. *Proc Natl Acad Sci USA.* (2014) 111:12008–12. doi: 10.1073/pnas.1402783111
217. Lin S, Qiu M, Chen J. IL-4 modulates macrophage polarization in ankylosing spondylitis. *Cell Physiol Biochem.* (2015) 35:2213–22. doi: 10.1159/000374026
218. Cheng W, Su J, Hu Y, Huang Q, Shi H, Wang L, et al. Interleukin-25 primed mesenchymal stem cells achieve better therapeutic effects on dextran sulfate sodium-induced colitis via inhibiting Th17 immune response and inducing T regulatory cell phenotype. *Am J Transl Res.* (2017) 9:4149–60.
219. Ullah M, Liu DD, Thakor AS. Mesenchymal stromal cell homing: mechanisms and strategies for improvement. *iScience.* (2019) 15:421–38. doi: 10.1016/j.isci.2019.05.004
220. Singer NG, Caplan AI. Mesenchymal stem cells: mechanisms of inflammation. *Annu Rev Pathol.* (2011) 6:457–78. doi: 10.1146/annurev-pathol-011110-130230
221. Bronckaers A, Hilkens P, Martens W, Gervois P, Ratajczak J, Struys T, et al. Mesenchymal stem/stromal cells as a pharmacological and therapeutic approach to accelerate angiogenesis. *Pharmacol Ther.* (2014) 143:181–96. doi: 10.1016/j.pharmthera.2014.02.013
222. Christy BA, Herzig MC, Montgomery RK, Delavan C, Bynum JA, Reddoch KM, et al. Procoagulant activity of human mesenchymal stem cells. *J Trauma Acute Care Surg.* (2017) 83(Suppl. 1):S164–9. doi: 10.1097/TA.0000000000001485
223. Li Y, Lin F. Mesenchymal stem cells are injured by complement after their contact with serum. *Blood.* (2012) 120:3436–43. doi: 10.1182/blood-2012-03-420612
224. Fischer UM, Harting MT, Jimenez F, Monzon-Posadas WO, Xue H, Savitz SI, et al. Pulmonary passage is a major obstacle for intravenous stem cell delivery: the pulmonary first-pass effect. *Stem Cells Dev.* (2009) 18:683–92. doi: 10.1089/scd.2008.0253
225. Masterson CH, Curley GF, Laffey JG. Modulating the distribution and fate of exogenously delivered MSCs to enhance therapeutic potential: knowns and unknowns. *Intensive Care Med Exp.* (2019) 7(Suppl. 1):41. doi: 10.1186/s40635-019-0235-4
226. Le Blanc K, Tammik C, Rosendahl K, Zetterberg E, Ringden O. HLA expression and immunologic properties of differentiated and undifferentiated mesenchymal stem cells. *Exp Hematol.* (2003) 31:890–6. doi: 10.1016/S0301-472X(03)00110-3

12

Non-Transcriptional and Translational Function of Canonical NF-κB Signaling in Activating ERK1/2 in IL-1β-Induced COX-2 Expression in Synovial Fibroblasts

*Rei Nakano[1,2,3], Taku Kitanaka[2,3], Shinichi Namba[2,3], Nanako Kitanaka[2,3], Yoko Suwabe[2], Tadayoshi Konno[3], Jun Yamazaki[4], Tomohiro Nakayama[2] and Hiroshi Sugiya[2,3]**

[1] Laboratory for Cellular Function Conversion Technology, RIKEN Center for Integrative Medical Sciences, Yokohama, Japan, [2] Laboratory of Veterinary Radiology, Department of Veterinary Medicine, College of Bioresource Sciences, Nihon University, Fujisawa, Japan, [3] Laboratory of Veterinary Biochemistry, Department of Veterinary Medicine, College of Bioresource Sciences, Nihon University, Fujisawa, Japan, [4] Laboratory of Veterinary Pharmacology, Department of Veterinary Medicine, College of Bioresource Sciences, Nihon University, Fujisawa, Japan

***Correspondence:**
Hiroshi Sugiya
sugiya.hiroshi@nihon-u.ac.jp

The pro-inflammatory cytokine interleukin 1β (IL-1β) induces the synthesis of prostaglandin E_2 by upregulating cyclooxygenase-2 (COX-2) in the synovial tissue of individuals with autoimmune diseases, such as rheumatoid arthritis (RA). IL-1β-mediated stimulation of NF-κB and MAPK signaling is important for the pathogenesis of RA; however, crosstalk(s) between NF-κB and MAPK signaling remains to be understood. In this study, we established a model for IL-1β-induced synovitis and investigated the role of NF-κB and MAPK signaling in synovitis. We observed an increase in the mRNA and protein levels of COX-2 and prostaglandin E_2 release in cells treated with IL-1β. NF-κB and ERK1/2 inhibitors significantly reduced IL-1β-induced COX-2 expression. IL-1β induced the phosphorylation of canonical NF-κB complex (p65 and p105) and degradation of IκBα. IL-1β also induced ERK1/2 phosphorylation but did not affect the phosphorylation levels of p38 MAPK and JNK. IL-1β failed to induce COX-2 expression in cells transfected with siRNA for p65, p105, ERK1, or ERK2. Notably, NF-κB inhibitors reduced IL-1β-induced ERK1/2 phosphorylation; however, the ERK1/2 inhibitor had no effect on the phosphorylation of the canonical NF-κB complex. Although transcription and translation inhibitors had no effect on IL-1β-induced ERK1/2 phosphorylation, the silencing of canonical NF-κB complex in siRNA-transfected fibroblasts prevented IL-1β-induced phosphorylation of ERK1/2. Taken together, our data indicate the importance of the non-transcriptional/translational activity of canonical NF-κB in the activation of ERK1/2 signaling involved in the IL-1β-induced development of autoimmune diseases affecting the synovial tissue, such as RA.

Keywords: rheumatoid arthritis, interleukin 1β (IL-1β), cyclooxygenase 2 (COX-2), NF-κB—nuclear factor kappa B, ERK1/2

INTRODUCTION

Rheumatoid arthritis (RA) is a chronic and progressive inflammatory autoimmune disease characterized by a dysregulated immune system in the synovial joint membrane, thereby causing severe damage and destruction of the cartilage and bone. Synovitis (inflammation of the synovial membrane) is a hallmark of RA. Pro-inflammatory cytokines, such as interleukin 1β (IL-1β) and tumor necrosis factor α (TNF-α), play a crucial role in the development of synovitis and progressive joint destruction (1, 2). The use of antibodies against IL-1 to treat patients with RA improves symptoms associated with RA and reduces joint erosions (3, 4). IL-1β induces the expression of prostaglandin E_2 by upregulating cyclooxygenase-2 (COX-2) in pro-inflammatory conditions. IL-1β activates numerous cellular signaling pathways, including nuclear factor-κB (NF-κB) and mitogen-activated protein kinase (MAPK) signaling.

NF-κB is a transcription factor that is important in regulating immune response and inflammation (5, 6). NF-κB consists of homo- and heterodimers of the Rel family of proteins, such as RelA (p65), RelB, c-Rel, p105/p50, and p100/p52 (6). The activity of NF-κB is primarily regulated by its interaction with inhibitory proteins, such as IκB, thereby enabling the cytoplasmic retention of these inactive complexes. NF-κB is activated upon the degradation of IκB that disrupts the interaction between IκB and NF-κB. Subsequently, the released NF-κB translocates into the nucleus where it induces the expression of immune and inflammatory genes by binding to their promoters (6). In response to the pro-inflammatory cytokine IL-1β, the heterotrimeric complex of NF-κB comprising p50, RelA (p65), and IκBα gets activated and results in canonical NF-κB signaling (5, 6).

MAPK signaling pathways are involved in the regulation of various cellular functions, including inflammation. MAPKs are serine-threonine kinases, such as c-Jun NH_2-terminal kinase (JNK), p38 MAPK, and extracellular signal-regulated kinase (ERK); all these kinases exist as isoforms in mammals. Depending on the stimulus and cell type, MAPKs are activated *via* multiple pathways, thereby phosphorylating a wide range of substrates, such as transcription factors and cytoskeletal proteins, and resulting in specific cellular responses (7–13). The MAPK signaling cascades consist of at least three sequential kinase components: MAPK kinase kinase, MAPK kinase, and MAPK. MAPK kinase kinases phosphorylate the serine/threonine residues of and activate MAPK kinases that phosphorylate the threonine/tyrosine residues in the activation loop of MAPKs, thereby stimulating MAPKs (14, 15). MAPK signaling activates NF-κB in synovial fibroblasts in other cellular models (16–21). Pro-inflammatory cytokines (*e.g.* IL-1β and TNF-α) stimulate the activation of NF-κB and MAPK signaling in synovial fibroblasts; however, the correlation between NF-κB and MAPK signaling remains to be elucidated (8, 9).

In this study, we have investigated IL-1β-induced expression of COX-2 and its role in the synthesis of prostaglandin E_2 in canine synovial fibroblasts. We observed crosstalk between NF-κB and ERK1/2 MAPK signaling. Canonical NF-κB signaling induced the activation of ERK1/2 in the presence of transcription and translation inhibitors. Taken together, our findings indicate that the non-transcriptional/translational function of canonical NF-κB signaling regulates the activation of ERK1/2 signaling in synovial fibroblasts.

MATERIALS AND METHODS

Materials

TRIzol and Lipofectamine 2000 were obtained from Life Technologies Co. (Carlsbad, CA). The Thermal Cycler Dice Real Time System II, TP900 DiceRealTime v4.02B, SYBR Premix Ex Taq II, PrimeScript RT Master Mix, and CELLBANKER 1 plus medium were purchased from TaKaRa Bio Inc. (Shiga, Japan). Rabbit monoclonal antibodies against human total JNK (t-JNK, EPR140 (2), Cat# ab110724, RRID : AB_10866293) and COX-1 (EPR5867, Cat# ab133319, RRID : AB_11157915), and rabbit polyclonal antibody against COX-2 (Cat# ab102005, RRID : AB_10972360) were procured from Abcam (Cambridge, UK). Anti-human phosphorylated p65 (Ser536) (p-p65, 93H1, Cat# 3033, RRID : AB_331284), anti-human total p65 (t-p65, D14E12, Cat# 8242, RRID : AB_10859369), anti-human total-IκBα (t-IκBα, I44D4, Cat# 4812, RRID : AB_10694416), anti-human phosphorylated p105 (Ser 933) (p-p105, 18E6, Cat# 4806, RRID : AB_2282911), anti-human total p105 (t-p105, D7H5M, Cat# 12540, RRID : AB_2687614), anti-rat total-ERK1/2 (t-ERK1/2, 137F5, Cat# 4695, RRID : AB_390779), anti-human phospho-ERK1/2 (Thr202/Tyr204) (p-ERK1/2, D13.14.4E, Cat# 4370, RRID : AB_2315112), anti-human total-p38 (t-p38, D13E1, Cat# 8690, RRID : AB_10999090), and anti-human phospho-p38 (Thr180/Tyr182) (p-p38, 3D7, Cat# 9215, RRID : AB_331762) rabbit monoclonal or polyclonal antibodies, horseradish peroxidase-conjugated anti-mouse (Cat# 7076, RRID : AB_330924) and anti-rabbit IgG antibodies (Cat# 7074, RRID : AB_2099233) were obtained from Cell Signaling Technology Japan, K.K. (Tokyo, Japan). Rabbit polyclonal antibody against phospho-JNK (Thr183/Tyr185) (p-JNK, Cat# V7931, RRID : AB_430864) was purchased from Promega, Co. (Madison, WI). BAY11-7082, TPCA-1, SKF86002, U0126, FR180204, SP600125, actinomycin D, cycloheximide, and mouse monoclonal anti-β-actin antibody (AC74, Cat# A5441, RRID : AB_476744) were procured from Sigma-Aldrich Inc. (St Louis, MO). ImageQuant LAS 4000 mini, protein A plus G Sepharose, and ECL Western blotting Analysis System were obtained from GE Healthcare (Piscataway, NJ). Mini-PROTEAN TGX gel and polyvinylidene difluoride membranes were purchased from Bio-Rad (Hercules, CA). Block Ace and Complete mini EDTA-free protease inhibitor mixture were purchased from Roche (Mannheim, Germany). Dulbecco's modified Eagle's medium supplemented with 1 g/L glucose (DMEM-LG) was obtained from Wako Pure Chemical Industries, Ltd. (Osaka, Japan). An enzyme-linked immunosorbent assay kit for prostaglandin E_2 was procured from Cayman Chemical Co. (Ann Arbor, MI). Canine recombinant IL-1β was purchased from Kingfisher Biotech,

Inc. (Saint Paul, MN). StatMate IV was obtained from ATMS (Tokyo, Japan). A freezing vessel (BICELL) was procured from Nihon Freezer Co., Ltd. (Tokyo, Japan).

Cell Culture

Canine synovial fibroblasts isolated from the synovium of the stifle joint were a kind gift from Ms. Aki Ohmori, Teikyo University School of Medicine. We used flow cytometry to characterize cells by their surface markers: positive for fibroblast markers CD29 (97.86 ± 1.23%), CD44 (97.40 ± 1.30%), and CD90 (97.50 ± 1.42%), and negative for hematopoietic cell markers CD14 (1.60 ± 0.50%), CD34 (1.12 ± 0.10%), CD45 (0.97 ± 0.13%), and HLA-DR (2.73 ± 1.45%) (9). Dissociated cells were maintained in static culture in DMEM-LG supplemented with 10% fetal bovine serum (FBS) in a 5% CO_2 incubator at 37°C. The medium was replaced once a week. Cells were cryopreserved and thawed as previously described (7–13, 22–26). Briefly, cells were harvested using 0.25% trypsin-EDTA once they were 90–95% confluent and resuspended in CELLBANKER 1 plus medium at a density of 2×10^6 cells/500 µl. The cell suspension (500 µl) was placed into sterilized serum tubes that were placed in a freezing vessel (BICELL) and cryopreserved at −80°C. Before performing the experiment, tubes were removed from the BICELL vessel and immersed in a water bath at 37°C. The thawed cell suspension was transferred into a centrifuge tube containing DMEM-LG with 10% FBS and centrifuged at 300×g for 3 min. The pellet was resuspended in DMEM-LG containing 10% FBS and transferred to a 75 cm^2 culture flask. Static cultures were maintained under the same conditions as prior to cryopreservation. Cells were harvested using 0.25% trypsin-EDTA once they were ~90% confluent; the collected cells were seeded at a density of 1×10^6 cells per 75 cm^2 culture flask. Experiments were performed with canine synovial fibroblasts from the fourth passage. Each experiment was performed with cells derived from a single donor.

Quantitative Reverse Transcription-Polymerase Chain Reaction

RT-qPCR was performed as previously described (7–13, 22–26). Total RNA was extracted from canine synovial fibroblasts using TRIzol. First-strand cDNA synthesis was performed using 500 ng of total RNA with the PrimeScript RT Master Mix. Real-time PCR was performed using 2 µl of the first-strand cDNA, SYBR Premix Ex Taq II, and primers specific for COX-1, COX-2, and TBP (TATA-binding protein; housekeeping internal control) in a total reaction volume of 25 µl (**Table 1**). Real-time PCR for no-template control was performed using 2 µl of RNase- and DNA-free water. Additionally, real-time PCR for the control for reverse transcription was performed using 2 µl of the RNAs. PCR was performed using the Thermal Cycler Dice Real Time System II with the following protocol: one cycle of denaturation at 95°C for 30 s, 40 cycles of denaturation at 95°C for 5 s, and annealing/extension at 60°C for 30 s. Data were analyzed using the second derivative maximum and comparative cycle threshold (ΔΔCt) methods using the real-time PCR analysis software. TBP amplification from the same amount of cDNA was used as the endogenous control, while amplification from feline synovial fibroblasts at 0 h was used as the calibration standard.

TABLE 1 | Primer sequences for RT-qPCR.

Gene Name	Gene bank ID	Primer sequences
COX-2	NM_001003354.1	F: 5′-TGTGTCTCATTAACCTGCATGTACC-3′
		R: 5′-CAGTGATATTTGCACCTGTGTCCTC-3′
COX-1	NM_001003023.2	F: 5′-ACGTGGCTGTGGAAACCATC-3′
		R: 5′-GGCATCAATGTCTCCATACAGCTC-3′
TBP	XM_863452	F: 5′-ACTGTTGGTGGGTCAGCACAAG-3′
		R: 5′-ATGGTGTGTACGGGAGCCAAG-3′

Western Blotting

Western blotting was performed as previously described (7–13, 22–26). Proteins were isolated by lysing cells with a lysis buffer containing 20 mM HEPES, 1 mM phenylmethanesulfonyl fluoride, 10 mM sodium fluoride, and a complete mini EDTA-free protease inhibitor cocktail at pH 7.4. Protein concentrations were measured using the Bradford method (27). Extracted proteins were boiled at 95°C for 5 min in sodium dodecyl sulfate buffer, loaded into separate lanes of 7.5 or 12% Mini-PROTEAN TGX gels, and electrophoretically separated. Separated proteins were transferred to polyvinylidene difluoride membranes. The membranes were treated with Block Ace for 50 min at room temperature and incubated with primary antibodies [COX-2 (1:1,000), COX-1 (1:100), p-p65 (1:1,000), t-p65 (1:1,000), p-p105 (1:1,000), t-p105 (1:1,000), t-IκBα (1:1,000), p-ERK1/2 (1:1,000), t-ERK1/2 (1:1,000), p-p38 (1:1,000), t-p38 (1:1,000), p-JNK (1:1,000), t-JNK (1:1,000), and *β*-actin (1:10,000)] for 2 h at room temperature. After washing, the membranes were incubated with horseradish peroxidase-conjugated anti-rabbit or anti-mouse IgG antibody (1:10,000) for 90 min at room temperature. The ECL Western Blotting Analysis System was used to detect immunoreactivity between the antibodies and blots. Chemiluminescent signals from the membranes were detected using the ImageQuant LAS 4000 mini system.

Immunocytochemistry

Immunocytochemistry was performed as previously described (10). Synovial fibroblasts were seeded at a density of 3×10^5 cells/ml culture medium into a 35-mm glass bottom dish (Iwaki, Tokyo, Japan) treated with IL-1*β*. The cells were fixed with 4% paraformaldehyde (Nacalai Tesque Inc., Kyoto, Japan) for 15 min and processed for immunocytochemistry to examine the intracellular localization of t-p65. The fixed cells were permeabilized by incubation with 0.2% Triton X-100 (Sigma-Aldrich Inc.) for 15 min at room temperature. Non-specific antibody reactions were blocked for 30 min with Block Ace (DS Pharma Biomedical, Osaka, Japan). The cells were then incubated for 90 min at room temperature with anti-t-p65 rabbit antibody [1:200]. After the cells were washed with PBS containing 0.2% polyoxyethylene (20) sorbitan monolaurate, they were incubated and visualized with Alexa Fluor 594-conjugated F(ab′)2 fragments of goat anti-rabbit IgG (H + L) [1:1,000] and TO-PRO-3-iodide [1:1,000] for 60 min in the dark at 25°C. These samples were washed thrice with PBS containing 0.2% polyoxyethylene (20) sorbitan monolaurate, dried, mounted with ProLong Gold Antifade Reagent, and visualized using a confocal laser scanning microscope (LSM-510; Carl Zeiss AG, Oberkochen, Germany). Co-localization analysis was performed using ZEN software (Carl Zeiss AG).

Immunoprecipitation

Total cell lysates (50 μg) were precleared with protein A/G plus Sepharose before incubation with specific antibodies, followed by addition of protein A/G plus Sepharose (10). The total cell lysate was incubated with 20 μg anti-p-p65 or p-pERK1/2 antibody at 4°C for 18 h. The precipitated proteins were dissolved and boiled at 95°C for 5 min in SDS buffer before electrophoresis. Finally, the precipitated proteins were analyzed by western blotting.

Prostaglandin E2 Assay

Synovial fibroblasts were seeded at a density of 3×10^5 cells/well in 6-well culture plates. The cells were stimulated with canine recombinant IL-1β after starvation for 24 h and culture supernatants were collected. To measure culture supernatant prostaglandin E_2 concentrations, we used an enzyme-linked immunosorbent assay kit according to the kit instructions.

siRNA Transfection

Canine synovial fibroblasts, seeded at a density of 1×10^5 cells per 35 mm dish or 5×10^5 cells per 90 mm dish, were transfected using Opti-MEM containing 5 μl per ml of Lipofectamine 2000 and 400 nM of p65, p105, ERK1, ERK2, or scramble siRNAs for 6 h (9, 26). **Table 2** lists siRNA sequences. siRNA efficiency was tested using western blotting with antibodies against t-p65 (1:1,000), t-p105 antibody (1:1,000), and t-ERK1/2 (1:1000).

Statistical Analysis

The data from all experiments have been presented as mean ± standard error of measurement. Statistical analyses were performed using StatMate IV. Data from immunoprecipitation and time-course studies were analyzed using the two-tailed Student's *t*-test and two-way analysis of variance, respectively. Data from other experiments were analyzed using one-way analysis of variance. Tukey's test was used during *post-hoc* analysis. *P*-values less than 0.05 were considered statistically significant.

RESULTS

IL-1β-Induced Secretion of Prostaglandin E_2 *via* Upregulation of COX-2 in Synovial Fibroblasts

We investigated the effect of IL-1β on the release of prostaglandin E_2 and expression of COX in canine synovial fibroblasts. IL-1β (100 pM) induced the time-dependent release of prostaglandin E_2 in synovial fibroblasts (**Figure 1A**). Secretion of prostaglandin E_2 increased with increasing concentrations of IL-1β (**Figure 1B**). Constitutive and inducible isoforms of COX (COX-1 and COX-2, respectively) are rate-limiting enzymes that are involved in the synthesis of prostaglandin E_2 from arachidonic acid (28, 29). IL-1β induced COX-2 mRNA expression in a time- (**Figure 1C**) and dose-dependent manner (**Figure 1D**), but had no effect on the expression of COX-1 (**Figure 1E**). The protein levels of COX-2 increased in IL-1β-treated synovial fibroblasts (**Figures 1F, G**), but those of COX-1 remained unchanged (**Figures 1F, H**). Taken together, IL-1β stimulated the secretion of prostaglandin E_2 *via* upregulated COX-2 expression in canine synovial fibroblasts.

TABLE 2 | Sequences for siRNA transfection.

Gene Name	Gene bank ID	siRNA sequences
p65	XM_014121307.2	GCAUCUCCCUGGUCACCAA
p105	AB183419.1	CUGCAAAGGUUAUUGUUCA
ERK1	NM_001252035.1	CCAATGTGCTCCACCGGGA
ERK2	NM_001110800.1	CCCAAATGCTGACTCGAAA

Role of Canonical NF-κB Signaling in IL-1β-Induced Expression of COX-2

Next, we used NF-κB inhibitors to determine the function of canonical NF-κB signaling in IL-1β-mediated prostaglandin E_2 release and COX-2 mRNA levels in canine synovial fibroblasts. Cells were pretreated with NF-κB inhibitors (10 μM BAY11-7082 or 10 μM TPCA-1) for 1 h and subsequently stimulated with IL-1β (100 pM) for 48 h. The NF-κB inhibitors significantly reduced the mRNA levels of COX-2 (**Figure 2A**) and IL-1β-mediated release of prostaglandin E_2 (**Figure 2B**). These results suggest that NF-κB signaling is involved in the expression of COX-2 and subsequent IL-1β-mediated release of prostaglandin E_2.

Pro-inflammatory cytokines, such as IL-1β, stimulate the phosphorylation of p65 and p105 subunits, which activate the transcriptional function of NF-κB (30–35). Thus, cells treated with IL-1β showed transient phosphorylation of p65 and p105 that reached peak levels at 15 min (**Figure 3A**). IκBα was found to degrade in IL-1β-treated cells in a time-dependent manner (**Figure 3A**). These observations strongly suggest that IL-1β activates NF-κB signaling.

Cells pretreated with NF-κB inhibitors BAY11-7082 or TPCA-1 for 1 h were stimulated using IL-1β for 15 min. Subsequently, we found a significant decrease in the IL-1β-mediated phosphorylation of p65 and p105 (**Figures 3B, C**). Then, we determined the role of p65 and p105 in IL-1β-mediated expression of COX-2. The protein levels of total p65 (t-p65) or p105 (t-p105) decreased significantly in cells transfected with siRNAs targeting p65 or p105 as compared to those in cells transfected with scramble siRNA (**Figures 4A, B**). We also observed that transfection of p65 or p105 siRNA had no effect of the expression of t-p105 or t-p65, respectively (**Figures 4A, B**). Cells depleted of p65 or p105 showed a reduction in IL-1β-induced COX-2 mRNA levels (**Figure 4C**); COX-2 mRNA levels did not significantly differ between cells depleted of p65 and p105. Thus, p65 and p105 play a role in IL-1β-induced expression of COX-2 in synovial fibroblasts.

Role of ERK1/2 Signaling in IL-1β-Induced Expression of COX-2

In mammalian cells, MAPK signaling is important in inflammation. Three MAPK signaling pathways have been characterized: ERK1/2, JNK, and p38 MAPK (36, 37). We investigated the contribution of

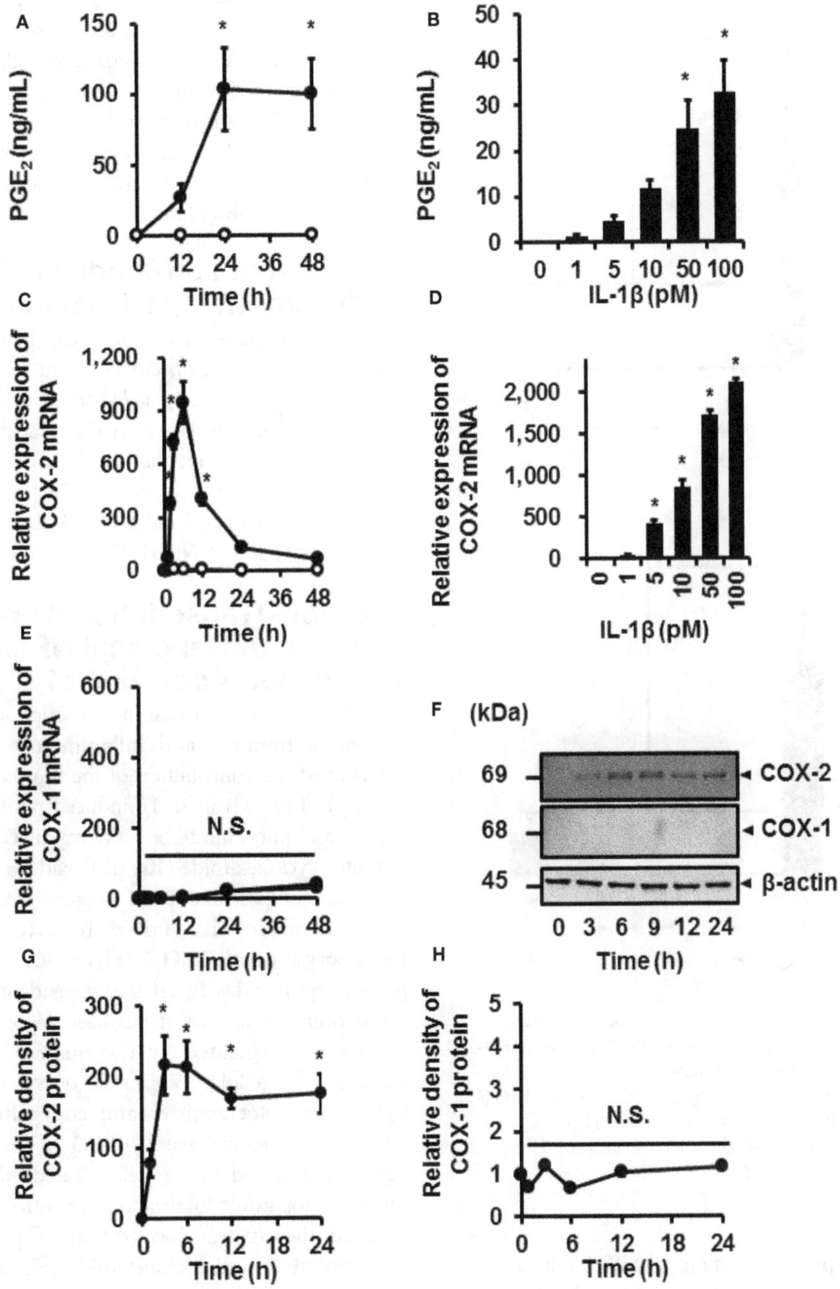

FIGURE 1 | IL-1β-induced prostaglandin E_2 release and COX-2 mRNA and protein levels in canine synovial fibroblasts. Cells treated with (closed circle) or without (open circle) canine recombinant IL-1β (100 pM) showed an increase in prostaglandin E_2 (PGE_2) release **(A)** and COX-2 mRNA levels **(C)** in a time-dependent manner, but did not affect COX-1 mRNA levels **(E)**. Cells were treated with the indicated concentrations of IL-1β for 48 h **(B)** or 6 h **(D)** and assayed for PGE_2 release **(B)** and COX-2 mRNA levels **(D)** in a dose-dependent manner. Cells treated with IL-1β (100 pM) for 0–48 h showed increased protein levels of COX-2 in a time-dependent manner (**F**; first row), but did not affect the protein levels of COX-1 (**F**; second row). The expression of COX-2 **(G)** and COX-1 **(H)** in IL-1β-stimulated cells were compared with the expression at 0 h. Results have been represented as mean ± standard error (SE) from biological triplicates. *$P < 0.05$. Cell lysates (10 μg protein) were used for immunoblotting. β-actin was used as the internal standard (**F**; third row).

MAPK signaling in the IL-1β-induced expression of COX-2 in canine synovial fibroblasts. Inhibitors of ERK1/2 and its upstream regulator MEK, FR180204 (50 μM) and U0126 (20 μM), respectively, decreased the IL-1β-induced expression of COX-2 (**Figure 5A**). However, inhibitors of JNK and p38, SP600125 (10 μM) and SKF86002 (10 μM), respectively did not significantly alter COX-2 mRNA levels. Inhibition of MEK or ERK reduced the IL-1β-induced release of prostaglandin E_2 (**Figure 5B**).

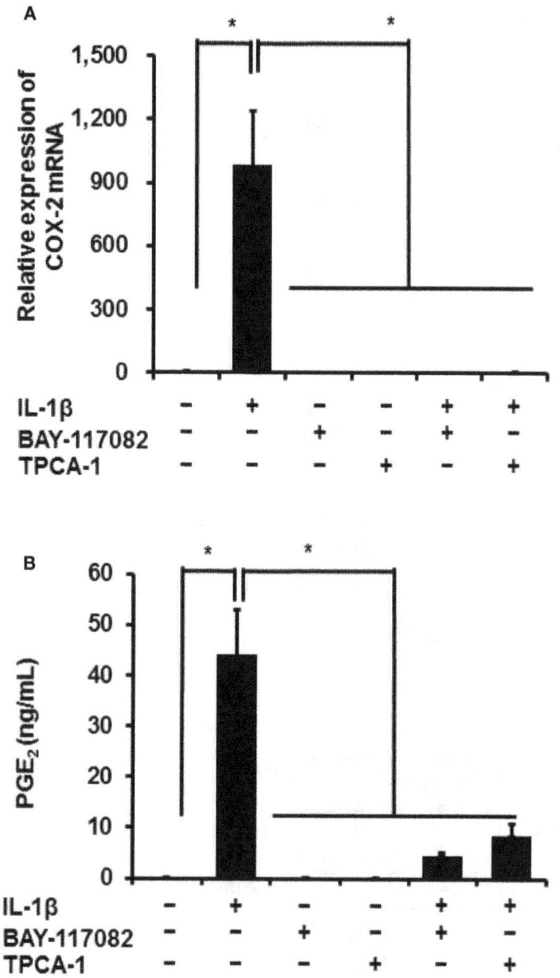

FIGURE 2 | Effect of NF-κB inhibitors on IL-1β-induced COX-2 expression. Synovial fibroblasts were pretreated with or without the NF-κB inhibitors BAY11-7082 (10 μM) and TPCA-1 (10 μM), for 1 h and subsequently stimulated with IL-1β (100 pM). After stimulation for 6 or 48 h, we analyzed COX-2 mRNA levels **(A)** and prostaglandin E_2 release **(B)**. The inhibitors decreased IL-1β-induced COX-2 expression and prostaglandin E_2 release. Results have been represented as mean ± SE from biological triplicates. $^*P < 0.05$.

IL-1β stimulated the phosphorylation of ERK1/2 in a time-dependent manner. However, the phosphorylation levels of p38 MAPK and JNK remained unchanged. Phosphorylation reached a peak 15 min after IL-1β stimulation (**Figure 6A**). Cells pretreated with MEK and ERK inhibitors showed a reduction in IL-1β-induced phosphorylation of ERK1/2 (**Figures 6B, C**). These results suggest that MEK/ERK1/2 signaling axes are dominantly involved in the IL-1β-induced expression of COX-2 in canine synovial fibroblasts. To confirm the role of ERK1/2 in IL-1β-induced COX-2 expression, we used siRNAs against ERK1 or ERK2 in the fibroblasts. We observed significant decreases in the ERK1 or ERK2 protein levels as compared to cells transfected with scramble siRNA (**Figures 7A, B**). We also observed that transfection of ERK1 or ERK2 siRNA had no effect of the expression of t-ERK2 or t-ERK1, respectively (**Figures 7A, B**). IL-1β-induced expression of COX-2 was attenuated in cells transfected with siRNAs for ERK1 or ERK2 as compared to mRNA levels of COX-2 in scramble siRNA-transfected cells (**Figure 7C**). The extent of reduction in the mRNA levels of IL-1β-induced COX-2 was similar in cells transfected with siRNAs targeting either ERK1 or ERK2 (**Figure 7C**). Taken together, our data indicate that ERK1/2 signaling is involved in the IL-1β-induced expression of COX-2 in canine synovial fibroblasts.

Inhibition of IL-1β-Induced ERK1/2 Activation Using NF-κB Inhibitors

Next, we determined the relationship between NF-κB and MEK/ERK signaling. In cells pretreated with NF-κB inhibitors, BAY 11-7082 and TPCA-1, IL-1β failed to induce the phosphorylation of ERK1/2, but had no effect on the total protein levels of ERK1/2 (**Figure 8A**). However, the use of MEK and ERK1/2 inhibitors, U0126 and FR180204, respectively, had no effect on IL-1β-induced phosphorylation of p65 and p105 (**Figure 8B**). These results suggest that the activation of NF-κB is pivotal for ERK1/2 signaling.

The Non-Transcriptional and Translational Function of Canonical NF-κB Regulates IL-1β-Induced Activation of ERK1/2

NF-κB plays a crucial role in transcriptionally and translationally regulating immune and inflammatory responses (5, 6). We determined the contribution of the transcriptional or translational function of NF-κB in IL-1β-induced phosphorylation of ERK1/2. The transcription inhibitor actinomycin D (1 μM) and translation inhibitor cycloheximide (100 μM) had no effect on IL-1β-induced activation of p65 and p105 (**Figure 9A**). Actinomycin D and cycloheximide also failed to attenuate IL-1β-induced phosphorylation of ERK1/2 (**Figure 9A**), suggesting that ERK1/2 phosphorylation by IL-1β is independent of transcriptional and translational regulation. It has been reported that the function of NF-κB was regulated by the nuclear localization. Then, we examined the cellular localization of NF-κB in IL-1β-treated cells by immunocytochemistry and co-localization analysis with a nucleic acid staining dye TO-PRO-3. The nuclear localization of p65 was observed in the cells treated with IL-1β, whereas p65 showed cytoplasmic localization in control cells (**Figure 9B**). IL-1β induced the nuclear localization of p65 in the presence of actinomycin D and cycloheximide (**Figure 9B**), suggesting that NF-κB acts as a transcription factor even in the presence of the inhibitors for transcription and translation.

To confirm the importance of NF-κB in the activation of ERK1/2, we depleted cells of p65 or p105 to observe a reduction in IL-1β-induced phosphorylation of ERK1/2 (**Figure 9C**). Then, we investigated the mechanism of the interaction between activated NF-κB and phosphorylated ERK1/2. As shown in **Figure 9D**, we detected that the levels of phosphorylated p65 or ERK1/2 in the fraction precipitated with anti-phosphorylated p65 or anti-phosphorylated ERK1/2, respectively, were increased. We observed that the levels of phosphorylated ERK1/2 in the fraction precipitated with anti-phosphorylated p65 increased in the cells treated with IL-1β. The increase in phosphorylated p65 in the fraction precipitated

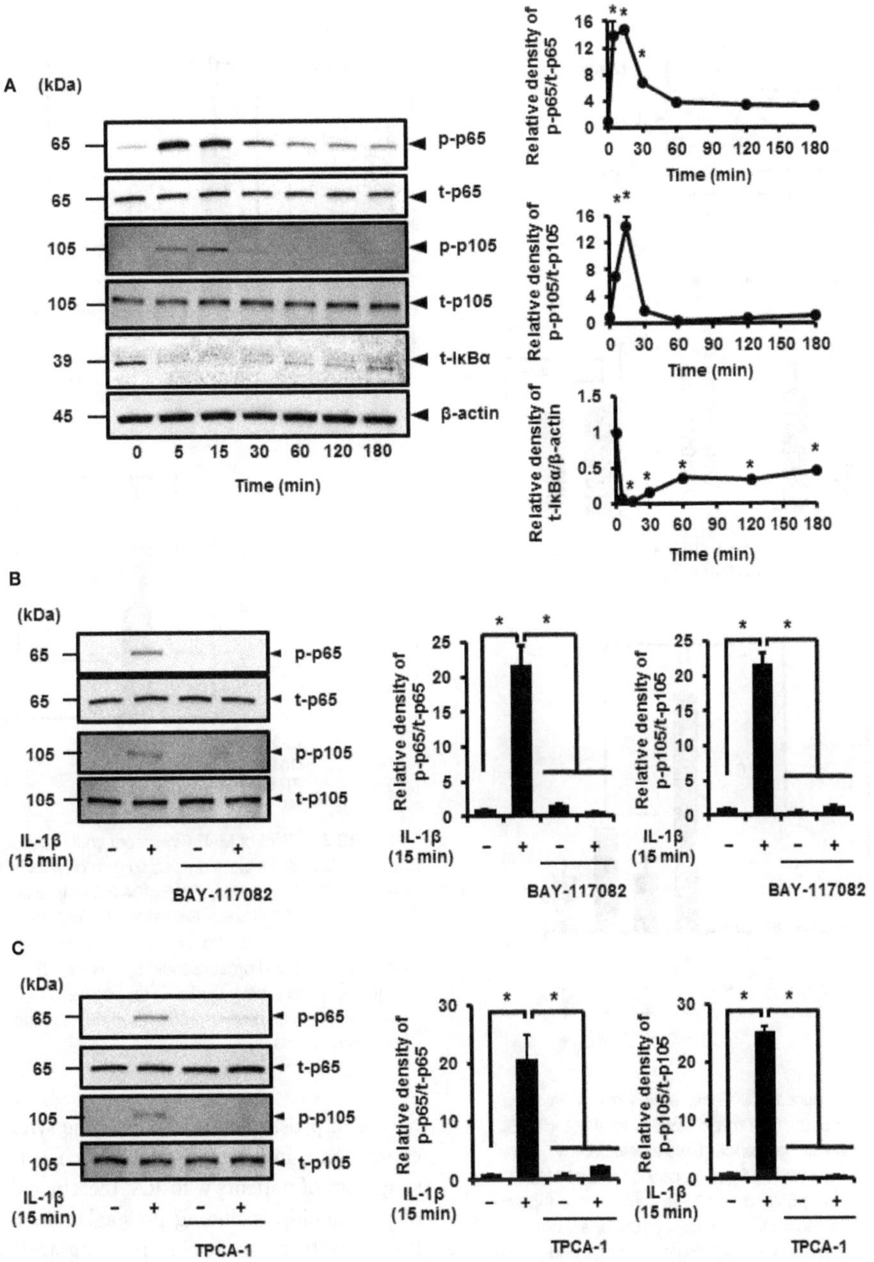

FIGURE 3 | IL-1β-induced activation of NF-κB signaling. **(A)** Western blotting for, the levels of phosphorylated p65 (p-p65), total p65 (t-p65), phosphorylated p105 (p-p105), total p105 (t-p105), and total IκBα (t-IκBα) in cells treated with IL-1β (100 pM). Relative expression of p-p65, p-p105, and t-IκBα as compared to the levels at 0 h (right panel). **(B, C)** Cells were pretreated with or without the NF-κB inhibitors BAY11-7082 (10 μM; **B**) and TPCA-1 (10 μM; **C**) for 1 h followed by stimulation with IL-1β for 15 min. The inhibitors reduced IL-1β-induced phosphorylation of p65 and p105. Relative levels of p-p65 and p-p105 compared with those in the absence of IL-1β (right panel). Results have been represented as mean ± SE from biological triplicates. *$P < 0.05$. For the immunoblotting, cell lysates (10 μg protein) were used for immunoblotting. β-actin was used as the internal standard **(A)**.

with anti-phosphorylated ERK1/2 was also detected (**Figure 9D**). Regarding the density of the IgG heavy chain (HC) band, there is no significant difference between control and the IL-1β-treated cells. These results suggest that the complex formation of activated NF-κB and phosphorylated ERK1/2 is induced by IL-1β. We further investigated whether phosphorylated p65 and phosphorylated ERK1/2 form a complex with phosphorylated MEK as an upstream regulator of ERK1/2. As shown in **Figure 9D**, we observed that the levels of phosphorylated MEK increased in the fraction precipitated with anti-phosphorylated p65 and ERK1/2, suggesting that phosphorylated MEK also forms a complex with NF-κB and ERK1/2 in the cells treated with IL-1β.

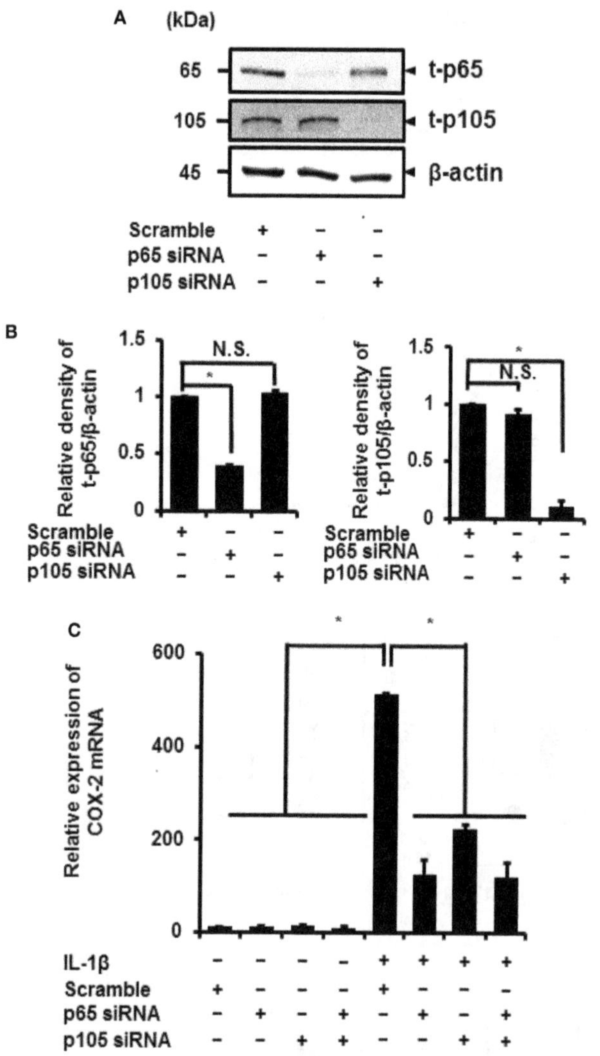

FIGURE 4 | Inhibition of IL-1β-induced COX-2 expression in synovial fibroblasts depleted of p65 and p105. **(A)** Protein levels of total p65 (t-p65), total p105 (t-p105), and β-actin (internal standard) were detected by immunoblotting in cells transfected with p65, p105, or scramble siRNAs (control). **(B)** The relative levels of t-p65 and t-p105 as compared to the levels in the control samples. **(C)** Cells transfected with p65, p105, or scramble siRNAs were stimulated with IL-1β for 6 h. Depleting cells of p65 and p105 inhibited IL-1β-induced COX-2 expression. Results have been represented as mean ± SE from biological triplicates. *$P < 0.05$. Cell lysates (10 µg protein) were used for immunoblotting.

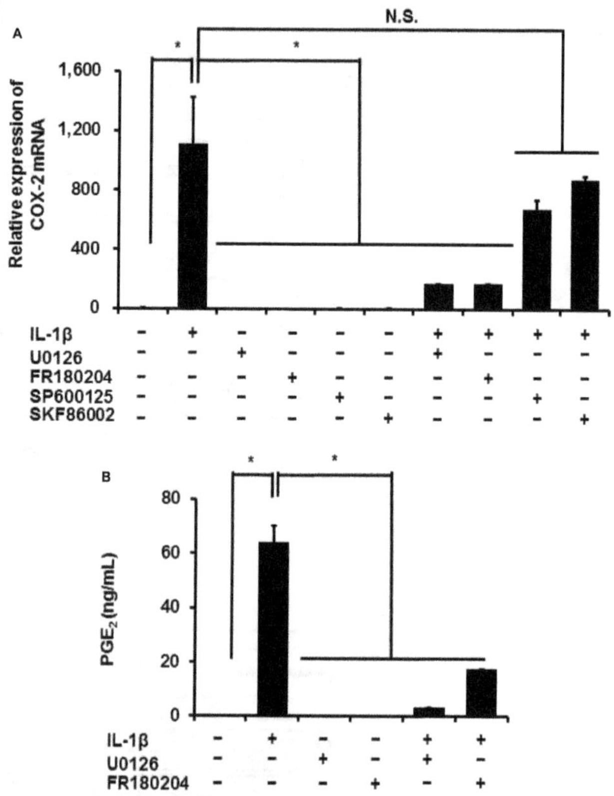

FIGURE 5 | Effect of MAPK inhibitors on IL-1β-induced COX-2 expression. Synovial fibroblasts were pretreated with or without the MEK inhibitor U0126 (20 µM), ERK1/2 inhibitor FR180204 (50 µM), JNK inhibitor SP600125 (10 µM), and p38 inhibitor SKF86002 (10 µM) for 1 h and subsequently stimulated with IL-1β. After stimulation for 6 h or 48 h, we determined COX-2 expression **(A)** and prostaglandin E_2 release **(B)**. IL-1β-induced COX-2 expression and prostaglandin E_2 release were significantly reduced by the inhibitors. Results have been represented as mean ± SE from biological triplicates. *$P < 0.05$.

Based on these results, we propose a model of atypical role of NF-κB signaling in the ERK1/2 regulation *via* the complex formation of NF-κB/MEK/ERK (**Figure 10**).

DISCUSSION

In this study, we have demonstrated that pro-inflammatory cytokine IL-1β-induced expression of COX-2 mediated the release of prostaglandin E_2 in canine synovial fibroblasts. COX-2 expression is induced by stimuli, such as IL-1β and TNF-α, in the synovium of patients with RA, thereby enhancing the production of prostanoids, including prostaglandin E_2, that are involved in inflammation. Synovial prostaglandin E_2 results in the manifestation of various pathological symptoms, including bone/cartilage degradation, inhibition of matrix synthesis, general discomfort, and body weight loss (38, 39). These studies suggest that the expression of COX-2 in the synovium plays a crucial role in the pathogenesis of RA *via* the synthesis of prostaglandins.

The NF-κB/p65/p105 axis was involved in IL-1β-mediated expression of COX-2 in synovial fibroblasts. NF-κB is a transcription factor important for the regulation of a wide range of target genes involved in physiological and pathological processes. The NF-κB family of proteins comprises five members: p65 (RelA), RelB, c-Rel, p50, and p52, that interact with each other to form homo- or heterodimers with distinct functions. Furthermore, NF-κB signaling can be classified into canonical and

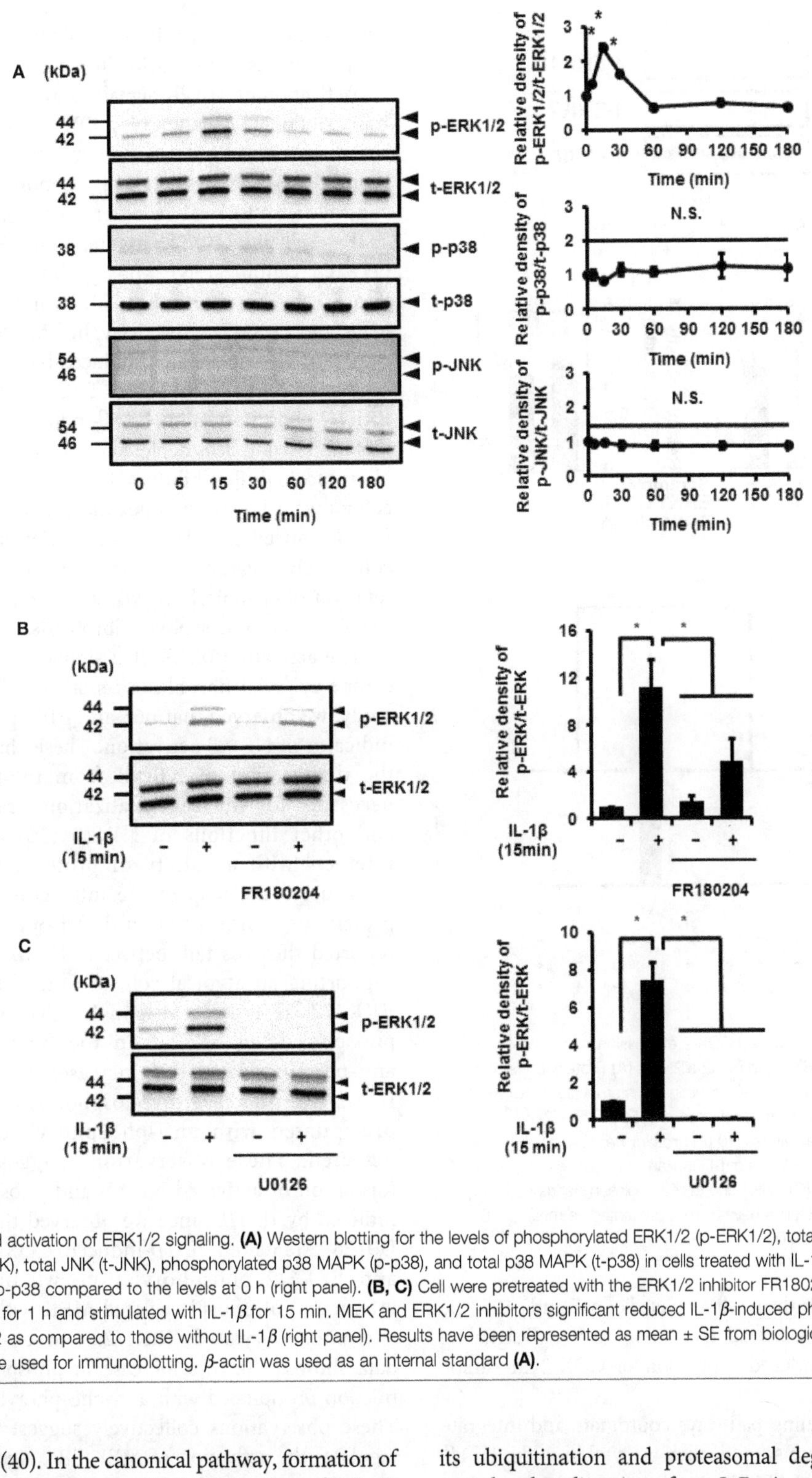

FIGURE 6 | IL-1β-induced activation of ERK1/2 signaling. **(A)** Western blotting for the levels of phosphorylated ERK1/2 (p-ERK1/2), total ERK1/2 (t-ERK1/2), phosphorylated JNK (p-JNK), total JNK (t-JNK), phosphorylated p38 MAPK (p-p38), and total p38 MAPK (t-p38) in cells treated with IL-1β (100 pM). Relative levels of p-ERK1/2, p-JNK, and p-p38 compared to the levels at 0 h (right panel). **(B, C)** Cell were pretreated with the ERK1/2 inhibitor FR180204 (50 μM; **B**) and MEK inhibitor U0126 (20 μM; C) for 1 h and stimulated with IL-1β for 15 min. MEK and ERK1/2 inhibitors significant reduced IL-1β-induced phosphorylation of ERK1/2. Relative levels of p-ERK1/2 as compared to those without IL-1β (right panel). Results have been represented as mean ± SE from biological triplicates. $^{*}P < 0.05$. Cell lysates (10 μg protein) were used for immunoblotting. β-actin was used as an internal standard **(A)**.

noncanonical signaling (40). In the canonical pathway, formation of the p50/p65 heterodimer is a key step in the activation of NF-κB (41, 42). In resting cells, p50 and p65 form an inactive complex with the inhibitory protein IκBα. IκB kinase is activated by exogenous signals, such as IL-1β, that phosphorylates IκBα, thereby inducing its ubiquitination and proteasomal degradation. The p50/p65 complex that dissociates from IκBα is transcriptionally active and induces the expression of the target genes of NF-κB (40). In this study, selective inhibitors of NF-κB, BAY11-7082, and TPCA-1 reduced IL-1β-mediated COX-2 expression. The expression of

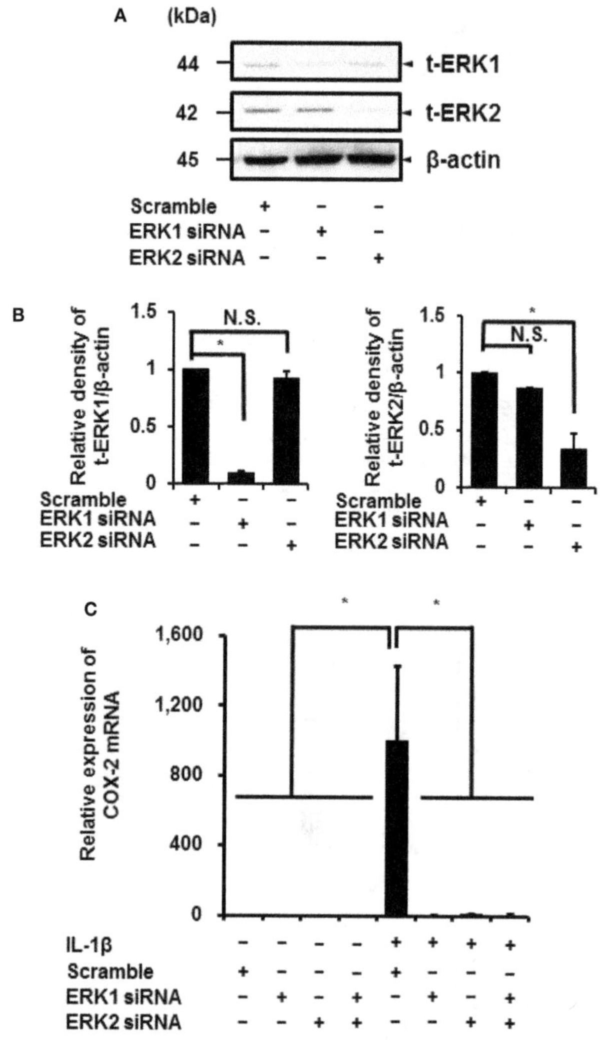

FIGURE 7 | Inhibition of IL-1β-induced COX-2 expression in synovial fibroblasts transfected with ERK1 and ERK2 siRNAs. **(A)** Protein levels of total ERK1 (t-ERK1), total ERK2 (t-ERK2), and β-actin (an internal standard) were detected by immunoblotting in cells transfected with ERK1, ERK2, or scramble siRNAs (control). Cell lysates (10 µg protein) were used for immunoblotting. **(B)** The relative levels of t-ERK1 and t-ERK2 as compared to the levels in the control cells. **(C)** ERK1 and ERK2 depletion decreased IL-1β-induced COX-2 expression. Results have been represented as mean ± SE from biological triplicates. $^{*}P < 0.05$.

COX-2 decreased significantly in cells depleted of p65 and p105 (the precursor of p50). Thus, the activation of canonical NF-κB signaling is important for IL-1β-induced expression of COX-2 in canine synovial fibroblasts.

Multiple MAPK signaling pathways coordinate and integrate cellular response to diverse stimuli, such as cytokines like IL-1β. However, the activation of MAPK signaling is highly dependent on cellular context. In this study, we have demonstrated that pharmacological inhibition of MEK and ERK1/2 drastically reduced IL-1β-induced COX-2 expression and prostaglandin E_2 release; IL-1β induced the activation of MEK/ERK1/2. Taken together, these results suggest that the activation of MEK/ERK1/2 signaling plays a crucial role in COX-2 expression and prostaglandin E_2 release in synovial fibroblasts that is important in the pathogenesis of synovitis in patients with RA.

Activation of MAPK signaling stimulates NF-κB that induces transcriptional regulation (43). ERK1/2 activates canonical NF-κB signaling in rat vascular smooth muscle cells that regulates IL-1β-induced gene expression (18). Canonical NF-κB signaling is controlled by ERK1/2 in other cells, *e.g.*, the human monocyte THP-1 cell line (20). Therefore, we investigated the interaction between canonical NF-κB signaling and ERK1/2 activation. Surprisingly, we found that U0126 and FR180204, inhibitors of MEK and ERK1/2, respectively, had no effect on the activation of canonical NF-κB signaling induced by IL-1β. In contrast, NF-κB inhibitors BAY 11-7082 and TPCA-1 inhibited IL-1β-induced ERK1/2 phosphorylation. IL-1β-induced ERK1/2 phosphorylation was inhibited in cells depleted of p65 and p105. Furthermore, the pharmacological inhibitors for transcription and translation, actinomycin D and cycloheximide, respectively, failed to inhibit IL-1β-induced ERK1/2 phosphorylation. These observations collectively suggest that the non-transcriptional/translational function of canonical NF-κB regulates the activation of ERK1/2 signaling in canine synovial fibroblasts.

The activation of ERK1/2 signaling by canonical NF-κB in canine synovial fibroblasts remains to be understood. In this study, we observed that p65 and p105 phosphorylation was an indicator of NF-κB activation. These changes are attributed to the dissociation of NF-κB from inhibitory IκBα and are necessary for nuclear localization, transcriptional activity, and other functions of NF-κB (38). Furthermore, NF-κB interacts with a variety of proteins (44, 45). Tieri et al. constructed the map of the interactome of NF-κB based on protein–protein interaction data from multiple databases and reported the crosstalk between NF-κB and MAPK signaling, supporting an atypical role of canonical NF-κB signaling in ERK1/2 activation (45). In this study, the level of phosphorylated ERK1/2 in the fraction precipitated with anti-phosphorylated p65 increased in the cells treated with IL-1β. The increase in phosphorylated p65 in the fraction precipitated with anti-phosphorylated ERK1/2 was also detected. These observations suggest that the complex formation of activated NF-κB and phosphorylated ERK1/2 is induced by IL-1β. Since we observed that the MEK inhibitor U0126 attenuated IL-1β-induced COX-2 mRNA expression and ERK1/2 phosphorylation, we further examined the interaction of phosphorylated MEK with phosphorylated p65 and phosphorylated ERK1/2. Our co-immunoprecipitation data showed that the increase in phosphorylated MEK in the fraction precipitated with anti-phosphorylated p65 and ERK1/2. These observations collectively suggest that NF-κB signaling regulates the activation of MEK/ERK signaling *via* the complex formation of NF-κB/MEK/ERK. Since the molecular feature of the NF-κB/MEK/ERK complex has been unclear, the detection of other components of NF-κB/MEK/ERK complex is currently underway in our laboratory. In addition, to confirm whether our proposed model is ubiquitously existed, studies targeting the atypical role of

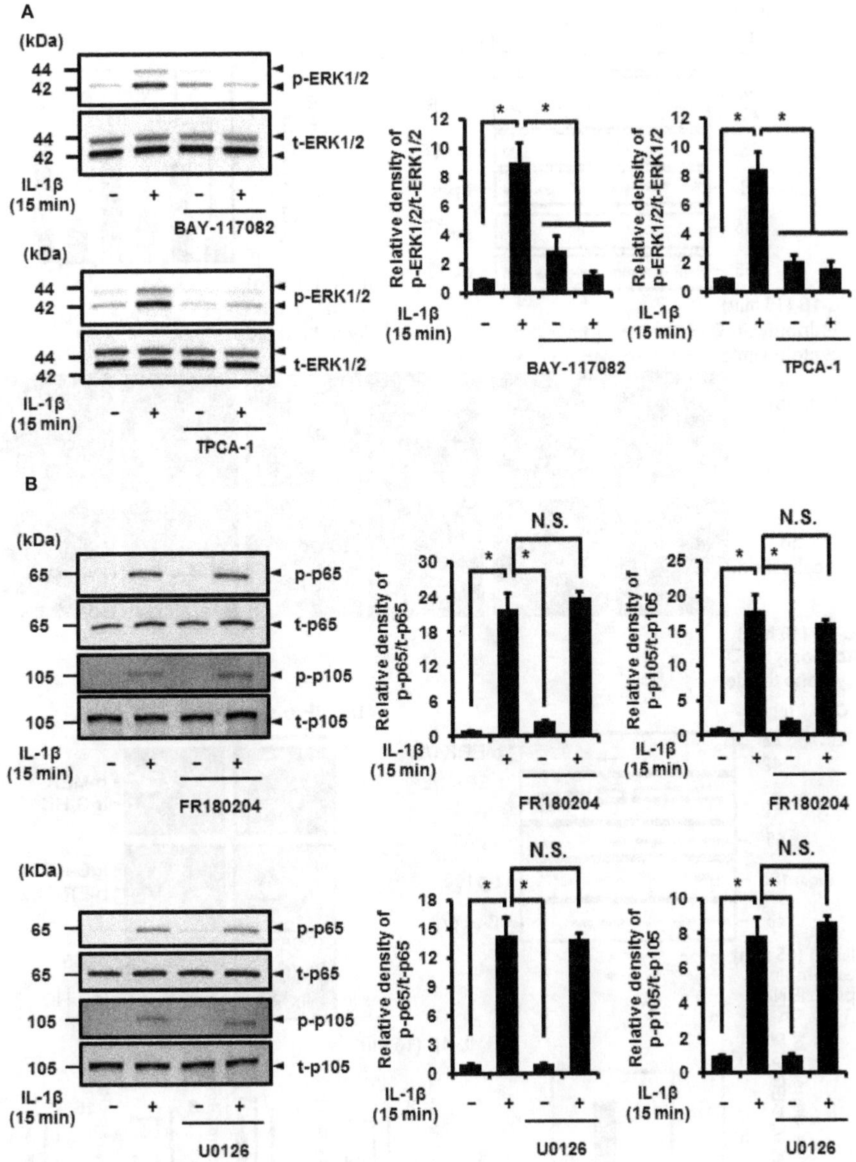

FIGURE 8 | Effect of NF-κB inhibitors on IL-1β-induced phosphorylation of ERK1/2. **(A)** Cells were pretreated with the NF-κB inhibitors BAY11-7082 (10 μM) and TPCA-1 (10 μM) for 1 h and stimulated with IL-1β for 15 min. NF-κB inhibitors significantly reduced IL-1β-induced phosphorylation of ERK1/2 as compared to phosphorylation in the absence of IL-1β. Representative blots and relative levels of p- and t-ERK1/2 have been illustrated in the left and right panels, respectively. **(B, C)** Cells were pretreated with the ERK1/2 inhibitor FR180204 (50 μM; **B**) and MEK inhibitor U0126 (20 μM; C) for 1 h followed by stimulation with IL-1β for 15 min. ERK1/2 and MEK inhibitors had no effect on IL-1β-induced phosphorylation of p65 and p105. Cell lysates (10 μg protein) were used for immunoblotting. Representative blots and relative levels of p- and t-p65 and p105 have been shown in the left and right panels, respectively. (Right) Results have been represented as mean ± SE from biological triplicates. *$P < 0.05$.

NF-κB signaling in the ERK1/2 regulation in several types of cells is indeed our next research subject.

In conclusion, we demonstrated that 1) canonical NF-κB signaling contributes to IL-1β-induced COX-2 expression and subsequent prostaglandin E_2 release in canine synovial fibroblasts, and 2) the activation of canonical NF-κB signaling non-transcriptionally and non-translationally activates ERK1/2 signaling. Based on our study findings, we propose a model highlighting the importance of IL-1β-induced NF-κB/ERK1/2/COX-2 signaling in canine synovial fibroblasts (**Figure 9C**). The atypical role of canonical NF-κB signaling in IL-1β-induced ERK1/2 activation may serve as promising molecular targets for the development of therapeutics in treating patients with RA and synovitis.

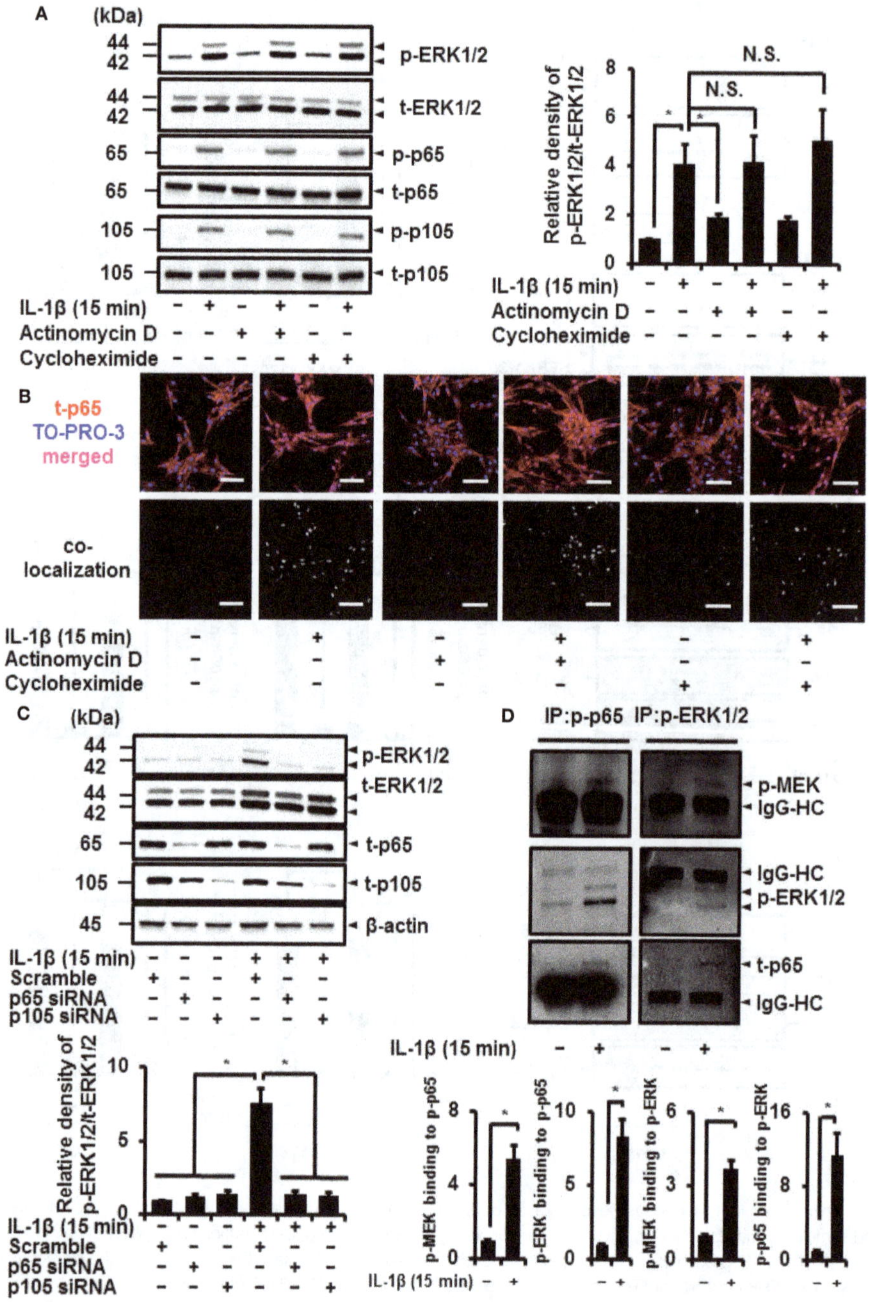

FIGURE 9 | Canonical NF-κB signaling non-transcriptionally and non-translationally regulates IL-1*β*-induced ERK1/2 activation. **(A)** Cells were pretreated with the transcription inhibitor actinomycin D (Act D; 1 μM) and translation inhibitor cycloheximide (CHX; 100 μM) for 6 h and stimulated with IL-1*β* for 15 min. ActD and CHX had no effect on IL-1*β*-induced phosphorylation of ERK1/2, p65 and p105. Representative blots and relative levels of p- and t-ERK1/2, p65 and p105 have been illustrated in the left and right panels, respectively. **(B)** Cells were pretreated with the transcription inhibitor actinomycin D (Act D; 1 μM) and translation inhibitor cycloheximide (CHX; 100 μM) for 6 h and stimulated with IL-1*β* for 15 min. Subsequently, immunocytochemistry and co-localization analysis with nuclear staining dye TO-PRO-3 were performed. The nuclear localization of t-p65 was detected in the cells treated with IL-1*β*, whereas t-p65 showed cytoplasmic localization in control cells. IL-1*β* induced the nuclear localization of t-p65 in the presence of actinomycin D and cycloheximide. **(C)** Western blotting for the levels of p-ERK1/2, t-ERK1/2, t-p65 and t-p105 in cells transfected p65, p105, or scramble siRNAs. Decreased IL-1*β*-induced phosphorylation of ERK1/2 was observed in p65 or p105 siRNA-transfected cells. Representative blots for the levels of p-ERK1/2, t-ERK1/2, t-p65, and t-p105 and relative expression of p-ERK1/2 have been compared with the levels in cells transfected with scramble siRNA in the left and right panels, respectively. Results have been represented as mean ± SE from biological triplicates. *$P < 0.05$. Cell lysates (10 μg protein) were used for immunoblotting. *β*-actin was used as an internal standard **(C)**. **(D)** Western blotting for the levels of p-MEK, p-ERK1/2 and p-p65 in the fraction precipitated with p-p65 and p-ERK1/2. Results have been represented as mean ± SE from biological triplicates. *$P < 0.05$. Cell lysates (50 μg protein) were used for co-immunoprecipitation experiments. IgG-heavy chain (IgG-HC) was used as an internal standard **(D)**.

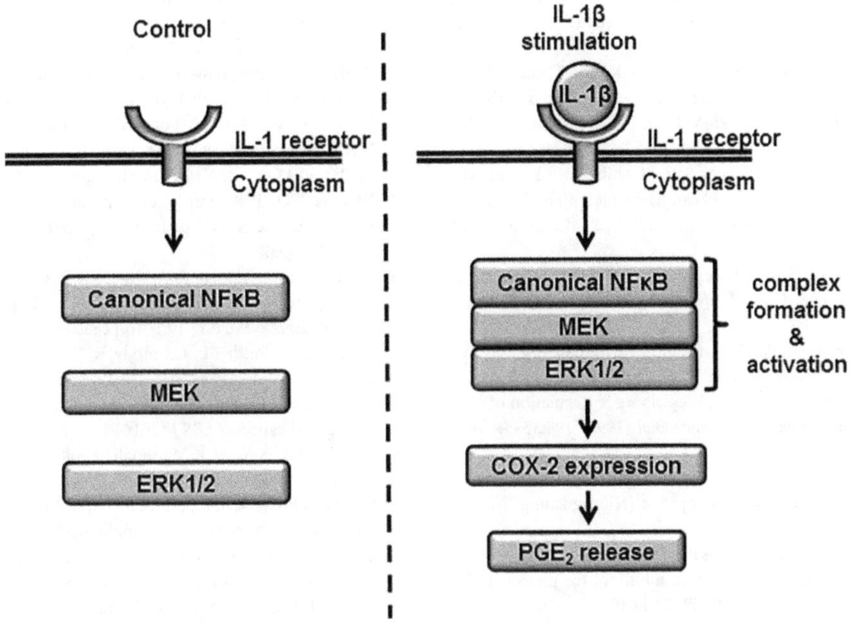

FIGURE 10 | The proposed model highlighting atypical role of NF-κB signaling in the ERK1/2 regulation *via* the complex formation of NF-κB/MEK/ERK in IL-1β-treated synovial fibroblasts. When the cells were stimulated with IL-1β, the complex formation of NF-κB/MEK/ERK was induced, which promoted the activation of ERK1/2, the expression of COX-2 and prostaglandin E_2 synthesis.

AUTHOR CONTRIBUTIONS

RN and HS designed and planned the experiments. RN, TKi, SN, NK, and YS prepared and measured samples. RN, TKi, SN, NK, YS, and TKo analyzed the data. RN, JY, TN, and HS interpreted the data and wrote the paper. All authors contributed to the article and approved the submitted version.

from the Ministry of Education, Science, Sports, and Culture of Japan (https://www.jsps.go.jp/j-grantsinaid/). The funders had no role in the study design, data collection and analysis, decision to publish, or preparation of the manuscript.

ACKNOWLEDGMENTS

We would like to thank Editage (www.editage.jp) for English language editing.

REFERENCES

1. Iwakura Y. Roles of IL-1 in the development of rheumatoid arthritis: consideration from mouse models. *Cytokine Growth Factor Rev* (2002) 13:341–55. doi: 10.1016/S1359-6101(02)00021-7
2. Ruscitti P, Cipriani P, Liakouli V, Carubbi F, Berardicurti O, Di Benedetto P, et al. The Emerging Role of IL-1 Inhibition in Patients Affected by Rheumatoid Arthritis and Diabetes. *Rev Recent Clin Trials* (2018) 13:210–4. doi: 10.2174/1574887113666180314102651
3. Gabay C, Lamacchia C, Palmer G. IL-1 pathways in inflammation and human diseases. *Nat Rev Rheumatol* (2010) 6:232–41. doi: 10.1038/nrrheum.2010.4
4. Gabay C. IL-1 inhibitors: novel agents in the treatment of rheumatoid arthritis. *Expert Opin Investig Drugs* (2000) 9:113–27. doi: 10.1517/13543784.9.1.113
5. Lawrence T. The nuclear factor NF-κB pathway in inflammation. *Cold Spring Harbor Pespect Biol* (2009) 1:a001651. doi: 10.1101/cshperspect.a001651
6. Hayden MS, Ghosh S. NF-κB, the first quarter-century: remarkable progress and outstanding questions. *Genes Dev* (2012) 26:203–34. doi: 10.1101/gad.183434.111
7. Tsuchiya H, Nakano R, Konno T, Okabayashi K, Narita T, Sugiya H. Activation of MEK/ERK pathways through NF-κB activation is involved in interleukin-1β-induced cyclooxygenase-2 expression in canine dermal fibroblasts. *Vet Immunol Immunopathol* (2015) 168:223–32. doi: 10.1016/j.vetimm.2015.10.003
8. Kitanaka T, Nakano R, Kitanaka N, Kimura T, Okabayashi K, Narita T, et al. JNK activation is essential for activation of MEK/ERK signaling in IL-1β-induced COX-2 expression in synovial fibroblasts. *Sci Rep* (2017) 7:39914. doi: 10.1038/srep39914
9. Namba S, Nakano R, Kitanaka T, Kitanaka N, Nakayama T, Sugiya H. ERK2 and JNK1 contribute to TNF-α-induced IL-8 expression in synovial fibroblasts. *PloS One* (2017) 12:e0182923. doi: 10.1371/journal.pone.0182923
10. Nakano R, Kitanaka T, Namba S, Kitanaka N, Sugiya H. Protein kinase Cε regulates nuclear translocation of extracellular signal-regulated kinase, which contributes to bradykinin-induced cyclooxygenase-2 expression. *Sci Rep* (2018) 8:8535. doi: 10.1038/s41598-018-26473-7

11. Kitanaka N, Nakano R, Sugiura K, Kitanaka T, Namba S, Konno T, et al. Interleukin-1β promotes interleulin-6 expression via ERK1/2 signaling pathway in canine dermal fibroblasts. *PloS One* (2019) 14:e0220262. doi: 10.1371/journal.pone.0220262
12. Kitanaka N, Nakano R, Sakai M, Kitanaka T, Namba S, Konno T, et al. ERK1/ATF-2 signaling axis contributes to interleukin-1β-induced MMP-3 expression in dermal fibroblasts. *PloS One* (2019) 14:e0222869. doi: 10.1371/journal.pone.0222869
13. Nakano R, Kitanaka T, Namba S, Kitanaka N, Sato M, Shibukawa Y, et al. All-trans retinoic acid induces reprogramming of canine dedifferentiated cells into neuron-like cells. *PloS One* (2020) 15:e0229892. doi: 10.1371/journal.pone.0229892
14. Imajo M, Tsuchiya Y, Nishida E. Regulatory mechanisms and functions of MAP kinase signaling pathways. *IUBMB Life* (2006) 58:312–7. doi: 10.1080/15216540600746393
15. Kim EK, Choi EJ. Compromised MAPK signaling in human diseases: an update. *Arch Toxicol* (2015) 89:867–82. doi: 10.1007/s00204-015-1472-2
16. Schulze-Osthoff K, Ferrari D, Riehemann K, Wesselborg S. Regulation of NF-κB activation by MAP kinase cascades. *Immunobiol* (1997) 198:35–49. doi: 10.1016/S0171-2985(97)80025-3
17. De Smaele E, Zazzeroni F, Papa S, Nguyen DU, Jin R, Jones J, et al. Induction of *gadd*45β by NF-κB downregulates pro-apoptotic JNK signalling. *Nature* (2001) 414:308–13. doi: 10.1038/35104560
18. García-García E, Sánchez-Mejorada G, Rosales C. Phosphatidylinositol 3-kinase and ERK are required for NF-κB activation but not for phagocytosis. *J Leukoc Biol* (2001) 70:649–58. doi: 10.1189/jlb.70.4.649
19. Vermeulen L, De Wilde G, Van Damme P, Vanden Berghe W, Haegeman G. Transcriptional activation of the NF-κB p65 subunit by mitogen- and stress-activated protein kinase-1 (MSK1). *EMBO J* (2003) 22:1313–24. doi: 10.1093/emboj/cdg139
20. Jiang B, Xu S, Hou X, Pimentel DR, Brecher P, Cohen RA. Temporal control of NF-κB activation by ERK differentially regulates interleukin-1β-induced gene expression. *J Biol Chem* (2004) 279:1323–9. doi: 10.1074/jbc.M307521200
21. Kim JH, Na HK, Pak YK, Lee YS, Lee SJ, Moon A, et al. Roles of ERK and p38 mitogen-activated protein kinases in phorbol ester-induced NF-κB activation and COX-2 expression in human breast epithelial cells. *Chem Biol Interact* (2008) 171:133–41. doi: 10.1016/j.cbi.2007.07.008
22. Nakano R, Edamura K, Sugiya H, Narita T, Okabayashi K, Moritomo T, et al. Evaluation of mRNA expression levels and electrophysiological function of neuron-like cells derived from canine bone marrow stromal cells. *Am J Vet Res* (2013) 74:1311–20. doi: 10.2460/ajvr.74.10.1311
23. Nakano R, Edamura K, Nakayama T, Teshima K, Asano K, Narita T, et al. Differentiation of canine bone marrow stromal cells into voltage- and glutamate-responsive neuron-like cells by basic fibroblast growth factor. *J Vet Med Sci* (2015) 77:27–35. doi: 10.1292/jvms.14-0284
24. Nakano R, Edamura K, Nakayama T, Narita T, Okabayashi K, Sugiya H. Fibroblast growth factor receptor-2 contributes to the basic fibroblast growth factor-induced neuronal differentiation in canine bone marrow stromal cells via phosphoinositide 3-kinase/Akt signaling pathway. *PloS One* (2015) 10: e0141581. doi: 10.1371/journal.pone.0141581
25. Konno T, Nakano R, Mamiya R, Tsuchiya H, Kitanaka T, Namba S, et al. Expression and function of interleukin-1β-induced neutrophil gelatinase-associated lipocalin in renal tubular cells. *PloS One* (2016) 11:e0166707. doi: 10.1371/journal.pone.0166707
26. Kitanaka N, Nakano R, Kitanaka T, Kitanaka N, Namba S, Konno T, et al. NF-κB p65 and p105 implicate in interleukin 1β-mediated COX-2 expression in melanoma cells. *PloS One* (2018) 13:e0208955. doi: 10.1371/journal.pone.0208955
27. Bradford MM. A rapid and sensitive method for the quantitation of microgram quantities of protein utilizing the principle of protein-dye binding. *Anal Biochem* (1976) 72:248–54. doi: 10.1016/0003-2697(76)90527-3
28. Smith WL, DeWit DL, Garavito RM. Cyclooxygeneses: structural, cellular, and molecular biology. *Annu Rev Biochem* (2000) 69:145–82. doi: 10.1146/annurev.biochem.69.1.145
29. Simmons DL, Botting RM, Hla T. Cyclooxygenese isozymes: the biology of prostaglandin synthesis and inhibition. *Pharmacol Rev* (2004) 56:387–437. doi: 10.1124/pr.56.3.3
30. Vermeulen L, De Wilde G, Notebaert S, Vanden Berghe W, Haegeman G. Regulation of the transcriptional activity of the NF-κB p65 subunit. *Biochem Pharmacol* (2002) 64:963–70. doi: 10.1016/S0006-2952(02)01161-9
31. Viatour P, Merville MP, Bours V, Chariot A. Phosphorylation of NF-κB and IκB proteins: implications in cancer and inflammation. *Trends Biochem Sci* (2005) 30:43–52. doi: 10.1016/j.tibs.2004.11.009
32. Perkins ND. Post-translational modifications regulating the activity and function of the NF-κB pathway. *Oncogene* (2006) 25:6717–30. doi: 10.1038/sj.onc.1209937
33. Huang B, Yang XD, Lamb A, Chen LF. Posttranslational modifications of NF-κB: another layer of regulation for NF-κB signaling pathway. *Cell Signal* (2010) 22:1282–90. doi: 10.1016/j.cellsig.2010.03.017
34. Christian F, Smith EL, Carmody RJ. The regulation of NF-κB subunits by phosphorylation. *Cells* (2016) 5:E12. doi: 10.3390/cells5010012
35. Cartwright T, Perkins ND, Wilson CL. NFKB1: a suppressor of inflammation, ageing and cancer. *FEBS J* (2016) 283:1812–22. doi: 10.1111/febs.13627
36. Kyriakis JM, Avruch J. Mammalian mitogen-activated protein kinase signal transduction pathways activated by stress and inflammation. *Physiol Rev* (2001) 81:807–69. doi: 10.1152/physrev.2001.81.2.807
37. Kyriakis JM, Avruch J. Mammalian MAPK signal transduction pathways activated by stress and inflammation: a 10-year update. *Physiol Rev* (2012) 92:689–737. doi: 10.1152/physrev.00028.2011
38. Akaogi J, Nozaki T, Satoh M, Yamada H. Role of PGE2 and EP receptors in the pathogenesis of rheumatoid arthritis and as a novel therapeutic strategy. *Endocr Metab Immune Disord Drug Targets* (2006) 6:383–94. doi: 10.2174/187153006779025711
39. Park JY, Pillinger MH, Abramson SB. Prostaglandin E_2 synthesis and secretion: the role of PGE_2 synthases. *Clin Immunol* (2006) 119:229–40. doi: 10.1016/j.clim.2006.01.016
40. Bonizzi G, Karin M. The two NF-κB activation pathways and their role in innate and adaptive immunity. *Trends Immunol* (2004) 25:280–8. doi: 10.1016/j.it.2004.03.008
41. Chen FE, Kempiak S, Huang DB, Phelps C, Ghosh G. Construction, expression, purification and functional analysis of recombinant NFκB p50/p65 heterodimer. *Protein Eng* (1999) 12:423–8. doi: 10.1093/protein/12.5.423
42. Phelps CB, sengchanthalangsy LL, Huxford T, Ghosh G. Mechanism of IκBα binding to NF-κB dimers. *J Biol Chem* (2000) 275:29840–6. doi: 10.1074/jbc.M004899200
43. Tak PP, Firestein GS. NF-κB: a key role in inflammatory diseases. *J Clin Invest* (2001) 107:7–11. doi: 10.1172/JCI11830
44. Hoesel B, Schmid JA. The complexity of NF-κB signaling in inflammation and cancer. *Mol Cancer* (2013) 12:86. doi: 10.1186/1476-4598-12-86
45. Tieri P, Termanini A, Bellavista E, Salvioli S, Capri M, Franceschi C. Charting the NF-κB pathway interactome map. *PloS One* (2012) 7:e32678. doi: 10.1371/journal.pone.0032678

13

Influence of *IL10* (rs1800896) Polymorphism and TNF-α, IL-10, IL-17A and IL-17F Serum Levels in Ankylosing Spondylitis

*Matheus Braga[1], Fernanda Formaggi Lara-Armi[1], Janisleya Silva Ferreira Neves[1], Marco Antônio Rocha-Loures[2], Mariana de Souza Terron-Monich[3], Larissa Danielle Bahls-Pinto[3], Quirino Alves de Lima Neto[1,3], Joana Maira Valentini Zacarias[1,3], Ana Maria Sell[1,3] and Jeane Eliete Laguila Visentainer[1,3]**

[1] Post Graduation Program in Biosciences and Physiopathology, Department of Clinical Analysis and Biomedicine, State University of Maringá, Paraná, Brazil, [2] Rheumatology Division, Department of Medicine, State University of Maringá, Paraná, Brazil, [3] Immunogenetics Laboratory, Department of Basic and Health Science, State University of Maringá, Paraná, Brazil

***Correspondence:**
Jeane Eliete Laguila Visentainer
jelvisentainer@uem.br

Ankylosing spondylitis (AS) is a chronic autoimmune inflammatory disease that mainly affects the axial and sacroiliac joints. Single-nucleotide polymorphisms (SNPs) in genes encoding cytokines have been associated with AS, which can interfere with the production of these cytokines and contribute to the development of AS. In order to contribute to a better understanding of the pathology of AS, our objective was to investigate a possible association of the *IL10* −1082 A>G SNP (rs1800896) with AS and to evaluate the serum levels of TNF-α, IL-10, IL-17A, and IL-17F in AS patients and controls comparing them with their respective genotypes (*TNF* rs1800629, *IL10* rs1800896, *IL17A* rs2275913, and *IL17F* rs763780). Patients and controls were selected from the Maringá University Hospital and the Maringá Rheumatism Clinic, in Paraná State, Southern Brazil, and they were diagnosed by the ASAS Criteria. In total, 149 patients and 169 controls were genotyped for the *IL10* −1082 A>G polymorphism using a polymerase chain reaction with sequence specific primers (PCR-SSP); the measurement of TNF-α serum levels was performed through the immunofluorimetric test and IL-10, IL-17A, and IL-17F using an ELISA test. There was a high frequency of the *IL10* −1082 G allele in AS patients compared with controls with an odds ratio of 1.83 and 95% confidence interval of 1.32 to 2.54, and a significant difference in the genotype frequencies of the *IL10* −1082 A/G+G/G between patients and healthy controls, with an odds ratio of 3.01 and 95% confidence interval of 1.75 to 5.17. In addition, increased serum levels of IL-10 were observed in AS patients: 2.38 (IQR, 0.91) pg/ml compared with controls 1.72 (IQR 0.93) pg/ml (P = 0.01). Our results also showed an association between *IL17F* rs763780 *C/T+T/T* genotypes and increased serum levels of IL-17F in patients with AS and also in controls. We can conclude that patients with the A/G and G/G genotypes for −1082 A>G (rs1800896) in the *IL10* gene are three times more likely to develop AS, that the serum level of IL-10 was higher in AS patients and that the *IL17F* rs763780 polymorphism can affect the levels of IL-17F in the serum of patients and controls in the same way.

Keywords: autoimmune disease, spondyloarthritis, rheumatological diseases, interleukin-10, interleukin-17, tumour necrosis factor alpha, single nucleotide polymorphisms, genetic polymorphism

INTRODUCTION

Ankylosing spondylitis (AS) is a chronic autoimmune inflammatory disease that mainly affects the axial and sacroiliac joints, causing severe pain. In more advanced cases, this inflammation can lead to fibrosis and calcification, spinal fusion, and consequently, a loss of flexibility (1, 2). Although the major histocompatibility complex (MHC) class I allele *HLA-B*27* is strongly associated with AS, genome-wide association studies have revealed a number of other risk factors for the disease, including several innate immune-related pathways and cytokines (3).

IL-10 is an immunomodulatory cytokine encoded by the *IL10* gene on chromosome 1q31–32, containing five exons separated by four introns (4). Polymorphisms located in the 5′-flanking region of the *IL10* gene, at positions −1082 A>G, −819 T>C, and −592 A>C, are known to be involved in regulating the production of IL-10, with the first being the best characterised of them (5).

Three single nucleotide polymorphisms (SNPs) in genes that encode inflammatory cytokines have been associated with AS, in a previous study by our research group (*TNF* rs1800629, *IL17A* rs2275913, and *IL17F* rs763780) (6). These polymorphisms can interfere with the level of production of these cytokines and contribute to the development of AS (7–10).

Inflammatory cytokines, such as tumour necrosis factor alpha (TNF-α) and interleukin 17 (IL-17), are known to be involved in AS (11, 12). TNF-α is a key component of the immune system and a potent pro-inflammatory cytokine that is highly produced after infection or tissue damage (13) and is present in high concentrations in patients with AS (12). IL-17 is a pro-inflammatory cytokine that contributes to the pathogenesis of several inflammatory diseases. The IL-17 family consists of six structurally related cytokines (IL-17A, IL-17B, IL-17C, IL-17D, IL-17E, and IL-17F) (14). In rheumatological diseases, this interleukin causes cartilage damage in an experimental animal model (15).

The pathogenesis of AS has not been fully elucidated, and some cytokines may play a key role in the disease. In order to elucidate the pathology of AS and identify new genetic markers, we investigated a possible association of the *IL10* SNP *−1082 A>G* (rs1800896) with AS, and evaluated the serum levels of TNF-α, IL-10, IL-17A, and IL-17F in AS patients and controls compared with their respective genotypes (*TNF* rs1800629, *IL17A* rs2275913, *IL17F* rs763780, and *IL10* rs1800896).

METHODOLOGY

Study Population

Unrelated patients were diagnosed by the ASAS Criteria 2009 (16) for axial spondyloarthritis (SpA) and the ASAS Criteria 2011 (17) for peripheral SpA. Patients were selected from the Maringá University Hospital-Maringá State University and the Maringá Rheumatism Clinic, in Paraná State, Southern Brazil. All patients had magnetic resonance imaging of the sacroiliac joints and were evaluated for the presence of *HLA-B*27*. In addition, individuals were selected to form the control group, following the criteria for inclusion: no autoimmune and/or rheumatic diseases, unrelated to the patient group, and belonging to the same ethnic group as the patients, and from the same region. This research was approved by the Standing Committee of Ethics of the State University of Maringá (CAAE 687.222/2014), and all participants signed an informed consent form.

Sample Collection and DNA Extraction

Peripheral blood was collected from case and control groups using tubes without anticoagulants for the determination of serum levels of cytokines and using EDTA-anticoagulant for DNA extraction. Genomic DNA was extracted from blood samples using the extraction kit Biopur® (BIOMETRIX Diagnostic, Curitiba, Paraná, Brazil), according to the manufacturer's recommendations.

Determination of *IL10* Gene Polymorphism

One hundred and forty-nine patients and 169 controls were genotyped for the *IL10* −1082 A>G polymorphism using a polymerase chain reaction with sequence specific primers (PCR-SSP), and a methodology adapted from (18). The primer sequences used are shown in **Table 1**.

The protocol was adapted to a final volume of 10 μL of the reaction mixture containing 50 ng of DNA template, 1.8 ng/μM of each *IL10* primer, 0.75 ng/μM of each Human growth hormone (HGH) for internal control, 0.19 mM of dNTP mixture, 1.5 mM of $MgCl_2$ for allele G reaction and 2.0 mM for allele A reaction, 0.47× Reaction Buffer, and 0.55 U of Taq DNA polymerase.

PCR conditions for amplification included an initial melting step of 5 min at 94°C, followed by 32 cycles of 40 s at 95°C, 50 s at 65°C, 40 s at 72°C, and a final elongation at 72°C for 7 min. After amplification, PCR products were visualised in a 2% agarose gel stained with SYBR™ Safe DNA Gel Stain dye (Invitrogen,

TABLE 1 | Primer sequences.

Primers	Sequence	Bp	Ref
IL10		550 bp	(18)
Common	5′-CAGCCCTTCCATTTTACTTTC-3′		
G allele	5′-TACTAAGGCTTCTTTGGGAG-3′		
A allele	5′-CTACTAAGGCTTCTTTGGGAA-3′		
HGH		431 bp	(19)
HGH F	5′-TGCCTTCCCAACCATTCCCTTA-3′		
HGH R	5′-CAACTCACGGATTTCTGTTGTGTTTC-3′		

Bp, base pairs; Ref, reference; HGH, human growth hormone.

Carlsbad, CA, USA) using the Quantum ultraviolet gel documentation system.

For methodology validation, samples previously genotyped in our laboratory using a commercial kit (One Lambda Cytokine Genotyping Primer Pack, One Lambda) were used as positive controls for each of the three genotypes obtained (A/A, G/A, and G/G) (**Figure 1**).

Determination of Serum Levels of Cytokines

The samples selected for cytokine measurement were randomly chosen, paired by age, gender, and genotype. For IL-10, 28 AS patients and 20 controls genotyped for *IL10* rs1800896 were selected, with 12 being A/A, and 16 being A/G+G/G for AS and 10 being A/A, and 10 being A/G+A/A for controls. *TNF, IL17A*, and *IL17F* gene polymorphisms were previously determined by our group for the same samples and the polymorphisms analysed were *TNF* rs1800629, *IL17A* rs2275913, and *IL17F* rs763780 (6). 35 patients were selected for the analysis of TNF-α levels, with 17 being G/G, and 20 being G/A+A/A for AS, and 15 controls were also included, of which 8 were G/G and 7 were G/A+A/A. For the IL-17A analysis, 45 AS patients, including 21 G/G and 24 G/A+A/A, and 15 controls, including 5 G/G and 10 G/A+A/A, were selected. For the IL-17F analysis, 40 patients were selected, with 24 being T/T, and 16 being C/T+C/C; for the 14 controls, there were seven T/T and seven C/T+C/C. The characteristics of AS patients and controls selected for measurement of cytokines are shown in **Table 2**. There were no significant differences between the patients with AS and controls for gender and age distribution for any group of cytokines ($P > 0.05$).

TABLE 2 | Characteristics of AS patients and controls selected for cytokines measurement.

Cytokine	Age		P value
	Patients	Controls	
TNF-α	44.32[a] ± 14.39	43.33[a] ± 11.02	0.33[b]
IL-10	46.03[a] ± 14.70	44.45[a] ± 11.74	0.30[b]
IL-17A	45[a] ± 14.96	42.87[a] ± 13.60	0.79[b]
IL-17F	43.73[a] ± 15.44	41.64[a] ± 9.20	0.05[b]
	Gender (M/F)		
	Patients	Controls	
TNF-α	22/15	8/7	0.68[c]
IL-10	19/15	15/5	0.99[c]
IL-17A	24/21	6/9	0.37[c]
IL-17F	21/19	8/6	0.76[c]

[a]Average age; ± standard deviation.
[b]Statistical analysis was performed by two-sample t test.
[c]Statistical analysis was performed by OpenEpi two-by-two tables χ^2 test.

The determination of serum levels of TNF-α was performed using the Kit Luminex Technology with the ProcartaPlex™ Immunoassay (Invitrogen, ThermoFisher Scientific, Inc., Burlington, Ontario, Canada). The determination of IL-10 serum levels was performed using the human IL-10 uncoated ELISA kit (Affymetrix eBioscience, North America, USA). The determination of serum levels of IL-17A was performed using the Human IL-17A platinum ELISA Kit (Affymetrix eBioscience, North America, USA), while the determination of serum levels of IL-17F cytokine was performed using the Human IL-17F ELISA Kit (Affymetrix eBioscience, North America, USA). The minimum detection limit for each kit was 0.5 picograms per ml (pg/ml) for TNF-α, 1.6 pg/ml for IL-10, 0.5 pg/ml for IL-17A, and 3.3 pg/ml for IL-17F.

Statistical Analysis

The QUANTO 1.2.4 software (http://biostats.usc.edu/software) was used to calculate the sample size using the following values: prevalence of the less frequent allele 0.30%, population risk

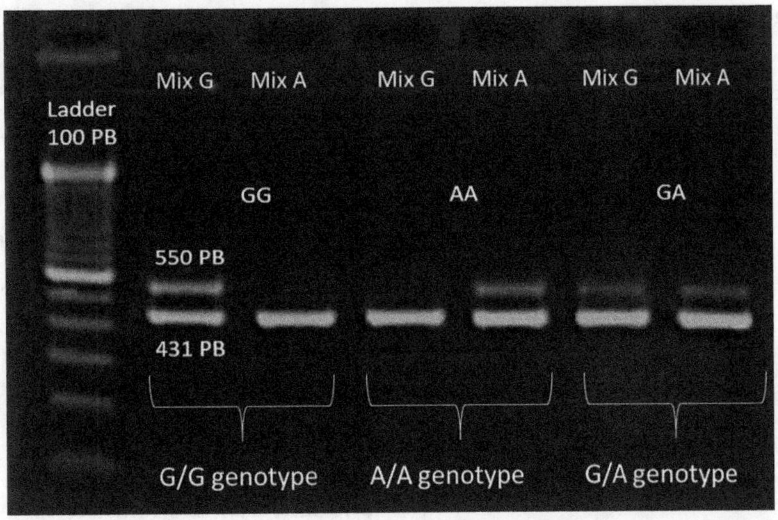

FIGURE 1 | Amplified products of the PCR-SSP assay for analysing the −1082 A>G polymorphism of *IL10* visualised in 2% agarose gel. Bands of 550 bp correspond to the *IL10* fragment and bands of 431 bp correspond to the *HGH* fragment, which was used as an internal control for the reaction.

0.01%, power 0.80, and OR >3.0. For genetic statistical analyses and to estimate the distribution of genotype frequencies according to the Hardy-Weinberg equilibrium (HWE), we applied the software SNPStats (available at: https://www.snpstats.net/start.htm) (20), which was also used for detecting the odds ratio balance, with a 95% confidence interval (CI) after adjustment for age and *HLA*B27* marker. The Akaike information criterion (AIC) was used to choose the inheritance model that best fits the data. The OpenEpi program was used to calculate the allele association using the two-by-two tables test (https://www.openepi.com/Menu/OE_Menu.htm) (21).

To compare the serum levels of cytokines with their respective genotypes, the BioEstat 5.0 program was used. The Shapiro-Wilk test was used to calculate the normality of the samples and the Mann-Whitney test to compare the samples. All values of serum concentration cytokines were expressed as median and Interquartile range (IQR); differences were considered statistically significant if P<0.05.

RESULTS

The characteristics and clinical data of individuals genotyped for the *IL10* −1082 A>G polymorphism are shown in **Table 3**. There were no significant differences between AS patients and controls for gender distribution (P>0.05). *HLA-B*27* was previously analysed using PCR-SSP according to the method published by our research group (22) and it was more frequent in patients with AS than in controls (P<0.0001).

Determination of the *IL10* gene polymorphism by PCR-SSP demonstrated an increased frequency of the −1082 G allele in AS patients compared to controls (**Table 4**). In addition, there was significant difference in the genotype frequency of the *IL10* −1082 A>G polymorphism between patients and controls. To estimate the association between the genotype and AS occurrence, the disease odds ratio (OR) and 95% confidence interval (CI) were assessed and adjusted for age and *HLA*B27* marker. The results suggest that the −1082 A/G and G/G genotypes were associated with disease in a dominant model with an increased risk for AS (OR, 3.01; 95% CI, 1.75–5.17). The *IL10* genotype frequency distributions were in Hardy-Weinberg equilibrium in patients and controls (P>0.05).

TABLE 3 | Characteristics of AS patients and healthy controls.

Characteristics	AS = 149	Controls = 169	P value
Gender (M/F)	72/77	69/100	0.17[b]
Age (years)	46.6 ± 15.4[a]	40.6 ± 12.1[a]	0.002[c]
HLA-B*27	64 (43%)	11 (6%)	<0.0001[b]
BASDAI (>4/<4)	110/39		
Sacroiliitis	133 (89%)		
Good response to NSAID	12 (8%)		
Family history of SpA	29 (19%)		
Elevated CRP	5 (3%)		
Arthritis	27 (18%)		
Enthesitis	56 (38%)		
Uveitis	5 (3%)		
Inflammatory bowel disease	6 (4%)		

[a]Mean ± standard deviation (all such values).
[b]Statistical analysis was performed by OpenEpi Two by Two tables χ^2- test.
[c]Statistical analysis was performed by two-sample t test.
AS, ankylosing spondylitis; BASDAI, bath ankylosing spondylitis disease activity index; NSAID, non-steroidal anti-inflammatory drugs; SpA, spondyloarthritis; CPR, c-reactive protein.

TABLE 4 | Allele and genotype frequency distribution for *IL10 −1082 A>G* and the association with the risk for ankylosing spondylitis, regardless of *HLA-B*27* marker and age in different genetic models.

IL10 −1082	AS N = 149	Controls N = 169	OR (95% CI)	P value	AIC
Codominant	n (f)	n (f)		0.0002	358.1
A/A	40 (0.27)	85 (0.5)			
A/G	83 (0.56)	63 (0.37)	3.05 (1.72–5.41)[a]		
G/G	26 (0.17)	21 (0.12)	2.87 (1.31–6.29)[a]		
Dominant	n (f)	n (f)		<0.0001	356.1*
A/A	40 (0.27)	85 (0.5)			
A/G – G/G	109 (0.73)	84 (0.50)	3.01 (1.75–5.17)[a]		
Recessive	n (f)	n (f)		0.23	371.5
A/A- A/G	124 (0.83)	147 (0.87)			
G/G	25 (0.17)	22 (0.13)			
Alleles	n (f)	n (f)		0.0002	
A	163 (0.55)	233 (0.69)			
G	135 (0.45)	105 (0.31)	1.83 (1.32–2.54)[b]		

*Best inheritance model defined according to 20.
[a]Statistical analysis was performed by SNPStats software.
[b]Statistical analysis was performed by OpenEpi Two by Two tables. f: genotype or allele frequency.
AS, ankylosing spondylitis; OR, odds ratio; CI, confidence interval; AIC, criterion Akaike information.

Results of the analysis of the association between *IL10* −1082 A>G (rs1800896) polymorphism with different clinical data of AS are shown in **Table 5**. There was no statistical difference between *IL10* genotypes or alleles in relation to clinical data of AS. The smaller number of patients in each subgroup could be related to these results.

The analyses of serum cytokine levels in AS patients and controls are shown in **Figure 2**. Higher serum levels of IL-10 were observed in patients, as the levels of IL-10 was 2.38 (IQR 0.91) pg/mL in patients and 1.72 (IQR, 0.93) pg/ml in controls (P=0.01) (**Figure 2B**). There were no statistically significant differences in the serum levels of the other cytokines when patients were compared to controls. The serum levels of the cytokines in patients were as follows: TNF-α 2.14 (IQR, 3.65) pg/ml, IL-17A 22.12 (IQR, 51.97) pg/ml, and IL-17F 100.13 (IQR, 1273.65) pg/ml. For controls, the serum levels were as follows: TNF-α 1.39 (IQR, 3.14) pg/ml; IL-17A 33.50 (IQR, 339) pg/ml, and IL-17F 251.04 (IQR, 765.45) pg/ml.

The analyses of TNF-α, IL-10, IL-17A, and IL-17F serum cytokine levels with genotypes in AS patients and controls are shown in **Figure 3**. Higher serum levels of IL-17F were observed in patients with the *IL17F* rs763780 T/C+C/C genotypes [796.04 (IQR, 1496.23) pg/ml compared to patients with the T/T genotype 43.77 (IQR, 384.1) pg/ml] (p=0.03) (**Figure 3H**). The same association was found for controls: T/C+C/C 570.10 (IQR, 1325.23) pg/ml compared with *T/T* 25.36 (IQR, 142.73) pg/ml (P=0.02) (**Figure 3I**).

No statistically significant difference was found for the other cytokines. TNF-α serum level in AS patients carrying *TNF* rs1800629 G/A+A/A was 1.70 pg/ml (IQR, 4.71) and 2.51 (IQR, 2.21) pg/ml for those carrying G/G (**Figure 3A**). For controls, it was 2.00 (IQR, 4.73) pg/ml for those carrying G/

TABLE 5 | Analysis of *IL10* gene polymorphisms (rs1800896) in AS patients separated according to clinical data.

Clinical data		Genotypes (n)				Alleles		
		AA	AG	GG	P1	A	G	P2
BASDAI (>4/<4)								
	> 4	28	62	20	0.70	118	102	0.53
	< 4	12	21	6		45	33	
Sacroiliitis								
	Positive	35	72	26	0.14	142	124	0.18
	Negative	5	11	0		21	11	
Good response to NSAID								
	Positive	1	8	3	0.30	10	14	0.18
	Negative	39	75	23		153	121	
Elevated CRP								
	Positive	1	3	1	0.93	5	5	0.76
	Negative	39	80	25		158	130	
Arthritis								
	Positive	7	15	5	0.98	29	25	0.87
	Negative	33	68	21		134	110	
Enthesitis								
	Positive	15	33	8	0.60	63	49	0.68
	Negative	25	49	18		99	85	
Uveitis								
	Positive	0	4	1	0.37	4	6	0.34
	Negative	40	79	25		159	129	
Inflammatory bowel								
	Positive	3	3	0	0.30	9	3	0.14
	Negative	37	80	26		154	132	

P1: Patients positive versus patients negative using 3×2 contingency table.
P2: Patients positive versus patients negative using 2×2 contingency table.
AS, ankylosing spondylitis; BASDAI, bath ankylosing spondylitis disease activity index; NSAID, non-steroidal anti-inflammatory drugs; SpA, spondyloarthritis; CPR, c-reactive protein.

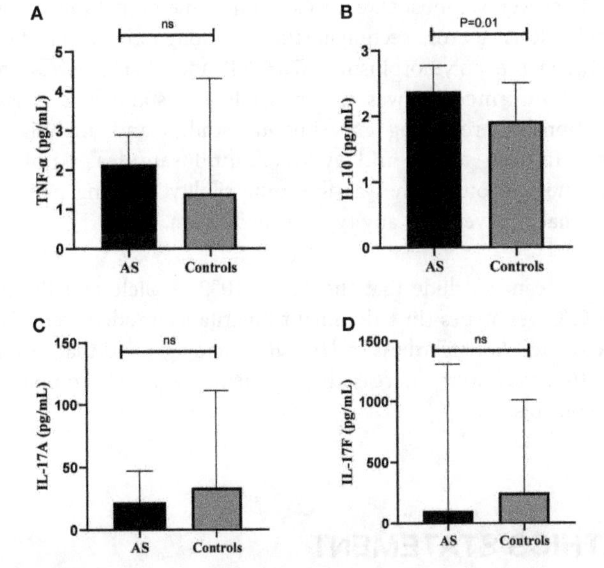

FIGURE 2 | Comparison between patients and controls for cytokine levels. **(A)** Comparison of TNF-α levels between patients and controls; **(B)** Comparison of IL-10 levels between patients and controls; **(C)** Comparison of IL-17A levels between patients and controls; **(D)** Comparison of IL-17F levels between patients and controls. AS, ankylosing spondylitis; ns, not significant.

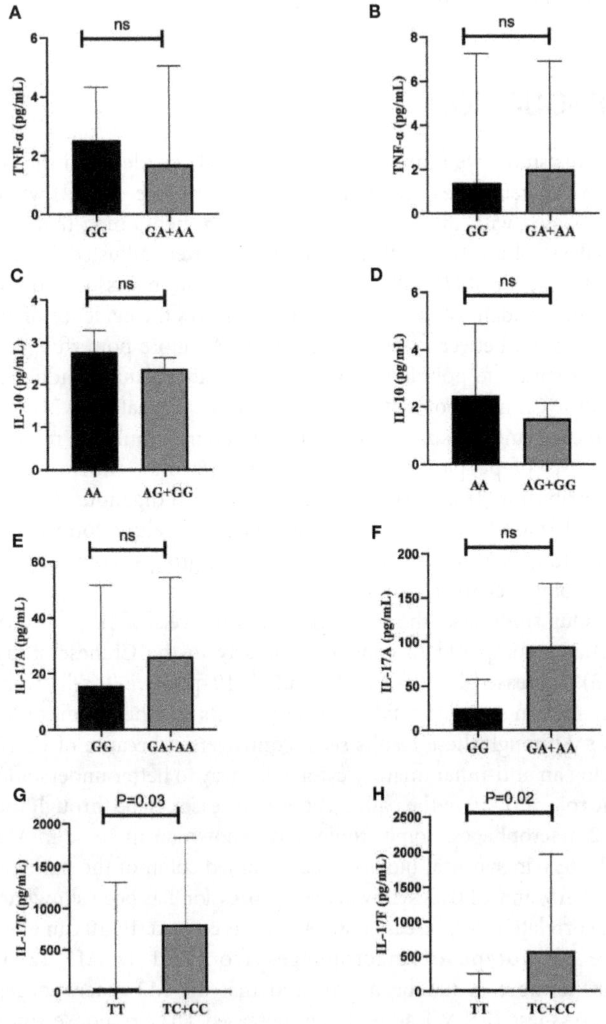

FIGURE 3 | Relation between serum cytokine levels and genotypes in AS patients and controls. **(A)** Comparison of TNF-α levels in patients with *TNF* rs1800629 G/G vs. G/A+AA genotypes. **(B)** Comparison of TNF-α levels in controls with *TNF* rs1800629 G/G *vs.* G/A+A/A genotypes. **(C)** Comparison of IL-10 levels in patients with *IL10* rs1800896 A/A *vs.* A/G+G/G genotypes. **(D)** Comparison of IL-10 levels in controls with *IL10* rs1800896 A/A *vs.* A/G+G/G genotypes. **(E)** Comparison of IL-17A levels in patients with *IL17A* rs2275913 G/A+A/A *vs.* G/G genotypes. **(F)** Comparison of IL-17A levels in controls with *IL17A* rs2275913 G/A+A/A *vs.* G/G genotypes. **(G)** Comparison of IL-17F levels in patients with *IL17F* rs763780 T/C+C/C *vs.* T/T genotypes. **(H)** Comparison of IL-17F levels in controls with *IL17F* rs763780 T/C+C/C *vs.* T/T genotypes; ns, not significant.

A+A/A and 1.39 (IQR, 1.37) pg/ml for G/G (**Figure 3B**). Serum levels of IL-10 in AS patients carrying *IL10* rs1800896 A/G +A/A were 2.38 (IQR, 0.45) pg/ml and 2.77 (IQR 0.91) pg/mL in those carrying A/A (**Figure 3C**); for controls carrying A/G +A/A, it was 1.58 (IQR, 0.68) pg/ml and for A/A 2.12 (IQR 1.19) pg/ml (**Figure 3D**). Serum levels of IL-17A were 26.00 (IQR, 51.6) pg/ml in AS patients carrying the *IL17A* rs2275913 G/A+A/A genotypes and 15.63 (IQR, 49.6) pg/ml for those carrying the G/G genotype (**Figure 3E**); for controls, it was 94.63 (IQR,

129.23) pg/ml for individuals carrying G/A+A/A and 24.37 (IQR, 30.43) pg/ml for those carrying G/G (**Figure 3F**).

DISCUSSION

In this study, we found that the *IL10* −1082 G allele and the A/G+G/G genotypes (in a dominant inheritance model) were associated with the risk of AS. It is worth mentioning that our analyses of the IL10 -1082 polymorphism were adjusted for age and presence of *HLA-B*27*, and that we found this association to be independent of these factors, which makes the evidence of an association between the IL10 gene and AS more powerful.

Despite the population difference, another study conducted with a Chinese population also found an association with the same polymorphism and AS (23). The Paraná population mainly consists of people of European origin (80.6%), with a small contribution from African (12.5%), and Indigenous (7.0%) populations (24, 25). Hence, patients and healthy controls in our study were classified as mixed ethnic groups, according to phenotypic characteristics.

Our study also showed higher serum levels of IL-10 in AS patients compared to controls, similarly to the Chinese study (23). Increased levels of IL-10 and IL-10–positive T cells were detected in synovial fluid from AS patients in other studies (26, 27). Although these results seem controversial because of IL-10 being an anti-inflammatory cytokine, a way to better understand the role of IL-10 in the pathogenesis of disease can be through the M2 macrophages. Some studies have shown an increase in M2 CD163+ in synovial biopsies and inflamed colon of the patients with AS, and CD163 synovial over-expression has been shown to be correlated with disease (28, 29); in this context, IL-10 can alter the phenotype of macrophages from M1 to M2 (30). Furthermore, it has been proposed that the M2 macrophages express less IFN-γ, leading to an increased Th17 response since IFN-γ can suppress IL-17 expression (31), and it has been reported that the IL-17 is one of the main cytokines involved in the pathogenesis of AS (28, 29).

In this study, we found no statistical differences between the levels of TNF-α, IL-17A, and IL-17F among patients and controls, despite some studies having shown an increase in inflammatory cytokines, such as IL-17 and TNF-α in AS (32, 33). We must take into account that our patients were being treated with non-steroidal anti-inflammatory drugs (NSAIDs), and anti-TNF therapy for longer than 6 months.

In order to better understand the influence of SNPs associated with AS, *IL10* rs1800896 in the present study, as well as *TNF* rs1800629, *IL17A* rs2275913, *IL17F* rs763780 that were associated with the risk of developing AS in a previous study by our group (6), we compared the serum levels of the cytokines between the risk genotypes and non-risk genotypes in patients and controls.

With regard to TNF-α, we found no differences in the serum levels of this cytokine between the *TNF* rs1800629 genotype G/G compared to the risk genotypes G/A+A/A. The G/A+A/A genotypes have also been reported to be major producers of TNF-α in congenital heart disease (34). The A allele was found to be the higher producer of TNF-α in an *in vitro* study (35). Although we did not observe this association, we should also consider the use of anti-TNF in the treatment.

Many studies show that the *IL10* *1082* genotypes A/G+G/G were the largest producers of IL-10 (23, 36–38). Despite the association of A/G+G/G genotypes with AS and increased levels of IL-10 in patients, we did not find any association between these genotypes and the levels of IL-10, suggesting that other SNPs could influence the production of the cytokine.

We also found no differences in the serum levels of IL-17A cytokine between G/G and G/A+A/A genotypes. The genotypes G/A and A/A have been reported to be associated with the increased production of IL-17A in a recent study on coronary disease (39). However, this relationship is controversial, as other studies have shown an increase in IL-17A in patients with the A/A genotype (40), a lack of association with this SNP and production (41), and high levels in individuals carrying the genotypes GG+GA (42). These differences could suggest that the polymorphism (rs2275913) does not influence IL-17A levels.

The assessment of the association between IL-17F levels and the *IL17F* T>C (rs763780) polymorphism showed an association between increased IL-17F production and the T/C+C/C genotypes in patients and controls. These results suggest that variations in the sequence of the specific nucleotides of *IL17F* can have a direct effect on the production of the encoded protein, IL-17F. Another study with psoriasis also reported a higher level of IL-17F in patients with the T/C+C/C genotypes (43).

However, we must take into account some limitations of our study. It is a cross-sectional study, although the association between the polymorphism (rs763780) and IL-17F levels has been confirmed. It was not possible to establish a causal relationship, requiring experimental studies and analysis of cytokines in tissue and synovial fluid samples. Another weakness of our study was the impossibility of using patients who had not yet used any type of medication.

We can conclude that the *IL10* −1082 G allele and the A/G+G/G genotypes (in a dominant inheritance model) were risk factors for AS, regardless of *HLA-B*27* and age, and that serum IL-10 levels were increased in patients with AS compared to controls.

ETHICS STATEMENT

This research was approved by the standing committee of ethics of the State University of Maringá (CAAE 687.222/2014). The patients/participants provided their written informed consent to participate in this study.

AUTHOR CONTRIBUTIONS

MB executed the research protocol, analyzed the data, and wrote the manuscript. MT-M, LB-P and JZ contributed to the writing and critical analysis of the manuscript. JN and MR-L contributed to the collection of data, sample and classification of patients. FL-A contributed to the implementation of the protocols. QN supervised the analyses and the execution of this research. AS and JV developed the original idea and provided intellectual input and critical analysis of the manuscript. All authors contributed to the article and approved the submitted version.

ACKNOWLEDGMENTS

The authors wish to thank the patients and volunteers for their valuable participation in the study, the Post-Graduation Program in Biosciences and Physiopathology, UEM, CAPES, Fundação Araucária-PR, and CNPq.

REFERENCES

1. Pedersen SJ, Maksymowych WP. The Pathogenesis of Ankylosing Spondylitis: An Update. *Curr Rheumatol Rep* (2019) 21:1–10. doi: 10.1007/s11926-019-0856-3
2. Zhu W, He X, Cheng K, Zhang L, Chen D, Wang X, et al. Ankylosing Spondylitis: Etiology, Pathogenesis, and Treatments. *Bone Res* (2019) 7:1–16. doi: 10.1038/s41413-019-0057-8
3. Vanaki N, Aslani S, Jamshidi A, Mahmoudi M. Role of Innate Immune System in the Pathogenesis of Ankylosing Spondylitis. *BioMed Pharmacother* (2018) 105:130–43. doi: 10.1016/j.biopha.2018.05.097
4. Moore KW, de Waal Malefyt R, Coffman RL, O'Garra A. Interleukin-10 and the interleukin-10 Receptor. *Annu Rev Immunol* (2001) 19:683–765. doi: 10.1146/annurev.immunol.19.1.683
5. Turner D, Williams DM, Sankaran D, Lazarus M, Sinnott PJ, Hutchinson IV. An Investigation of Polymorphism in the Interleukin-10 Gene Promoter. *Eur J immunogenetics* (1997) 24:1–8. doi: 10.1111/j.1365-2370.1997.tb00001.x
6. Rocha Loures MA, Macedo LC, Reis DM, Oliveira CF, Meneguetti JL, Martines GF, et al. Influence of TNF and IL17 Gene Polymorphisms on the Spondyloarthritis Immunopathogenesis, Regardless of HLA-B27, in a Brazilian Population. *Mediators Inflammation* (2018) 2018:1395823. doi: 10.1155/2018/1395823
7. Sode J, Bank S, Vogel U, Andersen PS, Sørensen SB, Bojesen AB, et al. Genetically Determined High Activities of the TNF-Alpha, IL23/IL17, and NFkB Pathways Were Associated With Increased Risk of Ankylosing Spondylitis. *BMC Med Genet* (2018) 19:1–16. doi: 10.1186/s12881-018-0680-z
8. Vargas-Alarcón G, Casasola-Vargas J, Rodríguez-Pérez JM, Huerta-Sil G, Pérez-Hernández N, Londoño J, et al. Tumor Necrosis Factor-α Promoter Polymorphisms in Mexican Patients With Spondyloarthritis. *Hum Immunol* (2006) 67:826–32. doi: 10.1016/j.humimm.2006.07.009
9. Romero-Sánchez C, Londoño J, Delgado G, Jaimes DA, De Avila J, Mora A, et al. Association of Tumor Necrosis Factor Alpha-308 Promoter Polymorphism With Spondyloarthritides Patients in Colombia. *Rheumatol Int* (2012) 32:2195–7. doi: 10.1007/s00296-011-1883-1
10. Yang B, Xu Y, Liu X, Huang Z, Wang L. Il-23R and IL-17A Polymorphisms Correlate With Susceptibility of Ankylosing Spondylitis in a Southwest Chinese Population. *Oncotarget* (2017) 8:70310. doi: 10.18632/oncotarget.20319
11. Shen H, Goodall JC, Hill Gaston JS. Frequency and Phenotype of Peripheral Blood Th17 Cells in Ankylosing Spondylitis and Rheumatoid Arthritis. *Arthritis Rheumatism: Off J Am Coll Rheumatol* (2009) 60:1647–56. doi: 10.1002/art.24568
12. Chou C-T, Huo A-P, Chang H-N, Tsai C-Y, Chen W-S, Wang H-P. Cytokine Production From Peripheral Blood Mononuclear Cells in Patients With Ankylosing Spondylitis and Their First-Degree Relatives. *Arch Med Res* (2007) 38:190–5. doi: 10.1016/j.arcmed.2006.09.008
13. Van Hauwermeiren F, Vandenbroucke RE, Libert C. Treatment of TNF Mediated Diseases by Selective Inhibition of Soluble TNF or TNFR1. *Cytokine Growth factor Rev* (2011) 22:311–9. doi: 10.1016/j.cytogfr.2011.09.004
14. Kawaguchi M, Adachi M, Oda N, Kokubu F, Huang S-K. IL-17 Cytokine Family. *J Allergy Clin Immunol* (2004) 114:1265–73. doi: 10.1016/j.jaci.2004.10.019
15. Koenders MI, Marijnissen RJ, Devesa I, Lubberts E, Joosten LAB, Roth J, et al. Tumor Necrosis Factor–Interleukin-17 Interplay Induces S100A8, Interleukin-1β, and Matrix Metalloproteinases, and Drives Irreversible Cartilage Destruction in Murine Arthritis: Rationale for Combination Treatment During Arthritis. *Arthritis Rheumatism* (2011) 63:2329–39. doi: 10.1002/art.30418
16. Rudwaleit M, van der Heijde D, Landewé R, Listing J, Akkoc N, Brandt J, et al. The Development of Assessment of SpondyloArthritis International Society Classification Criteria for Axial Spondyloarthritis (Part II): Validation and Final Selection. *Ann Rheumatic Diseases* (2009) 68:777–83. doi: 10.1136/ard.2009.108233corr1
17. Rudwaleit MV, van der Heijde D, Landewé R, Akkoc N, Brandt J, Chou CT, et al. The Assessment of SpondyloArthritis International Society Classification Criteria for Peripheral Spondyloarthritis and for Spondyloarthritis in General. *Ann Rheumatic Diseases* (2011) 70:25–31. doi: 10.1136/ard.2010.133645
18. Abdolrahim-Zadeh H, Hakkakian N, Asadollahi R, Gharesifard B, Sarvari J, Kamali-Sarvestani E, et al. Interleukin-10 Promoter Polymorphisms and Breast Cancer Risk in Iranian Women. *Iranian J Immunol* (2005) 2:158–65.
19. Silvestre APA, Zacarias JMV, Guelsin GAS, Visentainer JEL, Sell AM. Genetic Polymorphisms of Human Platelet Antigens in Euro-African and Japanese Descendants From Parana, Southern Brazil. *Platelets* (2017) 28:607–10. doi: 10.1080/09537104.2016.1257785
20. Solé X, Guinó E, Valls J, Iniesta R, Moreno V. Snpstats: A Web Tool for the Analysis of Association Studies. *Bioinformatics* (2006) 22:1928–9. doi: 10.1093/bioinformatics/btl268
21. Dean AG, Sullivan KM, Soe MM. *Openepi: Open Source Epidemiologic Statistics for Public Health, Version.* (2014). Available at: www.OpenEpi.com, updated 2013/04/06. (Accessed November 22, 2020).
22. Lara-Armi FF, Visentainer JEL, Alves HV, Rocha-Loures MA, Neves JSF, Colli CM, et al. Optimization of HLA-B* 27 ALLELE Genotyping by PCR-SSP. *Clinics* (2020) 75:e1840. doi: 10.6061/clinics/2020/e1840
23. Lv C, Wang Y, Wang J, Zhang H, Xu H, Zhang D. Association of Interleukin-10 Gene Polymorphisms With Ankylosing Spondylitis. *Clin Invest Med* (2011) 34:370–6. doi: 10.25011/cim.v34i6.15898
24. Probst CM, Bompeixe EP, Pereira NF, De O Dalalio MM, Visentainer JEL, Tsuneto LT, et al. HLA Polymorphism and Evaluation of European, African, and Amerindian Contribution to the White and Mulatto Populations From Paraná, Brazil. *Hum Biol* (2000) 72:597.
25. Reis PG, Ambrosio-Albuquerque EP, Fabreti-Oliveira RA, Moliterno RA, de Souza VH, Sell AM, et al. Hla-A,-B,-DRB1,-DQA1, and-DQB1 Profile in a Population From Southern Brazil. *Hla* (2018) 92:298–303. doi: 10.1111/tan.13368
26. Keller C, Webb A, Davis J. Cytokines in the Seronegative Spondyloarthropathies and Their Modification by TNF Blockade: A Brief Report and Literature Review. *Ann Rheumatic Diseases* (2003) 62:1128–32. doi: 10.1136/ard.2003.011023
27. Baeten D, Van Damme N, Van den Bosch F, Kruithof E, De Vos M, Mielants H, et al. Impaired Th1 Cytokine Production in Spondyloarthropathy Is Restored by Anti-TNFα. *Ann Rheumatic Diseases* (2001) 60:750–5. doi: 10.1136/ard.60.8.750
28. Baeten D, Kruithof E, De Rycke L, Boots AM, Mielants H, Veys EM, et al. Infiltration of the Synovial Membrane With Macrophage Subsets and

Polymorphonuclear Cells Reflects Global Disease Activity in Spondyloarthropathy. *Arthritis Res Ther* (2005) 7:R359. doi: 10.1186/ar1501

29. Ciccia F, Alessandro R, Rizzo A, Accardo-Palumbo A, Raimondo S, Raiata F, et al. Macrophage Phenotype in the Subclinical Gut Inflammation of Patients With Ankylosing Spondylitis. *Rheumatology* (2013) 53:104–13. doi: 10.1093/rheumatology/ket323
30. Deng B, Wehling-Henricks M, Villalta SA, Wang Y, Tidball JG. Il-10 Triggers Changes in Macrophage Phenotype That Promote Muscle Growth and Regeneration. *J Immunol* (2012) 189:3669–80. doi: 10.4049/jimmunol.1103180
31. Chu CQ, Swart D, Alcorn D, Tocker J, Elkon KB. Interferon-γ Regulates Susceptibility to Collagen-Induced Arthritis Through Suppression of Interleukin-17. *Arthritis Rheumatism* (2007) 56:1145–51. doi: 10.1002/art.22453
32. Mei Y, Pan F, Gao J, Ge R, Duan Z, Zeng Z, et al. Increased Serum Il-17 and IL-23 in the Patient With Ankylosing Spondylitis. *Clin Rheumatol* (2011) 30:269–73. doi: 10.1007/s10067-010-1647-4
33. Wang J, Zhao Q, Wang G, Yang C, Xu Y, Li Y, et al. Circulating Levels of Th1 and Th2 Chemokines in Patients With Ankylosing Spondylitis. *Cytokine* (2016) 81:10–4. doi: 10.1016/j.cyto.2016.01.012
34. Pan J, Hu J, Qi X, Xu L. Association Study of a Functional Variant of TNF-α Gene and Serum TNF-α Level With the Susceptibility of Congenital Heart Disease in a Chinese Population. *Postgraduate Med J* (2019) 95:547–51. doi: 10.1136/postgradmedj-2019-136621
35. Kroeger KM, Steer JH, Joyce DA, Abraham LJ. Effects of Stimulus and Cell Type on the Expression of the– 308 Tumour Necrosis Factor Promoter Polymorphism. *Cytokine* (2000) 12:110–9. doi: 10.1006/cyto.1999.0529
36. Miteva LD, Stanilov NS, Deliysky TS, Stanilova SA. Significance of -1082A/G Polymorphism of IL10 Gene for Progression of Colorectal Cancer and IL-10 Expression. *Tumour Biol* (2014) 35:12655–64. doi: 10.1007/s13277-014-2589-2
37. Fathy MM, Elsaadany HF, Ali YF, Farghaly MAA, Hamed ME, Ibrahim HE, et al. Association of IL-10 Gene Polymorphisms and Susceptibility to Juvenile Idiopathic Arthritis in Egyptian Children and Adolescents: A Case-Control Study. *Ital J pediatrics* (2017) 43:9. doi: 10.1186/s13052-017-0328-1
38. Azab SF, Abdalhady MA, Elsaadany HF, Elkomi MA, Elhindawy EM, Sarhan DT, et al. Interleukin-10-1082 G/A Gene Polymorphisms in Egyptian Children With CAP: A Case-Control Study. *Medicine* (2016) 95:e4013. doi: 10.1097/MD.0000000000004013
39. Ghaznavi H, Soltanpour MS. Association Study Between Rs2275913 Genetic Polymorphism and Serum Levels of IL-17A With Risk of Coronary Artery Disease. *Mol Biol Res Commun* (2020) 9:35–40. doi: 10.22099/mbrc.2020.35442.1463
40. Pasha HF, Tantawy EA, Youssef MA. Osteopontin and Interleukin-17A Genes Polymorphisms in Egyptian Systemic Lupus Erythematosus Patients: A Relation to Disease Activity and Severity. *Gene* (2019) 702:107–13. doi: 10.1016/j.gene.2019.02.100
41. Ocejo-Vinyals JG, de Mateo EP, Hoz MÁ, Arroyo JL, Agüero R, Ausín F, et al. The IL-17 G-152a Single Nucleotide Polymorphism Is Associated With Pulmonary Tuberculosis in Northern Spain. *Cytokine* (2013) 64:58–61. doi: 10.1016/j.cyto.2013.05.022
42. Huang H-T, Lu Y-L, Wang R, Qin H-M, Wang C-F, Wang J-L, et al. The Association of IL-17A Polymorphisms With Il-17a Serum Levels and Risk of Ischemic Stroke. *Oncotarget* (2017) 8:103499. doi: 10.18632/oncotarget.21498
43. Choi BG, Hong JY, Hong JR, Hur MS, Kim SM, Lee YW, et al. The IL17F His161arg Polymorphism, a Potential Risk Locus for Psoriasis, Increases Serum Levels of interleukin-17F in an Asian Population. *Sci Rep* (2019) 9:1–7. doi: 10.1038/s41598-019-55062-5

14

Association of CD40 Gene Polymorphisms with Systemic Lupus Erythematosus and Rheumatoid Arthritis in a Chinese Han Population

Qi Huang[1], Wang-Dong Xu[1], Lin-Chong Su[2], Xiao-Yan Liu[3] and An-Fang Huang[4*]*

[1] Department of Evidence-Based Medicine, School of Public Health, Southwest Medical University, Luzhou, China, [2] Department of Rheumatology and Immunology, Minda Hospital of Hubei Minzu University, Enshi, China, [3] Department of Nutrition and Food Hygiene, School of Public Health, Southwest Medical University, Luzhou, China, [4] Department of Rheumatology and Immunology, Affiliated Hospital of Southwest Medical University, Luzhou, China

***Correspondence:**
Wang-Dong Xu
loutch123@163.com
An-Fang Huang
loutch211@163.com

Systemic lupus erythematosus (SLE) and rheumatoid arthritis (RA) are complex autoimmune diseases. CD40 participates in inflammatory response, and promotes fibroblast proliferation, leading to occurrence and progression of SLE, RA. This study explores CD40 gene polymorphisms in SLE and RA patients from a Chinese Han population. Two hundred SLE patients, 340 RA patients, and 900 healthy controls were enrolled. Genomic DNA was extracted from peripheral blood, and six polymorphisms of CD40 gene (rs3765456, rs1569723, rs73115010, rs13040307, rs1883832, and rs4810485) were detected by KASP method. Frequencies of rs1569723 genotypes AA, AC, AA+AC were significantly higher in RA patients as compared to those in healthy controls ($P = 0.049$, $P = 0.024$, $P = 0.022$). Frequencies of genotypes CT, CC+CT of rs1883832, and GT, GG+GT of rs4810485 were significantly higher in RA patients as compared to those in healthy controls ($P = 0.012$, $P = 0.018$, $P = 0.009$, $P = 0.015$). RA patients carrying rs13040307 C allele and rs73115010 T allele showed increased number of swollen joints. Moreover, frequency of allele T of rs13040307 was lower in SLE patients with positive anti-dsDNA and hematuria as compared to that in patients without these parameters ($P = 0.038$, $P = 0.045$). There were increased frequencies of genotype TT, allele T for rs13040307 and lower frequencies of genotype TT, allele T for rs73115010 in lupus patients with myositis (all $P<0.05$). Interestingly, frequencies of rs1569723 A allele, rs4810485 T allele were higher in SLE patients with myositis, and frequencies of rs3765456 A allele, rs1883832 T allele were lower in SLE patients with myositis (All $P<0.05$). In conclusion, CD40 gene polymorphisms may associate with susceptibility to SLE and RA.

Keywords: CD40, polymorphism, systemic lupus erythematosus, rheumatoid arthritis, susceptibility, clinical features, disease activity parameters

INTRODUCTION

Systemic lupus erythematosus (SLE) and rheumatoid arthritis (RA) are inflammatory autoimmune diseases, with features of chronic inflammation. The main characteristics of RA are progressive joints lesion, synovial hyperplasia, and production of auto-antibodies. SLE relates to various tissues and organs damage, such as skin, blood vessels, kidney (1, 2). Etiology of these two diseases remains unclear. It is recognized that gene polymorphisms have been involved in these disorders pathogenesis (3, 4). To date, at least 88 genomic regions have been identified associated with SLE susceptibility, such as TNFSF4, STAT4, and TNIP1, and about 106 susceptible genes were reported to associate with RA, such as CD28, IL3-CSF2, NFKBIE (5, 6). However, finding out more risk polymorphisms for RA and SLE will be helpful to better elucidate the pathogenesis of these diseases.

CD40 is a glycoprotein with molecular weight 45 to 50 kDa, consisting of 277 amino acids. It is a member of the tumor necrosis factor family of transmembrane glycoproteins and is expressed in different cells, such as B cells, monocytes, dendritic cells, endothelial and epithelial cells, smooth muscle cells, fibroblasts (7). CD40 is a potent T-cell costimulatory factor. It interacts with ligand CD40L, and plays an important role in adaptive immune response, for example, induction of Th1 cell response (8). Human CD40 gene is composed of eight introns and nine exons, located on chromosome 20q11.2 to 13.2. To date, association of CD40 gene and autoimmune disorders has been discussed widely. Chen et al. analyzed three polymorphisms (rs1883832, rs4810485, and rs1569723) of CD40 gene and risk of SLE in a Chinese population. They found that rs1883832 related to development of SLE (9). Nie et al. found relation between rs4810485 and SLE risk in a Chinese population (10). In European origins, studies showed that rs4810485 polymorphism was a risk factor for SLE, RA, and rs3765456 polymorphism was related to RA susceptibility in Korea population (11–13). However, association of rs73115010, rs13040307, and rs1569723 polymorphisms with SLE and RA were discussed in different ethnicities, and showed inconsistent conclusions. Therefore, to better clarify the relationship between CD40 gene polymorphisms and SLE, RA susceptibility, we conducted the present study in a Chinese Han population to evaluate six polymorphisms (rs3765456, rs1569723, rs73115010, rs13040307, rs1883832, and rs4810485) with relation to SLE and RA patients by co-dominant, dominant, and recessive genetic models.

MATERIALS AND METHODS

Study Sample

This case-control study recruited 200 SLE patients (age, 38.0 [27.0–48.0] years), 340 RA patients (age, 56.0 [48.5–65.0] years) and 900 healthy controls (age, 38.0 [31.0–48.0] years) in Southern Chinese Han origin. All patients came from Department of Rheumatology and Immunology, Affiliated Hospital of Southwest Medical University. Healthy controls were from Physical Examination Center of Jiangyang District Center for Disease Control and Prevention in Luzhou city. RA and SLE patients were diagnosed according to the American College of Rheumatology and European League Against Rheumatism (ACR/EULAR) classification criteria (14, 15). RA patients disease activity was evaluated according to disease activity score 28 (DAS28) (16), and SLE patients disease activity was evaluated according to SLE disease activity index (SLEDAI) (17) (**Table 1**). This study was admitted by Ethic Research Committee of Southwest Medical University, and informed consent was collected from individual participant. Demographic and clinical characteristics of patients and controls were obtained as well. For instance, clinical characteristics myositis was diagnosed according to participants who had at least three of four items including clinical symptoms, serum creatine kinase level, electromyography, and muscle biopsy results (18).

Single Nucleotide Polymorphism Selection

A systemic exploration for previous studies about CD40 gene polymorphism was carried out. According to the online tools: 1000 genomes project (https://www.ncbi.nlm.nih.gov/variation/tools/1000genomes/), all candidate single nucleotide polymorphisms (SNPs) must conform to three standard: pairwise tagging of HapMap population with $r^2 \geq 0.8$; a minor allele frequency (MAF)≥5%; Chinese Han Beijing (CHB) ethnicity. Finally, a total of six SNPs including rs3765456, rs1569723, rs73115010, rs13040307, rs1883832, and rs4810485 were selected.

DNA Extraction and Genotyping

TIANamp Blood DNA kits (Tiangen, Beijing, China) were utilized for extracting genomic DNA. Genotyping of CD40 gene polymorphisms of these samples with qualified DNA concentration and purity was tested by Gene Company using KASP (Gene Company, Shanghai, China). KASP primers were summarized in **Supplementary Table 1**.

Statistics

Statistical Package for the Social Science (SPSS) version 17.0 (SPSS Inc., Chicago) was used for statistical analysis. Categorical data were presented as frequency, percentage and analyzed by chi-square test. If continuous data was normally distributed, mean ± standard deviation (SD) was displayed, and independent samples t test was adopted. Otherwise, we chose median (interquartile range) and Wilcoxon ranks sum test for comparison. Odds ratio (OR) and 95% confidence interval (CI) were analyzed by logistic regression model. To evaluate deviation of each polymorphism, Hardy-Weinberg equilibrium test was used for SLE patients, RA patients, and healthy controls. There are three inheritance models, including co-dominant model, dominant model, and recessive model. For rs1883832, the co-dominant model includes CC versus TT, CT versus TT, the dominant model is CC+CT versus TT, and the recessive model is CC versus CT+TT. For rs1569723, the co-dominant model includes AA versus CC, AC versus CC, the dominant model is AA+AC versus CC, and the recessive model is AA versus AC+CC. For rs4810485, the co-dominant model includes GG versus TT, GT versus TT, the dominant model is GG+GT versus TT, and the recessive model is GG versus GT+TT. For rs13040307,

TABLE 1 | Characteristics of patients and controls.

Characteristics	SLE	RA	Healthy controls	P_1	P_2
Male (%)/female (%)	13.50/86.5	23.20/76.80	13.70/86.30	0.950	<0.001
Age (years)	38.0 (28.0-48.0)	57.0 (49.00–65.00)	38.0 (31.0-48.0)	0.059	<0.001
Tender joints (n)	–	12.00 (4.00–24.00)	–	–	–
Swollen joints (n)	–	7.50 (2.00–16.00)	–	–	–
ESR (mm/H)	–	60.00 (35.00–93.00)	–	–	–
CRP (mg/L)	–	20.70 (5.23–55.55)	–	–	–
Self-evaluation	–	74.00 (65.00–80.00)	–	–	–
HAQ score	–	20.00 (9.75–27.25)	–	–	–
IgG (g/L)	–	13.01 (9.60–16.20)	–	–	–
IgA (mg/L)	–	2.34 (1.78–3.20)	–	–	–
IgM (mg/L)	–	1.32 (0.97–2.03)	–	–	–
anti-CCP (U/ml)	–	59.00 (28.80–115.45)	–	–	–
C3 (g/L)	–	1.27 (1.11–1.43)	–	–	–
C4 (g/L)	–	0.27 (0.22–0.32)	–	–	–
RF (IU/ml)	–	128.40 (37.95–235.00)	–	–	–
DAS28	–	3.37 (5.31–7.53)	–	–	–
SLEDAI	5.63 (4.81–6.40)	–	–	–	–
Arthritis, n (%)	92 (46.00)	–	–	–	–
Discoid rash, n (%)	83 (41.50)	–	–	–	–
Alopecia, n (%)	50 (25.50)	–	–	–	–
Oral ulcers, n (%)	24 (12.00)	–	–	–	–
Vasculitis	18 (9.00)	–	–	–	–
Pleurisy, n (%)	17 (8.50)	–	–	–	–
Pericarditis, n (%)	16 (8.00)	–	–	–	–
Myositis, n (%)	11(5.50)	–	–	–	–
Fever, n (%)	38 (19.00)	–	–	–	–
Hypocomplementemia, n (%)	100 (50.00)	–	–	–	–
ds-DNA (+), n (%)	48 (24.00)	–	–	–	–
Thrombocytopenia, n (%)	29 (14.50)	–	–	–	–
Leukopenia, n (%)	24 (12.00)	–	–	–	–
Hematuria, n (%)	65 (32.50)	–	–	–	–
Proteinuria, n (%)	96 (48.00)	–	–	–	–
Pyuria, n (%)	22 (11.00)	–	–	–	–

SLE, systemic lupus erythematosus; RA, rheumatoid arthritis; ESR, erythrocyte sedimentation rate; CRP, C-reactive protein; HAQ, health assessment questionnaire; RF, rheumatoid factor; DAS28, disease activity score 28; SLEDAI, SLE disease activity index.

[1]*Comparison between SLE and healthy controls.*

[2]*Comparison between RA and healthy controls.*

the co-dominant model includes CC versus TT, CT versus TT, the dominant model is CC+CT versus TT, and the recessive model is CC versus CT+TT. For rs3765456, the co-dominant model includes GG versus AA, GA versus AA, the dominant model is GG+GA versus AA, and the recessive model is GG versus GA+ AA. For rs73115010, the co-dominant model includes TT versus CC, TC versus CC, the dominant model is TT+TC versus CC, and the recessive model is TT versus TC+CC. Linkage disequilibrium (LD) and haplotype analysis were calculated by software: HaploView 4.2. A two-sided P value less than 0.05 was recognized as statistical significance.

RESULTS

Characteristics of All Participants

There was no significant difference in gender (P = 0.950) and age (P = 0.059) between SLE patients and healthy controls. Compared RA patients with healthy controls, the age and gender was significantly different (both P<0.05), therefore, when we discussed differences between RA patients and healthy controls for the polymorphism, age and gender were adjusted. Other clinical characteristics were summarized in **Table 1**. All six polymorphisms were in accordance with Hardy-Weinberg equilibrium (**Supplementary Table 2**).

Association Between CD40 Gene Polymorphisms and SLE

No differences for alleles and genotypes comparison of six SNPs between SLE patients and healthy controls were identified (**Table 2**). Subgroup analysis for association of CD40 gene polymorphisms and lupus patients by clinical features and laboratory parameters was carried out. Patients with positive anti-dsDNA had a lower frequency of rs13040307 allele T when compared to those with negative anti-dsDNA (P = 0.038). Patients with hematuria also showed a lower frequency of rs13040307 allele T as compared to that in patients without hematuria (P = 0.045). On the contrary, there was an increased frequency of genotype TT and allele T in lupus patients with myositis when compared to patients without the characteristic (P = 0.020, P = 0.002). A lower frequency of TT genotype and allele T for rs73115010 in lupus patients with myositis was

TABLE 2 | Allele and genotype frequencies of six polymorphisms in the CD40 gene in SLE patients, RA patients and healthy controls.

SNP	Analysed model	SLE, n (%)	RA, n (%)	Controls, n (%)	Before adjustment[a]				After adjustment[a]			
					OR_1 (95% CI)	P1	OR_2 (95% CI)	P_2	OR_1 (95% CI)	P_1	OR_2 (95% CI)	P_2
rs1883832	Gene types											
	CC	70 (45.0)	124 (36.5)	332 (36.9)	0.906 (0.568–1.447)	0.680	1.333 (0.900–1.974)	0.152	0.923 (0.578–1.476)	0.739	1.546 (0.964–2.479)	0.071
	CT	100 (50.0)	172 (50.6)	411 (45.7)	0.785 (0.502–1.229)	0.290	1.439 (1.022–2.181)	0.037	0.808 (0.515–1.266)	0.351	1.788 (1.135–2.817)	0.012
	TT	30 (15.0)	44 (12.9)	157 (17.4)	Reference		Reference		Reference		Reference	
	Allele											
	C	240 (60.0)	420 (61.8)	1075 (59.7)	1.012 (0.811–1.262)	0.918	1.089 (0.909–1.306)	0.354				
	T	160 (40.0)	260 (38.2)	725 (40.3)	Reference		Reference					
	Recessive model											
	CC	70 (45.0)	124 (36.5)	332 (36.9)	1.083 (0.786–1.494)	0.625	0.982 (0.758–1.273)	0.892	1.083 (0.786–1.494)	0.625	0.996 (0.726–1.366)	0.980
	CT+TT	130 (55.0)	216 (63.5)	568 (63.1)	Reference		Reference					
	Dominant model											
	CT+CC	170 (85.0)	296 (87.1)	743 (82.6)	0.835 (0.546–1.277)	0.465	1.422 (0.991–2.037)	0.055	0.855 (0.559–1.316)	0.473	1.681 (1.091–2.591)	0.018
	TT	30 (15.0)	44 (12.9)	157 (17.4)	Reference		Reference		Reference		Reference	
rs1569723	Gene types											
	AA	68 (34.0)	124 (36.5)	320 (35.6)	0.941 (0.594–1.492)	0.797	1.409 (0.951–2.087)	0.087	0.954 (0.601–1.515)	0.843	1.683 (1.002–2.571)	0.049
	AC	100 (50.0)	172 (50.6)	420 (46.6)	0.840 (0.542–1.301)	0.435	1.489 (1.021–2.173)	0.039	0.858 (0.553–1.332)	0.496	1.683 (1.072–2.642)	0.024
	CC	32 (16.0)	44 (12.9)	160 (17.8)	Reference		Reference		Reference		Reference	
	Allele											
	A	236 (59.0)	420 (61.8)	1060 (58.9)	1.005 (0.806–1.252)	0.967	1.128 (0.941-1.351)	0.193				
	C	164 (41.0)	260 (38.2)	740 (41.1)	Reference		Reference					
	Recessive model											
	AA	68 (34.0)	124 (36.5)	320 (35.6)	1.071 (0.776–1.479)	0.744	1.041 (0.803–1.349)	0.7764	1.069 (0.773–1.477)	0.680	1.083 (0.789–1.486)	0.623
	AC+CC	132 (66.0)	216 (63.5)	580 (64.4)	Reference		Reference		Reference		Reference	
	Dominant model											
	AC+AA	168 (84.0)	296 (87.1)	740 (82.2)	0.881(0.582–1.333)	0.607	1.453 (1.015–2.083)	0.040	0.898 (0.592–1.361)	0.610	1.650 (1.074–2.532)	0.022
	CC	32 (16.0)	44 (12.9)	160 (17.8)	Reference		Reference		Reference		Reference	
rs4810485	Gene types											
	GG	69 (34.5)	122 (35.9)	324 (36.0)	0.886 (0.554–1.416)	0.613	1.392 (0.937–2.069)	0.101	0.899 (0.562–1.438)	0.657	1.569 (0.975–2.523)	0.063
	GT	101 (50.5)	175 (51.5)	417 (46.3)	0.779 (0.498–1.218)	0.273	1.552 (1.061–2.270)	0.024	0.802 (0.512–1.255)	0.334	1.829 (1.160–2.884)	0.009
	TT	30 (15.0)	43 (12.6)	159 (17.7)	Reference		Reference		Reference		Reference	
	Allele											
	G	239 (59.7)	419 (61.6)	1065 (59.2)	1.024 (0.821–1.278)	0.830	1.108 (0.925–1.328)	0.267				
	T	161 (40.3)	261 (38.4)	735 (40.8)	Reference		Reference					
	Recessive model											
	GG	69 (34.5)	122 (35.9)	324 (36.0)	1.068 (0.774–1.473)	0.744	0.969 (0.767–1.290)	0.969	1.061 (0.768–1.465)	0.720	0.992 (0.723–1.362)	0.961
	GT+TT	131 (65.5)	218 (64.1)	576 (64.0)	Reference		Reference		Reference		Reference	
	Dominant model											
	GT+ GG	170 (85.0)	297 (87.4)	741 (82.3)	0.822(0.538–1.256)	0.408	1.481 (1.031–2.132)	0.033	0.894 (0.578–1.385)	0.427	1.715 (1.112–2.646)	0.015
	TT	30 (15.0)	43 (12.6)	159 (17.7)	Reference		Reference		Reference		Reference	
rs13040307	Gene types											
	CC	93 (46.5)	170 (50.0)	446 (49.5)	1.561(0.9652–2.527)	0.070	0.886 (0.580–1.354)	0.576	1.537 (0.948–2.492)	0.081	0.761 (0.445–1.301)	0.318
	CT	79 (39.5)	133 (39.1)	368 (40.9)	1.517 (0.928–2.478)	0.096	0.840 (0.545–1.296)	0.431	1.498 (0.915–2.451)	0.108	0.841 (0.487–1.451)	0.534
	TT	28 (14.0)	37 (10.9)	86 (9.6)	Reference		Reference		Reference		Reference	
	Allele											
	C	265 (66.3)	473 (69.6)	1260 (70.0)	0.841 (0.668–1.059)	0.141	0.979 (0.808–1.187)	0.831				

(Continued)

TABLE 2 | Continued

SNP	Analysed model	SLE, n (%)	RA, n (%)	Controls, n (%)	Before adjustment[a]				After adjustment[a]			
					OR_1 (95% CI)	P1	OR_2 (95% CI)	P_2	OR_1 (95% CI)	P_1	OR_2 (95% CI)	P_2
	T	135 (33.7)	207 (30.4)	540 (30.0)	Reference		Reference					
	Recessive model											
	CC	93 (46.5)	170 (50.0)	446 (49.5)	1.130 (0.831–1.536)	0.482	1.018 (0.793–1.306)	0.889	1.124 (0.826–1.529)	0.457	0.876 (0.647–1.186)	0.392
	CT+TT	107 (53.5)	170 (50.0)	454 (50.4)	Reference		Reference		Reference		Reference	
	Dominant model											
	CT+CC	172 (86.0)	303(89.1)	814 (90.4)	1.541(0.976–2.433)	0.072	0.865 (0.576–1.300)	0.486	1.520 (0.960–2.404)	0.074	0.796 (0.475–1.333)	0.387
	TT	28 (14.0)	37 (10.9)	86 (9.6)	Reference		Reference		Reference		Reference	
rs3765456	Gene types											
	GG	72 (36.0)	119 (35.0)	309 (34.3)	1.094 (0.708–1.690)	0.686	1.202 (0.818–1.767)	0.348	1.118 (0.722–1.730)	0.616	1.454 (0.913–2.315)	0.115
	GA	89 (44.5)	172 (50.6)	438 (48.7)	1.254 (0.825–1.907)	0.289	1.226 (0.850–1.770)	0.276	1.294 (0.849–1.973)	0.230	1.433 (0.921–2.229)	0.111
	AA	39 (19.5)	49 (14.4)	153 (17.0)	Reference		Reference		Reference		Reference	
	Allele											
	G	233 (58.3)	410 (60.3)	1056 (58.7)	0.983 (0.789–1.225)	0.878	1.070 (0.894–1.281)	0.462				
	A	167 (41.7)	270 (39.7)	744 (41.3)	Reference		Reference					
	Recessive model											
	GG	72 (36.0)	119 (35.0)	309 (34.3)	0.929 (0.675–1.280)	0.681	1.030 (0.793–1.338)	0.860	0.929 (0.670–1.280)	0.652	1.108 (0.805–1.525)	0.529
	GA+AA	128 (64.0)	221 (65.0)	591 (65.7)	Reference		Reference		Reference		Reference	
	Dominant model											
	GA+GG	161 (80.5)	291 (85.6)	747 (83.0)	1.182(0.800–1.748)	0.410	1.217 (0.896–1.724)	0.271	1.215 (0.820–1.799)	0.332	1.441 (0.947–2.193)	0.088
	AA	39 (19.5)	49 (14.4)	153 (17.0)	Reference		Reference		Reference		Reference	
rs73115010	Gene types											
	TT	89 (44.5)	155 (45.6)	423 (47.0)	1.451 (0.903–2.332)	0.124	0.941 (0.617–1.435)	0.777	1.430 (0.888–2.301)	0.141	0.808 (0.476–1.372)	0.430
	TC	82 (41.0)	148 (43.5)	382 (42.4)	1.422 (0.881–2.297)	0.150	0.995 (0.651–1.521)	0.981	1.415 (0.875–2.289)	0.157	1.055 (0.620–1.794)	0.844
	CC	29 (14.5)	37 (10.9)	95 (10.6)	Reference		Reference		Reference		Reference	
	Allele											
	T	260 (65.0)	458 (67.4)	1228 (68.2)	1.156 (0.920–1.452)	0.231	1.041 (0.862–1.256)	0.679				
	C	140 (35.0)	222 (32.6)	572 (31.8)	Reference		Reference					
	Recessive model											
	TT	89 (44.5)	155 (45.6)	423 (47.0)	1.106 (0.813–1.505)	0.532	0.945 (0.736–1.214)	0.657	1.094 (0.803–1.490)	0.569	0.773 (0.570–1.050)	0.099
	TC+CC	111 (55.5)	185 (54.4)	477 (53.0)	Reference		Reference		Reference		Reference	
	Dominant model											
	TC+TT	171 (85.5)	303 (89.1)	805 (89.4)	1.437(0.919–2.247)	0.137	0.966 (0.646–1.445)	0.868	1.422 (0.908–2.227)	0.123	0.919 (0.555–1.522)	0.743
	CC	29 (14.5)	37 (10.9)	95 (10.6)	Reference		Reference		Reference		Reference	

SNP, single-nucleotide polymorphism; SLE, systemic lupus erythematosus; RA, rheumatoid arthritis.

[a]Adjustment for age and sex; [1]comparison between SLE and controls; [2]comparison between RA and controls.

Description of alleles, genotypes of the six polymorphisms in SLE patients and healthy controls was listed as frequency, percentage. Differences of alleles, genotypes of the six polymorphisms between SLE patients and healthy controls were analyzed by chi-square test. Logistic regression calculated (adjusted) odds ratio and 95% confidence interval. Software SPSS 17.0 was used for the statistics.

obtained (P = 0.024, P = 0.004). Interestingly, higher frequencies of rs1569723 allele A, rs4810485 allele T and lower frequencies of rs3765456 allele A, rs1883832 allele T were noted in patients with myositis as compared to those in patients without the feature (P = 0.020, P = 0.030, P = 0.021, P = 0.032, respectively) (**Table 3** and **Supplementary Table 3**). SLEDAI was used to analyze disease activity for SLE patients, and association of genotypes for different polymorphisms and SLEDAI was evaluated. We found that none of the genotypes for the six polymorphisms associated with SLEDAI (**Supplementary Table 4**).

TABLE 3 | Analysis of CD40 gene polymorphisms (rs13040307, rs3765456, rs73115010) in SLE patients by clinical features.

Clinical features	rs13040307							rs3765456							rs73115010						
	Genotypefrequency (n)			P_1	Allele frequency (n)		P_2	Genotype frequency (n)			P_1	Allele frequency (n)		P_2	Genotype frequency (n)			P_1	Allele frequency (n)		P_2
	TT	TC	CC		T	C		AA	AG	GG		A	G		TT	TC	CC		T	C	
Arthritis																					
Positive	14	34	44	0.770	62	122	0.983	22	34	36	0.114	78	106	0.839	43	35	14	0.732	121	63	0.768
Negative	14	45	49		73	143		17	55	36		89	127		46	47	15		139	77	
Discoid rash																					
Positive	13	30	40	0.680	56	110	0.996	15	38	30	0.904	68	98	0.788	39	31	13	0.673	109	57	0.815
Negative	15	49	53		79	155		24	51	12		99	135		50	51	16		151	83	
Alopecia																					
Positive	7	21	22	0.907	35	65	0.760	10	22	18	0.994	42	58	0.953	22	20	8	0.949	64	36	0.809
Negative	28	58	71		100	200		29	67	54		125	175		67	62	21		196	104	
Oral ulcers																					
Positive	4	8	12	0.789	16	32	0.948	8	8	8	0.174	24	24	0.217	13	8	3	0.610	34	14	0.366
Negative	24	71	81		119	233		31	81	94		143	209		76	74	26		226	126	
Pleurisy																					
Positive	3	6	8	0.878	12	22	0.842	3	7	7	0.897	13	21	0.664	7	7	3	0.942	21	13	0.679
Negative	25	73	85		123	243		36	82	65		154	212		82	75	26		239	127	
Pericarditis																					
Positive	3	7	8	0.718	13	19	0.391	2	5	9	0.212	9	23	0.103	5	8	3	0.558	18	14	0.279
Negative	25	72	87		122	246		37	84	63		158	210		84	74	26		242	126	
Fever																					
Positive	7	13	18	0.608	27	49	0.716	8	15	15	0.786	31	45	0.850	16	15	7	0.778	47	29	0.593
Negative	21	66	75		108	216		31	74	57		136	188		73	67	22		213	111	
Hypocomplementemia																					
Positive	14	38	48	0.938	66	134	0.751	23	39	38	0.242	85	115	0.761	47	38	15	0.705	132	68	0.675
Negative	14	41	45		69	131		16	50	34		82	118		42	44	14		128	72	
ds-DNA(+)																					
Positive	5	14	29	0.086	24	72	0.038	12	23	13	0.281	47	49	0.100	26	15	7	0.244	67	29	0.259
Negative	23	65	64		111	193		27	66	59		120	184		63	67	22		193	111	
Thrombocytopenia																					
Positive	4	12	13	0.974	20	38	0.898	6	12	11	0.935	24	34	0.951	13	12	4	0.886	38	20	0.929
Negative	24	67	80		115	227		33	77	61		143	199		76	70	25		222	120	
Leukopenia																					
Positive	3	7	14	0.449	13	35	0.298	7	9	8	0.436	23	25	0.356	13	8	3	0.610	34	14	0.366
Negative	25	72	79		122	230		32	80	64		144	208		76	74	26		226	126	
Hematuria																					
Positive	8	19	38	0.057	35	95	0.045	17	25	23	0.225	59	71	0.306	34	23	8	0.310	91	39	0.146
Negative	20	60	55		100	170		22	64	49		108	162		55	59	21		169	101	
Proteinuria																					
Positive	17	34	45	0.273	68	124	0.498	21	38	37	0.393	80	112	0.974	44	35	17	0.336	123	69	0.706
Negative	11	45	48		67	141		18	51	35		87	121		45	47	12		137	71	
Pyuria																					
Positive	1	9	12	0.380	11	33	0.193	7	7	8	0.244	21	23	0.394	12	9	1	0.310	33	11	0.140
Negative	27	70	81		124	232		32	82	64		146	210		77	73	28		227	129	
Vasculitis																					
Positive	2	7	9	0.918	11	25	0.671	3	9	6	0.880	15	21	0.992	9	7	2	0.847	25	11	0.558
Negative	26	72	84		124	240		36	80	66		152	212		80	75	27		235	129	
Myositis																					
Positive	4	6	1	0.020	14	8	0.002	0	4	7	0.086	4	18	0.021	1	6	4	0.024	8	14	0.004
Negative	24	73	92		121	257		39	85	65		163	215		88	76	25		252	126	

P_1, Patients positive versus patients negative using 3×2 contingency table.
P_2, Patients positive versus patients negative using 2×2 contingency table.

TABLE 4 | Association of disease activity parameters in RA patients with CD40 gene polymorphisms (rs1569723, rs13040307).

Characteristics	rs13040307 [Median (P_{25}–P_{75})]			P_1	rs73115010 [Median (P_{25}–P_{75})]			P_2
	CC	CT	TT		TT	TC	CC	
Tender joints (n)	11.00 (4.00–23.75)	13.00 (5.00–24.00)	10.00 (4.00–26.00)	0.547	12.00 (4.00–23.25)	12.50 (5.00–27.00)	10.00 (2.50–23.75)	0.438
Swollen joints (n)	5.50 (1.00–16.00)	10.00 (2.00–16.00)	6.00 (1.00–14.00)	0.010	7.00 (2.00–14.00)	10.00 (2.00–20.00)	4.00 (0.00–12.00)	0.038
ESR (n)	63.50 (39.00–89.50)	62.00 (35.00–92.00)	52.00 (29.00–96.00)	0.798	60.00 (34.00–95.00)	60.00 (37.25–87.45)	67.50 (26.50–102.78)	0.635
CRP (mg/L)	12.60 (6.36–44.30)	24.70 (5.15–62.99)	18.10 (5.40–51.30)	0.792	18.90 (5.30–55.40)	20.95 (4.50–57.35)	26.00 (6.40–63.85)	0.631
Self-evaluation	79.00 (68.75–83.50)	70.00 (65.0–80.00)	75.00 (65.00–85.00)	0.806	75.00 (65.00–80.00)	70.00 (65.00–80.00)	75.00 (65.00–89.00)	0.416
HAQ score	20.00 (7.00–28.00)	20.00 (10.00–27.00)	20.00 (12.00–27.75)	0.906	20.00 (10.00–28.25)	20.00 (9.00–26.00)	20.00 (8.50–28.00)	0.753
IgG (g/L)	12.50 (11.34–16.64)	12.95 (9.41–16.35)	13.18 (9.58–16.27)	0.807	13.04 (9.41–18.19)	12.95 (9.72–16.49)	13.34 (9.53–15.71)	0.807
IgA (mg/L)	2.69 (2.08–4.58)	2.28 (1.75–3.12)	2.38 (1.78–3.20)	0.298	2.59 (1.79–3.76)	2.32 (1.78–3.01)	1.98 (1.74–2.75)	0.298
IgM (mg/L)	1.41 (1.05–1.86)	1.38 (0.99–2.01)	1.24 (0.91–2.07)	0.775	1.34 (0.97–1.98)	1.29 (1.00–2.05)	1.51 (0.80–2.07)	0.775
RF (IU/L)	110.20 (29.38–216.25)	122.65 (33.60–268.80)	139.00 (41.10–236.00)	0.683	140.85 (45.23–318.38)	121.00 (32.33–226.25)	97.60 (31.00–236.00)	0.613
anti-CCP (U/mL)	59.80 (25.40–91.00)	58.40 (30.20–139.90)	60.35 (29.10–121.35)	0.748	59.40 (26.53–107.88)	57.80 (30.60–149.00)	52.50 (25.53–137.00)	0.713
C3 (g/L)	1.25 (1.15–1.46)	1.22 (1.09–1.45)	1.28 (1.15–1.38)	0.644	1.28 (1.10–1.46)	1.24 (1.12–1.37)	1.28 (1.16–1.43)	0.644
C4 (g/L)	0.28 (0.23–0.37)	0.27 (0.22–0.32)	0.26 (0.21–0.36)	0.518	0.26 (0.21–0.34)	0.27 (0.22–0.31)	0.29 (0.19–0.37)	0.518
DAS28	6.38 (5.19–7.46)	6.50 (5.36–7.67)	6.06 (5.17–7.42)	0.694	6.27 (5.06–7.42)	6.50 (5.44–7.67)	6.06 (5.17–7.42)	0.679

Characteristics	rs4810485 [Median (P_{25}-P_{75})]			P_1	rs13040307 [Median (P_{25}-P_{75})]			P_2
	GG	TG	TT		CC	TC	TT	
Tender joints (n)	12.00 (3.00–23.50)	11.00 (5.00–27.00)	12.0 (4.00–24.00)	0.727	11.00 (4.00–23.75)	13.00 (5.00–24.00)	10.00 (4.00–26.00)	0.547
Swollen joints (n)	4.00 (0.00–12.00)	10.00 (2.00–20.00)	7.00 (2.00–16.00)	0.498	5.50 (1.00–16.00)	10.00 (2.00–16.00)	6.00 (1.00–14.00)	0.010
ESR (n)	55.50 (26.50–100.50)	60.00 (31.5–87.00)	61.00 (36.00–95.00)	0.761	63.50 (39.00–89.50)	62.00 (35.00–92.00)	52.00 (29.00–96.00)	0.798
CRP (mg/L)	26.00 (6.40–54.35)	19.90 (4.21–50.00)	21.05 (5.50–58.00)	0.479	12.60 (6.36–44.30)	24.70 (5.15–62.99)	18.10 (5.40–51.30)	0.792
Self-evaluation	70.00 (62.50–85.00)	75.00 (65.00–85.00)	72.50 (66.50–80.00)	0.300	79.00 (68.75–83.50)	70.00 (65.0–80.00)	75.00 (65.00–85.00)	0.806
HAQ score	20.00 (11.50–26.50)	20.00 (8.25–27.00)	20.00 (10.00–28.00)	0.458	20.00 7.00–28.00)	20.00 (10.00–27.00)	20.00 (12.00–27.75)	0.906
IgG (g/L)	13.34 (9.53–15.71)	12.95 (9.84–16.40)	13.04 (9.31–16.30)	0.688	12.50 (11.34–16.64)	12.95 (9.41–16.35)	13.18 (9.58–16.27)	0.807
IgA (mg/L)	1.98 (1.74–2.75)	2.40 (1.79–3.01)	2.34 (1.67–3.64)	0.140	2.69 (2.08–4.58)	2.28 (1.75–3.12)	2.38 (1.78–3.20)	0.298
IgM (mg/L)	1.51 (0.80–2.07)	1.27 (0.96–2.09)	1.36 (0.99–1.95)	0.632	1.41 (1.05–1.86)	1.38 (0.99–2.01)	1.24 (0.91–2.07)	0.775
RF (IU/L)	91.45 (34.98–268.78)	131.35 (36.67–232.25)	129.10 (38.15–258.95)	0.540	110.20 (29.38–216.25)	122.65 (33.60–268.80)	139.00 (41.10–236.00)	0.683
anti-CCP (U/mL)	63.00 (27.2–99.00)	58.40 (31.50–148.15)	58.75 (25.93–111.38)	0.577	59.80 (25.40–91.00)	58.40 (30.20–139.90)	60.35 (29.10–121.35)	0.748
C3 (g/L)	1.28 (1.16–1.43)	1.23 (1.12–1.37)	1.28 (1.10–1.46)	0.718	1.25 (1.15–1.46)	1.22 (1.09–1.45)	1.28 (1.15–1.38)	0.644
C4 (g/L)	0.29 (0.19–0.37)	0.27 (0.22–0.31)	0.26 (0.21–0.34)	0.330	0.28 (0.23–0.37)	0.27 (0.22–0.32)	0.26 (0.21–0.36)	0.518
DAS-28	6.14 (5.00–7.52)	6.49 (5.47–7.54)	6.70 (5.16–7.57)	0.963	6.38 (5.19–7.46)	6.50 (5.36–7.67)	6.06 (5.17–7.42)	0.694

ESR, erythrocyte sedimentation rate; CRP, C-reactive protein; HAQ, health assessment questionnaire; RF, rheumatoid factor; DAS28, disease activity score 28.
[1]CC+CT versus TT genotype for rs13040307; [2]TT+TC versus CC genotype for rs73115010.

Association Between CD40 Gene Polymorphisms and RA

Differences of alleles and genotypes of CD40 gene polymorphisms between RA patients and healthy controls were shown in **Table 2**. Frequencies of genotypes AA, AC, and AA+ AC of rs1569723 were different between RA patients and healthy controls after age and gender adjustment (AA vs CC, OR, 1.683; 95% CI, 1.002–2.571, P = 0.049; AC vs CC, OR, 1.683; 95% CI, 1.072–2.642, P = 0.024; AA+AC vs CC, OR, 1.650; 95% CI, 1.074–2.534; P = 0.022). Frequencies of genotypes CT, CT+CC of rs1883832 were different between RA patients and healthy controls after age and gender adjustment (CT vs TT; OR, 1.788; 95% CI, 1.135–2.817; P=0.012; CT+CC vs TT: OR, 1.681; 95% CI, 1.091–2.591; P = 0.018). For rs4810485, statistical significance was obtained for comparison of GT with TT, and GT+GG with TT after adjustment by age and gender (GT vs TT: OR, 1.829; 95% CI, 1.160–2.884; P = 0.009; GT+GG vs TT: OR, 1.715; 95% CI, 1.112–2.646; P=0.015). The other three polymorphisms were not related to RA risk.

Association of disease activity in RA patients with CD40 gene polymorphisms was displayed in **Table 4**. For rs13040307, number of the swollen joints between patients with CC+CT genotype and CC genotype was different (P = 0.010). RA patients carrying rs73115010 TT+TC genotype had higher number of swollen joints as compared to the patients carrying CC genotype (P = 0.038). Other polymorphisms were not related to RA clinical parameters (**Supplementary Table 5**, **Supplementary Table 6**).

CD40 Haplotype Analysis for RA and SLE

Considering linkage disequilibrium of genes, we performed haplotype analysis for CD40 gene polymorphisms. Two blocks were defined by 95% CI (19). The first one consists of four polymorphisms including rs1569723, rs13040307, rs1883832, and rs4810485, and the other one consists of rs3765456 and rs73115010 both for RA and SLE (**Figures 1A, B**). Results showed that there was no significant difference between patients and controls regarding different haplotypes (**Supplementary Table 7**).

DISCUSSION

This study explored association of CD40 gene polymorphisms with susceptibility to SLE and RA in a Southern Chinese Han population. A total of six polymorphisms, rs3765456, rs1569723, rs73115010, rs13040307, rs1883832, and rs4810485 were recruited. For RA, the co-dominant model and dominant model of rs1569723, rs1883832, and rs4810485 polymorphisms associated with increased susceptibility to RA. Number of swollen joints were increased in RA patients with genotypes CC+TC of rs13040307 and TT+TC of rs373115010. For SLE, rs13040307 of CD40 gene was related to clinic features, including hematuria and anti-dsDNA. Interestingly, the six polymorphisms may be related to SLE patients with myositis.

SLE and RA are autoimmune disorders with genetic pathogenesis. For rs3765456, this polymorphism may be a risk factor for SLE susceptibility and associated with disease activity in

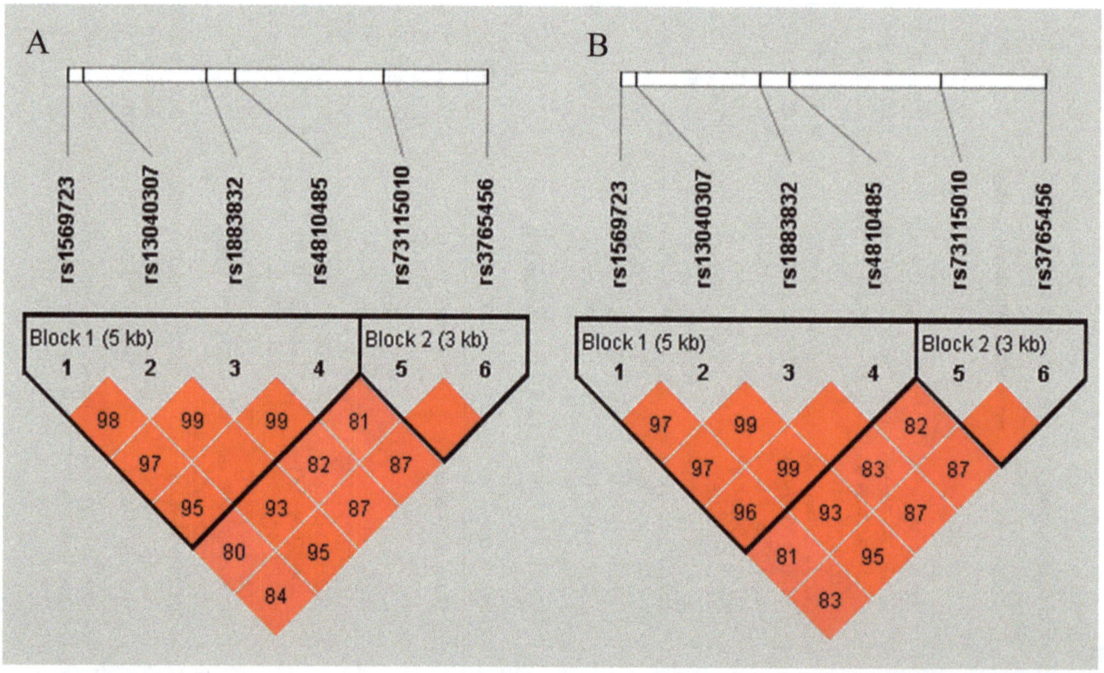

FIGURE 1 | Linkage disequilibrium(LD) of six single nucleotide polymorphisms. The intensity of linkage disequilibrium (LD) is reflected in the color and numeric value (D′) of each box. Bright red means D′ ≥0.95, LOD ≥2. Shade of red means D′<0.95, LOD≥2. **(A)** LD of RA patients and controls. **(B)** LD of SLE patients and controls. Both of them show that block 1 consists of four polymorphisms including rs1569723 A/C, rs13040307 T/C, rs1883832 T/C, and rs4810485 T/G, block 2 consists of rs3765456 A/G and rs73115010 T/C.

Korea population (12), whereas this polymorphism was not significantly related to SLE in Northern Chinese population (10). In our study, there was no significant difference regarding this polymorphism and SLE risk in Southern Chinese Han population. Interestingly, SLE patients with myositis associated with a lower frequency of rs3765456 allele A, suggesting that rs3765456 allele A may affect the patients complicated with this feature. To date, no study has discussed association of rs3765456 polymorphism with RA risk. In this study, we found that this polymorphism was not related to RA risk. For rs1569723, a previous genome-wide association study reported that there was relation between RA and rs1569732 in European population (20). In our study, we confirmed that this polymorphism related to Chinese RA patients. With respect to relationship between rs1569732 and SLE, a study in Chinese population showed that there was significant difference between rs1569723 and SLE (9). The present study did not find significant association of this polymorphism and SLE risk in our Southern Chinese Han population. However, higher frequency of rs1569723 allele A was related to SLE patients with myositis in this study. Regarding rs13040307 and rs73115010, there were limited studies evaluating association of the two polymorphisms with disease susceptibility, including lupus or arthritis. Wu et al. reported that these two polymorphisms may not associate with SLE in Chinese population by a relatively small sample size (21). By contrast, a study in Korea population indicated that rs73115010 may increase the risk of SLE (12). In this study, there was no significant association of these polymorphisms and SLE, RA risk in our Southern Chinese Han population. Interestingly, rs13040307 polymorphism was related to disease activity parameters of SLE, including anti-dsDNA, hematuria, and myositis. In addition, RA patients carrying genotype CC+CT of rs13040307 and genotype TT+TC of rs73115010 had higher number of swollen joints. However, further studies with larger sample size and different ethnicities are needed to illustrate the relationship of these two polymorphisms (rs13040307 and rs73115010) in SLE and RA.

For another two polymorphisms (rs1883832 and rs4810485), several studies have discussed the association with SLE, RA risk. Rs1883832 was significantly associated with SLE in a Tunisian population (22). However, a study in Egypt population and a study in Korea population did not find significant results (12, 23). For RA, there was no association of rs1883832 in Eastern Chinese and Iran population (24, 25) and the study published by Liu et al. showed that genotype TT versus CC+CT was significant in men (24). On the contrary, rs1883832 was related to RA risk in a Tunisian population (22). According to rs4810485, this polymorphism was confirmed related to SLE and RA risk in European population (11), but not in Korea and Tunisian population (12, 22). In the present study for Southern Chinese Han population, rs1883832 and rs4810485 was related to RA risk, whereas these two polymorphisms were not related to SLE by analyzing genetic models. However, these two polymorphisms were related to SLE patients complicated with myositis. Compared our findings with Liu et al., the differences may correlate with several reasons. First, Liu et al. genotyped the polymorphism by MALDI-TOF MS using the MassARRAY Nanodispenser, and we used KASP method. Second, we have larger sample size not only in RA patients but in healthy controls. Third, the author found a significant result regarding genotype TT versus CC+CT in men, while in our study, we did not find a significant result regarding genotype TT versus CC+CT in men (OR, 1.650; 95% CI, 0.651–4.180;P = 0.288), suggesting that whether this polymorphism may relate to RA risk either in all RA patients or male patients needs to be further discussed with larger sample size especially with larger men patients, the same genotyping method. Collectively, all these differences for SLE, RA risk as compared to our findings may relate to several possibilities. First, RA, SLE are complex diseases, and they have different pathogenesis, therefore, different polymorphisms may have distinct relation to SLE, RA risk, and it is possible that the same polymorphism may have different relation to SLE, RA. Second, different studies selected different methods to detect the polymorphisms may have distinct results. Third, different ethnicities may associate with different results.

Since CD40 gene polymorphisms may correlate with RA, SLE susceptibility, it is convinced that clarification of how polymorphism or what polymorphism of CD40 gene has affected mRNA expression and protein expression, and how does the protein perform in the pathogenesis of these diseases is meaningful and helpful. It is widely accepted that mRNA may be regulated by SNPs (26). Therefore, dysregulated expression of CD40 may be caused by upregulation of transcription and translation owing to mutated polymorphism. Studies showed that genotype TT, TC of rs1883832 associated with increased CD40 expression in Chinese and Egypt SLE patients (9, 23). Genotype GG of rs4810485 was related to increased CD40 expression in Greek and Turkish SLE patients (27, 28). CD40 is expressed on smooth muscle fibroblasts and synovial cells, which can be upregulated by pro-inflammatory cytokines, such as IFN-γ and TNFα. In turn, elevated expression of CD40 may further involve in the inflammatory response, leading to fibroblast proliferation, adhesion molecule upregulation, and generation of pro-inflammatory cytokines and chemokines, and finally causing diseases development and progression (7, 29). To date, several studies have showed that expression of CD40 was elevated in SLE, RA patients and associated with diseases activity (30–32). Therefore, mutation in CD40 gene may have affected CD40 expression, and promoted SLE, RA development. In our study, we did not discuss association of these polymorphism and CD40 expression in RA patients or SLE patients. Functional study in the future is necessary to elucidate how polymorphism regulates CD40 expression, especially the role in RA, SLE pathogenesis.

There are some limitations in the present study. First, selection bias cannot be avoided because patients were selected from a hospital. Second, this study focuses on association of SNPs with susceptibility to SLE, RA, however, exploring the process of transcription and translation of CD40 gene by the polymorphisms is of importance. Third, more SNPs of CD40 gene are needed to discuss association with SLE, RA risk, and discussion of gene-environment interaction should be investigated in the future. Fourth, we found association of myositis with the six polymorphisms, however, the conclusion is to take with caution because of the very low number of patients. Finally, replication of the results on other ethnics is lacking.

In conclusion, our study showed that CD40 gene polymorphisms may relate to SLE and RA susceptibility.

ETHICS STATEMENT

The studies involving human participants were reviewed and approved by Ethic Research Committee of Southwest Medical University. The patients/participants provided their written informed consent to participate in this study.

AUTHOR CONTRIBUTIONS

QH, W-DX, L-CS, X-YL, and A-FH designed and wrote this paper. All authors contributed to the article and approved the submitted version.

REFERENCES

1. Smolen JS, Aletaha D, McInnes IB. Rheumatoid arthritis [published correction appears in *Lancet* (2016) Oct 22;388(10055):1984]. *Lancet* (2016) 388(10055):2023–38. doi: 10.1016/S0140-6736(16)30173-8
2. Durcan L, O'Dwyer T, Petri M. Management strategies and future directions for systemic lupus erythematosus in adults. *Lancet* (2019) 393(10188):2332–43. doi: 10.1016/S0140-6736(19)30237-5
3. Aleman-Avila I, Jimenez-Morales M, Beltran-Ramirez O, Barbosa-Cobos RE, Jimenez-Morales S, Sanchez-Munoz F, et al. Functional polymorphisms in pre-miR146a and pre-miR499 are associated with systemic lupus erythematosus but not with rheumatoid arthritis or Graves' disease in Mexican patients. *Oncotarget* (2017) 8(54):91876–86. doi: 10.18632/oncotarget.19621
4. Zhao YL, Zhang TP, Wu J, Li BZ, Li XM, Pan HF, et al. Association of adiponectin and adiponectin receptor gene polymorphisms with rheumatoid arthritis in a Chinese population. *Postgrad Med J* (2020) 96(1133):149–55. doi: 10.1136/postgradmedj-2018-136372
5. Oparina N, Martinez-Bueno M, Alarcon-Riquelme ME. An update on the genetics of systemic lupus erythematosus. *Curr Opin Rheumatol* (2019) 31 (6):659–68. doi: 10.1097/BOR.0000000000000654
6. Amariuta T, Luo Y, Knevel R, Okada Y, Raychaudhuri S. Advances in genetics toward identifying pathogenic cell states of rheumatoid arthritis. *Immunol Rev* (2020) 294(1):188–204. doi: 10.1111/imr.12827
7. Karnell JL, Rieder SA, Ettinger R, Kolbeck R. Targeting the CD40-CD40L pathway in autoimmune diseases: Humoral immunity and beyond. *Adv Drug Deliv Rev* (2019) 141:92–103. doi: 10.1016/j.addr.2018.12.005
8. Nathan MJ, Mold JE, Wood SC, Csencsits K, Lu G, Eichwald EJ, et al. Requirement for donor and recipient CD40 expression in cardiac allograft rejection: induction of Th1 responses and influence of donor-derived dendritic cells. *J Immunol* (2004) 172:6626–33. doi: 10.4049/jimmunol.172.11.6626
9. Chen JM, Guo J, Wei CD, Wang CF, Luo HC, Wei YS, et al. The association of CD40 polymorphisms with CD40 serum levels and risk of systemic lupus erythematosus. *BMC Genet* (2015) 16:121. doi: 10.1186/s12863-015-0279-8
10. Nie D, Li H, Yan G, Wang Z, He Z, Zhou W. Gene-gene interaction between CD40 and CD226 gene on systemic lupus erythematosus in the Chinese Han population. *Rheumatol Int* (2016) 36(12):1657–62. doi: 10.1007/s00296-016-3570-8
11. Lee YH, Bae SC, Choi SJ, Ji JD, Song GG. Associations between the functional CD40 rs4810485 G/T polymorphism and susceptibility to rheumatoid arthritis and systemic lupus erythematosus: a meta-analysis. *Lupus* (2015) 24(11):1177–83. doi: 10.1177/0961203315583543
12. Joo YB, Park BL, Shin HD, Park SY, Kim I, Bae SC. Association of genetic polymorphisms in CD40 with susceptibility to SLE in the Korean population. *Rheumatol (Oxford)* (2013) 52(4):623–30. doi: 10.1093/rheumatology/kes339
13. Raychaudhuri S, Remmers EF, Lee AT, Hackett R, Guiducci C, Burtt NP, et al. Common variants at CD40 and other loci confer risk of rheumatoid arthritis. *Nat Genet* (2008) 40(10):1216–23. doi: 10.1038/ng.233
14. Hochberg MC. Updating the American College of Rheumatology revised criteria for the classification of systemic lupus erythematosus. *Arthrit Rheum* (1997) 40(9):1725. doi: 10.1002/art.1780400928
15. Neogi T, Aletaha D, Silman AJ, Naden RL, Felson DT, Aggarwal R, et al. The 2010 American College of Rheumatology/European League Against Rheumatism classification criteria for rheumatoid arthritis: Phase 2 methodological report. *Arthritis Rheum* (2010) 62(9):2582–91. doi: 10.1002/art.27580
16. Prevoo ML, van 't Hof MA, Kuper HH, van Leeuwen MA, van de Putte LB, van Riel PL. Modified disease activity scores that include twenty-eight-joint counts. Development and validation in a prospective longitudinal study of patients with rheumatoid arthritis. *Arthritis Rheumatol* (1995) 38(1):44–8. doi: 10.1002/art.1780380107
17. Bombardier C, Gladman DD, Urowitz MB, Caron D, Chang CH. Derivation of the SLEDAI. A disease activity index for lupus patients. The Committee on Prognosis Studies in SLE. *Arthritis Rheumatol* (1992) 35(6):630–40. doi: 10.1002/art.1780350606
18. Hoogendijk JE, Amato AA, Lecky BR, Choy EH, Lundberg IE, Rose MR, et al. 119th ENMC international workshop: trial design in adult idiopathic inflammatory myopathies, with the exception of inclusion body myositis, 10-12 October 2003, Naarden, The Netherlands. *Neuromuscul Disord* (2004) 14(5):337–45. doi: 10.1016/j.nmd.2004.02.006
19. Gabriel SB, Schaffner SF, Nguyen H, Moore JM, Roy J, Blumenstiel B, et al. The structure of haplotype blocks in the human genome. *Science* (2002) 296 (5576):2225–9. doi: 10.1126/science.1069424
20. Australia and New Zealand Multiple Sclerosis Genetics Consortium (ANZgene). Genome-wide association study identifies new multiple sclerosis susceptibility loci on chromosomes 12 and 20. *Nat Genet* (2009) 41(7):824–8. doi: 10.1038/ng.396
21. Wu CJ, Guo J, Luo HC, Wei CD, Wang CF, Lan Y, et al. Association of CD40 polymorphisms and haplotype with risk of systemic lupus erythematosus. *Rheumatol Int* (2016) 36(1):45–52. doi: 10.1007/s00296-015-3345-7
22. Soussi M, Kallel A, Ben Wafi S, Ben Halima M, Sanhaji H, Mourali MS, et al. Associations of rs1883832 and rs4810485 polymorphisms of CD40 gene with myocardial infarction in the Tunisian population. *Biomarkers* (2019) 24 (6):530–7. doi: 10.1080/1354750X.2019.1602168
23. Mousa TG, Omar HH, Emad R, Salama MI, Omar W, Fawzy M, et al. The association of CD40 polymorphism (rs1883832C/T) and soluble CD40 with the risk of systemic lupus erythematosus among Egyptian patients. *Clin Rheumatol* (2019) 38(3):777–84. doi: 10.1007/s10067-018-4349-y
24. Liu R, Xu N, Wang X, Shen L, Zhao G, Zhang H, et al. Influence of MIF, CD40, and CD226 polymorphisms on risk of rheumatoid arthritis. *Mol Biol Rep* (2012) 39(6):6915–22. doi: 10.1007/s11033-012-1518-y
25. Hosseini N, Tahoori MT, Mohammadzadeh A, Zarei Jaliani H, Bitaraf Sani M, Soleimani Salehabadi H. IRAK1 Gene Polymorphism in Rheumatoid Arthritis. *Immunol Invest* (2021) 50(2–3):304–21. doi: 10.1080/08820139.2020.1764028
26. Lu YF, Mauger DM, Goldstein DB, Urban TJ, Weeks KM, Bradrick SS. IFNL3 mRNA structure is remodeled by a functional non-coding polymorphism associated with hepatitis C virus clearance. *Sci Rep* (2015) 5:16037. doi: 10.1038/srep16037
27. Vazgiourakis VM, Zervou MI, Choulaki C, Bertsias G, Melissourgaki M, Yilmaz N, et al. A common SNP in the CD40 region is associated with systemic lupus erythematosus and correlates with altered CD40 expression:

implications for the pathogenesis. *Ann Rheum Dis* (2011) 70:2184–90. doi: 10.1136/ard.2010.146530

28. Tapia-Llanos R, Muñoz-Valle JF, Román-Fernández IV, Marín-Rosales M, Salazar-Camarena DC, Cruz A, et al. Association of soluble CD40 levels with -1 C > T CD40 polymorphism and chronic kidney disease in systemic lupus erythematosus. *Mol Genet Genomic Med* (2019) 7(12):e1014. doi: 10.1002/mgg3.1014
29. Peters AL, Stunz LL, Bishop GA. CD40 and autoimmunity: the dark side of a great activator. *Semin Immunol* (2009) 21(5):293–300. doi: 10.1016/j.smim.2009.05.012
30. Perper SJ, Westmoreland SV, Karman J, Twomey R, Seagal J, Wang R, et al. Treatment with a CD40 Antagonist Antibody Reverses Severe Proteinuria and Loss of Saliva Production and Restores Glomerular Morphology in Murine Systemic Lupus Erythematosus. *J Immunol* (2019) 203(1):58–75. doi: 10.4049/jimmunol.1900043
31. Chamberlain C, Colman PJ, Ranger AM, Burkly LC, Johnston GI, Otoul C, et al. Repeated administration of dapirolizumab pegol in a randomised phase I study is well tolerated and accompanied by improvements in several composite measures of systemic lupus erythematosus disease activity and changes in whole blood transcriptomic profiles. *Ann Rheum Dis* (2017) 76 (11):1837–44. doi: 10.1136/annrheumdis-2017-211388
32. Ota Y, Niiro H, Ota S, Ueki N, Tsuzuki H, Nakayama T, et al. Generation mechanism of RANKL(+) effector memory B cells: relevance to the pathogenesis of rheumatoid arthritis. *Arthritis Res Ther* (2016) 18:67. doi: 10.1186/s13075-016-0957-6

15

Plasma C4d Correlates with C4d Deposition in Kidneys and with Treatment Response in Lupus Nephritis Patients

Myriam Martin[1,2], Rebecca Trattner[1,2], Sara C. Nilsson[1], Albin Björk[3], Agneta Zickert[3,4], Anna M. Blom[1,2†] and Iva Gunnarsson[3,4†]*

[1] Department of Translational Medicine, Section of Medical Protein Chemistry, Lund University, Malmö, Sweden, [2] Region Skåne, Laboratory Medicine, Clinical Chemistry, Malmö, Sweden, [3] Department of Medicine, Division of Rheumatology, Karolinska Institutet, Stockholm, Sweden, [4] Rheumatology, Karolinska University Hospital, Stockholm, Sweden

***Correspondence:**
Anna M. Blom
anna.blom@med.lu.se

† These authors have contributed equally to this work

Objective: To examine whether C4d plasma levels correlate with treatment response and C4d kidney deposition in systemic lupus erythematosus (SLE) with lupus nephritis (LN).

Methods: C4d plasma levels were analyzed by a unique assay specifically detecting C4d arising from complement activation and C4 plasma levels were quantified with competitive ELISA. SLE patients with LN (71) and active SLE patients without LN (22) plus 145 controls were included. For 52 LN patients samples were available both at baseline and after immunosuppressive treatment. C4d kidney deposition was detected using immunohistochemistry in two matching kidney biopsies of 12 LN patients.

Results: In comparison to population-based controls, plasma C4d levels were significantly increased in SLE patients (0.33 mg/L versus 0.94 mg/ml, $p < 0.0001$) with significantly higher levels in LN patients (1.02 mg/L) than in non-renal SLE patients (0.57 mg/L, $p = 0.004$). The C4d/C4 ratio was also significantly higher in LN (11.2) than in non-renal SLE patients (2.5, $p = 0.0002$). According to ROC curve analysis, C4d was found to be an accurate marker to discriminate LN from non-renal SLE patients ($p = 0.004$). The C4d/C4 ratio displayed even higher specificity, sensitivity and overall accuracy as marker for LN than C4d and C4 alone. At baseline, C4d levels correlated significantly with urine-albumin to creatinine ratio ($r_S = 0.43$, $p = 0.011$) and with renal activity index ($r_S = 0.37$, $p = 0.002$). Immunohistochemical staining showed glomerular deposits of C4d in kidney biopsies, which strikingly correlated with plasma C4d levels ($r_S = 0.7$, $p = 0.0002$). Plasma C4d declined significantly after treatment in patients that experienced favorable clinical and histopathological response ($p < 0.0001$), while levels remained mainly unchanged in non-responders.

Conclusion: Plasma C4d discriminates LN from active non-renal SLE, correlates with C4d kidney deposits and appears valuable in monitoring responsiveness to various treatments. The C4d/C4 ratio might be superior to C4d alone.

Keywords: systemic lupus erythematosus, complement, C4d, lupus nephritis, treatment response, kidney deposition

INTRODUCTION

Systemic lupus erythematosus (SLE) is a chronic autoimmune disorder with heterogeneous manifestations. Despite advanced treatment strategies, lupus nephritis (LN) remains one of the most common organ-threatening manifestations with significant morbidity and mortality (1). Early diagnosis and initiation of treatment is of uttermost importance for the prognosis. Renal biopsy is the gold standard to diagnose and classify LN as well as to guide therapy (2–4). The overarching treatment goal is to prevent renal failure and optimally to achieve complete clinical remission and maintain it long-term (5). To monitor responsiveness to immunosuppressive treatment, different scoring systems mainly based on the reduction of proteinuria can be applied (2, 6).

Repeated renal biopsies have been suggested to improve the evaluation of treatment response in LN (7). The downside is that renal biopsies are invasive and bear the risk of complications. Thus, less invasive biomarkers for renal disease activity are desirable. We previously showed that C4d, which is the final cleavage fragment of C4 arising from complement activation, is a superior marker to C4 in identifying LN flares and that C4d, but not C3 and C4, can forecast recurrence of LN (8). Levels of C3 and C4 are the net result of complement activation and rate of synthesis, whereas C4d is exclusively generated upon complement activation, which strengthens its suitability as biomarker. Further, it has a favorable half-life compared to other complement activation products such as C3a or C5a. C4d measurement is robust, easy and highly specific with our assay (9).

In the current study, we confirmed the value of C4d as a biomarker for LN in an independent SLE cohort. We revealed that plasma C4d levels correlate with C4d deposited in kidney biopsies of LN patients and that plasma C4d levels associate with both histopathological and clinical treatment response at follow-up. Thus, the simple measurement of C4d plasma levels might be used to improve the evaluation of treatment outcome.

MATERIALS AND METHODS

SLE Patients and Control Populations

In total, 93 patients with diagnosed SLE and classified according to the American College of Rheumatology classification criteria and/or the Systemic Lupus International Collaboration Clinics (SLICC) classification criteria were included in the study (10, 11). In 71 patients, samples were obtained at the time-point of renal biopsy. The renal biopsies were classified according to the International Society of Nephrology/Renal Pathology Society (ISN/RPS) classification (see **Table 1**) (12). Activity and chronicity index were evaluated in the renal biopsies (13). There were two patients with ISN/RPS class II (mesangial LN), 51 patients with a proliferative pattern (class III and IV$\pm$V) and 18 patients with a pure membranous LN (class V). In 52 of the patients with LN, repeated biopsies were collected after three to fourteen (median eight) months to evaluate the histopathological response.

TABLE 1 | Classification of renal biopsies according to the International Society of Nephrology/Renal Pathology Society (ISN/RPS) classification.

ISN/RPS class	Baseline	Post-treatment
I-II	0	14
III (A)	9	0
III (A/C)	5	5
III (A)+V	5	1
III (A/C)+V	1	0
III (C)	0	5
IV-S (A)	4	1
IV-S (A/C)	3	0
IV-S (A/C)+V	1	0
IV-G (A)	7	1
IV-G (A/C)	4	1
IV-G (A)+V	2	1
IV-G (A/C)+V	0	1
V	11	19
V+II	0	3

ISN/RPS, International Society of Nephrology/Renal Pathology Society.

Twenty-two of the SLE patients had active SLE with no signs of renal involvement and were used as non-renal SLE controls. Disease activity in the non-renal SLE patients was estimated using the SLE Disease Activity Index 2000 (SLEDAI-2K) (14). The median score was 8 (range 2–18).

As disease controls, fourteen patients with biopsy-proven IgA nephropathy were included. Blood samples from 145 population-based controls were also included. Demographics of all participants are shown in **Table 2**.

Collection of samples and healthy control subjects was performed according to the Declaration of Helsinki and approved by the Regional Ethical Review Boards in Stockholm (Dnr. 2012/1550, 2014/1337) with all participants providing written consent to participate in the study.

Enzyme Immunoassay for Assessment of Complement C4d

Plasma C4d levels were measured with Complement C4d assay (#COMPL C4d RUO, SVAR Life Science) according to the manufacturer's instruction. The normal reference range is defined as 0.03–0.15 mg/L. Absorbance was measured in Cytation-5 multi-mode reader (BioTek).

Competitive Immunoassay for Assessment of Complement C4

Plasma C4 levels were determined with Human Complement C4 ELISA Kit (#ab108824, Abcam) according to the manufacturer's instruction. The normal reference range is defined as 160–480 mg/L. Absorbance was measured as above. Values below the detection limit were set to 3.15 mg/L for statistical calculations.

Immunohistochemical Staining of C4d in Kidney Biopsies

In order to test the specificity of the antibody, Daudi cells coated with C4b and C4d were prepared. The cells were incubated

TABLE 2 | Demographics of patients and controls.

Characteristics	Controls *n* = 145	IgAN *n* = 14	LN (SLE) *n* = 71	Non-renal (SLE) *n* = 22
Age	41 (16–79)	48 (20–72)	33 (18–79)	46 (18–65)
Females, n (%)	114 (79%)	7 (50%)	62 (86%)	22 (100%)
C4d (mg/L)	0.33 (0–1.55)	0.30 (0.05–1.39)	1.02 (0.15–3.03)	0.57 (0–1.71)
C3 (g/L)	n. d.	n. d.	0.57 (0.12–1.38) 9 missing	0.82 (0.41–1.24)
C4 (mg/L)	n. d.	n. d.	86 (3.15–554)	231 (3.15–441)
C4d/C4 ratio	n. d.	n. d.	11.2 (0.47–930)	2.49 (0–527)
Creatinine (μmol/L)	n. d.	n. d.	75 (32–188)	64 (55–161)
Activity index	n. d.	n. d.	5 (0–12)	n.d.
Chronicity index	n. d.	n. d.	0 (0–7)	n.d.
Urine-albumin to creatinine ratio (mg/mmol)	n.d.	n.d.	124 (0–556) 37 missing	n.d.
Urine-albumin >0.5 g/day, n (%)	n.d.	n.d.	56 (79%)	n.d.
Anti-dsDNA-Ab positive, n (%)	n. d.	n. d.	49 (78%) 8 missing	17 (77%)
Prednisolone, n (%) (mg/day)	n.d.	8 (57.1%) 5 (0–30)	45 (63%) 7.5 (0–60)	11 (50%) 2.5 (0–30)
DMARD, n (%)	n. d.	Any 3 (21.4%), AZA 1, CYC 1, INF 1	Any 14 (20%), AZA 6, MMF 4, CYC 2, MTX 2	Any 9 (41%), AZA 3, MMF 2, CYC 3, MTX 1
Antimalarials, n (%)	n. d.	0	19 (27%)	12 (55%)

Values are presented as median (range) unless otherwise stated. AZA, azathioprine; CYC, cyclophosphamide; DMARD, disease-modifying anti-rheumatic drugs; MMF, mycophenolate mofetil; MTX, methotrexate; IFN, infliximab; n.d., not determined.

in DGVB^{++} (2.5 mM veronal buffer pH 7.3, 72 mM NaCl, 140 mM glucose, 0.1% gelatin, 1 mM $MgCl_2$, and 0.15 mM $CaCl_2$) with 1 μM recombinantly expressed OmCI (to prevent lysis of cells), 50 μg/ml ofatumumab recognizing CD20 expressed on cells (GlaxoSmithKline) and 5% normal human serum, 5% heat-inactivated human serum or 5% factor I depleted human serum (Complement Tech). The cells were then formalin-fixed and paraffin-embedded. Normal human serum was prepared as previously described (15) with approval of the Regional Ethical Review Boards in Lund (Dnr. 2013/846). Heat-inactivated was achieved by incubation at 56°C for 30 min. Paraffin-embedded kidney biopsies and controls were cut in 4 μm sections and pre-treated using the PT-link system (Dako) with antigen retrieval at pH 9 (Envision Flex high pH kit, Dako). C4d deposition was detected with the same anti-C4d-neo monoclonal Ab (dilution 1:5000, SVAR Life Science) as used in the C4d assay. Biopsies were stained for 30 min using Envision Flex (Dako) reagents in an Autostainer Plus system according to the manufacturer's protocol (Dako). Intensity of the staining in glomeruli was scored from zero (negative) to three (high) by two researchers and one pathologist in a blinded manner. Kidney biopsies were only scored if at least two glomeruli were present. Kidney C4d scores for individual patients are presented in **Table 3**.

Standard Laboratory Tests and Reference Values

Plasma creatinine was analyzed according to clinical routine at the Karolinska University Hospital and expressed as micromole/liter. Renal function was estimated using the Modification of Diet in Renal Disease (MDRD) study equation for estimating glomerular filtration rate (16).

For analysis of albuminuria, either 24-h urinary collections (grams/24 h) or urine-albumin to creatinine ratios (u-ACR) (mg/mmol) were performed. Being a retrospective study, methods for estimation of albuminuria have changed over time and some data regarding u-ACR for the entire cohort is thereby missing. In order to analyze response to therapy, we have thus estimated the grade of proteinuria (<0.2 g/day or < 0.5 g/day) by the method available at the biopsy time-point.

Anti-dsDNA antibodies were analyzed according to CLIFT, ELISA or multiplex methods used as routine at the Department of Clinical Immunology at the Karolinska University Hospital, method depending on the analysis available at the inclusion time-point. As different methods were used, we chose to define anti-dsDNA as positive or negative.

Definitions of Response to Treatment

We defined complete clinical response (CR) as having an inactive urinary sediment, proteinuria ≤0.2 g/day and normal glomerular filtration rate >90 mL/min or stable (within 10% of normal if previously abnormal) renal function. Partial response (PR) was defined by having an inactive sediment, proteinuria ≤0.5 g/day and normal or stable (<10% deterioration from baseline if previously abnormal) renal function. Patients not reaching the above criteria were regarded as clinical non-responders (NR) (2).

Using repeated renal biopsies for evaluation of response, we defined histopathological response (HR) as transformation into class I, II or III/IV-C whereas persistent class III/IV-A or III/IV-A/C and persistent, or transformation into,

TABLE 3 | Comparison of plasma C4d levels, kidney C4d score and LN classes.

	Baseline			Post-treatment		
Patient #	**C4d (mg/L)**	**Kidney score**	**ISN/RPS class**	**C4d (mg/L)**	**Kidney score**	**ISN/RPS class**
P1	0.686	2	V	1.208	3	V
P2	3.033	2	IV-S (A)	0.385	0	I
P3	1.154	2	IV-G (A)+V	0.551	3	V
P4	1.002	3	V	1.881	3	III (A)+V
P5	2.104	2	IV-G (A)	0.279	0	II
P6	2.928	3	IV-G (A)+V	0.746	3	IV-G (A)+V
P7	0.807	2	III (A)	0.225	0	II
P8	0.706	1	III (A)	0.315	1	II
P9	1.173	0	III (A/C)	0.293	0	V
P10	1.386	2	IV-G (A)	0.590	1	V
P11	0.789	1	IV-S (A/C)	0.272	1	II
P12	1.100	1	III (A)	0.354	0	II

LN, lupus nephritis; ISN/RPS, International Society of Nephrology/Renal Pathology Society.

class V was considered as histopathological non-response (HNR) (17).

Statistical Analyses

The control and patient data did not pass the normality test, thus nonparametric statistics were applied. Mann-Whitney U and Kruskal-Wallis rank-sum tests were used to calculate statistical significance of nonparametric continuous data, which are displayed as median with 25–75% quantiles plus whisker and listed as median (range). Wilcoxon matched-pairs signed rank test was applied for comparison of baseline and post-treatment measurements. Spearman's rank-order correlation test was used to analyze correlations of nonparametric data. ROC curve analysis was used to categorize C4d and C4 levels. To evaluate accuracy, the AUC of ROC curves as well as sensitivity, specificity, positive predictive values (PPVs) and negative predictive values (NPVs) were determined. McNemar's test was used for comparison of two markers in terms of accuracy. To estimate the relative risk, odds ratios (ORs) and 95% confidence intervals (CIs) were calculated by logistic regression. A statistical significance level (p value) < 0.05 was defined as statistically significant. Analyses were carried out using JMP Pro 12 (SAS Institute) and IBM SPSS Statistics 25 (IBM) software.

RESULTS

Plasma C4d Levels Are Higher in Lupus Nephritis Patients Than in Non-renal SLE Patients

Plasma C4d levels were determined by a commercial complement C4d assay, which is a further development of our in-house ELISA (9). The median C4d level of population-based controls was 0.33 mg/L (0–1.55 mg/L) (**Figure 1A**). Fourteen IgA nephropathy patients were included as disease controls and showed C4d levels in the same range (0.30 mg/L, 0.05–1.39 mg/L). In comparison to the population-based controls, C4d levels were significantly increased in SLE patients ($p < 0.0001$), with significantly higher C4d levels in LN patients (1.02 mg/L, 0.15–3.03 mg/L) than in non-renal SLE patients (0.57 mg/L, 0–1.71 mg/L, $p = 0.004$). As expected, LN patients had significantly lower C4 levels (86 mg/L, 3.15–554 mg/L) than non-renal SLE patients (231 mg/L, 3.15–441 mg/L, $p = 0.003$) (**Figure 1B**). The C4d/C4 ratio was additionally calculated and displayed significant difference between LN (11.2, 0.47–930) and non-renal SLE patients (2.49, 0–527, $p = 0.0002$) (**Figure 1C**).

C4d Levels Correlate With LN

ROC curve analysis showed that C4d likewise C3 and C4 exhibited statistically significant accuracy as markers for LN. The AUC of the C4d/C4 ratio was higher than for C4d or C4 alone, but slightly lower than for C3 (**Figure 1D**). C4d, C4 and the C4d/C4 ratio were categorized according to the ROC curve analyses. Routine clinical reference values were applied to categorize C3. C4d levels above 0.67 mg/L were defined as high. Applying this cut-off, 79% of LN patients, 32% of non-renal SLE patients and less than 18% of the controls had high C4d levels, confirming the validity of this cut-off. C4 levels below 154 mg/L were defined as low and C4d/C4 ratios above 4.19 were defined as high.

Validating the suitability as biomarker for LN further, we found that high C4d levels exhibited higher sensitivity, specificity, positive predictive value (PPV), negative predictive value (NPV) and overall accuracy than low C3 and C4 levels (**Figure 1E**). However, according to McNemar's test, high C4d levels alone were not statistically superior to low C4 levels ($p = 0.31$), but high C4d/C4 ratios, which were even more sensitive and specific than high C4d levels alone, exhibited statistically superior accuracy as a marker for LN than low C4 ($p = 0.012$) and similar to high C4d ($p = 0.58$). McNemar's test could not be performed for comparisons to low C3 levels, since C3 levels were not determined for nine LN patients. OR analysis revealed that high C4d (OR 8.0, $p = 0.0001$), low C3 (OR 5.03, $p = 0.002$) and low C4 (OR 5.1, $p = 0.002$) levels as well as high C4d/C4 ratios (OR 13.1, $p < 0.0001$) all associated significantly with LN and that high

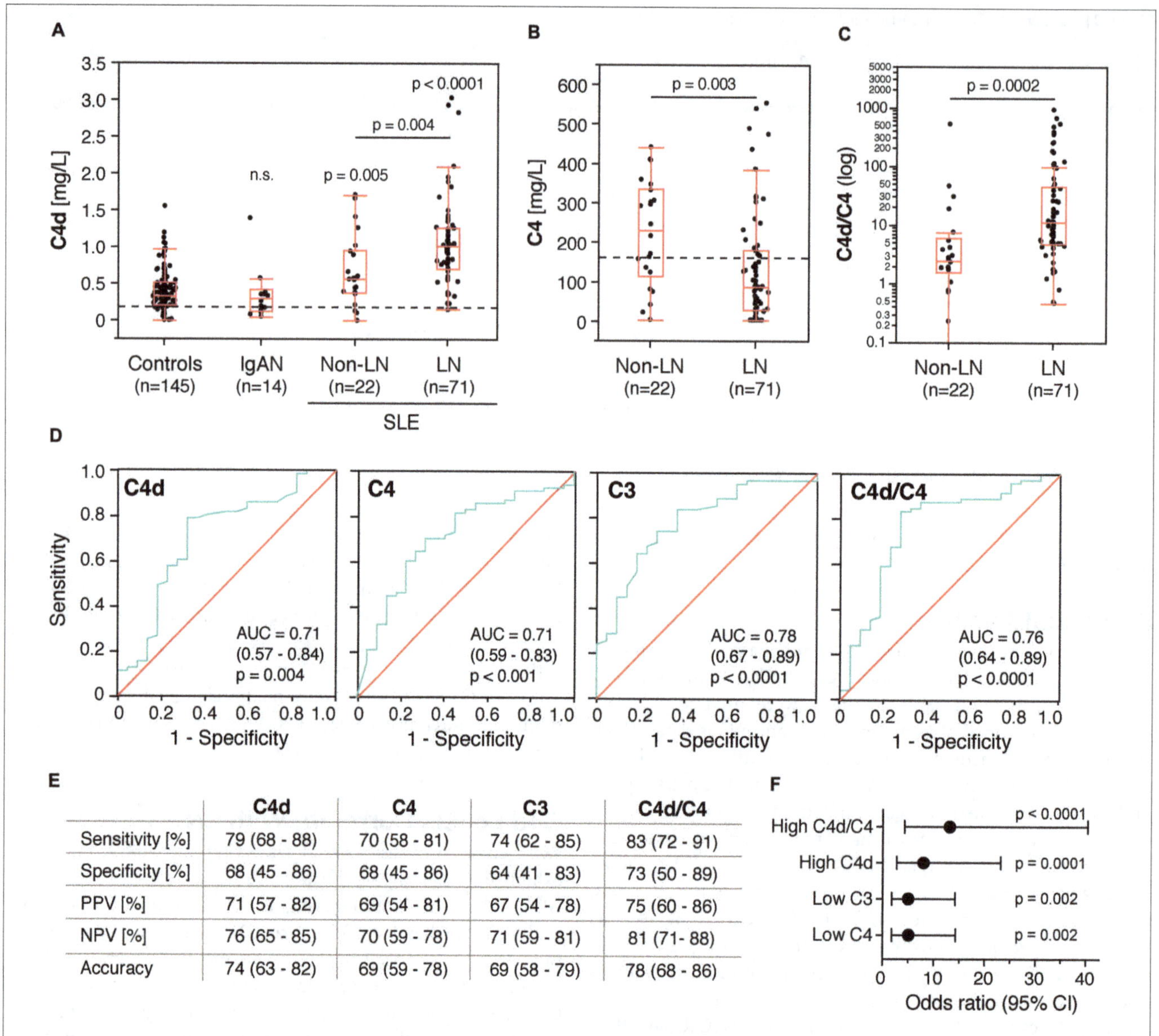

	C4d	C4	C3	C4d/C4
Sensitivity [%]	79 (68 - 88)	70 (58 - 81)	74 (62 - 85)	83 (72 - 91)
Specificity [%]	68 (45 - 86)	68 (45 - 86)	64 (41 - 83)	73 (50 - 89)
PPV [%]	71 (57 - 82)	69 (54 - 81)	67 (54 - 78)	75 (60 - 86)
NPV [%]	76 (65 - 85)	70 (59 - 78)	71 (59 - 81)	81 (71- 88)
Accuracy	74 (63 - 82)	69 (59 - 78)	69 (58 - 79)	78 (68 - 86)

FIGURE 1 | Plasma C4d levels are increased in patients with systemic lupus erythematosus (SLE) and discriminate lupus nephritis (LN) from non-renal SLE patients. **(A)** C4d levels in control subjects, IgA nephropathy patients (IgAN) and SLE patients without and with lupus nephritis. **(B,C)** C4 levels and C4d/C4 ratio in non-renal SLE patients and LN patients. Data are presented as medians with 25–75% quantiles plus whiskers, and significance was calculated using Kruskal-Wallis rank-sum and Mann–Whitney U tests. The C4d/C4 ratio for one of the non-renal SLE patients is zero and can thus not be displayed on a logarithmic scale. Dotted lines indicate the upper normal reference range for C4d (0.15 mg/L) and the lower normal reference range for C4 (160 mg/L). **(D)** Area under the ROC curve analysis showing accuracy of C4d, C3, C4, and C4d/C4 ratio as markers for LN. **(E)** Sensitivity, specificity, positive predictive value (PPV), negative predictive value (NPV) and overall accuracy for C4d, C3, C4, and C4d/C4 ratio as markers for LN. The disease prevalence was set to 50%. Data are presented with 95% CIs. **(F)** Association of high C4d (>0.67 mg/L), low C3 (<0.77 g/L), low C4 (<154 mg/L) and high C4d/C4 ratios (>4.19) with LN. Significance was calculated using binary logistics, and ORs are indicated with a dot connected to the 95% CI.

C4d/C4 ratios exhibited the highest relative odds to occur if the patient has LN (**Figure 1F**).

Correlation of Plasma C4d Levels With Other Clinical Variables

At baseline, C4d correlated negatively with C3 ($r_s = -0.37$, $p = 0.0005$, values for nine LN patients were not determined) and C4 ($r_s = -0.38$, $p = 0.0002$) in all 93 SLE patients (**Figures 2A,B**). Interestingly, C4d did not correlate significantly with C3 ($r_s = -0.07$, $p = 0.76$) and C4 ($r_s = -0.41$, $p = 0.057$) in the 22 non-renal SLE patients, but only in the 71 LN patients [C3 ($r_s = -0.31$, $p = 0.014$), C4 ($r_s = -0.26$, $p = 0.031$)] (**Figures 2A,B**).

Data regarding urine-albumin to creatinine ratio (u-ACR) was available in 34 of the LN patients, either at baseline in patients with repeated biopsies ($n = 25$) or among LN patients with single renal biopsy samples only ($n = 9$). In these, C4d correlated

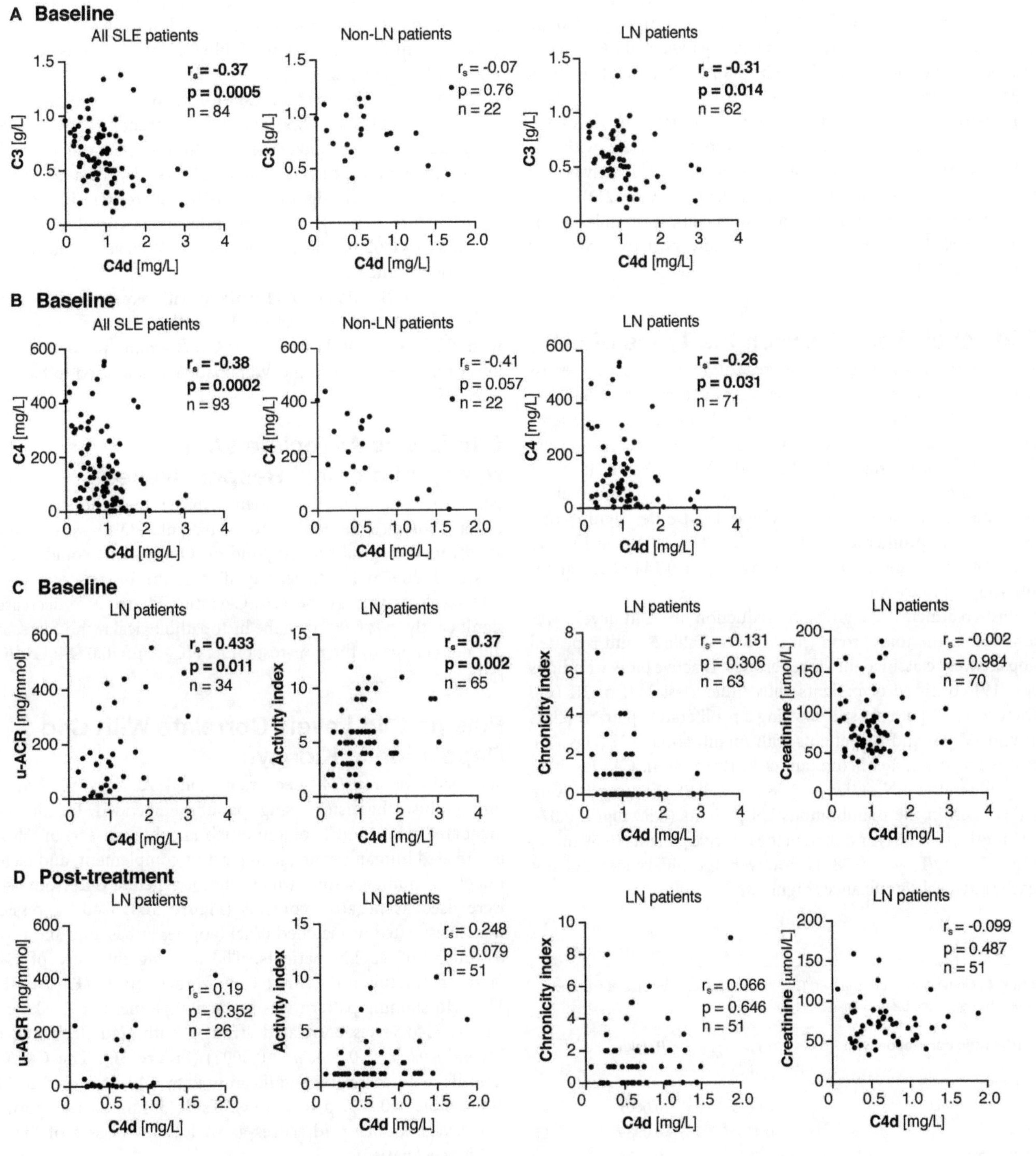

FIGURE 2 | Correlations of plasma C4d levels with clinical variables. **(A,B)** Correlations of plasma C4d with C3 **(A)** and C4 **(B)** in all 93 SLE patients as well as split up in the 22 non-LN and 71 LN patients at baseline. **(C,D)** Correlation of plasma C4d with u-ACR, activity and chronicity index as well as creatinine at baseline **(C)** and post-treatment **(D)**. **(A–D)** Not all variables were determined for all patients; therefore n is shown in each correlation graph separately. Significant correlation coefficients and *p* values are bold. Significance was calculated using Spearman's rank-order correlation test. u-ACR, urine-albumin to creatinine ratio.

strongly with u-ACR ($r_s = 0.433$, $p = 0.011$). Additionally, C4d correlated significantly with the renal activity index ($r_s = 0.37$, $p = 0.002$), but not with chronicity index or creatinine level (**Figure 2C**).

In all SLE patients as well as in the LN patients at baseline, neither prednisolone, antimalarial or disease-modifying anti-rheumatic drugs influenced C4d levels. However, in the non-renal SLE patients, patients on disease-modifying anti-rheumatic drugs had significantly lower C4d levels than patients not receiving this medication (0.39 mg/L versus 0.66 mg/L, $p = 0.042$). C4d levels were slightly, but insignificantly higher in LN patients with occurrence of anti-dsDNA-Abs than in LN patients without (1.05 mg/L versus 0.86 mg/L, $p = 0.175$).

Post-treatment, data on u-ACR was available in 26 of the 52 patients. In these, C4d levels did not correlate with the u-ACR. Furthermore, there was no association with activity and chronicity index, or with the creatinine levels (**Figure 2D**).

Correlations of the C4d/C4 ratio with clinical variables of the 52 re-biopsied LN patients at baseline and post-treatment are listed in **Table 4**.

C4d Levels Vary Between the Types of LN

In order to investigate C4d in regard to the responsiveness to various treatments, C4d levels were determined at baseline and post-treatment in 52 LN patients. At baseline, all patients had an active LN and according to biopsies, 41 cases were classified as proliferative LN (class III/IV ± V) and 11 cases as pure membranous LN (class V) (for detailed information see **Table 1**). At baseline, C4d levels did not differ significantly between the proliferative (1.1 mg/L, 0.36–3.03 mg/L) and membranous (1 mg/L, 0.23–1.95 mg/L, $p = 0.244$) LN patient subgroups (**Figure 3A**).

Post-treatment, a significant reduction in C4d levels was observed in the total group ($p < 0.0001$, **Table 5**) and repeated biopsies were classified into three groups. Inactive biopsy findings ($n = 19$) consisted of patients with either class I, II or III (C). There were 11 patients still showing a proliferative pattern (class III and IV±V) and 22 patients with membranous LN (class V). In three of these, a concomitant class II was seen. C4d levels in the proliferative LN patients (0.78 mg/L, 0.28–1.88 mg/L) were higher than in the membranous LN patients (0.57 mg/L, 0.07–1.44 mg/L, $p = 0.064$) and than in the inactive patients (0.59 mg/L, 0.18–1.28 mg/L, $p = 0.085$). However, the differences did not reach statistical significance (**Figure 3A**).

TABLE 4 | Correlation of plasma C4d/C4 ratio with clinical variables at first and second biopsy of the 52 re-biopsied LN patients.

C4d/C4 ratio correlation with	r_s	P Value	n
Baseline			
C3	−0.475	**0.0007**	47
u-ACR	0.415	**0.0389**	25
Activity index	0.261	0.0674	50
Chronicity index	−0.330	**0.0192**	50
Creatinine	0.044	0.7595	51
Post-treatment			
C3	−0.532	**0.0002**	44
u-ACR	0.062	0.7630	26
Activity index	0.191	0.1798	51
Chronicity index	0.003	0.9841	51
Creatinine	−0.078	0.5868	51

All statistical p-values (p < 0.05) are bold.

The C4d levels of the 11 patients with remaining PLN findings post-treatment were not significantly lower than for the 41 patients with PLN at baseline (**Table 5**). The same was observed for the MLN patients.

At baseline, the median C4d/C4 ratio was also higher in proliferative (14.5, 1.5–929) than in membranous (9.8, 0.5–251) LN patients. However, likewise for C4d levels, the difference did not reach significance ($p = 0.426$) (**Figure 3B**). Post-treatment, the C4d/C4 ratio was significantly higher in proliferative LN than in inactive patients ($p = 0.039$) and than in membranous LN patients ($p = 0.025$), where differences in C4d levels alone did not reach significance.

The C4d/C4 ratio of the 11 patients with remaining PLN post-treatment was not significantly lower than for the 41 patients with PLN at baseline. However, the C4d/C4 ratio was significantly lower post-treatment in the MLN patients compared to baseline levels (**Table 5**).

C4d Levels Associate With Histopathological Responsiveness

Following treatment, 34 patients (65%) met the criteria of histopathological response and 17 patients (33%) were defined as histopathological non-responders. One patient could not be classified due to insufficient quality of the biopsy. Strikingly, C4d levels as well as the C4d/C4 ratio (**Figure 3C**) decreased significantly ($p < 0.0001$) in the histopathological responders, but did not change in the non-responders (C4d, $p = 0.0714$; C4d/C4 ratio, $p = 0.2842$).

Plasma C4d Levels Correlate With C4d Deposition in Kidneys

Specificity of anti-C4d-neo monoclonal Ab was verified by immunohistochemistry using paraffin-embedded Daudi cells incubated with OmCI, ofatumumab and human serum. Heat-inactivated human serum lacking active complement, and factor I depleted human serum, which cannot generate C4d from C4b, were used as negative controls (**Figure 3D**). C4d expression was investigated in matched renal biopsies at baseline and post-treatment of 12 LN patients. The staining intensity of C4d in the glomeruli was scored from zero to three (**Figure 3E**). The C4d staining pattern was segmental glomerular. Strikingly, plasma C4d levels correlated strongly with C4d deposited in LN kidneys ($r_s = 0.696$, $p = 0.0002$) (**Figure 3F**). The C4d/C4 ratio likewise correlates significantly with C4d deposited in LN kidneys ($r_s = 0.637$, $p = 0.0011$). **Table 3** summarizes plasma C4d levels, kidney C4d scores as well as LN classes of the 12 re-biopsied patients.

Plasma C4d Levels Associate With Clinical Responsiveness

Twenty-five patients (48%) met the definition of complete clinical response, 10 patients (19%) of partial clinical response and 17 patients (33%) were categorized as clinical non-responders. C4d levels decreased most significantly in the clinical complete responders ($p < 0.0001$) and strongly in the clinical partial responders ($p = 0.002$), whereas the decrease in the

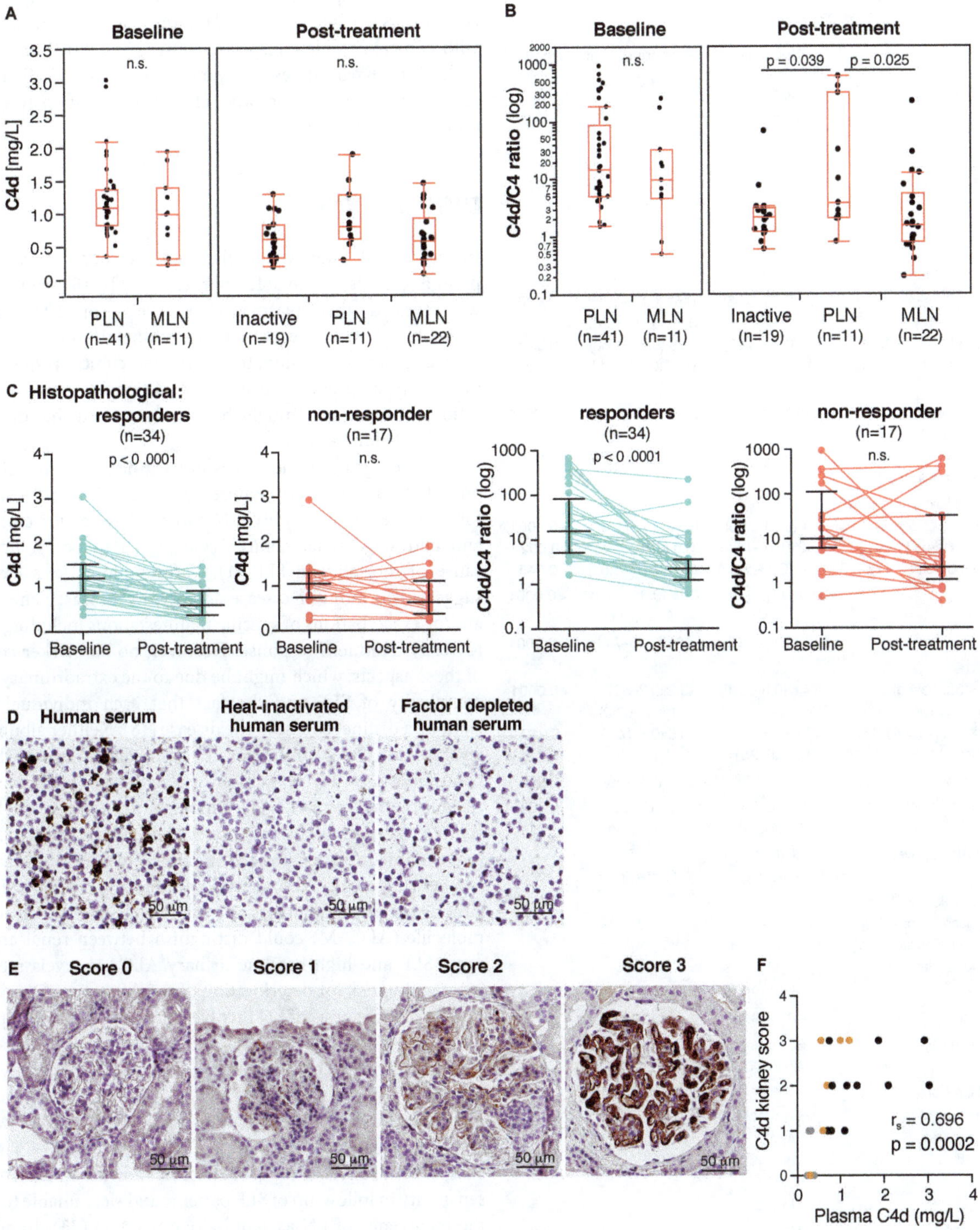

FIGURE 3 | In lupus nephritis (LN) patients, C4d levels associate with histopathological responsiveness to treatment and plasma C4d levels correlate with C4d deposited in kidney biopsies. **(A)** C4d levels and **(B)** C4d/C4 ratio at baseline and post-treatment of LN subgroups. Inactive patients represent ISN class I, II and III C. **(C)** C4d levels and C4d/C4 ratio at baseline and post-treatment in histopathological responders and non-responders. Each patient sample plus the medians and interquartile ranges are shown. **(D)** Specificity of C4d staining with anti-C4d-neo monoclonal Ab was determined by immunohistochemistry of Daudi cell pellets incubated with OmCl, ofatumumab and 5% human serum. Heat-inactivated human serum (5%) and 5% factor I depleted sera were applied as negative controls not able to generate C4d. **(E)** Scoring of C4d levels in kidney biopsies of LN patients. Representative images for each score at 40× magnification are presented. **(F)** Correlation of C4d plasma levels with C4d deposition in kidney biopsies. PLN samples are shown in black, MLN samples in orange and inactive samples in gray. Significance was calculated using Kruskal-Wallis rank-sum and Mann–Whitney U tests **(A,B)**, Wilcoxon matched-pairs signed rank test **(C)** and Spearman's rank-order correlation test **(F)**. PLN, proliferative LN; MLN, membranous LN.

TABLE 5 | Clinical, laboratory and histopathological characteristics at first and second biopsy of the 52 re-biopsied LN patients.

Characteristics	Baseline	Post-treatment	*P* Value
Age	31.5 (18–62)		
Females, n (%)	45 (87%)		
Ethnicity, n			
Caucasian	40		
African	1		
Asian	5		
Hispanic	3		
Middle East	3		
C4d (mg/L)			
LN all (*n* = 52, paired)	1.1 (0.23–3.03)	0.61 (0.07–1.88)	**<0.0001**
Inactive (*n* = 0/19)	–	0.59 (0.18–1.28)	–
Proliferative LN (*n* = 41/11)	1.1 (0.36–3.03)	0.78 (0.28–1.88)	0.059
Membranous LN (*n* = 11/22)	1 (0.23–1.95)	0.57 (0.07–1.44)	0.123
C4d (mg/L)			
Histopathological responders (*n* = 35)	1.15 (0.24–3.03)	0.59 (0.07–1.44)	**<0.0001**
Histopathological non-responders (*n* = 16)	1.04 (0.23–2.93)	0.66 (0.21–1.88)	0.071
C4d (mg/L) – Clinical response			
Complete responders (*n* = 25)	1.1 (0.33-3.03)	0.54 (0.23–1.44)	**<0.0001**
Partial responders (*n* = 10)	1.12 (0.67–1.82)	0.6 (0.18–1.09)	**0.002**
Non-responders (*n* = 17)	1.07 (0.23–2.93)	0.66 (0.07–1.88)	**0.045**
C3 (g/L)	0.54 (0.12–1.38) 5 missing	0.77 (0.34–1.31) 8 missing	**<0.0001**
C4 (mg/L)	85 (3.15–554)	281 (3.15–744)	**<0.0001**
C4d/C4 ratio			
LN all (*n* = 52, paired)	14.5 (0.5–929)	2.2 (0.2–597)	**<0.0001**
Inactive (*n* = 0/19)	–	2.1 (0.6–67.3)	–
Proliferative LN (*n* = 41/11)	14.5 (1.5–929)	3.8 (0.8–597)	0.219
Membranous LN (*n* = 11/22)	9.8 (0.5–251)	1.55 (0.2–217)	**0.023**
Creatinine (μmol/L)	75 (32–173)	71 (33–159)	0.089
Urine-albumin to creatinine ratio (mg/mmol)	126 (0.8–556) 27 missing	5.6 (0–503) 26 missing	0.064
Anti-dsDNA Ab positive, n (%)	36 (84%) 9 missing	22 (73%) 17 missing	
Renal histology (ISN/RPS), n			
Inactive [class I, II or III (C)]	0	19	
Proliferative [class III/IV ± V]	41	11	
Membranous [class V]	11	22	
Activity index	5 (0–12)	1 (0–10)	**<0.0001**
Chronicity index	0 (0–6)	1 (0–9)	**0.017**
Prednisolone, n (%) (mg/day)	36 (69%) 7.5 (0–60)	51 (1%) 10 (0–40)	
Antimalarials, n (%)	17 (33%)		
DMARD at biopsy, n (%)	Any 14 (27%) AZA 7 MMF 4 CYC 1 MTX 2		
Treatment after first biopsy	MMF 17 CYC 19 MMF/CYC switched 4 RTX 7 RTX combined with other DMARD 4 AZA 1		

All statistical significant p-values (p < 0.05) are bold. Values are presented as median (range) unless otherwise stated. LN, lupus nephritis; AZA, azathioprine; CYC, cyclophosphamide; DMARD, disease-modifying anti-rheumatic drugs; MF, mycophenolate mofetil; MTX, methotrexate; RTX, rituximab; n.d., not determined.

clinical non-responders just reached significance ($p = 0.045$) (**Figure 4A**). Also, the C4d/C4 ratio associated most strongly with clinical complete responsiveness ($p = 0.0013$) and strongly with clinical partial responsiveness ($p = 0.0078$) (**Figure 4B**). However, no association with clinical non-responsiveness was observed ($p = 0.051$).

DISCUSSION

In the current study, we confirm our previous observation that plasma C4d is a valuable marker for LN (8). Furthermore, we revealed that plasma C4d levels correlate with the intensity of C4d deposition in kidney biopsies and that they associate with histopathological and clinical responsiveness to immunosuppressive treatment. Additionally, we show that the ratio of C4d over C4 might be even more valuable than either C4d or C4 alone as a marker for LN.

Despite significant advances in treatment options, LN is still one of the most severe manifestations in SLE and it accounts for an increased morbidity. LN patients have a worse prognosis and end stage renal failure is suggested to be an important cause of mortality in SLE (1). Various biomarkers have been suggested to monitor disease activity, to forecast general flares and/or exacerbations of specific manifestations including LN and to verify treatment response. However, no biomarker covers all of these aspects, which might be due to the extraordinary clinical complexity of SLE and the fact that each individual patient exhibits a distinct course of the disease (18). Neither albuminuria, levels of anti-DNA antibodies nor complement levels, which are commonly used for evaluation of renal response, proved to be reliable biomarkers in LN (7). Among biomarkers, serum levels of soluble Axl were recently proposed as useful marker to reflect the grade of inflammation and tissue damage in the kidneys as well as to assess histological response to immunosuppression in LN (19). Among urinary biomarkers, the activated leucocyte cell adhesion molecule (ALCAM) could distinguish between renal and non-renal SLE and high baseline urinary ALCAM levels seemed to increase the risk for deterioration of renal function (20).

The pathogenesis of LN involves immune complex deposition (21), which strongly activate complement and thus incite inflammatory mechanisms contributing to the severity of the disease. Importantly, low levels of C3 and C4 are included in the SLE disease activity index 2000 (SLEDAI-2K), which is commonly used to monitor SLE (14). However, C3 and C4 exhibit wide reference ranges in healthy individuals (22), have low sensitivity in follow-up of SLE patients and were unable to predict the recurrence of LN as stand-alone markers (23). In addition, low C3 and C4 levels do not accurately mirror complement activation, since their levels are also affected by the rate of synthesis, which further increases during inflammation. We have previously introduced a unique assay to quantify plasma levels of C4d, which is the final cleavage fragment of C4 exclusively arising from complement activation (9). This specificity is achieved by a neoepitope-specific antibody that is directed against a very short linear epitope in the cleavage site of C4d that becomes exposed solely after complement-mediated cleavage of C4b, and

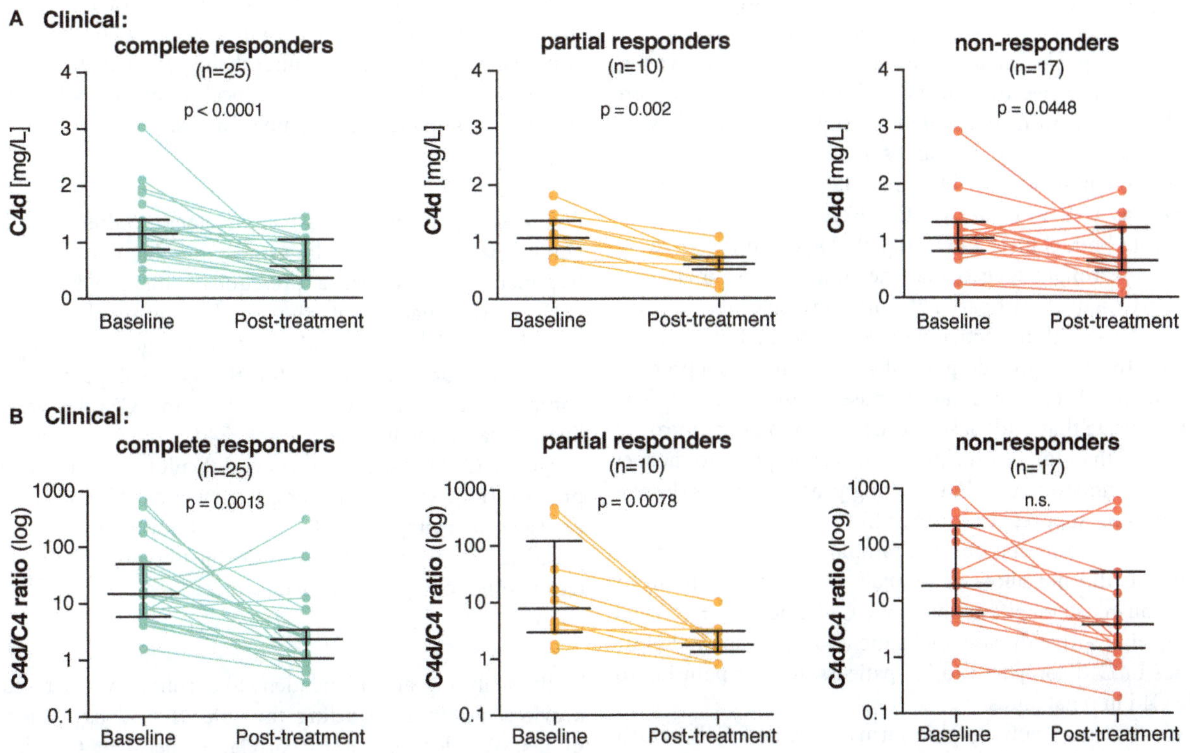

FIGURE 4 | In lupus nephritis patients, C4d levels associate with clinical responsiveness to treatment. **(A)** C4d levels as well as **(B)** C4d/C4 ratios at baseline and post-treatment in clinical complete, partial and non-responders. Each patient sample plus the medians and interquartile ranges are shown. Significance was calculated using Wilcoxon matched-pairs signed rank test.

that cannot be mimicked by non-proteolytic events (9). By the use of this assay, we could confirm that C4d levels are increased in LN patients and that C4d is a valuable marker to discriminate LN from non-renal SLE. Previously, we showed that C4d levels were negligible in healthy individuals that were sampled under optimal conditions (8). In the current study, population-based controls were used for comparison and the C4d levels were as expected higher than in previously determined healthy controls, but still significantly lower than in SLE patients. Considering that these control individuals could have other diseases than SLE, and thus represent a more representative control cohort, the results show that C4d associates with SLE and especially with LN in relevant settings.

Previously, we discovered that C4d, but not C3 or C4, was an accurate marker to distinguish between remission and flare, as well as to predict future LN flares in relapsing patients in a cross-sectional SLE cohort (8). C4d levels were significantly higher in LN patients than in patients without renal involvement (8). This observation was confirmed in the current study. However, high C4d levels alone, even though exhibiting higher sensitivity, specificity, PPV, NPV and overall accuracy than low C4, were not statistically superior to low C4 levels, as it was the case in the previous study.

A clear strength of the current study is that all LN cases were biopsy verified and repeated biopsies allowed us to determine both histopathological and clinical outcome. Clinical responsiveness was defined using established outcome measures (2), although no general definition of histopathological outcome has been generally introduced. Applying similar histopathological response criteria from studies on repeat renal biopsies (7), we have previously identified high interferon lambda levels as a marker of poor treatment response (17) and now C4d levels associate even more strongly with treatment outcome.

According to the current treatment guidelines, LN patients should be treated with corticosteroids in combination with aggressive immunosuppressive drugs (4). Furthermore, angiotensin converting enzyme inhibitors (ACEi) or angiotensin receptor blockers (ARB) are generally recommended. Apart from being anti-hypertensive, ACEi/ARB reduce the amount of proteinuria, which in turn may influence the evaluation of renal response, proteinuria being one of the main clinical measures in the established response criteria (2). Thus, firm evaluation of response may be hampered by therapy itself, further stressing the need for a reliable biomarker that may reflect ongoing inflammation. At baseline biopsies, we found a clear correlation between C4d and the grade of albuminuria, most probably reflecting the renal activity. The lack of association at repeated biopsy could be explained by the use of ACEi/ARB, which lower the albuminuria to various degrees and thereby interfere with the evaluation of clinical response.

Here, we report that plasma C4d levels, as well as the C4d/C4 ratio, declined in LN patients with favorable clinical and histopathological response, but remained mostly unchanged in non-responders. This strongly suggests that C4d and the C4d/C4 ratio might be useful markers to study the responsiveness to immunosuppressive treatments. Although renal biopsies are the gold standard to diagnose and classify LN (24), follow-up biopsies after induction of immunosuppressive therapy are not and carry potential risks for bleeding complications (25). Since C4d levels as well as C4d/C4 ratios were shown to associate strongly with both clinical and histopathological responsiveness, our findings strongly suggest that the simple determination of plasma C4d might at least partially replace invasive biopsies. C4d levels correlated with the activity index at baseline but not post-treatment. Interestingly, despite effective immunosuppressive treatment, the chronicity index increased post-treatment. The findings indicate that C4d plasma levels may be a better measure for active LN than for chronic presentation and point to the fact that the inflammatory and thus scarring process persists despite intense immunosuppressive treatment.

The diverse manifestations and sample size in the non-renal SLE controls did not allow us to analyze associations between specific non-renal manifestations and C4d findings. However, despite having active disease, this patient group displayed clear difference in C4d compared to LN patients, further pointing to the role C4d in renal lupus.

C4 exists in two polymorphic forms, C4A and C4B, which exhibit distinct chemical reactivities. Partial C4 deficiency can arise due to copy number variations (C4 null alleles) as well as mutations (26). Notably, this does not only occur in SLE patients, but also in approximately 35% of the general population. However, deficiencies or low copy numbers of either total C4 or C4A are a risk factor for SLE development (27). In the case of partial C4 deficiency, low C4 levels are a consequence of decreased synthesis rather than increased complement activation. Accordingly, quantifying the C4d/C4 ratio might correct for this phenomenon. In a recent study of severe LN patients, that included patients on combination therapy of rituximab and belimumab, the C4d/C4 ratio correlated better with levels of anti-dsDNA and anti-C1q antibodies than stand-alone measurement of C4d or C4 (28). None of these markers correlated with the renal outcome criteria of proteinuria. However, the change in C4d/C4 ratio from baseline to post-treatment correlated to the change in proteinuria and outperformed sole quantification of C4d or C4. Importantly, no repeated biopsies were performed and thus no data on histopathological response are available.

The limitation of our study is the retrospective nature and that methods for detection of anti-dsDNA antibody levels were determined with various methods and missing data in a proportion of patients. Thus it is reasonable that we only detected a weak association of C4d levels with anti-dsDNA antibody occurrence in this study, whereas we previously found a strong association (8). Another limitation of the current study is that proteinuria was also quantified with different methods.

C4d is frequently used as a biomarker for antibody-mediated renal graft rejection (29). Besides the presence of donor-specific antibodies and histopathological evidence of tissue injury, C4d deposition in peritubular capillaries has become the cornerstone diagnostic parameter in graft rejection (30). In contrast to the peritubular deposition, we now found expected distinct glomerular C4d expression in LN patients. Although complement activation is an underlying pathogenetic mechanism in the two renal conditions, the localization of C4d differs and thus targets separate renal compartments.

Increasing numbers of complement inhibitors are in clinical trials and reliable assays for the determination of treatment response are a prerequisite for conclusive studies (31). Determination of the soluble terminal complement complex (sTCC) is a good measure for general complement activation, but not specific for the classical pathway. Other complement biomarkers, such as C3a and C5a are very short lived. Measurement of cell-bound C4d and C3d was previously suggested (32) but these assays are difficult to perform in clinical practice (flow cytometry using fresh patient blood). Thus, our cleavage neoepitope specific C4d antibody used in a fast and practical C4d assay might be a valuable tool not only in SLE, but also in other complement-mediated diseases.

By analyzing an independent SLE cohort, we here confirm previous findings regarding the role of C4d as a biomarker in LN. We demonstrate a correlation between C4d levels in plasma and C4d levels in kidney biopsies, as well as showing C4d as being a marker of treatment response, both at a clinical and histopathological level. If confirmed in larger studies, measurement of circulating C4d could contribute to assessment of LN activity and may lessen the need of renal biopsies in the future.

ETHICS STATEMENT

The studies involving human participants were reviewed and approved by Regional Ethical Review Board in Stockholm. The patients/participants provided their written informed consent to participate in this study.

AUTHOR CONTRIBUTIONS

MM, RT, and SN performed the experiments and analyzed the results. IG and AZ acquired and analyzed clinical parameters. AB organized and diluted the samples. IG recruited patients and supervised the study together with MM and AMB, who also interpreted the data. MM drafted the manuscript together with AMB. All authors have read, revised and approved the final manuscript.

ACKNOWLEDGMENTS

The authors would like to acknowledge all patients and their physicians and thank Dr. Ben King for language revision.

REFERENCES

1. Reppe Moe SE, Molberg O, Strom EH, Lerang K. Assessing the relative impact of lupus nephritis on mortality in a population-based systemic lupus erythematosus cohort. *Lupus.* (2019) 28:818–25. doi: 10.1177/0961203319847275
2. Gordon C, Jayne D, Pusey C, Adu D, Amoura Z, Aringer M, et al. European consensus statement on the terminology used in the management of lupus glomerulonephritis. *Lupus.* (2009) 18:257–63. doi: 10.1177/0961203308100481
3. Hahn BH, McMahon MA, Wilkinson A, Wallace WD, Daikh DI, Fitzgerald JD, et al. American College of Rheumatology guidelines for screening, treatment, and management of lupus nephritis. *Arthritis Care Res (Hoboken).* (2012) 64:797–808.
4. Fanouriakis A, Kostopoulou M, Alunno A, Aringer M, Bajema I, Boletis JN, et al. 2019 update of the EULAR recommendations for the management of systemic lupus erythematosus. *Ann Rheum Dis.* (2019) 78:736–45.
5. Almaani S, Meara A, Rovin BH. Update on lupus nephritis. *Clin J Am Soc Nephrol.* (2017) 12:825–35.
6. Liang MH, Schur PH, Fortin P, Clair EWS, Balow JE, Costenbader K, et al. The American College of Rheumatology response criteria for proliferative and membranous renal disease in systemic lupus erythematosus clinical trials. *Arthritis Rheum.* (2006) 54:421–32. doi: 10.1002/art.21625
7. Zickert A, Sundelin B, Svenungsson E, Gunnarsson I. Role of early repeated renal biopsies in lupus nephritis. *Lupus Sci Med.* (2014) 1:e000018. doi: 10.1136/lupus-2014-000018
8. Martin M, Smolag KI, Bjork A, Gullstrand B, Okroj M, Leffler J, et al. Plasma C4d as marker for lupus nephritis in systemic lupus erythematosus. *Arthritis Res Ther.* (2017) 19:266.
9. Blom AM, Osterborg A, Mollnes TE, Okroj M. Antibodies reactive to cleaved sites in complement proteins enable highly specific measurement of soluble markers of complement activation. *Mol Immunol.* (2015) 66:164–70. doi: 10.1016/j.molimm.2015.02.029
10. Tan EM, Cohen AS, Fries JF, Masi AT, McShane DJ, Rothfield NF, et al. The 1982 revised criteria for the classification of systemic lupus erythematosus. *Arthritis Rheum.* (1982) 25:1271–7. doi: 10.1002/art.1780251101
11. Petri M, Orbai AM, Alarcon GS, Gordon C, Merrill JT, Fortin PR, et al. Derivation and validation of the Systemic Lupus International Collaborating Clinics classification criteria for systemic lupus erythematosus. *Arthritis Rheum.* (2012) 64:2677–86.
12. Weening JJ, D'Agati VD, Schwartz MM, Seshan SV, Alpers CE, Appel GB, et al. The classification of glomerulonephritis in systemic lupus erythematosus revisited. *J Am Soc Nephrol.* (2004) 15:241–50. doi: 10.1097/01.asn.0000108969.21691.5d
13. Austin HA III, Muenz LR, Joyce KM, Antonovych TA, Kullick ME, Klippel JH, et al. Prognostic factors in lupus nephritis. Contribution of renal histologic data. *Am J Med.* (1983) 75:382–91.
14. Gladman DD, Ibanez D, Urowitz MB. Systemic lupus erythematosus disease activity index 2000. *J Rheumatol.* (2002) 29:288–91.
15. Happonen KE, Sjoberg AP, Morgelin M, Heinegard D, Blom AM. Complement inhibitor C4b-binding protein interacts directly with small glycoproteins of the extracellular matrix. *J Immunol.* (2009) 182:1518–25. doi: 10.4049/jimmunol.182.3.1518
16. Levey AS, Coresh J, Greene T, Stevens LA, Zhang YL, Hendriksen S, et al. Using standardized serum creatinine values in the modification of diet in renal disease study equation for estimating glomerular filtration rate. *Ann Intern Med.* (2006) 145:247–54. doi: 10.7326/0003-4819-145-4-200608150-00004
17. Zickert A, Oke V, Parodis I, Svenungsson E, Sundstrom Y, Gunnarsson I. Interferon (IFN)-lambda is a potential mediator in lupus nephritis. *Lupus Sci Med.* (2016) 3:e000170. doi: 10.1136/lupus-2016-000170
18. Ahearn JM, Manzi S, Liu CC. The lupus biomarker odyssey: one experience. *Methods Mol Biol.* (2014) 1134:17–35. doi: 10.1007/978-1-4939-0326-9_2
19. Parodis I, Ding H, Zickert A, Cosson G, Fathima M, Gronwall C, et al. Serum Axl predicts histology-based response to induction therapy and long-term renal outcome in lupus nephritis. *PLoS One.* (2019) 14:e0212068. doi: 10.1371/journal.pone.0212068
20. Parodis I, Gokaraju S, Zickert A, Vanarsa K, Zhang T, Habazi D, et al. ALCAM and VCAM-1 as urine biomarkers of activity and long-term renal outcome in systemic lupus erythematosus. *Rheumatology (Oxford).* (2019) 59:2237–49. doi: 10.1093/rheumatology/kez528
21. Lech M, Anders HJ. The pathogenesis of lupus nephritis. *J Am Soc Nephrol.* (2013) 24:1357–66.
22. Ritchie RF, Palomaki GE, Neveux LM, Navolotskaia O, Ledue TB, Craig WY. Reference distributions for complement proteins C3 and C4: a practical, simple and clinically relevant approach in a large cohort. *J Clin Lab Anal.* (2004) 18:1–8. doi: 10.1002/jcla.10100
23. Birmingham DJ, Irshaid F, Nagaraja HN, Zou X, Tsao BP, Wu H, et al. The complex nature of serum C3 and C4 as biomarkers of lupus renal flare. *Lupus.* (2010) 19:1272–80. doi: 10.1177/0961203310371154
24. Luciano RL, Moeckel GW. Update on the native kidney biopsy: core curriculum 2019. *Am J Kidney Dis.* (2019) 73:404–15. doi: 10.1053/j.ajkd.2018.10.011
25. Sun YS, Sun IT, Wang HK, Yang AH, Tsai CY, Huang CJ, et al. Risk of complications of ultrasound-guided renal biopsy for adult and pediatric patients with systemic lupus erythematosus. *Lupus.* (2018) 27:828–36. doi: 10.1177/0961203317751048
26. Kamitaki N, Sekar A, Handsaker RE, de Rivera H, Tooley K, Morris DL, et al. Complement genes contribute sex-biased vulnerability in diverse disorders. *Nature.* (2020) 582:577–81. doi: 10.1038/s41586-020-2277-x
27. Wu YL, Yang Y, Chung EK, Zhou B, Kitzmiller KJ, Savelli SL, et al. Phenotypes, genotypes and disease susceptibility associated with gene copy number variations: complement C4 CNVs in European American healthy subjects and those with systemic lupus erythematosus. *Cytogenet Genome Res.* (2008) 123:131–41. doi: 10.1159/000184700
28. Kraaij T, Nilsson SC, van Kooten C, Okroj M, Blom AM, Teng YO. Measuring plasma C4D to monitor immune complexes in lupus nephritis. *Lupus Sci Med.* (2019) 6:e000326. doi: 10.1136/lupus-2019-000326
29. Feucht HE, Schneeberger H, Hillebrand G, Burkhardt K, Weiss M, Riethmuller G, et al. Capillary deposition of C4d complement fragment and early renal graft loss. *Kidney Int.* (1993) 43:1333–8. doi: 10.1038/ki.1993.187
30. Racusen LC, Colvin RB, Solez K, Mihatsch MJ, Halloran PF, Campbell PM, et al. Antibody-mediated rejection criteria – an addition to the Banff 97 classification of renal allograft rejection. *Am J Transplant.* (2003) 3:708–14.
31. Mastellos DC, Ricklin D, Lambris JD. Clinical promise of next-generation complement therapeutics. *Nat Rev Drug Discov.* (2019) 18:707–29. doi: 10.1038/s41573-019-0031-6
32. Kao AH, Navratil JS, Ruffing MJ, Liu CC, Hawkins D, McKinnon KM, et al. Erythrocyte C3d and C4d for monitoring disease activity in systemic lupus erythematosus. *Arthritis Rheum.* (2010) 62:837–44. doi: 10.1002/art.27267

16

Integrative Clinical, Molecular and Computational Analysis Identify Novel Biomarkers and Differential Profiles of Anti-TNF Response in Rheumatoid Arthritis

Maria Luque-Tévar [1†], Carlos Perez-Sanchez [1†], Alejandra Mª Patiño-Trives [1†], Nuria Barbarroja [1], Ivan Arias de la Rosa [1], Mª Carmen Abalos-Aguilera [1], Juan Antonio Marin-Sanz [1], Desiree Ruiz-Vilchez [1], Rafaela Ortega-Castro [1], Pilar Font [1], Clementina Lopez-Medina, Montserrat Romero-Gomez [1], Carlos Rodriguez-Escalera [2], Jose Perez-Venegas [3], Mª Dolores Ruiz-Montesinos [3], Carmen Dominguez [3], Carmen Romero-Barco [4], Antonio Fernandez-Nebro [5], Natalia Mena-Vazquez [5], Jose Luis Marenco [6], Julia Uceda-Montañez [6], Mª Dolores Toledo-Coello [7], M. Angeles Aguirre [1], Alejandro Escudero-Contreras [1‡], Eduardo Collantes-Estevez [1‡] and Chary Lopez-Pedrera [1‡]*

[1] Instituto Maimónides de Investigación Biomédica de Córdoba (IMIBIC), Hospital Reina Sofia, Universidad de Cordoba, Córdoba, Spain, [2] Hospital Universitario de Jaen, Jaén, Spain, [3] Hospital Universitario Virgen Macarena, Sevilla, Spain, [4] Hospital Clínico Universitario, Malaga, Spain, [5] Hospital Regional Universitario de Malaga, Malaga, Spain, [6] Hospital Universitario Virgen de Valme, Sevilla, Spain, [7] Hospital Universitario de Jerez de la Frontera, Cádiz, Spain

***Correspondence:**
Chary Lopez-Pedrera
rosario.lopez.exts@juntadeandalucia.es

† These authors share first authorship

‡ These authors share last authorship

Background: This prospective multicenter study developed an integrative clinical and molecular longitudinal study in Rheumatoid Arthritis (RA) patients to explore changes in serologic parameters following anti-TNF therapy (TNF inhibitors, TNFi) and built on machine-learning algorithms aimed at the prediction of TNFi response, based on clinical and molecular profiles of RA patients.

Methods: A total of 104 RA patients from two independent cohorts undergoing TNFi and 29 healthy donors (HD) were enrolled for the discovery and validation of prediction biomarkers. Serum samples were obtained at baseline and 6 months after treatment, and therapeutic efficacy was evaluated. Serum inflammatory profile, oxidative stress markers and NETosis-derived bioproducts were quantified and miRNomes were recognized by next-generation sequencing. Then, clinical and molecular changes induced by TNFi were delineated. Clinical and molecular signatures predictors of clinical response were assessed with supervised machine learning methods, using regularized logistic regressions.

Results: Altered inflammatory, oxidative and NETosis-derived biomolecules were found in RA patients vs. HD, closely interconnected and associated with specific miRNA profiles. This altered molecular profile allowed the unsupervised division of three clusters of RA patients, showing distinctive clinical phenotypes, further linked to the TNFi effectiveness. Moreover, TNFi treatment reversed the molecular alterations in parallel to the clinical outcome. Machine-learning algorithms in the discovery cohort identified both, clinical and molecular signatures as potential predictors of response to TNFi treatment with high accuracy, which was further increased when both features were integrated in a mixed model (AUC: 0.91). These results were confirmed in the validation cohort.

Conclusions: Our overall data suggest that: 1. RA patients undergoing anti-TNF-therapy conform distinctive clusters based on altered molecular profiles, which are directly linked to their clinical status at baseline. 2. Clinical effectiveness of anti-TNF therapy was divergent among these molecular clusters and associated with a specific modulation of the inflammatory response, the reestablishment of the altered oxidative status, the reduction of NETosis, and the reversion of related altered miRNAs. 3. The integrative analysis of the clinical and molecular profiles using machine learning allows the identification of novel signatures as potential predictors of therapeutic response to TNFi therapy.

Keywords: rheumatoid arthritis, anti-TNF agents, inflammation, NEtosis, microRNAs, machine learning, predictors, efficacy

INTRODUCTION

Rheumatoid arthritis (RA) is a systemic inflammatory autoimmune disease identified by continuous joint inflammation promoting cartilage and bone damage, incapacity and eventually systemic complications. Prompt treatment can preclude severe disability and bring significant benefits to patients, although the lack of therapeutic efficacy in a substantial number of patients is still challenging (1).

In the last years, advances in the understanding of RA pathogenesis by identifying key cells and cytokines have allowed the development of new targeted disease-modifying antirheumatic drugs (2). In the late 1990s, the introduction of anti-tumor necrosis factor alpha drugs (TNF inhibitors, TNFi) greatly improved the medical management of RA patients, although some of them were reported to be ineffective.

A recent observational study has found that nowadays anti-TNF drugs are the first-line treatment in 96% of patients who fail methotrexate therapy. Besides, patients who do not reach their treatment targets (3) are forced to cycle through multiple anti-TNF drugs while their disease has time to progress. As all anti-TNF drugs target similar molecular and inflammatory pathways, it is not surprising that most patients who are primary non-responders to their initial anti-TNF therapy fail to achieve their treatment targets when cycled through alternative anti-TNFs. This suggests that primary non-responders should be switched to an alternative therapy rather than enduring anti-TNF cycling. Thus, the development of a personalized medicine approach to identify primary non-responders to anti-TNFs prior to treatment would allow significantly more patients to reach their treatment target by treating them with alternative therapies as first-line therapies.

Nowadays, the number of robust treatment response predictors in RA is very limited, so that it has been demonstrated that pathophysiological biomarkers have insufficient discriminating power. Hence, several studies have identified a number of potential clinical biomarkers of RA response to biological therapies, including age, sex, disease duration and activity, smoking status, presence of comorbidities, tender joint counts (TJC), concomitant methotrexate therapy, etc. (4–7). Yet, those studies were inconsistent and contradictory results have been published.

Besides, none of these studies have evaluated the molecular mechanisms underlying the distinctive response to TNF-inhibitors (TNFi) among RA patients and their potential as predictors of treatment response.

In the last years, relevant findings in the field of RA pathogenesis have been described, among which new insights come from studies on synovial fibroblasts and cells belonging to the innate and adaptive immune system, which have documented the aberrant production of inflammatory mediators, oxidative stress and NETosis, along with relevant alterations of the genome and on the regulatory epigenetic and posttranslational mechanisms. Moreover, emerging studies by several groups, including ours, have demonstrated that the pharmacological therapy with biological disease modifying anti-rheumatic drugs (bDMARDs) such as TNF or IL-6 receptor inhibitors, or anti-CD20 antibodies promotes, in parallel to their clinical efficacy, a specific and significant alteration in several of these altered molecular mechanisms (8–12).

The complexity of the treatment response in a given patient and the significant differences between patients suggest that the combination of biomarkers may be more helpful than studying them separately. Therefore, the development of matrices containing clinical and laboratory parameters related to diagnosis or prognosis might help to select the best treatment for each patient.

Integrative biology by advanced computational analysis is a fast-expanding field that can be expected to identify combinations of parameters capable of predicting the response to various drugs (13).

In this study, we developed an integrative clinical and molecular longitudinal study in RA patients to explore changes in serologic parameters related to inflammation, NETosis, oxidative stress and regulating microRNAs (miRNAs) following TNFi treatment. Besides, by using machine-learning algorithms, we aimed at the prediction of TNFi response based on the combination of clinical and molecular profiles of RA patients.

PATIENTS AND METHODS

Study Design and Patients

In a prospective multicenter study, a total of 104 RA patients and 29 healthy donors (HD), from two independent cohorts, were recruited (during a 48-months period). These cohorts attended the Reina Sofia University Hospital of Córdoba, the Virgen Macarena Hospital of Sevilla, The Virgen del Valme Hospital of Sevilla, the Virgen de la Victoria University hospital of Malaga, Jerez de la Frontera University Hospital, and the University Hospital of Jaen. All patients fulfilled the American College of Rheumatology revised criteria for RA (14).

Approval from the ethics committees was obtained, and subjects provided written informed consent.

Clinical/laboratory parameters of RA patients and HD from the discovery cohort are displayed in **Table 1** while clinical data of RA patients belonging to the independent validation cohort are displayed in **Supplementary Table 1**.

All patients had an inadequate response to at least two disease-modifying antirheumatic drugs (DMARDs) and received TNFi in combination therapy with DMARDs. All patients were naïve to TNFi treatment.

Within the discovery cohort, 22 patients were given infliximab (3 mg/kg/day intravenous infusion at times 0, 2, and 6 weeks, and every 8 weeks thereafter), 39 patients received etanercept (50 mg subcutaneously every week), 12 patients were treated with adalimumab (40 mg subcutaneously every 2 weeks), 4 with golimumab (50 mg subcutaneously every month) and 2 with certolizumab (400 mg at times 0, 2, and 4 weeks, and 200 mg every 2 weeks thereafter).

Within the validation cohort, 5 patients were given infliximab, 10 patients received etanercept, 8 patients were treated with adalimumab, 1 with golimumab and 1 with certolizumab.

Clinical assessment, before and after 3 and 6 months of TNFi therapy, included swollen joint count (SJC), tender joint count (TJC), 28-joint disease activity score (DAS28), clinical disease activity index (CDAI), simple disease activity index (SDAI), and health assessment questionnaire (HAQ). Serological evaluation, performed by clinical laboratory routine analysis, included analysis of rheumatoid factor (RF, U/mL), anti-cyclic citrullinated peptide antibodies (ACPAs, U/mL), C-reactive protein (CRP, mg/L) and erythrocyte sedimentation rate (ESR, mm/h).

Response to TNFi treatment was assessed by the European League Against Rheumatism (EULAR) criteria, based on the changes in DAS28 score, and the patients were categorized into responders and non-responders to TNFi. An improvement in DAS28 over $\geq$1.2 and a DAS28 value $\leq$ 3.2 after 6 months of treatment was considered a good response; a DAS28 value after 6 months between 3.2 and 5.1 and a reduction between 0.6 and 1.2 was considered a moderate response. Both of them were categorized as responders to the therapy. Patients who exhibited a DAS28 score at T6 > 5.1 or a reduction in DAS28 under 0.6 were considered a non-responders.

TABLE 1 | Clinical and molecular profiles of rheumatoid arthritis patients and healthy donors recruited to the study.

Clinical parameters	HD (n = 29)	RA patients (n = 79)	p
Gender (female/male)	19/10	64/15	0.12
Age, years (mean ± SD)	47 ± 17	51.2 ± 10.5	0.056
Disease evolution, years (mean ± SD)		11.5 ± 9.1	
TJC (mean ± SD)		8.1 ± 6.0	
SJC (mean ± SD)		5.9 ± 4.9	
DAS28 (mean ± SD)		4.7 ± 1.2	
SDAI (mean ± SD)		29.6 ± 13.3	
CDAI (mean ± SD)		27.9 ± 11.9	
HAQ (mean ± SD)		1.4 ± 0.7	
Smoking (n, %)	5/29 (17%)	19/79 (24%)	0.323
Arterial hypertension (n, %)	0/29 (%)	17/79 (21%)	0.005
Diabetes (n, %)	0/29 (%)	7/79 (8%)	0.186
Hypercholesterolemia (n, %)	16/29 (%)	35/79 (44%)	0.197
Extra-articular manifestations (n, %)		13/79 (16%)	
Radiological involvement (n, %)		29/79 (37%)	
Eroded joints (mean ± SD)		1.3 ± 2.3	
Laboratory parameters			
CRP, mg/mL (mean ± SD)	1.6 ± 2.2	15.8 ± 26.2	0.000
ESR, mm/h (mean ± SD)	8.1 ± 5.8	23.7 ± 17.9	0.000
ACPAs, IU/mL (mean ± SD)		343.3 ± 762.6	
RF, IU/mL (mean ± SD)		112.9 ± 205.8	
Treatments			
NSAIDS (n, %)		59/79 (74%)	
Corticosteroids (n, %)		73/79 (92%)	
Statins (n, %)		8/79 (10%)	
Vit D (n, %)		24/79 (30%)	
Osteoporosis treatment (n, %)		18/79 (22%)	
Antiplatelet (n, %)		2/79 (2%)	
Anticoagulants (n, %)		2/79 (2%)	
Methotrexate (n, %)		48/79 (61%)	
Leflunomide (n, %)		50/79 (63%)	
Dolquine (n, %)		46/79 (58%)	
Salazopyrine (n, %)		16/79 (20%)	

Blood Collection

Whole blood from HD and RA patients was collected by direct venous puncture either, into tubes with ethylenediaminetetraacetic acid (EDTA) as an anticoagulant, or into specific tubes for obtaining serum.

Blood samples were obtained before and after 6 months of TNFi treatment. To avoid blood composition changes promoted by diet and circadian rhythms, samples were always collected in the early hours in the morning and after a fasting period of 8 h. The blood was processed by spinning at 2,000 × g for 10 min at room temperature. Then, serum was transferred to a fresh RNase-free tube and stored at −80°C.

To avoid differences related to the origin of samples and their processing all the blood samples were collected and processed following the same protocol. In this multicenter study, our lab was the reference center. Thus, tubes for obtaining blood were sent to all the hospitals that collaborated on recruitment, and serum purification and storage were developed under the same conditions. Hence, all the samples coming from external centers were processes in our lab following the same procedures, which ensured the homogeneity of the downstream analysis.

Assessment of Circulating Inflammatory Profile and Oxidative Stress Markers

The inflammatory profile was analyzed in the serum of HD and RA patients both, before and after 6 months of TNFi therapy, by using a multiplex-type immunoassay—Bioplex (*Bio-Rad, CA, USA*)—in which a panel of 27 cytokines was evaluated.

Oxidative stress parameters were determined through the evaluation of oxidation of both lipids and proteins, along with the analysis of the total antioxidant capacity. Assays of lipid peroxidation levels were carried out using the Thiobarbituric acid reactive substances (TBARS) assay kit (Canvax Biotech, Córdoba, Spain), following the manufacturer's recommendations.

Protein nitrosylation was measured by using the Nitrotyrosine ELISA kit (Abcam, Cambridge, UK), following the manufacturer's recommendations. Serum total antioxidant capacity (TAC) was measured by quantitative colorimetric determination, using TAC Assay kit (Biovision, Mountain View, CA, USA) following the instructions provided by the manufacturer.

NETosis-Derived Products Assessment

To analyze NETosis-derived products, circulating levels of both elastase and nucleosomes were evaluated. Cell-free elastase levels were measured in RA patients' and HDs' serum using the Human PMN Elastase ELISA Kit (Abcam, Cambridge, UK) following the manufacturer's recommendations.

Likewise, cell-free nucleosomes were measured using the human cell death detection ELISAPLUS kit (Roche, Sigma-Aldrich, St Louis, MO, USA) following the manufacturer's recommendations. In this assay, monoclonal antibodies against DNA (double and single strand) and histones (H1, H2A, H2B, H3, and H4) were used to detect mono- and oligo nucleosomes in serum from RA patients. Quantification of nucleosomes was performed by photometrical determination of the absorbance at 405 nm, using as reference wavelength 492 nm.

MicroRNA Isolation, Profiling, and Quantitative Real-Time PCR

Total serum RNA—including the miRNA fraction—was extracted using the QIAzol miRNeasy kit (*Qiagen, Valencia, CA, USA*) with some modifications. A total of 200 µl of serum were thawed on ice and lysed in 1 mL QIAzol Lysis Reagent (*Qiagen*). Samples in QIAzol were incubated at room temperature for 5 min to inactivate RNases. To adjust for variations in RNA extraction and/or copurification of inhibitors, 5 fmol of spike-in non-human synthetic miRNA (*C. elegans* miR-39 miRNA mimic: 5′-UCACCGGGUGUAAAUCAGCUUG-3′) were added to the samples after the initial denaturation. The remaining extraction protocol was performed according to the manufacturer's instruction. Total RNA was eluted in 14 µl of RNase-free water.

To identify the profiles of miRNAs in the serum of HDs and RA patients, an array was performed in an exploratory cohort -including 6 samples from clinically representative RA patients and 3 from HDs- using the HTG EdgeSeq miRNA whole transcriptome assay (*miRNA WTA*), which enabled to measure the expression of 2,083 human miRNA transcripts using next generation sequencing (NGS) (HTG Molecular technologies, Tucson, AZ, USA).

All differentially regulated miRNAs and fold changes were imported into the web-based bioinformatics tool QIAGEN's Ingenuity Pathway Analysis (IPA) (Ingenuity Systems, http://www.INGENUITY.com) to perform a functional classification and identify potential mRNA targets. The right-tailed Fisher's exact test was used to calculate the *p*-value determining the statistical probability that the association between a set of molecules and a pathway or function might be due to chance alone. IPA analysis also allowed the selection of altered miRNAs that exhibited an enrichment in mRNA targets involved in the pathogenesis of RA for their validation in the whole cohort by real time PCR (RT-PCR) using a LightCycler® Thermal Cycler System (Roche Diagnostics, Indianapolis, Indiana, USA). Specifically, 3 µl of RNA eluate were reverse transcribed in 10 µl reactions using the miRCURY LNATM Universal RT mi-RNA PCR, Polyadenylation and cDNA synthesis kit (Exiqon, Vedbaek, Denmark). RT-PCR was carried out with 4 µL cDNA diluted 20x and 6 µL of reaction mixture [5 µL of SYBR Green master mix (Exiqon) and 1 µL of the corresponding PCR primer mix (microRNAs LNATM PCR primer set, Exiqon)]. After an initial hold of 10 min at 94°C, samples were cycled 40 times at 95°C for 10 s and at 60°C for 1 min. The expression levels of miRNAs were normalized to the mean of spiked-in miRNA Cel-miR-39. The expression levels of miRNA were calculated using the 2-$\Delta\Delta$Ct method. All measurements were performed in duplicate. Controls consisting of reaction mixture without cDNA were negative in all runs. List of miRNA sequences is displayed in **Supplementary Table 2**.

Machine Learning Analysis

Three different logistic models (15) were made to study clinical and molecular variables groups before starting therapy, looking for patients' best classification as responders or non-responders, using Python library Scikit-Learn (16). A logistic regression model with L2 penalty (all variables used) was made for clinical variables group. Training set (75%) and test set (25%) were settled for model validation. Identical approach was developed for molecular variables group. To study combined effect of both variables' groups, the same approach was used changing only to L1 penalty (variables selection) (**Supplementary Figure 1**).

Statistical Analyses

Statistical analysis and graphical representation of results were performed using GraphPad Prism 8 software (San Diego CA,

USA). The normal distribution of the variables to characterize the differences in the analyzed parameters was assessed using the Kolmogorov-Smirnov test.

Based on this test, comparisons between quantitative and qualitative variables were made using the Student's *t*-test, or alternatively, using a non-parametric test (Mann-Whitney U).

Paired samples within the same subjects were compared by Wilcoxon signed-rank test. Differences among groups of treatment were analyzed by repeated measures ANOVA. Correlations were assessed by Spearman's rank correlation. Differences were considered significant at $P < 0.05$.

When considering clinical and analytical measures, missing data values were <1% either, at baseline and after 3 and 6 months of therapy.

Regarding molecular measures, missing data values at baseline were around 5%.

Because of a number of patients were not willing to donate blood samples after 6 months of therapy, and/or bleeding was not recommended by clinicians at this time, we achieved molecular data from approximately 75% of patients included in the study.

RESULTS

MicroRNA Profile, Inflammatory, Oxidative Stress and NETosis-Derived Serum Parameters, Are Deregulated, Interrelated and Associated With the Clinical Profile of RA Patients

Whole miRNome profiling in serum samples identified altered levels of 223 miRNAs in RA patients before TNFi, when compared to HDs (cut-off: 2-fold change), of which 137 resulted to be upregulated and 86 downregulated (**Figure 1A** left panel).

By using the IPA software, the functional classification of these miRNAs revealed their association with clinical features of the RA physiopathology. Thus, the altered miRNAs signature in RA was enriched for biological processes such as connective tissue disorders, inflammatory response, infection, immunological, hematological, metabolic, respiratory and skeletal and muscular disorders, among others (**Figure 1A** central panel).

In order to validate the results in the whole cohort of RA patients and HDs, we performed an *in-silico* analysis that allowed the identification of a set of microRNAs as potential modulators of the expression of key targets involved in the pathology of RA. We identified a panel of 5 microRNAs including miR- 106a-5p, 143-5p, 148b-3p, 199a-5p, and 346 that showed potential targets molecules related to pro-inflammatory cytokines, chemokines, metalloproteinases, adhesion factors and critical immune receptors (BMP3, CCL-4, CCL-5, CCL-20, CXCL6, CXCL8, ITGA5, IL-6, IL6ST, IL-1RL1, MMP3, MMP13, TLR7, TNF, VCAM1, VEGFA, etc), along with a high number of molecules that regulate intracellular pathways associated with inflammatory and autoimmune processes (DKK-1,−2,−3, IKBKB, JAK1, MAPK14, MAP2K1, MAP3K5, NFKB1, NFßKBIA, PI3K3C2A, SOCS3, STAT3, WNT7, WNT2, WNT9B, etc.) (**Supplementary Figure 2**).

The expression of the 5 selected miRNAs was further analyzed by RT-PCR in the entire cohort, thus showing that the relative expression of all the selected circulating miRNAs was significantly altered in serum from RA patients when compared to HDs ($p < 0.05$) (**Figure 1A** right panel).

An inflammatory profile was also demonstrated in the serum of RA patients, including over-expression of a number of interleukins (IL-1β,−1RA,−2,−4,−5,−6,−8,−12,−13,−15 and−17) (**Figure 1B**), cytokines, chemokines and growth factors (Eotaxin, FGFbasic, GCSF, GM-CSF, IFNγ, MCP-1, MIP-1α, PDGF-BB, TNFα, and VEGF) (**Figure 1C**).

In addition, direct predicted miRNA-target interactions were identified between those deregulated miRNAs and several altered pro-inflammatory molecules (**Supplementary Figure 3**).

Increased NETs extrusion and enhanced oxidative status were also demonstrated by enlarged neutrophil cell-free elastase and Nucleosomes serum levels in RA patients (**Figure 1E**), along with increased levels of LPO and reduced N-Tyr and TAC (**Figure 1D**).

Correlation studies demonstrated a strong relationship among the levels of all the parameters evaluated, including inflammatory and oxidative stress markers, as well as with NETosis-derived products and microRNAs (**Supplementary Figure 4**).

Unsupervised Cluster Analysis of the Integrated Serum Molecular Signatures Stratified RA Patients According to Their Disease Status

By using self-organizing map (SOM) clustering analysis in the RA cohort, 3 clusters were distinguished, representing different serum molecular profile groups with respect to the circulating levels of inflammatory, oxidative and netotic mediators along with those of validated microRNAs (**Figures 2A,C**). Principal component analyses (PCA) confirmed a well-defined separation between these molecular clusters (**Figure 2B**). The clinical and laboratory profiles of each cluster were then evaluated (**Figures 2C,E**).

Briefly, cluster 1 (22% of the clustered cohort) was described on average by medium disease activity scores and low radiologic involvement, low prevalence of smokers and reduced prevalence of cardiovascular risk factors such as hypercholesterolemia.

On the contrary, cluster 3 (23% of the clustered cohort) comprised the patients with highest disease activity scores, along with a higher percentage of smokers and an enlarged prevalence of hypercholesterolemia.

Cluster 2 (55% of the clustered cohort) represented an intermediate clinical phenotype, though closer to cluster 3 in relation to disease activity scores, radiologic involvement, percentage of smokers and incidence of hypercholesterolemia.

No differences among clusters were found in relation to age, sex, positivity for autoantibodies, and disease duration.

Molecular analyses further recognized differential inflammatory, netotic, oxidative and miRNA profiles in RA patients' serum among clusters, on which patients belonging to clusters 1 and 3 displayed the most specific and distinctive expression patterns of interleukins, chemokines and growth factors, along with distinctive levels of oxidative stress markers such as lipoperoxides and N-Tyr, products of NETosis, including Elastase and Nucleosomes, and microRNAs (**Figure 2D**).

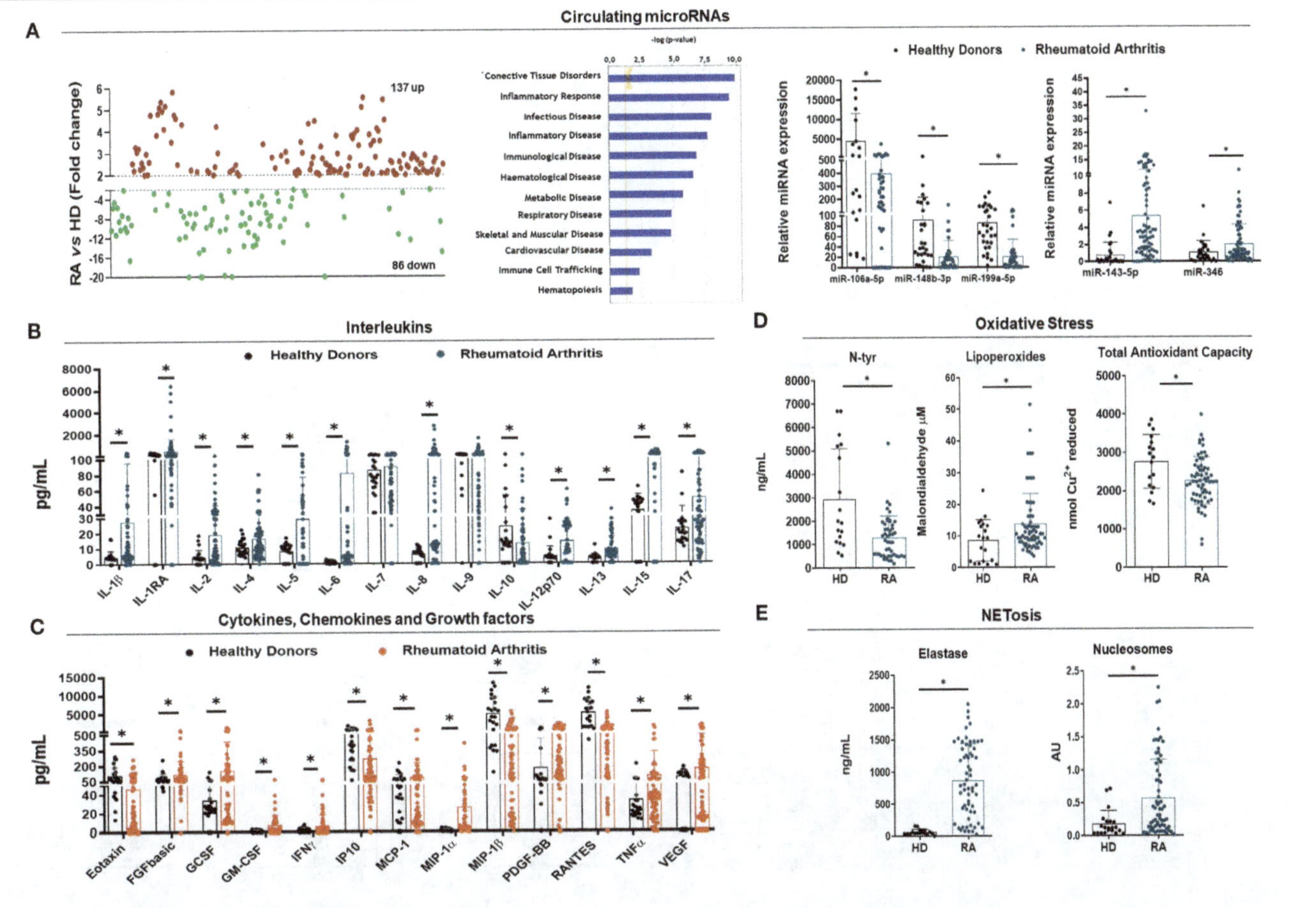

FIGURE 1 | Molecular characterization of rheumatoid arthritis patients. **(A)** Whole circulating microRNA (miRNA) expression profile in plasma of Rheumatoid Arthritis (RA) patients ($n = 6$) and healthy donors (HDs) ($n = 3$) by HTG EdgeSeq Assay showing miRNAs up-regulated in red and miRNAs downregulated in green (Fold Change >2 or <-2) (Left panel). Functional classification of altered miRNAs according biological functions and diseases following Ingenuity Pathway Analysis (central panel). RT-PCR validation of selected miRNAs associated with the pathogenesis of RA (right panel). **(B)** Interleukin profile of RA patients and HDs in serum by Luminex Assay (Bio-Plex). **(C)** Cytokine, chemokine and growth factor profile of RA patients and HDs in serum by Luminex Assay (Bio-Plex). **(D)** Oxidative stress markers in serum of RA patients and HDs including Nitrotyrosine (N-Tyr), Lipoperoxides and Total Antioxidant Capacity (TAC). **(E)** NETosis-derived products in serum of RA patients and HDs including neutrophil elastase and nucleosome levels. Analyses were performed on the whole cohort of RA patients ($n = 79$) and HD ($n = 29$). *$p < 0.05$.

Clinical Profile of RA Patients and Response to TNFi Therapy

At the start of the TNFi therapy all subjects showed medium-high disease activity, reflected by a mean DAS28 of 4.75 (2.05–7.5). A 74% of patients took non-steroidal anti-inflammatory drugs (NSAIDS) daily, and 92% received steroid treatment (range 2.5–30 mg/d prednisone). Methotrexate alone or in combination with other DMARD was further administered in 61% of subjects.

According to DAS28 response criteria, at 3 months of treatment, 28 (35%), 25 (32%), and 26 (33%) RA patients showed good, moderate, and no response to TNFi therapy, respectively (**Figure 3A**). All the clinical parameters evaluated, including DAS28, SDAI and CDAI scores, along with HAQ, number of swollen and tender joints improved significantly. In addition, acute phase reactants were also reduced (**Figure 3B**). Interestingly, most of good responders at 3 months remained responsive to therapy at 6 months. Besides, a significant number of moderate responders shifted to good responders in relation to those that remained as moderate or changed to non-responders (**Figure 3A**).

All five biological agents had a favorable influence on the evolution of those parameters, so that changes were not influenced by treatment with monoclonal antibodies nor with soluble receptor (**Supplementary Figure 5A**). Considering the clinical response more consolidated at 6 months of treatment, we selected this time after starting therapy to assess serum molecular changes and to search for potential biomarkers as predictors of response.

TNFi Changes on Serum Molecular Profile of RA Patients Were Specific of the Cluster Evaluated and Associated With the Clinical Response

According to EULAR response criteria, all patients belonging to cluster 1 showed clinical response after 6 months of therapy. In

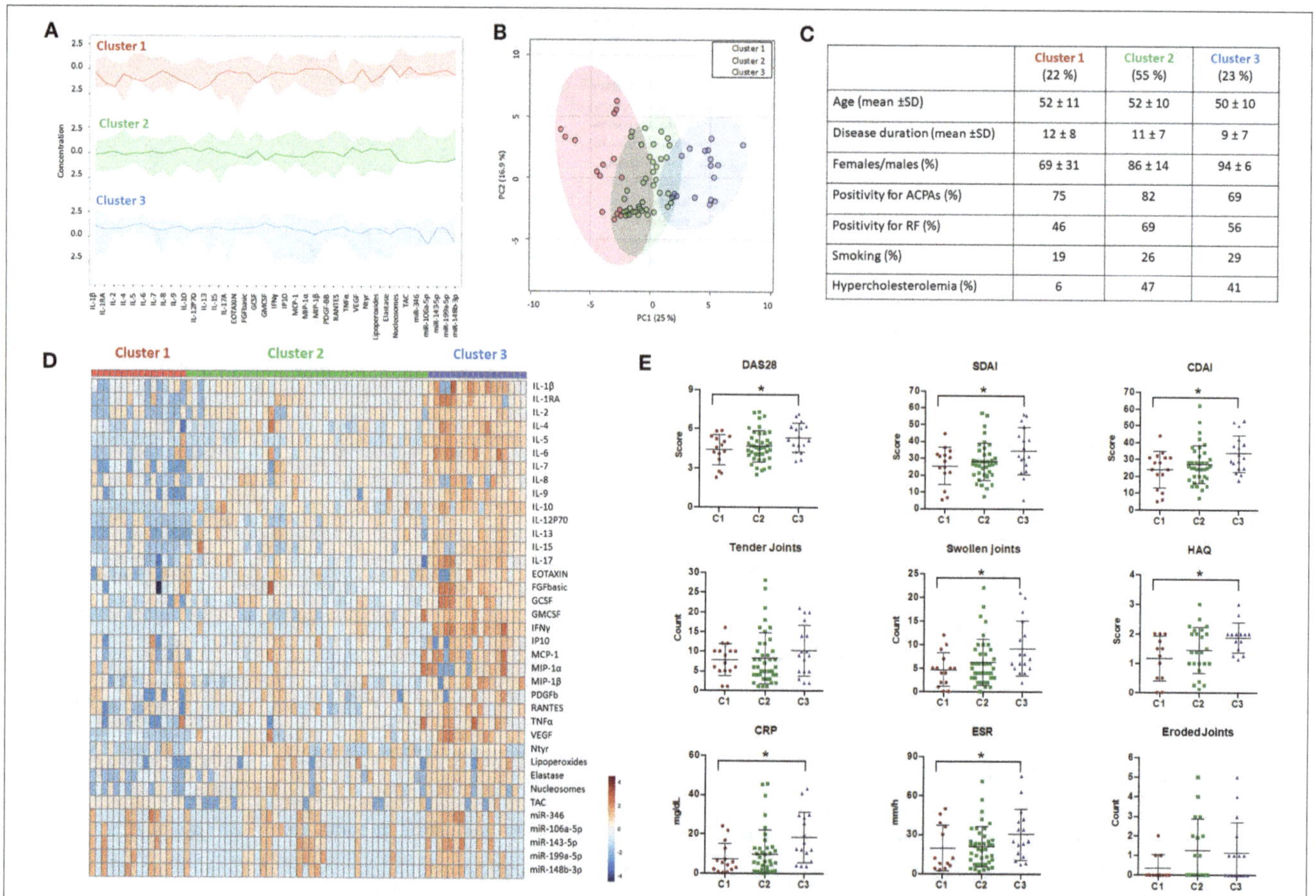

FIGURE 2 | Cluster analysis of molecular features in rheumatoid arthritis patients. **(A)** Overview plot of the differential molecular profiles of Rheumatoid Arthritis (RA) patients ($n = 74$) using Self Organization Map (SOM) clustering analysis from MetaboAnalyst 4.0. The darker lines represent the median intensities of each cluster. **(B)** Principal component analysis (PCA) summarizing the differences in the molecular profile of each cluster. **(C)** Table of demographic and laboratory parameters of RA patients characterizing each cluster (Cluster 1 = 16; Cluster 2 = 41; Cluster 3 = 17). **(D)** Heatmap of the molecular profile of each cluster showing the normalized levels of all the biomolecules analyzed in RA patients. **(E)** Clinical features associated with each cluster including Disease Activity Score (DAS28), Simple Disease Activity index (SDAI), Clinical Disease Activity Index (CDAI), Tender and Swollen Joints, Health Assessment Questionnaire (HAQ), C-reactive protein (CRP), Erythrocyte Sedimentation Rate (ESR), and Bone Erosion. $^{*}p < 0.05$.

clusters 2 and 3, 67% of patients were responders and a 33% of them were non-responders (**Figure 4A**). Thus, considering the similarity of these clusters concerning both, the clinical and molecular profiles and the response to treatment, and in order to identify molecular mechanisms of non-response, we decided to evaluate jointly the molecular changes occurred in these clusters after TNFi therapy.

As a general feature, we identified two main distinctive molecular profiles among RA patients responders to TNFi, involving, on one hand, low-medium baseline levels of inflammatory, oxidative and netotic mediators in those belonging to cluster 1, and on the other hand, high baseline levels of these parameters in responders belonging to the other two clusters.

Accordingly, in cluster 1 we observed few or no changes in the levels of these parameters after 6 months of therapy. On the contrary, the clinical response to TNFi in clusters 2 and 3 was found linked to a significant reduction in levels of a number of inflammatory mediators, oxidative stress markers, and products of NETosis, along with the restoration in the levels of microRNAs. These changes were not observed in patients that did not display clinical response to therapy (**Figure 4**).

Moreover, we observed that in responders patients to TNFi therapy, the levels of most of these parameters reached the ranks found in healthy donors after 6 months of therapy, while in non-responders, these parameters remained significantly elevated (**Figure 5**).

It must be noted that changes observed in molecular parameters were similar among patients treated with either, monoclonal anti-TNF antibodies or soluble receptor, independently of both, the cluster on which patients were included and the clinical response to therapy (**Supplementary Figure 5B**).

In support for these results, we further observed a significant positive correlation among the changes arisen in the levels of these molecules and the improvement of the disease activity, identified by DAS28 score (**Figure 6**).

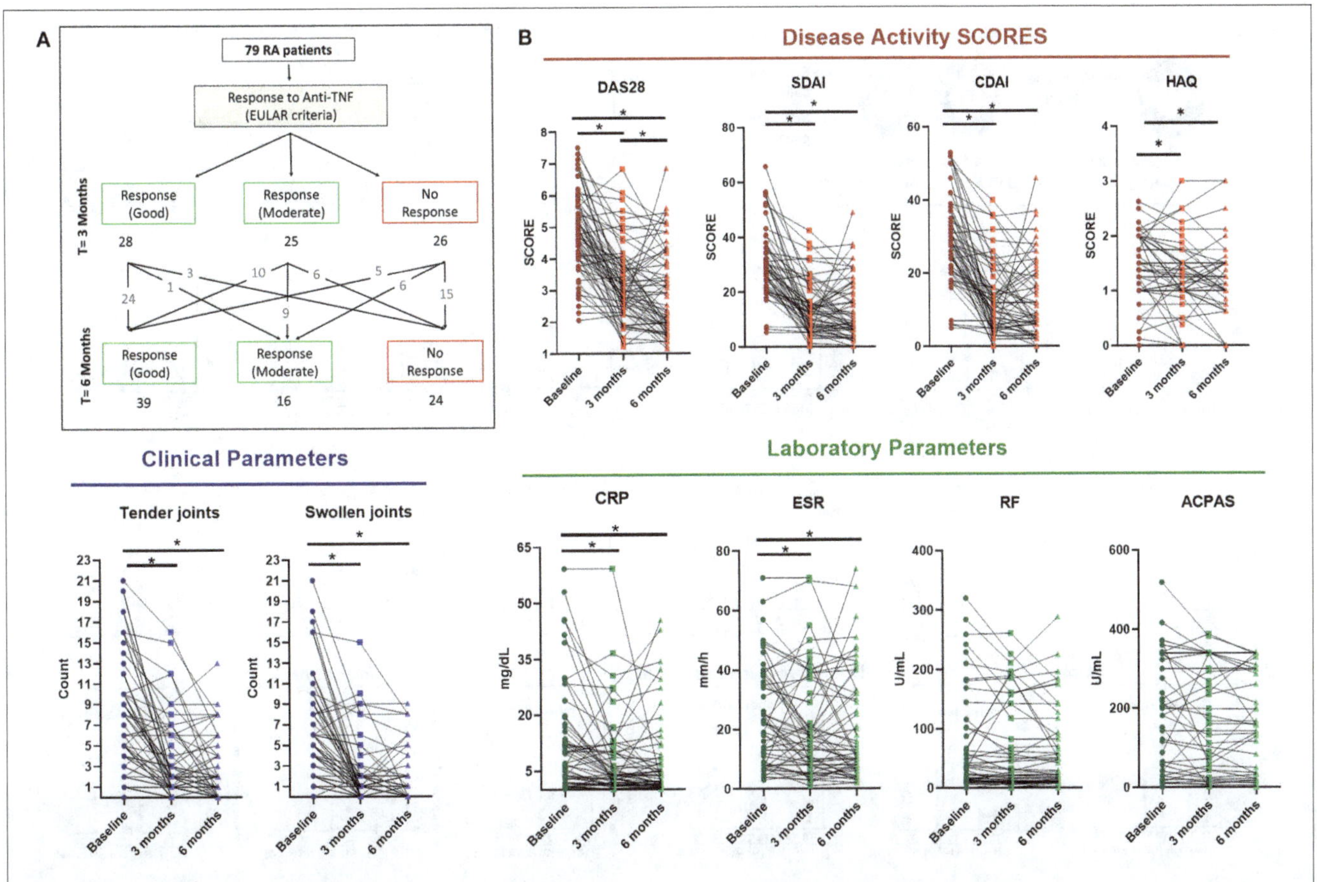

FIGURE 3 | Clinical response to anti-TNF therapy in rheumatoid arthritis patients. **(A)** Flow diagram representing the clinical response at 3 and 6 months of anti-TNF therapy following EULAR criteria. **(B)** RA patients' ($n = 79$) changes in clinical features at 3 and 6 months of anti-TNF therapy including Disease Activity Score (DAS28), Simple Disease Activity index (SDAI), Clinical Disease Activity Index (CDAI), Tender and Swollen Joints, Health Assesment Questionnaire (HAQ), C-reactive protein (CRP), erythrocyte Sedimentation Rate (ESR), Rheumatoid Factor (RF) and Anticitrullinated protein antibodies (ACPAS). $^{*}p < 0.05$.

Machine Learning Algorithms Allowed the Identification of Potential Predictors of TNFi Response

By using machine-learning algorithms such as logistic regression models, we searched for potential predictors of TNFi response based on clinical and molecular profiles of RA patients before starting therapy.

Firstly, we identified the clinical and molecular parameters that significantly distinguished among responder and non-responder patients, based on EULAR criteria (**Figures 7A,B**). Then, the identified parameters were split in clinical and molecular groups and logistic models were performed.

Among clinical groups, logistic model identified as good response factors, higher levels of creatinine, complement C4, total IgM, number of swollen joints, longer disease duration and complementary therapy with vitamin D, showed by odd ratio (OR) coefficients > 1. ROC curve analyses demonstrated that the combined model of these parameters identified responder patients with high accuracy (AUC = 0.81) (**Figure 7C**).

Among molecular parameters, logistic model identified as good response factors, high levels of nucleosomes, IL-10, miR106a-5p and IL-13, (OR > 1). Yet, high levels of lipoperoxides, IL-15 and IL-12p70 were predictors of non response (OR < 1). Likewise, ROC curve analysis with the combined model of molecular variables identified responder patients with similar accuracy (AUC = 0.807) (**Figure 7D**).

Interestingly, in the mixed model, combining clinical and molecular features, ROC curve showed better discriminative capacity than each single model (AUC = 0.909), thus supporting the relevance of combining both, clinical and molecular features to allow an accurate prediction of TNFi response (**Figure 7E**).

Moreover, similar prediction patterns were found when compared the treatments with soluble receptor vs. monoclonal antibodies. In fact, predictive models that mixed clinical and molecular features fit well for both types of TNFi, displaying areas under the curve close to 0.9 (**Supplementary Figure 6**). This data reinforces the potential clinical utility of this mixed model.

Likewise, when we evaluated the performance of these models in an independent cohort of 25 patients (invonving 14 responders and 11 non-responder patients to TNFi), we could validate their capacity to predict the response to TNFi before therapy. Thus, the mixed model integrating clinical and molecular features predicted the response with an AUC of 0.83, which was significantly higher compared to separated clinical and molecular models as in the case of the discovery cohort (**Figures 7F–H**).

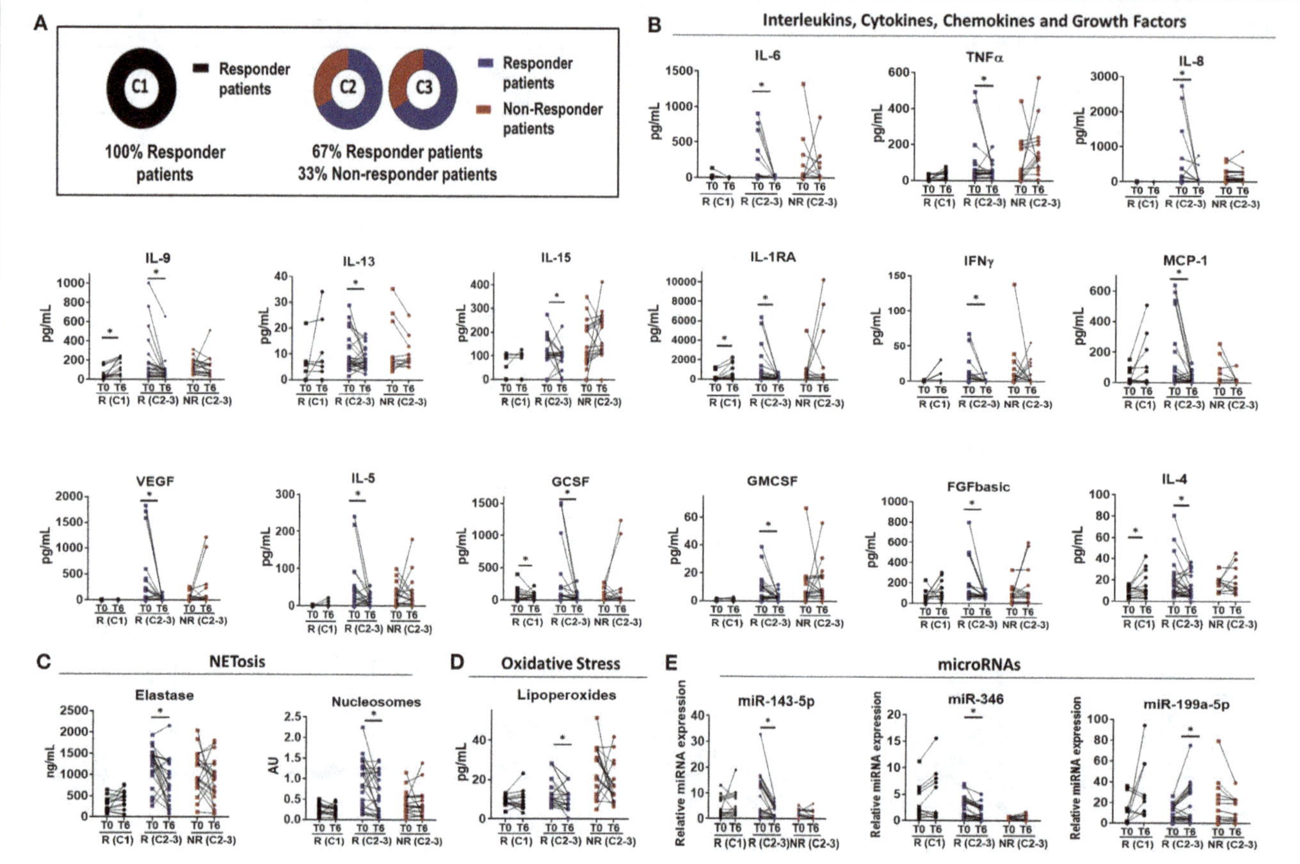

FIGURE 4 | Molecular response to anti-TNF therapy in rheumatoid arthritis patients. **(A)** Diagram showing the distribution of EULAR responder and non-responder patients among the different molecular clusters that characterized Rheumatoid Arthritis (RA) patient at baseline. Cluster 1 was characterized by responder patients while non-responder patients were identified only in cluster 2 and 3. **(B–E)** Individual changes in the level of biomolecules related to inflammation **(B)**, NETosis **(C)**, oxidative stress **(D)**, and microRNAs **(E)** before and after 6 months of Anti-TNF-therapy between responders and non-responder patients. *$p < 0.05$. R (C1), Responder patients of Cluster 1 ($n = 16$); R (C2-3), Responder patients of Cluster 2 and 3 ($n = 25$); NR (C2-3), Non-Responder patients of Cluster 2 and 3 ($n = 17$).

DISCUSSION

Continuous updating of the knowledge on molecular processes associated to the pathogenesis of RA, and on the specific effects of bDMARDs in the correction of their dysregulation, are essential in the early and correct approach to the treatment of this complex autoimmune disorder. RA is a dissimilar disease, involving multiple clinical manifestations and pathogenic mechanisms among individuals with the same diagnosis and/or throughout different disease stages. These traits support the complexity of the disease and the involvement of numerous factors in the trigger and the evolution of RA (17).

The present longitudinal study has elucidated the effects of TNFi treatment at the molecular level. In addition, a comprehensive analysis that combines data from different molecular categories and detailed clinical parameters has allowed a better understanding of molecular systems linked to disease severity effects of drugs treatment. Therefore, we demonstrated that, in parallel to the clinical response, TNFi promoted the re-establishment in the levels of circulating inflammatory and oxidative stress mediators, a significant reduction of NETosis-derived bioproducts and a substantial reversal of altered miRNAs.

It has been suggested that the diversity of biological processes underlying the pathogenesis of RA implies that their clinical phenotypes represent jointly altered pathways rather than exemplify the outcomes of single altered entities. Accordingly, different biological therapies have demonstrated numerous beneficial molecular effects that modulate pathological processes of the disease in RA (18). In the present study we identified a number of molecular alterations that develops jointly in these patients and are intimately associated to distinctive clinical phenotypes.

Firstly, clustering analysis based on molecular profiles before TNFi therapy, allowed the unsupervised division of three groups of RA patients, showing distinctive clinical phenotypes, further linked to the effectiveness of TNFi treatment. Thus, cluster 1 comprised patients 100% responders to therapy, who displayed a less prominent inflammatory status at baseline. On the contrary, on clusters 2 and 3, RA responders' patients to TNFi therapy were characterized by a high inflammatory status that paralleled a high disease activity. Patients from cluster 1 did not show

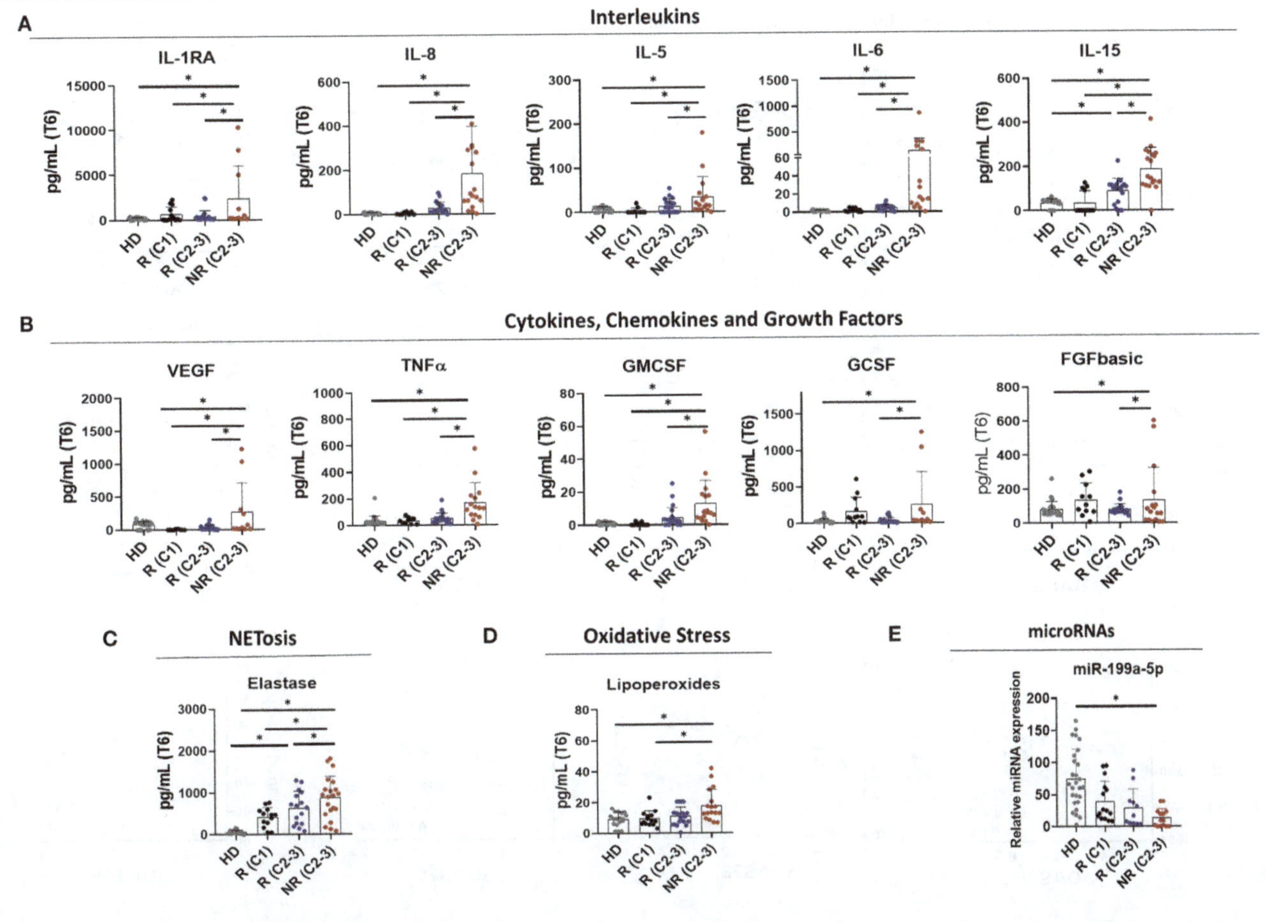

FIGURE 5 | Increased levels of altered biomolecules in non-responder patients to anti-TNF therapy after 6 months of treatment. Level of Interleukins **(A)**, Cytokines, Chemokines and Growth Factors **(B)**, NETosis-derived products **(C)**, oxidative stress markers **(D)**, and circulating microRNAs **(E)** in the plasma of Healthy donors (HDs) and responder and non-responder patients after 6 months of Anti-TNF therapy. $^*p < 0.05$. R (C1), Responder patients of Cluster 1 ($n = 16$); R (C2-3), Responder patients of Cluster 2 and 3 ($n = 25$); NR (C2-3), Non-Responder patients of Cluster 2 and 3 ($n = 17$).

changes in the molecular panel evaluated. However, the fact that all of them achieved a clinical response suggests that changes in other inflammatory mediators might be responsible for the therapy effectiveness. In these patients from cluster 2 and 3, therapy promoted a clear inflammatory response, involving the downregulation of cytokines, chemokines, growth factors, NETosis bioproducts and oxidative stress molecules. Quite the reverse, in non-responder patients belonging to these two clusters, the high levels found of inflammatory mediators and other altered metabolites were not reduced by TNFi, remaining increased after 6 months of therapy. Similar results have been published in previous works, including ours (19). Although core mechanisms remain to be clarified, this is the first study that identifies two sets of patients with distinctive molecular profiles at baseline that share a good response to TNFi therapy, underlying a heterogeneity in these patients that most probably derives of numerous clinical, genetic and environmental factors awaiting to be clarified.

In addition, our data strengths the relevance of integrating molecular and clinical studies in these patients, in order to identify potential predictors of treatment response. Hence, by using machine-learning algorithms (i.e., logistic regression models) we searched for potential predictors of TNFi response based on clinical and molecular profiles of RA patients. Our results identified signatures involving both clinical and molecular parameters that might predict the response to TNFi, which was further independent of the TNF inhibitor used, either monoclonal antibody or soluble receptor. Thus, several inflammatory cytokines, along with bioproducts of NETosis, oxidative stress and microRNAs, whose altered levels have been previously demonstrated to be altered in RA patients and modified by bDMARDs, were predictors of response to TNFi. Consistently, among clinical parameters, longer disease evolution, high number of swollen joints, and increased serum levels of creatinine, triglycerides, complement C4 and IgM, along with the concomitant treatment with vitamin D, were associated to the response to TNFi after 6 months of treatment.

Preceding studies demonstrated that these parameters were linked to the altered autoimmune and inflammatory status of RA patients (i.e., inflamed joints, elevated IgM and complement C4) (20, 21), and/or were indicative of an active metabolic status (i.e., high creatinine) (22). Moreover, available evidence indicates

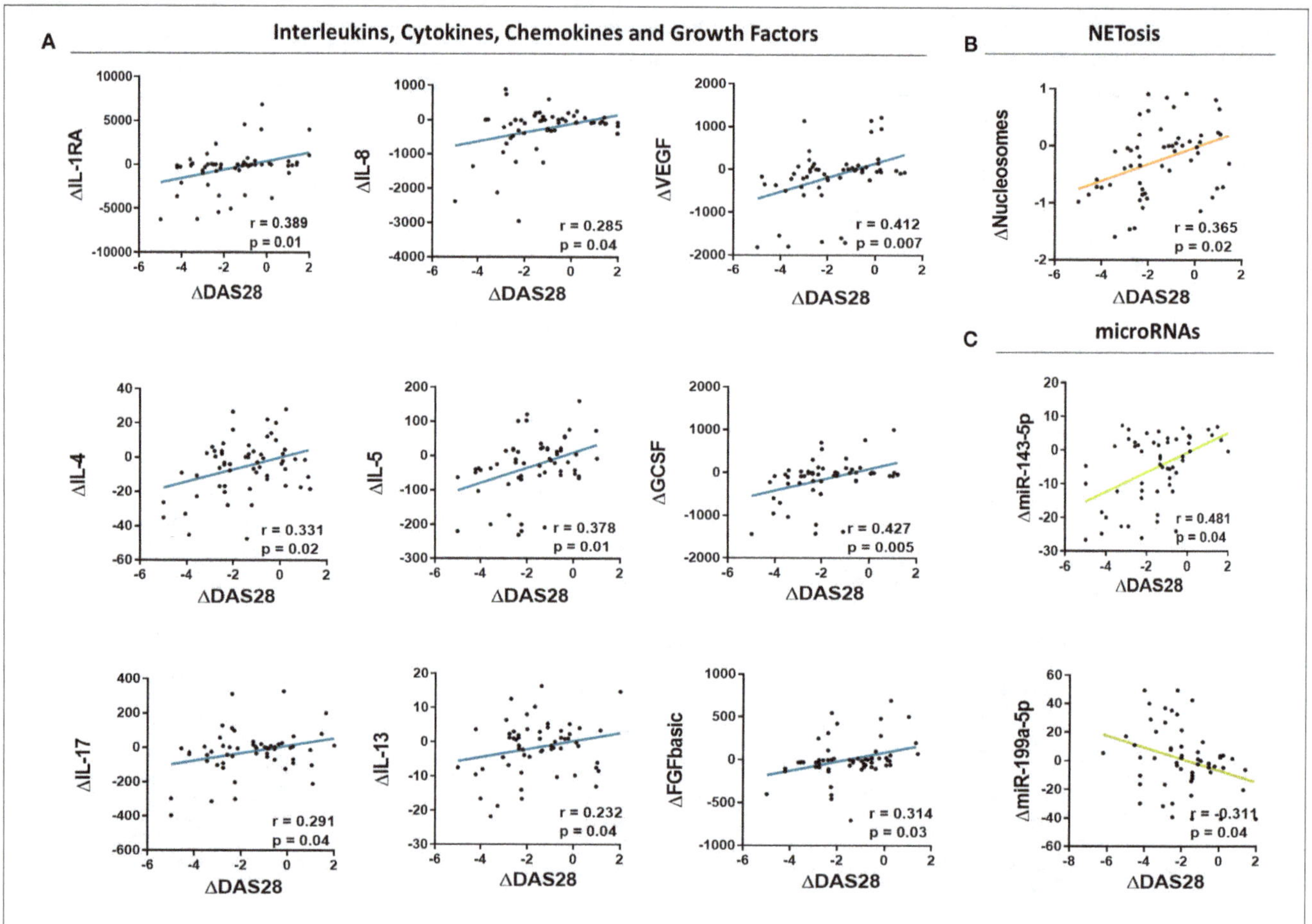

FIGURE 6 | Correlations among changes in the levels of altered biomolecules and the clinical response induced by anti-TNF therapy in rheumatoid arthritis patients. Correlation analysis among changes in the levels of inflammatory mediators **(A)**, NETosis markers **(B)** and microRNAs **(C)** in the serum of Rheumatoid Arthritis patients after 6 months of anti-TNF Therapy and changes in the disease activity score (DAS28).

that high inflammation interferes with lipid metabolism, so that hyperlipidemia is frequently associated to the adverse clinical outcome of the disease, and good control of the chronic inflammatory state may positively influence the lipid profile (23).

Additionally, several studies have shown that supplementary vitamin D can effectively control the DAS28, TJC and ESR levels in RA patients, mainly due to its anti-inflammatory properties (24). Correspondingly, in our hands, patients having a supplemental vitamin D treatment showed a better response to TNFi. Similar results have been also shown in other inflammatory diseases such Inflammatory Bowel Disease where higher levels of Vitamin D are associated with greater odds of remission with TNFi (25).

Hence, in our cohort, signatures involving clinical and molecular parameters associated to a more significantly altered inflammatory and metabolic status at baseline, and a concomitant therapy with a compound with anti-inflammatory properties -such as vitamin D-, seems to identify those patients who could benefit more from TNFi treatment.

Machine learning is a new field gaining attention in Rheumatology (26). Thus, two recent studies have shown their potential to predict TNFi response using clinical or molecular data. Guan et al., showed that large collection of clinical data at baseline along with a Gaussian process regression model correctly classified 78% of responder patients (27). In line with this, Tao et al. showed the capacity of gene expression and DNA methylation to predict TNFi response in RA using random forest algorithms with an accuracy of 85% (28).

In our study, we demonstrated for the first time that the combination of molecular and clinical data using machine learning exhibited a greater capacity to predict the clinical response to TNFi therapy in RA patients than each one separately. This finding could pave the way for the development of larger and independent validation studies aimed to achieve a precision medicine model to predict TNFi in RA and related diseases. Likewise, future analysis of predictors of therapy response using other biological drugs with different mechanism of action (Anti-CD20, Anti-IL6, JAK-inhibitors etc.) will be also required for the development of a wide approach of personalized medicine in RA patients in which all the available drugs are included.

Limitations of the study: Firstly, since we did not perform a complete serum profile involving inflammatory mediators, oxidative stress markers, NETotic bioproducts and miRNAs,

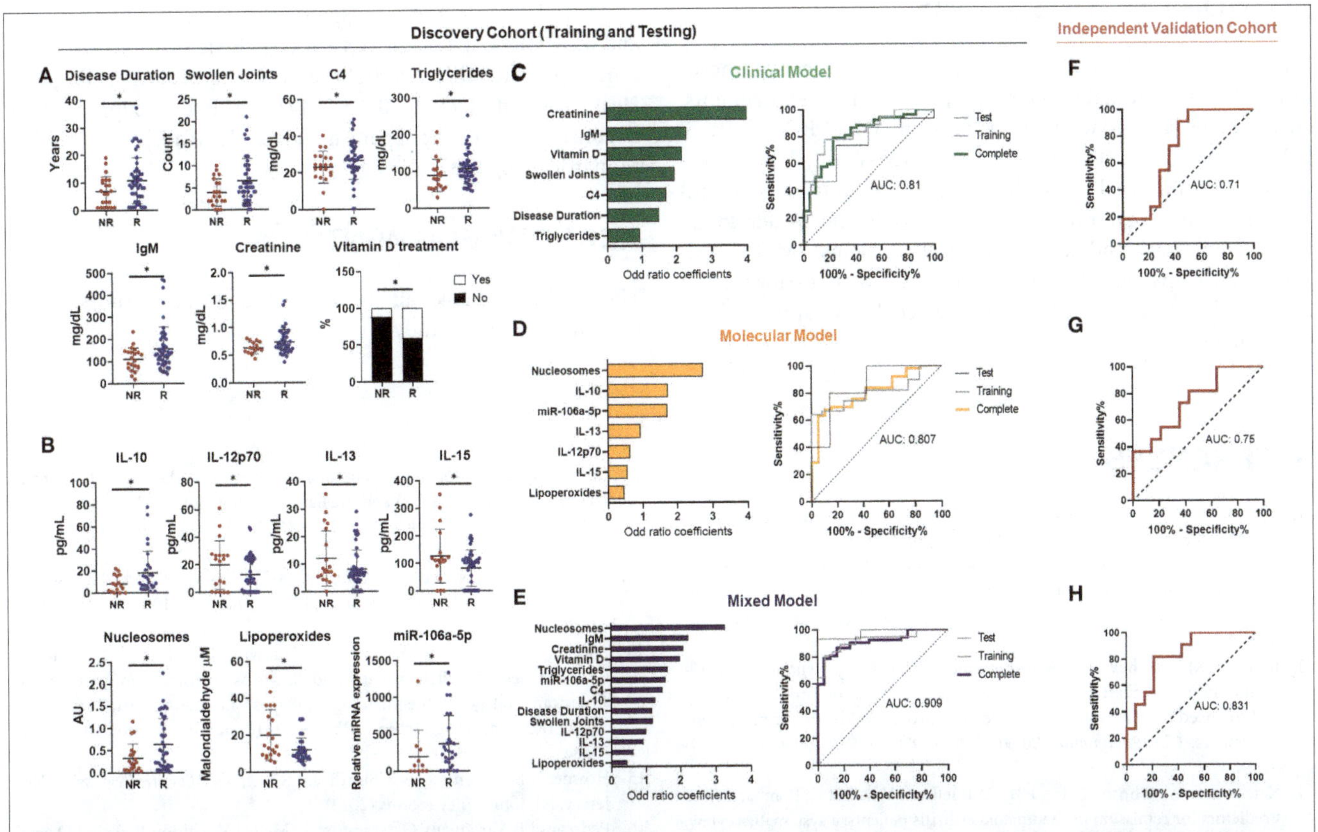

FIGURE 7 | Biomarkers predictors of anti-TNF response in rheumatoid arthritis by using machine learning. **(A)** Baseline clinical variables associated with the EULAR clinical response to Anti-TNF in Rheumatoid Arthritis (RA) patients after 6 months ($n = 74$, including 52 R and 22 NR). **(B)** Baseline molecular variables associated with the EULAR clinical response in RA patients after 6 months. **(C)** ROC curve of the machine learning model predictor of clinical response (left panel) using only clinical variables and their individual contribution represented by the odd ratio coefficients (right panel). **(D)** ROC curve of the machine learning model predictor of clinical response (left panel) using only molecular variables and their individual contribution represented by the odd ratio coefficients (right panel). **(E)** ROC curve of the machine learning model predictor of clinical response (left panel) using the best combination of clinical and molecular variables and their individual contribution represented by the odd ratio coefficients (right panel). **(F)** ROC curve of the machine learning model predictor of clinical response in an independent validation cohort. **(G)** ROC curve of the machine learning model predictor of molecular response in an independent validation cohort. **(H)** ROC curve of the machine learning model predictor using both clinical and molecular variables. (validation cohort: $n = 25$, including 14 R and 11 NR). *$p < 0.05$. R, responders; NR, non responders; AUC, area under the curve.

we cannot exclude the complementary role of other circulating biomolecules, -including non-evaluated inflammatory molecules or miRNAs, among others- in the response to treatment. In addition, due to the clinical heterogeneity of RA patients and the relatively small number of patients analyzed in this study, data must be confirmed in larger cohorts. Moreover, specific analyses on the mechanisms underlying the altered expression of these molecules after TNFi therapy, as well as the identification of cellular sources of these circulating biomolecules are still required.

Taken together, our overall data suggest that:

1. RA patients undergoing anti-TNF-therapy conform distinctive clusters based on altered molecular profiles, which are directly linked to their clinical status at baseline.
2. Clinical effectiveness of anti-TNF therapy was divergent among these molecular clusters and associated with a specific modulation of the inflammatory response, the reestablishment of the altered oxidative status, the reduction of NETosis, and the reversion of related altered miRNAs.
3. Through a systematic and comprehensive study design including discovery and validation phases, we have developed an integrative analysis of the clinical and molecular profiles of RA patients using machine learning, which allowed the identification of novel signatures as potential predictors of therapeutic response to TNFi therapy.

Our overall data pave the way for the development of large prospective and validation studies, needed to achieve a personalized medicine approach for RA patients.

ETHICS STATEMENT

The studies involving human participants were reviewed and approved by Ethics Committee of Reina Sofia Hospital. The patients/participants provided their written informed consent to participate in this study.

AUTHOR CONTRIBUTIONS

ML-T, CP-S, AE-C, EC-E, and CL-P formed the hypothesis, directed and coordinated the project, designed the experiments, analyzed the data and wrote the manuscript. DR-V, RO-C, MR-G, CR-E, JP-V, MR-M, CD, CR-B, AF-N, NM-V, JM, JU-M, MT-C, and MA followed up with patients and contributed useful discussion and suggestions. NB, MA-A, AP-T, and IA developed the *in vivo* assays and solved technical problems. JM-S CL-M, and PF were involved in statistical analysis and discussing related results. All authors contributed to the article and approved the submitted version.

manera de hacer Europa, Spain, the Spanish Inflammatory and Rheumatic Diseases Network (RIER), Instituto de Salud Carlos III (RD16/0012/0015) and the Andalusian Regional Health System (ref. PI-0285-2017). CL-P was supported by a contract from the Spanish Junta de Andalucía (Nicolas Monardes program).

ACKNOWLEDGMENTS

The authors thank all patients and healthy subjects for participation in the study.

REFERENCES

1. McInnes IB, Schett G. The pathogenesis of rheumatoid arthritis. *N Engl J Med.* (2011) 365:2205–19. doi: 10.1056/NEJMra1004965
2. Chen Z, Bozec A, Ramming A, Schett G. Anti-inflammatory and immune regulatory cytokines in rheumatoid arthritis. *Nat Rev Rheumatol.* (2019) 15:9–17. doi: 10.1038/s41584-018-0109-2
3. Johnson KJ, Sanchez HN, Schoenbrunner N. Defining response to TNF-inhibitors in rheumatoid arthritis: the negative impact of anti-TNF cycling and the need for a personalized medicine approach to identify primary non-responders. *Clin Rheumatol.* (2019) 38:2967–976. doi: 10.1007/s10067-019-04684-1
4. Katchamart W, Johnson S, Lin HJL, Phumethum V, Salliot C, Bombardier C. Predictors for remission in rheumatoid arthritis patients: a systematic review. *Arthrit Care Res.* (2010) 62:1128–43. doi: 10.1002/acr.20188
5. Callaghan C, Boyter A, Mullen A, McRorie E. Biological therapy for rheumatoid arthritis: is personalised medicine possible? *Eur J Hosp Pharm.* (2014) 21:229–37. doi: 10.1136/ejhpharm-2013-000386
6. Vastesaeger N, Kutzbach AG, Amital H, Pavelka K, Lazaro MA, Moots RJ, et al. Prediction of remission and low disease activity in disease-modifying anti-rheumatic drug-refractory patients with rheumatoid arthritis treated with golimumab. *Rheumatology.* (2016) 55:1466–76. doi: 10.1093/rheumatology/kew179
7. Ganhão S, Bernardes M, Lucas R, Fonseca J, Rosa-Gonçalves D, Madeira N, et al. Remission and low disease activity matrix tools: results in real-world rheumatoid arthritis patients under anti-tnfa therapy. *Acta Reumatol Portuguesa.* (2019) 45:245–52.
8. Smallwood MJ, Nissim A, Knight AR, Whiteman M, Haigh R, Winyard PG. Oxidative stress in autoimmune rheumatic diseases. *Free Radic Biol Med.* (2018) 125:3–14. doi: 10.1016/j.freeradbiomed.2018.05.086
9. Grayson PC, Kaplan MJ. At the bench: neutrophil extracellular traps (NETs) highlight novel aspects of innate immune system involvement in autoimmune diseases. *J Leukoc Biol.* (2016) 99:253–64. doi: 10.1189/jlb.5BT0615-247R
10. Pérez-Sánchez C, Ruiz-Limón P, Aguirre MA, Jiménez-Gómez Y, Arias-de la Rosa I, Ábalos-Aguilera MC, et al. Diagnostic potential of NETosis-derived products for disease activity, atherosclerosis and therapeutic effectiveness in rheumatoid arthritis patients. *J Autoimmun.* (2017) 82:31–40. doi: 10.1016/j.jaut.2017.04.007
11. Perez-Sanchez C, Cecchi I, Barbarroja N, Patino-Trives AM, Luque-Tevar M, Perez-Sanchez L, et al. Early restoration of immune and vascular phenotypes in systemic lupus erythematosus and rheumatoid arthritis patients after B cell depletion. *J Cell Mol Med.* (2019) 23:6308–18. doi: 10.1111/jcmm.14517
12. Ruiz-Limón P, Ortega R, Arias de la Rosa I, Ábalos-Aguilera MDC, Pérez-Sánchez C, Jiménez-Gómez Y, et al. Tocilizumab improves the proatherothrombotic profile of rheumatoid arthritis patients modulating endothelial dysfunction, NETosis, and inflammation. *Transl Res.* (2017) 183:87–103. doi: 10.1016/j.trsl.2016.12.003
13. Sanchez-Pinto LN, Luo Y, Churpek MM. Big data and data science in critical care. *Chest.* (2018) 154:1239–48. doi: 10.1016/j.chest.2018.04.037
14. Aletaha D, Neogi T, Silman AJ, Funovits J, Felson DT, Bingham CO 3rd, et al. 2010 rheumatoid arthritis classification criteria: an American College of Rheumatology/European League Against Rheumatism collaborative initiative. *Arthritis Rheum.* (2010) 62:2569–81. doi: 10.1002/art.27584
15. Hosmer Jr DW, Lemeshow S, Sturdivant RX. *Applied Logistic Regression.* New Jersey, NJ: John Wiley & Sons (2013).
16. Pedregosa F, Varoquaux G, Gramfort A, Michel V, Thirion B, Grisel O, et al. Scikit-learn: machine learning in python. *J Mach Learn Res.* (2011) 12:2825–30.
17. Smolen JS, Aletaha D, Barton A, Burmester GR, Emery P, Firestein GS, et al. Rheumatoid arthritis. *Nat Rev Dis Primers.* (2018) 4:18001. doi: 10.1038/nrdp.2018.1
18. Conigliaro P, Triggianese P, De Martino E, Fonti GL, Chimenti MS, Sunzini F, et al. Challenges in the treatment of rheumatoid arthritis. *Autoimmun Rev.* (2019) 18:706–13. doi: 10.1016/j.autrev.2019.05.007
19. Castro-Villegas C, Pérez-Sánchez C, Escudero A, Filipescu I, Verdu M, Ruiz-Limón P, et al. Circulating miRNAs as potential biomarkers of therapy effectiveness in rheumatoid arthritis patients treated with anti-TNFalpha. *Arthritis Res Ther.* (2015) 17:49. doi: 10.1186/s13075-015-0555-z
20. Lin Y-J, Anzaghe M, Schülke S. Update on the pathomechanism, diagnosis, and treatment options for rheumatoid arthritis. *Cells.* (2020) 9:880. doi: 10.3390/cells9040880
21. Vignesh P, Rawat A, Sharma M, Singh S. Complement in autoimmune diseases. *Clin Chim Acta.* (2017) 465:123–30. doi: 10.1016/j.cca.2016.12.017
22. Kapoor SR, Filer A, Fitzpatrick MA, Fisher BA, Taylor PC, Buckley CD, et al. Metabolic profiling predicts response to anti-tumor necrosis factor α therapy in patients with rheumatoid arthritis. *Arthritis Rheum.* (2013) 65:1448–56. doi: 10.1002/art.37921
23. Cacciapaglia F, Anelli MG, Rinaldi A, Serafino L, Covelli M, Scioscia C, et al. Lipid profile of rheumatoid arthritis patients treated with anti-tumor necrosis factor-alpha drugs changes according to disease activity and predicts clinical response. *Drug Dev Res.* (2014) 75:S77–80. doi: 10.1002/ddr.21203
24. Jeffery LE, Raza K, Hewison M. Vitamin D in rheumatoid arthritis—towards clinical application. *Nat Rev Rheumatol.* (2016) 12:201–10. doi: 10.1038/nrrheum.2015.140

25. Winter RW, Collins E, Cao B, Carrellas M, Crowell AM, Korzenik JR. Higher 25-hydroxyvitamin D levels are associated with greater odds of remission with anti-tumour necrosis factor-α medications among patients with inflammatory bowel diseases. *Aliment Pharmacol Ther.* (2017) 45:653–9. doi: 10.1111/apt.13936
26. Pandit A, Radstake TR. Machine learning in rheumatology approaches the clinic. *Nat Rev Rheumatol.* (2020) 16:69–70. doi: 10.1038/s41584-019-0361-0
27. Guan Y, Zhang H, Quang D, Wang Z, Parker SC, Pappas DA, et al. Machine learning to predict anti–tumor necrosis factor drug responses of rheumatoid arthritis patients by integrating clinical and genetic markers. *Arthritis Rheumatol.* (2019) 71:1987–96. doi: 10.1002/art.41056
28. Tao W, Concepcion AN, Vianen M, Marijnissen AC, Lafeber FP, Radstake TR, et al. Multi-omics and machine learning accurately predicts clinical response to adalimumab and etanercept therapy in patients with rheumatoid arthritis. *Arthritis Rheumatol.* (2020). doi: 10.1002/art.41516. [Epub ahead of print].

17

Identification of a Novel Serum Proteomic Signature for Primary Sjögren's Syndrome

Guillaume Padern [1], Claire Duflos [2], Rosanna Ferreira [1], Said Assou [1], Philippe Guilpain [1,3], Alexandre Thibault Jacques Maria [1,3], Radjiv Goulabchand [4], Pascale Galea [5], Maja Jurtela [2], Christian Jorgensen [1] and Yves-Marie Pers [1]*

[1] IRMB, University of Montpellier, INSERM, CHU Montpellier, Montpellier, France, [2] Clinical Research and Epidemiology Unit, CHU Montpellier, Montpellier University, Montpellier, France, [3] Internal Medicine and Multi-Organic Diseases Department, Hôpital Saint Éloi, CHU Montpellier, Montpellier, France, [4] Internal Medicine Department, Caremeau University Hospital, Nîmes, France, [5] BioRad Laboratory, Research and Development Department, Montpellier, France

***Correspondence:**
Yves-Marie Pers
ym-pers@chu-montpellier.fr

Context: Primary Sjögren's syndrome (pSS) is a complex heterogeneous autoimmune disease (AID) which can mimic rheumatoid arthritis (RA) or systemic lupus erythematosus (SLE). Our exploratory study investigated serum biomarkers that may discriminate pSS from RA and SLE.

Methods: Serum concentrations of 63 biomarkers involved in immune cell trafficking, inflammatory response, cellular movement, and cell-to-cell signaling were measured in AID patients, included prospectively into the study at the Montpellier University Hospital. A multivariate analysis by multiple logistic regression was performed, and discriminative power assessed using logistic regression adjusted on significant demographic factors.

Results: Among the 95 patients enrolled, 42 suffered from pSS, 28 from RA, and 25 from SLE. Statistical analysis showed that concentrations of BDNF (OR = 0.493 with 95% CI [0.273–0.891]; p = 0.0193) and I-TAC/CXCL11 (OR = 1.344 with 95% CI [1.027–1.76]; p = 0.0314) can significantly discriminate pSS from RA. Similarly, greater concentrations of sCD163 (OR = 0.803 with 95% CI [0.649–0.994]; p = 0.0436), Fractalkine/CX3CL1 (OR = 0.534 with 95% CI [0.287–0. 991]; p = 0.0466), MCP-1/CCL2 (OR = 0.839 with 95% CI [0.732–0.962]; p = 0.0121), and TNFa (OR = 0.479 with 95% CI [0.247–0.928]; p = 0.0292) were associated with SLE diagnosis compared to pSS. In addition, the combination of low concentrations of BDNF and Fractalkine/CX3CL1 was highly specific for pSS (specificity 96.2%; positive predictive value 80%) compared to RA and SLE, as well as the combination of high concentrations of I-TAC/CXCL11 and low concentrations of sCD163 (specificity 98.1%; positive predictive value 75%).

Conclusion: Our study highlights biomarkers potentially involved in pSS, RA, and SLE pathophysiology that could be useful for developing a pSS-specific diagnostic tool.

Keywords: primary Sjögren syndrome, systemic lupus erythematosus, rheumatoid arthritis, biomarkers, proteomics

INTRODUCTION

Primary Sjögren's syndrome (pSS) is a complex heterogeneous autoimmune disease (AID) characterized by salivary and/or ocular dryness (sicca syndrome) related to lymphoid infiltration of exocrine glands. pSS is distinguished from secondary Sjögren's syndrome (sSS), which often coexists with systemic lupus erythematosus (SLE) and rheumatoid arthritis (RA) (1). While pSS, RA, and SLE have distinct clinical and pathophysiological features (2–4), patients may initially present with sicca symptoms, and over the course of the disease, the specific underlying condition will then manifest (5, 6). Accurate diagnosis is often challenging in patients with overlapping disease entities. In addition, the lack of specificity of lymphocytic sialadenitis and anti-SSa/b antibodies (7, 8) can complicate pSS diagnosis. Glandular epithelial cells play a central pathophysiological role in the development of autoimmune epithelitis, especially concerning antigen presentation of Ro/SSA- and La/SSB-protein complexes. Both the innate and the adaptive immune system are involved in the disease initiation and maintenance of the immune response. An "interferon signature" is observed in the salivary glands and T-cell derived cytokines (Th1/Th2 polarization, Th17, and regulatory T cells) play a central role in the pathophysiology of pSS. Moreover, through activation of various CD4+ T-helper cell subsets, B cells are involved in auto-antibody production and the formation of ectopic germinal center-like structures associated with malignant transformation to Non-Hodgkin lymphoma (9).

Identifying new biomarkers involved in these AIDs and developing pSS diagnosis or prognosis methods is urgently needed (10). Single biomarker approaches are overwhelmed by their limitations and the complexity of AID physiopathology. Proteomic techniques consider the multifactorial processes involved, and their more global approach may provide a more complete picture of the disease (11). Multiplex immunoassays are promising and have allowed for the identification of interesting biomarkers in AIDs (12–15). Such an approach may soon be available in clinical practice despite limitations such as interference by highly concentrated proteins and cross-reactivity (16).

Several recently launched research initiatives are attempting to identify clinical and immunological signatures in pSS patients (17). Furthermore, many potential biomarkers of pSS have emerged for several years (18–22), but none of them have been validated yet (23). In comparisons with RA and SLE, a better characterization of the pathophysiological mechanisms involved in pSS seems useful to better discriminate these AIDs. Therefore, we conducted a proteomic study investigating the concentration of several serum biomarkers in pSS, RA, and SLE patients.

PATIENTS AND METHODS

Study Population

This transversal study was conducted in the Rheumatology and Internal Medicine departments of Montpellier University Hospital. Patients were recruited consecutively and prospectively during 5 months between October 2016 and February 2017. They all met the international classification criteria for pSS (2), RA (3), or SLE (24). RA and SLE patients with sSS were excluded. Written informed consent was obtained from all patients, after which a blood sample was collected. The local ethics committee approved all procedures in accordance with international Helsinki regulations (Comité de Protection des Personnes Sud Méditerranée IV: DC-2015-2584).

Data Collection

On the day of inclusion, the following data were obtained from each patient's computerized medical record: age, gender, smoking status, date of diagnosis, articular and extra-articular autoimmune symptoms, disease severity, accessory salivary gland biopsy results (pSS only), autoantibody presence and specificity, cardiovascular risk factors (diabetes, hypertension, smoking, dyslipidemia, and chronic renal failure with a glomerular filtration rate below 30ml/min), bone erosions, C-reactive protein (CRP) levels, and ongoing specific AID therapy. At the time of inclusion, measurement of disease activity was performed using ESSDAI score (25) for pSS, DAS28-CRP score (26) for RA and SLEDAI score (27) for SLE. Low disease activity was defined by an ESSDAI score 5, a DAS28-CRP score 3.2, or a SLEDAI score ≤5. Moderate disease activity was defined by an ESSDAI score between 5 and 13 inclusive, a DAS28-CRP score 3.2 and 5.1, or a SLEDAI score between 6 and 10 inclusive. High disease activity was defined by an ESSDAI score 13, a DAS28-CRP score 5.1, or a SLEDAI score >10.

Determination of Biomarkers Serum Concentration

Blood samples were stored for 30 min at room temperature (RT) before being centrifuged (2,000g, 10min, RT), frozen at −80°C, and stored in the biological resource center of Montpellier University Hospital (Pr Sylvain LEHMANN, NFS 96-900 and ISO 9001 standards, BB-0033-00031) until their use in the biomarkers assay.

Serum protein concentrations of 63 biomarkers were measured using Bio-Plex Pro™ Human Chemokine 40-plex Panel (Bio-Rad) for CCL1, CCL2 (Monocyte Chemoattractant Protein 1 or MCP-1), CCL3, CXCL5, CCL7, CCL8, CCL11 (Eotaxin), CCL13, CCL15, CCL17 (Thymus- and Activation-Regulated Chemokine or TARC), CCL19, CCL20, CCL21, CCL22, CCL23, CCL24, CCL25 (Eotaxin-2), CCL26 (Eotaxin-3), CCL27, CXCL1, CXCL2, CXCL6, CXCL9, CXCL10, CXCL11 (Inducible T-cell Alpha Chemoattractant or I-TAC), CXCL12, CXCL13, CXCL16, CX3CL1, Granulocyte-macrophage colony-stimulating factor (GM-CSF), IL1-beta, IL-2, IL-4, IL-6, IL-8, IL-10, IL-16, Macrophage migration Inhibitory Factor (MIF), Tumor Necrosis Factor Alpha (TNFa), and Interferon gamma (IFNg). Quality control was validated for 34 biomarkers, and data for the six non-validated biomarkers were rejected (CCL-26, IL1-beta, IL-2, IL-6, IL-10, and IFNg). The Bio-Plex Pro™ Human Inflammation Panel 1, 37-Plex (Bio-Rad) was validated for the dosage of A Proliferation-Inducing Ligand (APRIL), B

Cell Activating Factor (BAFF), sCD30, sCD163, Chitinase 3-like 1, soluble IL-6 Receptor alpha (sIL-6Ra), soluble IL-6 Receptor beta (sIL-6Rb or gp130), Matrix Metalloproteinase-2 (MMP-2), Matrix Metalloproteinase-3 (MMP-3), Osteocalcin, Osteopontin (SPP1), Pentraxin-3, soluble TNF Receptor 1 (sTNF-R1), soluble TNF Receptor 2 (sTNF-R2), and TNF-related Weak inducer of apoptosis (TWEAK). Enzyme-linked immunosorbent assay (ELISA) kits were used for the remaining biomarkers: galectin binding protein 3 (LGalS3P) form Abnova, Fatty Acid-Binding Protein 4 (FABP4) from Biovendor, Hydroxyproline (HDP) from Cusabio, pre-Haptoglobin 2 (preHp2), from Bio-Rad (28), Oxidized low-density lipoprotein (OxLDL) from Mercodia, Secreted Phosphoprotein 1 (SPP1), Thrombospondin 2 (TPS2), adiponectin, hyaluronic acid (HA), Cathepsin S (CTSS), Brain Derived Neurotrophic Factor (BDNF), Secreted Protein Acidic Rich Cysteine (SPARC), haptoglobin, sCD14, and Mannose Binding Lectin 2 (MBL2) from R&D Systems. The osteopontin assay (SPP1) was performed using two different kits: an ELISA kit (R&D systems) whose result is reported under "SPP1", and the Bio-Plex kit Pro™ Human Inflammation Panel 1, 37-Plex (BioRad) whose result is reported under "osteopontin" (**Table S1, Supplemental Data**). Reproducibility and sensitivity of all ELISA kits were first validated before performing serum biomarker assays with patient samples. Biomarker assays were performed in duplicate for each sample according to the recommendations of manufacturers.

The top canonical pathways and the gene ontology analysis of the 63 biomarkers were functionally categorized using the ingenuity pathway analysis (IPA) software (QIAGEN Inc., https://www.qiagenbioinformatics.com/products/ingenuitypathway-analysis) (29). A large portion of this list is involved in hematological system development and function, immune cell trafficking, inflammatory response, cellular movement, and cell-to-cell signaling (**Figure 1**).

Statistical Analysis

A simple descriptive analysis was performed on the entire study population and then by group. Groups were initially compared using univariate tests. Age and sex were considered clinically pertinent confounding factors and were included in our principal analysis if they were statistically significant in the univariate analysis.

The association between biomarkers and the risk of presenting with pSS rather than RA was assessed using separate logistic regressions for each biomarker. When the log-linearity hypothesis was met, to provide readable odds ratios (OR), biomarkers were specified in the model using the most convenient unit of concentration, ranging from 10 to 10,000 original units, depending on the biomarker. When the log-linearity hypothesis was not met, biomarkers were specified in the model as categorical variables. Thresholds were the quantiles determining six balanced groups. Finally, classes with comparable OR were grouped together.

The association between biomarkers and the risk of presenting with pSS rather than SLE was assessed using the same method. In addition, since the SLE patients were clinically and statistically younger than pSS patients, the logistic regressions were adjusted on age.

Samples were removed from the analysis if the concentration of a biomarker varied by more than 20% between technical duplicates (coefficient of variation > 20%) or if the concentration was outside the test detection range (**Table S2, Supplemental Data**). All statistical tests were two-tailed with a Type I error of 0.05. Analyses were performed using SAS® Version 7.12 HF4 software.

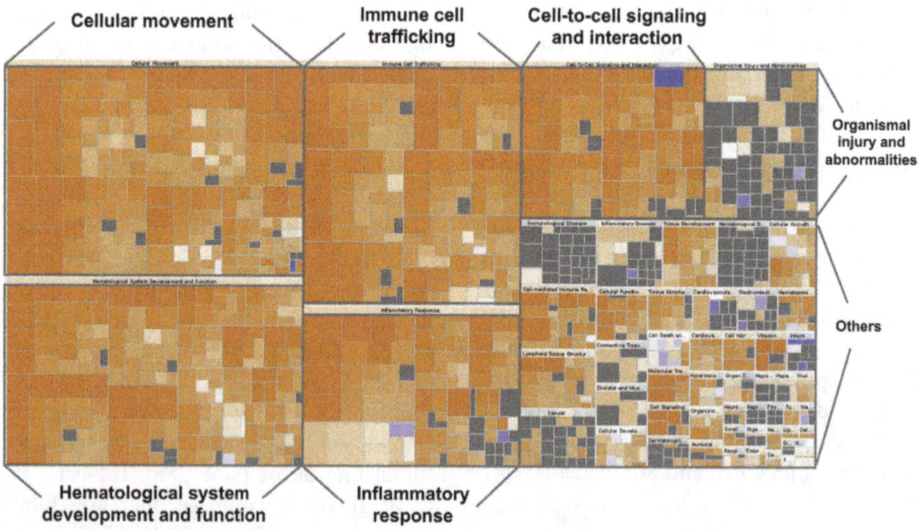

FIGURE 1 | Heatmap representing the classification of diseases and functions by ingenuity pathway analysis (IPA). The visualization is a hierarchical heat map of functional categories generated by IPA software in which the major boxes represent a family (or category) of related functions. Within each box, each individual rectangle is a sub-function linked to the biological function of a group of proteins. The size of a rectangle is correlated with increasing overlap significance among the proteins members of the related function and the query proteins. The color scheme shown is based on z-scores, with activation in orange, inhibition in blue and undetermined functions in gray. Darker shades indicate higher absolute z-score heat map. For instance, most 'Inflammatory response', 'Cellular movement', 'Immune cell trafficking', 'Cell-to-cell signaling and interaction', 'Hematological system development and function' proteins were over-represented.

RESULTS

Study Population

Ninety-five patients were prospectively enrolled in the study between October 2016 and February 2017: 42 pSS patients, 28 RA patients, and 25 SLE patients. Population characteristics are summarized in **Table 1**, and biological diagnostic criteria in **Supplemental Table S3**. The median age of pSS patients (62.5 years) did not differ from those in the RA group (60.5 years), while both pSS and RA patients were significantly older than those in the SLE group (40 years, Q25: 31.5 – Q75: 50.5; p<0.001). Mean disease duration was significantly shorter in pSS patients (9.2 ± 8.6 years) compared to RA patients (15.8 ± 9.3 years; p<0.01) but did not differ in comparison with the SLE patients (12.1 ± 9.7 years; p = 0.53). Low disease activity was common in all three groups: 76.2% in pSS patients, 58.3% in RA patients, and 76% in SLE patients. As expected, more patients were treated by biologic drugs in the RA group compared to the pSS and SLE groups (p<0.001). Corticosteroid treatment did not differ among groups (p = 0.62). SLE patients were more often treated by synthetic Drug Modifying Anti-Rheumatic Diseases (DMARDs) than the others (p = 0.04). Likewise, SLE patients were treated by mycophenolate mofetil (MMF) or azathioprine (AZA) more than pSS and RA patients (for MMF p<0.001; for AZA p = 0.02). In contrast, the RA group included significantly more patients treated with methotrexate (p = 0.01) and fewer patients treated with hydroxychloroquine (p = 0.02) compared to the pSS and SLE groups.

Biomarkers Associated With pSS *Versus* RA

Identification of markers distinguishing pSS versus RA or SLE was determined by logistic regression analysis. The analysis was age-adjusted for the comparison with SLE patient samples. Results are presented as a function of the increase in each biomarker concentration. All results are available in **Table 2**.

The serum concentration of four of the 63 tested biomarkers could statistically discriminate pSS patients from RA patients. A 10,000 pg/ml greater concentration of BDNF was significantly associated with a decreased likelihood of pSS diagnosis compared to RA (OR = 0.493 and 95% CI [0.273–0.891]; p = 0.0193). While greater concentrations of haptoglobin (10,000 ng/ml) and I-TAC/CXCL11 (10 pg/ml) were significantly associated

TABLE 1 | Characteristics of patients included in the study.

Characteristics	pSS	RA	SLE	p
Patients (n)	42	28	25	NA
Female gender (%)	40 (95.2%)	24 (85.7%)	24 (96%)	0.35
Median age (year; IQR)	62.5 (54.7;71.2)	60.5 (53; 73.5)	40 (31.5; 50.5)	< 0.01
Smoking patients (%)	4 (8.3%)	3 (10.3%)	5 (18.5%)	0.45
Mean BMI (kg/m2 ± SD)	27.6 ± 7.5	26.2 ± 5.7	25.4 ± 5.8	0.52
Cardiovascular risk factor				
No cardiovascular risk factor	22 (52.4%)	9 (32.1%)	11 (44%)	0.25
1 or 2 cardiovascular risk factors	17 (40.5%)	14 (50%)	12 (48%)	0.70
3 or 4 cardiovascular risk factors	3 (7.1%)	5 (17.9%)	2 (8%)	0.39
SSa and/or SSb positivity (%)	16 (38.1%)	0 (0%)	8 (32%)	< 0.01
Mean disease duration (year ± SD)	9.2 ± 8.6	15.8 ± 9.3	12.1 ± 9.7	0.01
Disease status				
Low disease activity	32 (76.2%)	14 (58.3%)	19 (76%)	0.25
Moderate disease activity	6 (14.3%)	8 (33.3%)	6 (24%)	0.26
High disease activity	4 (9.5%)	2 (8.3%)	0	0.36
Medications				
No treatment (%)	9 (27.3%)	2 (7.7%)	8 (32%)	0.08
Steroids (%)	8 (24.2%)	7 (26.9%)	4 (16%)	0.62
All synthetic DMARDs (%)	21 (63.6%)	15 (57.7%)	22 (88%)	0.04
Methotrexate (%)	6 (18.2%)	12 (46.2%)	3 (12%)	0.01
Sulfasalazine (%)	3 (9.1%)	1 (3.8%)	0	0.38
Leflunomide (%)	2 (6.1%)	1 (3.8%)	0	0.77
Hydroxychloroquine (%)	9 (27.3%)	1 (3.8%)	9 (36%)	0.02
Ciclosporin (%)	1 (3%)	0	0	> 0.99
Mycophenolate (%)	0	0	6 (24%)	0.01
Azathioprine (%)	0	0	3 (12%)	0.02
Tacrolimus (%)	0	0	1 (4%)	0.30
All biologic DMARDs (%)	3 (9.1%)	19 (73.1%)	1 (4%)	< 0.01
Rituximab (%)	3 (9.1%)	3 (11.5%)	1 (4%)	0.70
TNF inhibitors (%)	0	6 (23.1%)	0	0.01
Tocilizumab (%)	0	7 (27%)	0	0.01
Abatacept (%)	0	3 (11.5%)	0	0.05

Representation of the three autoimmune diseases groups: pSS, RA, and SLE. Comparisons between groups were done using either a Kruskall-Wallis test or a Chi-2 test (or a Fisher's exact test when conditions necessary for Chi-2 were not met). Results from these tests are in column "p".

pSS, primary Sjogren syndrome; RA, rheumatoid arthritis; SLE, systemic lupus erythematosus; IQR, interquartile range (Q1–Q3); DMARDs, Disease Modifying Anti-Rheumatic Drugs; NA, Not Applicable.

TABLE 2 | Likelihood of primary Sjogren syndrome (pSS) diagnosis versus rheumatoid arthritis (RA) or Systemic Lupus Erythematosus (SLE) as a function of an increase in biomarker concentration.

Biomarker name / Value of unit increase in serum concentration		pSS probability vs RA		pSS probability vs SLE	
		OR [95% CI]	p	OR [95% CI]	p
SPP1 / +10 ng/ml		1.067 [0.876–1.299]	0.5193	1.035 [0.787–1.36]	0.8076
HDP / +100 ng/ml		1.057 [0.974–1.147]	0.1835	0.9 [0.817–0.991]	0.0318
TPS2 / +10 ng/ml		1.059 [0.716–1.567]	0.7737	0.697 [0.433–1.122]	0.1371
preHp2 / +100 ng/ml		1.019 [0.877–1.183]	0.8066	0.859 [0.686–1.074]	0.1827
LGalS3P/ +1,000 ng/ml		1.116 [0.982–1.268]	0.092	1.029 [0.886–1.196]	0.7042
Adiponectin / +1,000 ng/ml		0.954 [0.87–1.047]	0.3191	0.958 [0.845–1.086]	0.5009
oxLDL/ +10,000 mU/ml		1.034 [0.822–1.301]	0.7737	1.093 [0.815–1.465]	0.5538
Hyaluronic Acid / +10 ng/ml		0.936 [0.863–1.015]	0.1109	1.137 [0.948–1.363]	0.1662
RA: FABP4 / +10 ng/ml	SLE: FABP4 Tertile 1	1.033 [0.9–1.186]	0.6408	0.32 [0.063–1.631]	0.1704
	SLE: FABP4 Tertile 2			0.459 [0.086–2.459]	0.3632
RA: CTSS / +1000pg/ml	SLE: CTSS Classes 0, 1, 2	0.939 [0.771–1.143]	0.5289	3.123 [0.563–17.314]	0.1925
	SLE: CTSS Classes 3, 4			14.064 [1.56–126.806]	0.0185
BDNF / +10,000pg/ml		0.493 [0.273–0.891]	0.0193	0.817 [0.406–1.647]	0.5728
RA: SPARC / +100ng/ml	SLE: SPARC Classes 0, 1, 2	1.065 [0.877–1.293]	0.5263	0.311 [0.031–3.173]	0.3246
	SLE: SPARC Class 3	1.794 [0.073–44.11]	0.7205		
	SLE: SPARC Class 4	0.035 [0.002–0.66]	0.0253		
Haptoglobin / +10,000 ng/ml		1.015 [1.002–1.029]	0.0262	1.004 [0.991–1.018]	0.5438
RA: sCD14 Tertile 1	SLE: sCD14+10,000 pg/ml	0.825 [0.245–2.783]	0.757	0.99 [0.975–1.005]	0.1907
RA: sCD14 Tertile 2		0.779 [0.243–2.501]	0.675		
MBL2 / +100 ng/ml		1.032 [0.976–1.09]	0.2679	1.055 [0.959–1.161]	0.2691
APRIL/TNFSF13 / +10,000 pg/ml		1.059 [0.952–1.177]	0.2921	0.995 [0.931–1.063]	0.8788
BAFF/TNFSF13B / +10,000 pg/ml		0.745 [0.53–1.047]	0.0898	0.704 [0.408–1.215]	0.2076
sCD30/TNFRSF8 / +100 pg/ml		1.045 [0.841–1.3]	0.6903	0.806 [0.631–1.03]	0.0848
sCD163 / +10,000 pg/ml		1.138 [0.96–1.35]	0.1364	0.803 [0.649–0.994]	0.0436
Chitinase 3 like / +1,000 pg/ml		0.972 [0.922–1.025]	0.3004	0.949 [0.881–1.023]	0.1699
gp130/sIL-6Rb / +1,000 pg/ml		1.031 [0.98–1.084]	0.2383	1.007 [0.948–1.069]	0.8271
sIL-6Ra / +1,000 pg/ml		0.901 [0.803–1.012]	0.0776	0.856 [0.698–1.049]	0.1329
MMP-2 / +1,000 pg/ml		1.025 [0.975–1.077]	0.3314	1.009 [0.947–1.075]	0.7793
MMP-3 / +1,000 pg/ml		1.007 [0.898–1.13]	0.9025	1.043 [0.899–1.209]	0.579
Osteocalcin / +100 pg/ml		0.96 [0.903–1.02]	0.1886	0.981 [0.919–1.047]	0.5574
Osteopontin / +1000 pg/ml		0.994 [0.957–1.033]	0.7697	1.001 [0.962–1.04]	0.9794
Pentraxin-3 / +10 pg/ml		1.003 [0.972–1.035]	0.8548	0.981 [0.945–1.018]	0.3007
sTNFR1 / +1,000 pg/ml		1.784 [0.882–3.607]	0.1072	0.929 [0.617–1.4]	0.7255
sTNFR2 / +1,000 pg/ml		1.317 [0.969–1.79]	0.0785	0.79 [0.588–1.06]	0.1162
TWEAK/TNSF12 / +10 pg/ml		1.03 [0.955–1.112]	0.4429	0.983 [0.883–1.095]	0.7539
6Ckine/CCL21 / +1,000 pg/ml		1.104 [0.703–1.733]	0.6669	0.63 [0.366–1.086]	0.0964
BCA-1/CXCL13 / +10 pg/ml		0.984 [0.921–1.051]	0.6347	0.931 [0.802–1.081]	0.3501
CTACK/CCL27 / +100 pg/ml		1.001 [0.931–1.076]	0.9865	0.534 [0.287–0.991]	0.5596
ENA-78/CXCL5 / +100 pg/ml		1.052 [0.984–1.126]	0.1393	1.029 [0.977–1.083]	0.2799
Eotaxin/CCL11 / +10 pg/ml		0.964 [0.858–1.084]	0.5408	0.895 [0.767–1.043]	0.1556
Eotaxin-2/CCL24 / +100 pg/ml		1.036 [0.971–1.105]	0.2819	0.889 [0.811–0.974]	0.0117

(Continued)

TABLE 2 | Continued

Biomarker name / Value of unit increase in serum concentration		pSS probability vs RA		pSS probability vs SLE	
		OR [95% CI]	p	OR [95% CI]	p
RA: Fractalkine/CX3CL1 Tertile 1	SLE: Fractalkine/CX3CL1 / +100 pg/ml	0.467 [0.138–1.583]	0.2213		0.0466
RA: Fractalkine/CX3CL1 Tertile 2		0.52 [0.148–1.825]	0.3075		
GCP-2/CXCL6 / +10 pg/ml		1.03 [0.881–1.204]	0.7122	0.971 [0.816–1.156]	0.743
GM-CSF / +10 pg/ml		1.065 [0.909–1.249]	0.4347	0.898 [0.753–1.071]	0.2329
RA: Gro-a/CXCL1 / +10 pg/ml	SLE: Gro-a/CXCL1 Tertile 1	1.018 [0.977–1.06]	0.3973	3.931 [0.901–17.155]	0.0686
	SLE: Gro-a/CXCL1 Tertile 2	1.663 [0.292–9.463]			0.5662
Gro-b/CXCL2 / +100 pg/ml		1.057 [0.938–1.192]	0.3636	0.965 [0.867–1.074]	0.5118
I-309/CCL1 / +10 pg/ml		1.025 [0.786–1.338]	0.8544	0.962 [0.728–1.272]	0.787
IL-4 / +10 pg/ml		0.623 [0.317–1.226]	0.1709	0.632 [0.293–1.363]	0.2422
IL-8 / +10 pg/ml		0.966 [0.883–1.056]	0.4444	0.904 [0.602–1.357]	0.6257
IL-16 / +100 pg/ml		1.027 [0.847–1.245]	0.7891	0.87 [0.645–1.175]	0.3641
IP-10/CXCL10 / +100 pg/ml		0.973 [0.781–1.213]	0.8105	0.808 [0.596–1.095]	0.1689
I-TAC/CXCL11 / +10 pg/ml		1.344 [1.027–1.76]	0.0314	0.932 [0.844–1.028]	0.1572
RA: MCP-1/CCL2 Tertile 1	SLE: MCP-1/CCL2 / +10 pg/ml	1.925 [0.568–6.519]	0.2927	0.839 [0.732–0.962]	0.0121
RA: MCP-1/CCL2 Tertile 2		2.2 [0.681–7.102]	0.1873		
MCP-2/CCL8 / +10 pg/ml		1.011 [0.883–1.157]	0.8734	0.92 [0.794–1.067]	0.2699
MCP-3/CCL7 / +10 pg/ml		0.935 [0.809–1.08]	0.3612	0.898 [0.738–1.094]	0.2856
MCP-4/CCL13 / +100 pg/ml		1.122 [0.579–2.175]	0.7337	0.712 [0.277–1.832]	0.4808
MDC/CCL22 / +100 pg/ml		1.013 [0.914–1.122]	0.8056	0.869 [0.749–1.008]	0.0633
MIF / +1000 pg/ml		0.942 [0.87–1.02]	0.141	1.329 [0.872–2.026]	0.1853
MIG/CXCL9 / +100 pg/ml		1.077 [0.962–1.206]	0.1965	0.956 [0.85–1.075]	0.4536
MIP-1a/CCL3 / +10 pg/ml		0.93 [0.778–1.111]	0.4215	0.601 [0.323–1.12]	0.1088
MIP-1d/CCL15 / +1,000 pg/ml		1.05 [0.985–1.119]	0.1313	0.963 [0.904–1.026]	0.24
MIP-3a/CCL20 / +10 pg/ml		0.977 [0.622–1.533]	0.9179	0.664 [0.355–1.244]	0.2013
RA: MIP-3b/CCL19 Classe 0	SLE: MIP-3b/CCL19 / +100 pg/ml	2.571 [0.361–18.325]	0.3459	0.928 [0.753–1.144]	0.4858
RA: MIP-3b/CCL19 Classes 1, 2, 3		0.429 [0.106–1.736]	0.2352		
RA: MIP-3b/CCL19 Classe 4		3.142 [0.45–21.952]	0.2483		
MPIF-1/CCL23 / +100 pg/ml		1.051 [0.82–1.348]	0.6944	0.887 [0.638–1.234]	0.4762
SCYB16/CXCL16 / +100 pg/ml		1.066 [0.848–1.341]	0.5843	0.934 [0.697–1.252]	0.6477
SDF-1a+b/CXCL12 / +1,000 pg/ml		0.954 [0.562–1.621]	0.8631	0.651 [0.345–1.23]	0.1864
RA: TARC/CCL17 Tertile 1	SLE: TARC/CCL17 / +100 pg/ml	0.706 [0.2–2.487]	0.5878	0.913 [0.678–1.23]	0.5507
RA: TARC/CCL17 Tertile 2		0.227 [0.065–0.793]	0.0202		
TECK/CCL25 / +100 pg/ml		1.002 [0.755–1.331]	0.9866	0.824 [0.566–1.2]	0.3125
TNFa / +10 pg/ml		0.798 [0.506–1.258]	0.3316	0.479 [0.247–0.928]	0.0292

Odds Ratios (OR), and their 95% confidence intervals (CI), for the likelihood of pSS diagnosis versus RA or SLE, in separate logistic regressions for each biomarker, are represented. ORs comparing pSS versus SLE were age-adjusted. For biomarkers specified as categorical variables in the models, the reference level was the highest class.

with moderate increases in the likelihood of pSS diagnosis over RA (haptoglobin: OR = 1.015 and 95% CI [1.002–1,029]; p = 0.0262; I-TAC/CXCL11: OR = 1.344 and 95% CI [1.027–1.76]; p = 0.0314). TARC/CCL17 concentration in the second tertile, compared to the third tertile, was associated with a decreased likelihood of pSS diagnosis compared to RA (OR = 0.227 and 95% CI [0.065–0.793]; p = 0.0202). However, a lower concentration of this biomarker (first tertile) did not significantly alter the likelihood of pSS diagnosis, suggesting a potentially spurious association.

Biomarkers Associated With pSS *Versus* SLE

Serum concentrations of eight biomarkers could statistically discriminate samples from pSS versus SLE patients (**Table 2**). A 100 ng/ml greater concentration of HDP was associated with a moderate decrease in the likelihood of pSS compared to SLE (OR = 0.9 and 95% CI [0.817–0.991]; p = 0.0318). CTSS concentration in classes 3 and 4, rather than in class 5, was strongly associated with an increased likelihood of pSS compared to SLE (OR = 14.064 and 95% CI [1.56–126.806]; p = 0.0185). However, lower concentrations of this marker (in classes 0, 1, or 2) could not significantly distinguish pSS from SLE. Similarly, SPARC concentration in class 4, rather than class 5, was associated with an increased likelihood of pSS compared to SLE (OR = 0.035 and 95% CI [0.002–0.66]; p = 0.0253), while at lower concentrations (in classes 0, 1, 2, or 3) there were no significant differences between the two AIDs. A 10,000 pg/ml greater concentration of sCD163 was significantly associated with a moderate decrease in the likelihood of pSS compared to SLE diagnosis (OR = 0.803 and 95% CI [0.649–0.994]; p = 0.0436). A 100 pg/ml greater concentration of Eotaxin-2/CCL24 was associated with a moderate decrease in the likelihood of pSS compared to SLE (OR = 0.889 and 95% CI [0.811–0.974]; p = 0.0117). A 100 pg/ml greater concentration of Fractalkine/CX3CL1 almost halved the likelihood of pSS compared to SLE (OR = 0.534 and 95% CI [0.287–0.991]; p = 0.0466). Lastly, a 10 pg/ml greater concentration of MCP-1/CCL2 was associated with a moderate decrease in the likelihood of pSS compared to SLE (OR = 0.839 and 95% CI [0.732–0.962]; p = 0.0121), while a 10 pg/ml greater concentration of TNFa was strongly associated with a decreased likelihood of pSS compared to SLE diagnosis (OR = 0.479 and 95% CI [0.247–0.928]; p = 0.0292).

Specific Proteomic Signature in pSS

None of the studied biomarkers could simultaneously discriminate pSS from RA and SLE. We therefore determined the positive predictive value (PPV), sensitivity, and specificity of different combinations of BDNF, I-TAC/CXCL11, sCD163 and Fractalkine/CX3CL1 concentrations. These biomarkers were chosen because they were those most strongly associated with distinguishing pSS from the other AIDs (OR < 0.8 or OR > 1.2, and p<0.05), thus constituting a specific proteomic signature of pSS compared to RA and SLE (**Table 3**). Concentrations of these biomarkers were considered low or high based on their median concentration in the whole cohort. We observed that a combination of low BDNF and high Fractalkine concentrations was very specific for pSS (96.2%) with a PPV of 80% but weakly sensitive (19%). Conversely, a combination of high I-TAC concentration and low sCD163 concentration was strongly specific for pSS (98.1%), with a PPV of 75%, but with very low sensitivity (7.1%). Other biomarkers associations had significantly lower statistical performance (**Table 3**).

In addition, we investigated the association between expression of the four main biomarkers (BDNF, I-TAC/CXCL11, sCD163 and Fractalkine/CX3CL1) and disease activity (**Table S4, Supplemental Data**). A significant negative correlation was observed between pSS activity according to the ESSDAI score and serum sCD163 concentrations (r = −0.33859; p = 0.0283). In the SLE group, SLEDAI disease activity was significantly and positively correlated with serum BDNF concentrations (r = 0.49541; p = 0.0138). For the other biomarkers, there was no statistically significant correlation between their serum concentration and pSS, RA or SLE disease activity.

Regulatory Roles of the Identified Biomarkers and Pathways Involved

Using IPA, we identified the top canonical pathways among the list of the 63 biomarkers that were enriched including BDNF, I-TAC/CXCL11, sCD163, and Fractalkine/CX3CL1. **Figure 2** displays the top networks found to be enriched in this list. Each network shows interactions *via* major signaling pathway proteins, including Extracellular signal-Regulated Kinases 1/2 (ERK1/2), Nuclear Factor-kappa B (NF-kB), IL-17, and interferon. Functions associated with the top networks

TABLE 3 | Statistical performance of biomarker combinations to discriminate primary Sjögren's syndrome (pSS) from rheumatoid arthritis (RA) and systemic lupus erythematosus (SLE).

	Low BDNF	HighI-TAC	Low sCD163	Low Fractalkine	pSS patients (n)	No-pSS patients (n)	PPV % (pSS)	Se % (pSS)	Spe % (pSS)
2 BMKs	X	X			2	3	40.0	4.8	94.3
	X		X		3	4	42.9	7.1	92.5
	X			X	8	2	80.0	19.0	96.2
		X	X		3	1	75.0	7.1	98.1
		X		X	1	3	25.0	2.4	94.3
			X	X	2	6	25.0	4.8	88.7
3 BMKs	X	X	X		4	2	66.7	9.5	96.2
	X	X		X	1	2	33.3	2.4	96.2
	X		X	X	4	8	33.3	9.5	84.9
		X	X	X	0	0	–	–	–
4 BMKs	X	X	X	X	0	1	0	0	98.1

Estimation of the positive predictive value (PPV), sensitivity (Se), and specificity (Spe) of different biomarker (BMKs) combinations to discriminate pSS (primary Sjogren Syndrome) from RA (Rheumatoid Arthritis) and SLE (Systemic Lupus Erythematosus). In contrast to other biomarkers, BDNF, I-TAC, sCD163 and Fractalkine serum concentrations were significantly associated with pSS diagnosis compared to RA or SLE (OR < 0.8 or > 1.2). Concentrations of these biomarkers were considered high or low relative to their median concentration in the whole cohort.

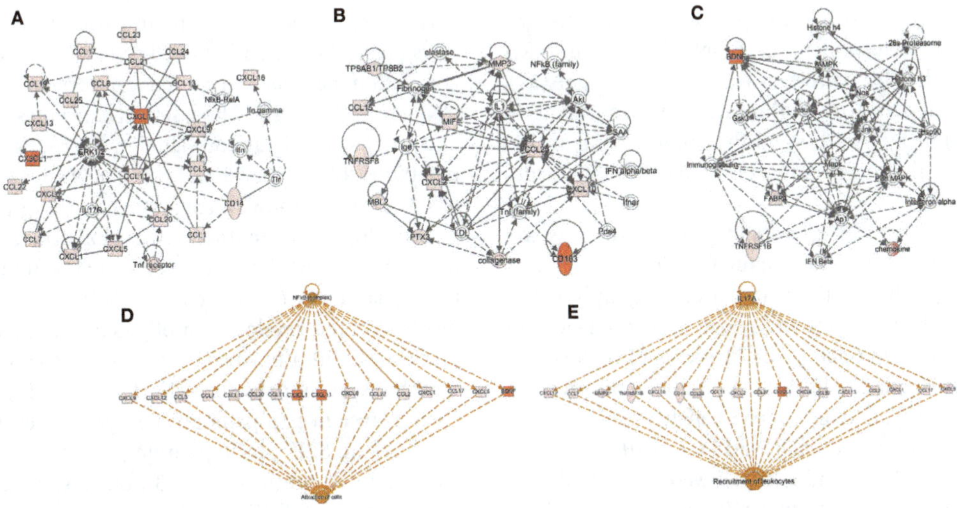

FIGURE 2 | Functional and upstream regulatory networks. The most significant networks included proteins related to: **(A)** Cell-to-cell signaling and interaction, and cellular movement, **(B)** immune cell trafficking and inflammatory response, **(C)** organismal functions, hematological disease, and metabolic disease, **(D, E)** top-scoring network of regulator effects activated in the list of 63 biomarkers. Protein interaction networks were constructed using the ingenuity pathway analysis (IPA) software. Nodes shaded in pink represent proteins present in the list of 63 biomarkers; red nodes are proteins that are CXCL11 (I-TAC), CX3CL1 (Fractalkine), Brain Derived Neurotrophic Factor (BDNF), and sCD163; and proteins that are not found in the list of 63 biomarkers are in white. Dotted lines indicate indirect molecular interactions between proteins and continuous lines between nodes indicate direct functional interactions between connected proteins. Orange lines lead to activation.

include cellular movement, cell interaction, and inflammatory response. The I-TAC/CXCL11-centered network displayed a functional interaction with several cytokines and forming a tightly connected network with ERK1/2 (**Figure 2A**). Fractalkine/CX3CL1 was also related to ERK1/2 and displayed direct interaction with this pathway. Moreover, the network (**Figure 2B**) shows interactions between sCD163 and the TNF family, suggesting an operative role of TNF signaling pathways. In addition, BDNF displayed a tightly connected network with functional interaction with immunoglobulins, histones, and 26s proteasomes (**Figure 2C**). Finally, the upstream regulator analysis in IPA identified NF-kB and IL17A as key regulators of I-TAC/CXCL11, Fractalkine/CX3CL1, BDNF, and multiple cytokines that are implicated in the attraction of cells and recruitment of leukocytes (**Figures 2D, E**).

DISCUSSION

Our study compared the serum concentration of 63 biomarkers in patients with an established diagnosis of pSS to patients with established RA or SLE without secondary SS. We observed that differences in the concentration of BDNF, haptoglobin, and I-TAC/CXCL11 may allow discrimination of pSS from RA patients. Similarly, differences in the concentration of HDP, sCD163, Eotaxin-2/CCL24, Fractalkine/CX3CL1, MCP-1/CCL2, and TNFa may discriminate pSS from SLE. In addition, we observed that combinations of low BDNF and high Fractalkine/CX3CL1 concentrations, as well as high I-TAC and low sCD163 concentrations, were associated with high PPV and specificity for pSS. These four biomarkers may constitute a new and potentially useful specific signature for distinguishing pSS compared to RA and SLE. Indeed, our approach of screening a large number of biomarkers was also intended to highlight new lines of research, which could improve knowledge of pSS physiopathology, may differentiate pSS patients from patients with SLE or RA, and may provide future therapeutic targets.

Pathway analysis in which BDNF, Fractalkine/CX3CL1, and I-TAC/CXCL11 are linked strongly implies a potential functional role of NF-kB and IL-17 signaling pathways (**Figure 2**). Our results are consistent with previous reports of NF-kB pathway involvement in pSS pathophysiology. Indeed, its expression is increased in human salivary glands cells from pSS patients compared to controls (30). Polymorphisms of NF-kB target or regulatory genes are also associated with increased susceptibility to pSS (31) and pSS-related lymphoma (32–34). In addition, activation of the NF-kB pathway in Peripheral Mononuclear Blood Cells (PMBCs) from pSS patients may lead to IL-17 production through Toll-Like Receptor 2 (TLR2) activation (35), and NF-kB activation by TLR9 signaling appears to be facilitated in B lymphocytes of pSS patients (36). Therefore, the NF-kB pathway might be crucial in pSS pathophysiology through its activation in innate or acquired immunity cells, or even in epithelial cells, leading to an inflammatory response and activation of other inflammatory pathways such as IL-17, which is also involved in pSS development and progression (37).

To the best of our knowledge, our study is the first to compare serum BDNF levels in patients with pSS to those in patients with

RA and SLE. Changes in BDNF concentration may depend on age or platelet levels (38). However, these two parameters were similar between the pSS and RA groups. Our study, therefore, suggests a different involvement of BDNF in pSS and RA physiopathology, either by its role in the nervous system (39), where BDNF is involved in proliferation and survival of nervous tissue (40) or by its action on the immune system (41) where BDNF affects the proliferation of T- and B-lymphocytes (42, 43).

I-TAC/CXCL11 is an IFNg-inducible chemokine, as are CXCL9 and CXCL10 (44), whose main function is to attract CXCR3-expressing cells (mainly activated T-lymphocytes, Natural Killer lymphocytes, and monocytes/macrophages) to the inflammatory site. Although CXCL11 seems to be involved in pSS salivary gland lesions (45–47), we did not find previous data regarding circulating CXCL11 in pSS patients. Furthermore, while serum concentrations of CXCL9 and CXCL10, two IFNg-induced chemokines able to bind CXCR3, were correlated with CXCL11 exclusively in the pSS group ($p<0.0001$), they could not discriminate pSS from RA or SLE (see **Table 2**). Therefore, it is possible that among the three ligands of CXCR3, only CXCL11 is differentially regulated in both RA and pSS, highlighting the role of IFNg in pSS.

sCD163 is derived from proteolytic cleavage of the extracellular portion of CD163 (48, 49), which is a membrane receptor found on anti-inflammatory M2 macrophages. Although sCD163 possesses anti-inflammatory activity (50), it is also considered a macrophage activation marker (51–54). Here, an increase in serum sCD163 concentration was significantly associated with a decreased likelihood of pSS compared to SLE. Corticosteroid could increase $CD163^+$ cell counts and impact sCD163 circulating levels, although this has not yet been demonstrated (55). Here, the number of patients receiving corticosteroid was comparable between groups. However, the action of synthetic DMARDs or biologic drugs on sCD163 concentrations remains to be studied (55). Furthermore, sCD163 concentration may be associated with cardiovascular disease risk (56, 57). However, we did not find differences between SLE and pSS groups concerning the number of cardiovascular comorbidities. Thus, from a pathophysiological perspective, our results suggest either a different role of CD163+ macrophage lineage or a divergent regulation of sCD163 production in pSS and SLE.

Another molecule differentiating pSS from SLE is Fractalkine/CX3CL1, the latter being a membrane form chemokine released by proteolytic cleavage (58). In addition to Fractalkine's chemotactic activity on monocytes and T-lymphocytes, it can facilitate the extravasation of leukocytes toward the inflammatory site (59). Fractalkine seems particularly involved in the pathophysiology of Sjogren sialadenitis (60–62) and lupus nephritis (63–65). Here, we observed an increase in serum Fractalkine concentration approximately halved the probability of pSS compared to SLE. We found only one study that analyzed serum Fractalkine concentration in SLE, RA, and pSS patients, with results consistent with ours (66). Fractalkine could therefore be involved in pSS and SLE pathophysiology, but with different regulation patterns and degrees of importance. As with I-TAC/CXCL11, Fractalkine is a chemokine induced by IFNg, which further emphasizes the primordial role of IFNg in pSS physiopathology. In addition, Lee et al. (61) found a significant correlation between serum concentrations of Fractalkine and TNFa in pSS patients. Here, serum concentrations of Fractalkine and TNFa were highly correlated in all groups (pSS: $r = 0.689$ and $p<0.0001$; RA: $r = 0.608$ and $p = 0.0005$; SLE: $r = 0.563$ and $p = 0.003$; data not shown), suggesting a strong pathophysiological relationship between these two biomarkers. TNFa is a pro-inflammatory cytokine involved in many autoimmune or auto-inflammatory diseases such as RA (67). While TNFa may be involved in the development of pSS in murine models (68), TNF inhibitors did not show efficacy in the treatment of pSS symptoms in humans (69–71). Thus, this cytokine may not be a key player in pSS pathophysiology. However, TNFa could be involved in SLE physiopathology, although its specific role remains to be specified (72, 73); our results are consistent with such a role of TNFa as we observed that greater serum concentrations of TNFa decreased the likelihood of pSS compared to SLE. Based on our data and those available in the literature, integration of serum TNFa concentration into a strategy to discriminate pSS from SLE appears premature.

Finally, we found that variation in serum concentrations of haptoglobin, HDP, MCP-1/CCL2, and Eotaxin-2/CCL24, were weakly associated with the likelihood of pSS compared to RA or SLE ($0.8 < OR < 1.2$). Despite statistically significant results, it is unlikely that these biomarkers could provide any clinical benefit. Similarly, we observed that at least one of the TARC/CCL17, CTSS, and SPARC concentration classes statistically discriminated pSS from one of the other AIDs. However, since pSS probability does not vary linearly across concentration classes, and given the small number of patients in SLE and RA groups, it is difficult to reach strong conclusions on these biomarkers' discriminative abilities.

Our study has several limitations. First, heterogeneity in patient characteristics between each group could potentially influence the serum concentrations of the different biomarkers. For example, SLE patients were significantly younger than pSS and RA patients, disease duration was shorter in pSS group (and also in the chronic phase), and treatments differed among groups, particularly for biologic drugs. The potential confounding bias of age was corrected in logistic regression when necessary. Furthermore, the effect of immunomodulatory therapies on serum biomarker concentrations remains to be identified. We performed additional statistical analysis and the concomitant use of biologic drugs was not associated with significant changes in the expression of the four main biomarkers (BDNF, Fractalkine/CX3CL1, I-TAC/CXCL11 and sCD163). In addition, we did not find significant variations between patients with and without steroids except for the sCD163 biomarker where we observed lower levels in steroid-treated patients (**Table S5, Supplemental Data**). Another potential limitation is a lack of statistical power arising from the relatively small number of patients in RA and SLE groups, with sample sizes further reduced in some analyses by the exclusion of patients with no exploitable biological data (biomarker concentration outside the kit detection capabilities or variation of more than 20% between technical duplicates, **Table S2 Supplemental Data**). However, the number of patients does not seem so low when compared to previous studies recently published in the field (<100 patients) (21–23). Indeed, our results need to be reproduced and validated in a larger and independent cohort as suggested by Chau et al. (74), since only few of our candidate biomarkers may prove relevant, and we did not correct the alpha risk for multiple analyses. Finally, approximately 70% of our patients had a low disease activity, while a small minority of patients had a high disease activity (none in the SLE group). This restricted disease activity spectrum ensured a good comparison between groups. However, having a larger number of patients with a higher level of disease activity would probably improve biomarker identification and discriminatory ability.

In conclusion, serum concentrations of 63 immunological biomarkers in pSS, RA, and SLE patients showed that four biomarkers were relevant to discriminate pSS from RA (BDNF and I-TAC/CXCL11), and pSS from SLE (sCD163, Fractalkine/CX3CL1). The next steps are to validate the markers with a larger and more homogeneous population and then investigate how these four molecules contribute to the physiopathology of pSS. The NF-kB, IL-17, and interferon pathways seem to be implicated, consistent with the mechanisms already known in pSS.

ETHICS STATEMENT

The studies involving human participants were reviewed and approved by Comité de Protection des Personnes Sud Méditerranée IV: DC-2015-2584. The patients/participants provided their written informed consent to participate in this study.

AUTHOR CONTRIBUTIONS

CJ, PGa, and Y-MP designed the experiments. RF, PGu, AM, RG, CJ, and Y-MP collected clinical data. Experimental works were performed by PGa and SA, and data were analyzed by GP, CD, MJ, SA, and Y-MP. GP and Y-MP prepared the manuscript. All authors have contributed to revising the manuscript and final approval. All authors contributed to the article and approved the submitted version.

ACKNOWLEDGMENTS

We gratefully acknowledge the Bio-Rad laboratory for support of biological tests, the Biological Resource Center for collecting samples, the University of Montpellier, and University Hospital of Montpellier.

REFERENCES

1. Theander E, Jacobsson LTH. Relationship of Sjögren's syndrome to other connective tissue and autoimmune disorders. *Rheum Dis Clin North Am* (2008) 34(4):935–47, viii–ix. doi: 10.1016/j.rdc.2008.08.009
2. Shiboski CH, Shiboski SC, Seror R, Criswell LA, Labetoulle M, Lietman TM, et al. American College of Rheumatology/European League Against Rheumatism Classification Criteria for Primary Sjögren's Syndrome: A Consensus and Data-Driven Methodology Involving Three International Patient Cohorts. *Arthritis Rheumatol* (20162017) 69(1):35–45. doi: 10.1002/art.39859
3. Aletaha D, Neogi T, Silman AJ, Funovits J, Felson DT, Bingham CO, et al. Rheumatoid arthritis classification criteria: An American College of Rheumatology/European League Against Rheumatism collaborative initiative. *Arthritis Rheumatol* (20102010) 62(9):2569–81.
4. Aringer M, Costenbader K, Daikh D, Brinks R, Mosca M, Ramsey-Goldman R, et al. European League Against Rheumatism/American College of Rheumatology classification criteria for systemic lupus erythematosus. *Ann Rheum Dis* (20192019) 78(9):1151–9. doi: 10.1136/annrheumdis-2018-214819
5. McDonagh JE, Isenberg DA. Development of additional autoimmune diseases in a population of patients with systemic lupus erythematosus. *Ann Rheum Dis* (2000) 59(3):230–2. doi: 10.1136/ard.59.3.230
6. Lazarus MN, Isenberg DA. Development of additional autoimmune diseases in a population of patients with primary Sjögren's syndrome. *Ann Rheum Dis* (2005) 64(7):1062–4. doi: 10.1136/ard.2004.029066
7. Carrozzo M, Scally K. Oral manifestations of hepatitis C virus infection. *World J Gastroenterol WJG* (2014) 20(24):7534–43. doi: 10.3748/wjg.v20.i24.7534
8. Franceschini F, Cavazzana I. Anti-Ro/SSA and La/SSB antibodies. *Autoimmunity* (2005) 38(1):55–63. doi: 10.1080/08916930400022954
9. Nocturne G, Mariette X. Advances in understanding the pathogenesis of primary Sjögren's syndrome. *Nat Rev Rheumatol* (2013) 9(9):544–56. doi: 10.1038/nrrheum.2013.110
10. Bautista-Vargas M, Vivas AJ, Tobón GJ. Minor salivary gland biopsy: Its role in the classification and prognosis of Sjögren's syndrome. *Autoimmun Rev* (2020) 19:102690. doi: 10.1016/j.autrev.2020.102690
11. Laborde CM, Castro-Santos P, Díaz-Peña R. Contribution of Multiplex Immunoassays to Rheumatoid Arthritis Management: From Biomarker Discovery to Personalized Medicine. *J Pers Med* (2020) 10(4):202. doi: 10.3390/jpm10040202
12. Ruiz-Romero C, Lam MPY, Nilsson P, Önnerfjord P, Utz PJ, Van Eyk JE, et al. Mining the Proteome Associated with Rheumatic and Autoimmune Diseases. *J Proteome Res* (2019) 18(12):4231–9. doi: 10.1021/acs.jproteome.9b00360
13. Moreno-Quispe LA, Serrano J, Virto L, Sanz M, Ramírez L, Fernández-Castro M, et al. Association of salivary inflammatory biomarkers with primary Sjögren's syndrome. *J Oral Pathol Med Off Publ Int Assoc Oral Pathol Am Acad Oral Pathol* (2020) 49(9):940–7. doi: 10.1111/jop.13070
14. Eastman PS, Manning WC, Qureshi F, Haney D, Cavet G, Alexander C, et al. Characterization of a multiplex, 12-biomarker test for rheumatoid arthritis. *J Pharm BioMed Anal* (2012) 70:415–24. doi: 10.1016/j.jpba.2012.06.003

15. Casey KA, Smith MA, Sinibaldi D, Seto NL, Playford MP, Wang X, et al. Modulation of cardiometabolic disease markers by type I interferon inhibition in systemic lupus erythematosus. *Arthritis Rheumatol Hoboken NJ* (2020). doi: 10.1002/art.41518
16. Ward G, Simpson A, Boscato L, Hickman PE. The investigation of interferences in immunoassay. *Clin Biochem* (2017) 50(18):1306–11. doi: 10.1016/j.clinbiochem.2017.08.015
17. Tzioufas AG, Bootsma H, Pers J-O. EULAR Sjögren's syndrome study group: an eSSential way to address the unmet needs of the disease. *Clin Exp Rheumatol* (2020) 38 Suppl 126(4):23–4.
18. Baldini C, Ferro F, Elefante E, Bombardieri S. Biomarkers for Sjögren's syndrome. *Biomark Med* (2018) 12(3):275–86. doi: 10.2217/bmm-2017-0297
19. Martín-Nares E, Hernández-Molina G. Novel autoantibodies in Sjögren's syndrome: A comprehensive review. *Autoimmun Rev* (2019) 18(2):192–8. doi: 10.1016/j.autrev.2018.09.003
20. Ramponi G, Folci M, Badalamenti S, Angelini C, Brunetta E. Biomarkers and Diagnostic Testing for Renal Disease in Sjogren's Syndrome. *Front Immunol* (2020) 11:2226. doi: 10.3389/fimmu.2020.562101
21. Tasaki S, Suzuki K, Nishikawa A, Kassai Y, Takiguchi M, Kurisu R, et al. Multiomic disease signatures converge to cytotoxic CD8 T cells in primary Sjögren's syndrome. *Ann Rheum Dis* (2017) 76(8):1458–66. doi: 10.1136/annrheumdis-2016-210788
22. Nishikawa A, Suzuki K, Kassai Y, Gotou Y, Takiguchi M, Miyazaki T, et al. Identification of definitive serum biomarkers associated with disease activity in primary Sjögren's syndrome. *Arthritis Res Ther* (2016) 18(1):106. doi: 10.1186/s13075-016-1006-1
23. Jonsson R, Brokstad KA, Jonsson MV, Delaleu N, Skarstein K. Current concepts on Sjögren's syndrome – classification criteria and biomarkers. *Eur J Oral Sci* (2018) 126(Suppl Suppl 1):37–48. doi: 10.1111/eos.12536
24. Petri M, Orbai A-M, Alarcón GS, Gordon C, Merrill JT, Fortin PR, et al. Derivation and Validation of Systemic Lupus International Collaborating Clinics Classification Criteria for Systemic Lupus Erythematosus. *Arthritis Rheumatol* (2012) 64(8):2677–86. doi: 10.1002/acr.21649
25. Seror R, Bootsma H, Saraux A, Bowman SJ, Theander E, Brun JG, et al. Defining disease activity states and clinically meaningful improvement in primary Sjögren's syndrome with EULAR primary Sjögren's syndrome disease activity (ESSDAI) and patient-reported indexes (ESSPRI). *Ann Rheum Dis* (2016) 75(2):382–9. doi: 10.1002/art.1780350606
26. Anderson J, Caplan L, Yazdany J, Robbins ML, Neogi T, Michaud K, et al. Rheumatoid arthritis disease activity measures: American College of Rheumatology recommendations for use in clinical practice. *Arthritis Care Res* (2012) 64(5):640–7. doi: 10.1002/acr.21649
27. Bombardier C, Gladman DD, Urowitz MB, Caron D, Chang CH. Derivation of the SLEDAI. A disease activity index for lupus patients. The Committee on Prognosis Studies in SLE. *Arthritis Rheumatol* (1992) 35(6):630–40. doi: 10.1002/art.1780350606
28. Flanagan JJ, Arjomandi A, Delanoy ML, Du Paty E, Galea P, Laune D, et al. Development of monoclonal antibodies to pre-haptoglobin 2 and their use in an enzyme-linked immunosorbent assay (ELISA). *J Immunol Methods* (2014) 406:34–42. doi: 10.1016/j.jim.2014.02.009
29. Krämer A, Green J, Pollard J, Tugendreich S. Causal analysis approaches in Ingenuity Pathway Analysis. *Bioinforma Oxf Engl* (2014) 30(4):523–30. doi: 10.1093/bioinformatics/btt703
30. Vakrakou AG, Polyzos A, Kapsogeorgou EK, Thanos D, Manoussakis MN. Impaired anti-inflammatory activity of PPARγ in the salivary epithelia of Sjögren's syndrome patients imposed by intrinsic NF-κB activation. *J Autoimmun* (2018) 86:62–74. doi: 10.1016/j.jaut.2017.09.007
31. Reksten TR, Lessard CJ, Sivils KL. Genetics in Sjögren Syndrome. *Rheum Dis Clin North Am* (2016) 42(3):435–47. doi: 10.1016/j.rdc.2016.03.003
32. Papageorgiou A, Mavragani CP, Nezos A, Zintzaras E, Quartuccio L, De Vita S, et al. A BAFF receptor His159Tyr mutation in Sjögren's syndrome-related lymphoproliferation. *Arthritis Rheumatol Hoboken NJ* (2015) 67(10):2732–41. doi: 10.1002/art.39231
33. Nocturne G, Tarn J, Boudaoud S, Locke J, Miceli-Richard C, Hachulla E, et al. Germline variation of TNFAIP3 in primary Sjögren's syndrome-associated lymphoma. *Ann Rheum Dis* (2016) 75(4):780–3. doi: 10.1136/annrheumdis-2015-207731
34. Nezos A, Gkioka E, Koutsilieris M, Voulgarelis M, Tzioufas AG, Mavragani CP. TNFAIP3 F127C Coding Variation in Greek Primary Sjogren's Syndrome Patients. *J Immunol Res* (2018) 2018:6923213. doi: 10.1155/2018/6923213
35. Kwok S-K, Cho M-L, Her Y-M, Oh H-J, Park M-K, Lee S-Y, et al. TLR2 ligation induces the production of IL-23/IL-17 via IL-6, STAT3 and NF-kB pathway in patients with primary Sjogren's syndrome. *Arthritis Res Ther* (2012) 14(2):R64. doi: 10.1186/ar3780
36. Sun J-L, Zhang H-Z, Liu S-Y, Lian C-F, Chen Z-L, Shao T-H, et al. Elevated EPSTI1 promote B cell hyperactivation through NF-κB signalling in patients with primary Sjögren's syndrome. *Ann Rheum Dis* (2020) 79(4):518–24. doi: 10.1136/annrheumdis-2019-216428
37. Verstappen GM, Corneth OBJ, Bootsma H, Kroese FGM. Th17 cells in primary Sjögren's syndrome: Pathogenicity and plasticity. *J Autoimmun* (2018) 87:16–25. doi: 10.1016/j.jaut.2017.11.003
38. Naegelin Y, Dingsdale H, Säuberli K, Schädelin S, Kappos L, Barde Y-A. Measuring and Validating the Levels of Brain-Derived Neurotrophic Factor in Human Serum. *eNeuro* (2018) 5(2):R262–264. doi: 10.1523/ENEURO.0419-17.2018
39. Bathina S, Das UN. Brain-derived neurotrophic factor and its clinical implications. *Arch Med Sci AMS* (2015) 11(6):1164–78. doi: 10.5114/aoms.2015.56342
40. Thomas K, Davies A. Neurotrophins: a ticket to ride for BDNF. *Curr Biol CB* (2005) 15(7):R262–264. doi: 10.1016/j.cub.2005.03.023
41. Vega JA, García-Suárez O, Hannestad J, Pérez-Pérez M, Germanà A. Neurotrophins and the immune system. *J Anat* (2003) 203(1):1–19. doi: 10.1046/j.1469-7580.2003.00203.x
42. De Santi L, Cantalupo L, Tassi M, Raspadori D, Cioni C, Annunziata P. Higher expression of BDNF receptor gp145trkB is associated with lower apoptosis intensity in T cell lines in multiple sclerosis. *J Neurol Sci* (2009) 277 (1–2):65–70. doi: 10.1016/j.jns.2008.10.006
43. Dubanet L, Bentayeb H, Petit B, Olivrie A, Saada S, de la Cruz-Morcillo MA, et al. Anti-apoptotic role and clinical relevance of neurotrophins in diffuse large B-cell lymphomas. *Br J Cancer* (2015) 113(6):934–44. doi: 10.1038/bjc.2015.274
44. Groom JR, Luster AD. CXCR3 ligands: redundant, collaborative and antagonistic functions. *Immunol Cell Biol* (2011) 89(2):207–15. doi: 10.1038/icb.2010.158
45. Ogawa N, Ping L, Zhenjun L, Takada Y, Sugai S. Involvement of the interferon-gamma-induced T cell-attracting chemokines, interferon-gamma-inducible 10-kd protein (CXCL10) and monokine induced by interferon-gamma (CXCL9), in the salivary gland lesions of patients with Sjögren's syndrome. *Arthritis Rheumatol* (2002) 46(10):2730–41. doi: 10.1002/art.10577
46. Ogawa N, Kawanami T, Shimoyama K, Ping L, Sugai S. Expression of interferon-inducible T cell alpha chemoattractant (CXCL11) in the salivary glands of patients with Sjögren's syndrome. *Clin Immunol Orlando Fla* (2004) 112(3):235–8. doi: 10.1016/j.clim.2004.03.008
47. Aota K, Yamanoi T, Kani K, Nakashiro K, Ishimaru N, Azuma M. Inverse correlation between the number of CXCR3+ macrophages and the severity of inflammatory lesions in Sjögren's syndrome salivary glands: A pilot study. *J Oral Pathol Med* (2018) 47(7):710–8. doi: 10.1111/jop.12756
48. Timmermann M, Högger P. Oxidative stress and 8-iso-prostaglandin F (2alpha) induce ectodomain shedding of CD163 and release of tumor necrosis factor-alpha from human monocytes. *Free Radic Biol Med* (2005) 39(1):98–107. doi: 10.1016/j.freeradbiomed.2005.02.031
49. Zhi Y, Gao P, Xin X, Li W, Ji L, Zhang L, et al. Clinical significance of sCD163 and its possible role in asthma. *Mol Med Rep* (2017) 15(5):2931–9. doi: 10.3892/mmr.2017.6393
50. Frings W, Dreier J, Sorg C. Only the soluble form of the scavenger receptor CD163 acts inhibitory on phorbol ester-activated T-lymphocytes, whereas membrane-bound protein has no effect. *FEBS Lett* (2002) 526(1–3):93–6. doi: 10.1016/S0014-5793(02)03142-3
51. Cui Y, Zhang Y, Rong Q, Zhu Y. [Changes and significance of soluble CD 163 in sepsis and severe sepsis in children]. *Zhonghua Er Ke Za Zhi Chin J Pediatr* (2012) 50(9):653–6. doi: 10.1111/j.1365-2036.2012.05134.x
52. Zanni MV, Burdo TH, Makimura H, Williams KC, Grinspoon SK. Relationship between monocyte/macrophage activation marker soluble CD163 and insulin resistance in obese and normal-weight subjects. *Clin Endocrinol (Oxf)* (2012) 77(3):385–90. doi: 10.1111/j.1365-2265.2011.04284.x

53. Grønbaek H, Sandahl TD, Mortensen C, Vilstrup H, Møller HJ, Møller S. Soluble CD163, a marker of Kupffer cell activation, is related to portal hypertension in patients with liver cirrhosis. *Aliment Pharmacol Ther* (2012) 36(2):173–80. doi: 10.1111/j.1365-2036.2012.05134.x
54. Shaked I, Hanna DB, Gleißner C, Marsh B, Plants J, Tracy D, et al. Macrophage inflammatory markers are associated with subclinical carotid artery disease in women with human immunodeficiency virus or hepatitis C virus infection. *Arterioscler Thromb Vasc Biol* (2014) 34(5):1085–92. doi: 10.1161/ATVBAHA.113.303153
55. Jude C, Dejica D, Samasca G, Balacescu L, Balacescu O. Soluble CD163 serum levels are elevated and correlated with IL-12 and CXCL10 in patients with long-standing rheumatoid arthritis. *Rheumatol Int* (2013) 33(4):1031–7. doi: 10.1007/s00296-012-2459-4
56. Aristoteli LP, Møller HJ, Bailey B, Moestrup SK, Kritharides L. The monocytic lineage specific soluble CD163 is a plasma marker of coronary atherosclerosis. *Atherosclerosis* (2006) 184(2):342–7. doi: 10.1016/j.atherosclerosis.2005.05.004
57. David C, Divard G, Abbas R, Escoubet B, Chezel J, Chauveheid MP, et al. Soluble CD163 is a biomarker for accelerated atherosclerosis in systemic lupus erythematosus patients at apparent low risk for cardiovascular disease. *Scand J Rheumatol* (2019) 2:1–5. doi: 10.1080/03009742.2019.1614213
58. Clark AK, Staniland AA, Malcangio M. Fractalkine/CX3CR1 signalling in chronic pain and inflammation. *Curr Pharm Biotechnol* (2011) 12(10):1707–14. doi: 10.2174/138920111798357465
59. Jones B, Koch AE, Ahmed S. Pathological role of fractalkine/CX3CL1 in rheumatic diseases: a unique chemokine with multiple functions. *Front Immunol* (2011) 2:82. doi: 10.3389/fimmu.2011.00082
60. Astorri E, Scrivo R, Bombardieri M, Picarelli G, Pecorella I, Porzia A, et al. CX3CL1 and CX3CR1 expression in tertiary lymphoid structures in salivary gland infiltrates: fractalkine contribution to lymphoid neogenesis in Sjogren's syndrome. *Rheumatol Oxf Engl* (2014) 53(4):611–20. doi: 10.1093/rheumatology/ket401
61. Lee JH, Kwok S-K, Jung SM, Lee J, Lee J-S, Baek SY, et al. Role of fractalkine in the pathogenesis of primary Sjögren syndrome: increased serum levels of fractalkine, its expression in labial salivary glands, and the association with clinical manifestations. *J Rheumatol* (2014) 41(12):2425–38. doi: 10.3899/jrheum.130892
62. Zhao L, Xu W, Chen Z, Zhang H, Zhang S, Lian C, et al. Aberrant distribution of CD3+CD56+ NKT-like cells in patients with primary Sjögren's syndrome. *Clin Exp Rheumatol* (2020) 33:520–23.
63. Yoshimoto S, Nakatani K, Iwano M, Asai O, Samejima K, Sakan H, et al. Elevated levels of fractalkine expression and accumulation of CD16+ monocytes in glomeruli of active lupus nephritis. *Am J Kidney Dis Off J Natl Kidney Found.* (2007) 50(1):47–58. doi: 10.1053/j.ajkd.2007.04.012
64. You Y, Liao P, Qin Y, Lin X, Li J. [Blood and renal fractalkine expression in patients with lupus nephritis and its significance]. *Nan Fang Yi Ke Da Xue Xue Bao* (2013) 33(4):520–3. doi: 10.1136/ard.2005.051276s
65. Olaru F, Döbel T, Lonsdorf AS, Oehrl S, Maas M, Enk AH, et al. Intracapillary immune complexes recruit and activate slan-expressing CD16+ monocytes in human lupus nephritis. *JCI Insight* (2018) 3(11):907–16. doi: 10.1172/jci.insight.96492
66. Sato E, Iikuni N, Yoshio T, Minota S, Kamatani N, Okamoto H. Soluble fractalkine in the cerebrospinal fluid of patients with neuropsychiatric lupus. *Ann Rheum Dis* (2006) 65(9):1257–9. doi: 10.1136/ard.2005.051276
67. Choy EH, Panayi GS. Cytokine pathways and joint inflammation in rheumatoid arthritis. *N Engl J Med* (2001) 344(12):907–16. doi: 10.1056/NEJM200103223441207
68. Zhou J, Kawai T, Yu Q. Pathogenic role of endogenous TNF-α in the development of Sjögren's-like sialadenitis and secretory dysfunction in non-obese diabetic mice. *Lab Investig J Tech Methods Pathol* (2017) 97(4):458–67. doi: 10.1038/labinvest.2016.141
69. Sankar V, Brennan MT, Kok MR, Leakan RA, Smith JA, Manny J, et al. Etanercept in Sjögren's syndrome: a twelve-week randomized, double-blind, placebo-controlled pilot clinical trial. *Arthritis Rheumatol* (2004) 50(7):2240–5. doi: 10.1002/art.20299
70. Mariette X, Ravaud P, Steinfeld S, Baron G, Goetz J, Hachulla E, et al. Inefficacy of infliximab in primary Sjögren's syndrome: results of the randomized, controlled Trial of Remicade in Primary Sjögren's Syndrome (TRIPSS). *Arthritis Rheumatol* (2004) 50(4):1270 6. doi: 10.1002/art.20146
71. Moutsopoulos NM, Katsifis GE, Angelov N, Leakan RA, Sankar V, Pillemer S, et al. Lack of efficacy of etanercept in Sjögren syndrome correlates with failed suppression of tumour necrosis factor alpha and systemic immune activation. *Ann Rheum Dis* (2008) 67(10):1437–43. doi: 10.1136/ard.2007.077891
72. Aringer M, Smolen JS. The role of tumor necrosis factor-alpha in systemic lupus erythematosus. *Arthritis Res Ther* (2008) 10(1):202. doi: 10.1186/ar2341
73. Postal M, Appenzeller S. The role of Tumor Necrosis Factor-alpha (TNF-α) in the pathogenesis of systemic lupus erythematosus. *Cytokine* (2011) 56(3):537–43. doi: 10.1016/j.cyto.2011.08.026
74. Chau CH, Rixe O, McLeod H, Figg WD. Validation of analytic methods for biomarkers used in drug development. *Clin Cancer Res Off J Am Assoc Cancer Res* (2008) 14(19):5967–76. doi: 10.1158/1078-0432.CCR-07-4535

18

Monocytes from Patients with Macrophage Activation Syndrome and Secondary Hemophagocytic Lymphohistiocytosis are Hyperresponsive to Interferon Gamma

Antonia Pascarella[1], Claudia Bracaglia[2], Ivan Caiello[1], Alessia Arduini[2], Gian Marco Moneta[1], Marianna Nicoletta Rossi[1], Valentina Matteo[1], Manuela Pardeo[2], Fabrizio De Benedetti[2] and Giusi Prencipe[1]*

[1] Division of Rheumatology, IRCCS Ospedale Pediatrico Bambino Gesù, Rome, Italy, [2] Laboratory of Immuno-Rheumatology, IRCCS Ospedale Pediatrico Bambino Gesù, Rome, Italy

***Correspondence:**
Fabrizio De Benedetti
fabrizio.debenedetti@opbg.net

Objective: To investigate the activation of the IFNγ signaling pathway in monocytes of patients with secondary hemophagocytic lymphohistiocytosis (sHLH)/macrophage activation syndrome (MAS) and to evaluate whether levels of phosphorylated STAT1 represent a biomarker for the identification of patients at early stages of the disease.

Methods: Fresh whole blood samples from pediatric patients with active sHLH/MAS, not receiving (n=10) and receiving glucocorticoids (n=14) at time of sampling, were prospectively collected. As disease control groups, patients with active systemic juvenile idiopathic arthritis (sJIA) without MAS, patients with sHLH/MAS in remission and patients with other rheumatic diseases were also sampled. Whole blood cells were left unstimulated or stimulated with increasing concentrations of IFNγ for 10 minutes and the intracellular Tyrosine (701)-phosphorylated STAT1 (pSTAT1) levels were evaluated in monocytes by flow cytometry.

Results: Monocytes from untreated sHLH/MAS patients showed significantly higher basal levels of pSTAT1 compared to those observed in monocytes from glucocorticoid-treated sHLH/MAS patients and from all the other disease controls. In addition, a significant increase in responsiveness to IFNγ, as assessed by increased levels of pSTAT1 following *ex vivo* stimulation, was observed in monocytes from untreated sHLH/MAS patients. pSTAT1 levels in monocytes distinguished patients with sHLH/MAS not treated with glucocorticoids from patients with active sJIA or with other rheumatic diseases [AUC, 0.93; 95% confidence interval 0.85-1.00, $p<0.001$]. Statistically significant correlations between *IFNG* mRNA levels in whole blood cells, circulating IFNγ levels and pSTAT1 levels in sHLH/MAS monocytes were found.

Conclusion: Our data demonstrating higher basal levels of pSTAT1 as well as a hyperreactivity to IFNγ stimulation in monocytes from patients with sHLH/MAS point to perturbations in the activation of downstream IFNγ signaling pathway as a contributor to the hyperinflammation occurring in these patients. Finally, the observation that glucocorticoids affect pSTAT1 levels *in vivo*, makes it difficult to consider the measurement of pSTAT1 levels as a biomarker to identify patients at early stages of sHLH/MAS in clinical practice.

Keywords: hemophagocytic lymphohistiocytosis, IFNγ, STAT1, macrophage activation syndrome, monocytes

INTRODUCTION

Hemophagocytic lymphohistiocytosis (HLH) is a life-threatening syndrome characterized by hyperinflammation caused by uncontrolled activation of immune cells, particularly monocytes/macrophages and CD8+ T cells. It is classified into primary and secondary forms, depending on whether they are inherited or acquired (1). Indeed, while primary HLH (pHLH) is caused by loss-of-function mutations in genes encoding proteins involved in the cytolytic secretory functions of natural killer (NK) cells and cytotoxic T lymphocytes, secondary HLH forms (sHLH)/macrophage activation syndrome (MAS) often occur as complication of malignancies, infections and rheumatic diseases (2).

A growing body of evidence demonstrated the involvement of IFNγ in the pathogenesis of primary and secondary HLH as a major regulator of macrophage hyperactivation and hemophagocytosis (3–6). Further pointing to the role of IFNγ in the development of sHLH, elevated levels of IFNγ and IFNγ-regulated chemokines CXCL9 and CXCL10 have been found in the blood and in target tissues of patients and animal models (5, 7–10). Therapeutic neutralization of IFNγ has been shown to be efficacious in the treatment of primary and secondary HLH forms (11–13).

IFNγ is a pleiotropic cytokine with a key role in the regulation of innate and adaptive immune responses. It is mainly produced by activated NK and T cells and is involved in the activation of macrophages and NK cells, as well as in the differentiation and proliferation of T cells (14). IFNγ exerts its biological effects by activation of the Janus kinase (JAK)/signal transducer and activator of transcription (STAT) signal transduction pathway (15). Upon binding of IFNγ to its receptor, JAK1 and JAK2 are recruited and phosphorylated at the intracellular domain of the receptor. This event allows the recruitment of STAT1 and its activation *via* the JAKs-mediated phosphorylation of the tyrosine 701 residue (Y701). Finally, activated STAT1 translocates into the nucleus and initiates the transcription of IFNγ inducible genes (16).

In this study, we evaluated the activation of the IFNγ signaling pathway in monocytes of patients with sHLH/MAS, by assessing the intracellular levels of STAT1-Y701 phosphorylation (pSTAT1), under both basal conditions and following *ex vivo* stimulation with IFNγ. We aimed to investigate the activation of the IFNγ signaling pathway in monocytes of patients with sHLH/MAS and to evaluate whether levels of pSTAT1 could be used in a clinical setting to identify patients at early stages of HLH/MAS.

METHODS AND PATIENTS

Patients

Patients were classified as follows. sJIA patients were diagnosed according to the ILAR criteria (17, 18). The 2016 classification criteria for MAS in sJIA were used to define patients with MAS in the context of sJIA (19). The 2004-HLH diagnostic guidelines were used to define those with sHLH (20). Patients who experienced an episode of MAS or sHLH, but were in clinical and laboratory remission at the time of whole blood collection, were also enrolled in the study. Since there are no criteria available to define disease remission of sHLH and MAS, we used those applied in the context of the clinical trial with the anti- IFNγ monoclonal antibody (emapalumab) in primary HLH and in MAS in the context of sJIA, respectively (11, 21).

The study was reviewed and approved by the local Institutional Ethical Committee of Bambino Gesù Children's Hospital (number 1649/2018). Written informed consent to participate in this study was provided by the participants' legal guardian/next of kin.

Flow Cytometry

Fresh peripheral whole blood cells were left unstimulated or stimulated with different concentrations of human recombinant IFNγ (0.01, 0.1, 1, 10 ng/ml) (R&D Systems) for 10 minutes at 37°C. Anti-CD3, anti-CD14 and anti-CD16 (all from Becton Dickinson) staining was performed for 20 minutes at 4°C, in order to discriminate the monocyte, neutrophil, natural killer and T cell subpopulations. Whole blood cells where then fixed with Lyse/Fix Buffer 10 min at 37°C and further incubated 10 min at RT with FcBlock 1:200 in Stain Buffer (all from Becton Dickinson). After permeabilization with Perm Buffer II (BD PhosFlow) 20 min at 4°C, samples were stained with antibodies against phosphorylated Tyrosine (701) STAT1 (pSTAT1) and total STAT1 (all from Becton Dickinson) for 20 min at 4°C. Isotype-matched control mAbs were used to determine non-specific background staining. Samples were run on a BD LSRFortessa X-20 instrument (BD Biosciences) and data were analyzed with FlowJo software, version 8.3 (Tree Star). Results were expressed as Delta mean fluorescence intensity (ΔMFI, calculated by subtracting MFI values of isotype controls from sample MFI values).

Real-Time PCR

Whole blood samples were collected in Tempus Tube (Applied Biosystems). RNA was extracted with Tempus Spin RNA isolation kit (Applied Biosystems). Total RNA was reverse-transcribed with Superscript VILO cDNA synthesis Kit (Invitrogen). Gene expression levels were evaluated by quantitative polymerase chain reaction (qPCR) (ABI Prism 7900 HT sequence detection platform, Applied Biosystems), with Taqman Universal PCR Mastermix and Gene-expression Assays (Applied Biosystems; *IFNG*, Hs00989291_m1). The results, determined using the $2^{-\Delta Ct}$ method, were normalized using GAPDH (Hs99999905_m1; Applied Biosystems) as endogenous control.

IFNγ Measurements

Plasma levels of IFNγ were measured using the IFNγ quantikine Elisa Kit (R&D Systems Inc.). The detection limit of the assays was 15.6 pg/ml.

Statistical Analysis

Normality was tested using the Kolmogorov-Smirnov test. For normally distributed data, differences between groups were analyzed by one-way or two-way analysis of variance (ANOVA) test with Bonferroni's correction. Data are expressed as mean ± standard error of the mean (SEM). For non-normally distributed data, differences between groups were analyzed by the nonparametric Mann–Whitney U test and data are expressed as median and interquartile range (IQR). Correlations were tested using Spearman's rank order test. Significance level for all statistical tests was at $^{*}p < 0.05$, $^{**}p < 0.01$, $^{***}p < 0.001$ and $^{****}p < 0.0001$ values. Graphpad Prism 9 software was used for statistical analysis and graphs.

RESULTS

Patients

Sixty-one patients were enrolled from 2017 to 2019 at Ospedale Pediatrico Bambino Gesù: patients with active sJIA (n=12; age 10.3 years, IQR 5.7-14.2; 4/12 treated with glucocorticoids), patients with sHLH/MAS not treated with glucocorticoids (n=10; age 7.1 years, IQR 5.1-14.04/12; 0/10 treated with glucocorticoids), patients with sHLH/MAS treated with glucocorticoids (n=14; age 6.3 years, IQR 2.5-14.9; 14/14 treated with glucocorticoids), patients with sHLH/MAS in remission phase (n=12; age 11.8 years, IQR 5.7-17.8; 2/12 treated with glucocorticoids), patients with other rheumatic diseases (n=13; age 6.2 years, IQR 4.3-12.7; 0/13 treated with glucocorticoids). Between 26 patients with sHLH/MAS enrolled, 13 patients experienced MAS in sJIA and 13 patients experienced sHLH, of which 5 secondary to infections, 4 secondary to inflammatory disorders, 2 secondary to malignancy, 2 of unknown origin. Between 13 patients with other rheumatic diseases enrolled, 2 patients with polyarticular juvenile idiopathic arthritis (JIA) antinuclear antibodies (ANA) positive, 5 patients with oligoarticular JIA (3 of whom with ANA positive and 2 with ANA negative), 1 with chronic non-bacterial osteomyelitis, 3 with undefined autoinflammatory diseases, 1 with undefined orbital granulomatous lesions and 1 with Kikuchi-Fujimoto disease. Patients' laboratory parameters are shown in **Table 1**.

Increased Levels of Phosphorylated STAT1 in Monocytes From Untreated sHLH/MAS Patients

To evaluate the *in vivo* activation of the IFNγ pathway in patients with sHLH/MAS and to investigate whether levels of activated STAT1 represent a biomarker for the identification of patients at early stages of the disease, we measured basal activated Tyrosine (701) phosphorylated STAT1 (pSTAT1) levels in monocytes of patients with sHLH/MAS at time of blood sampling. These levels were compared with those of patients with active sJIA without MAS, with sHLH/MAS in remission phase, and with other inflammatory rheumatic diseases. sHLH/MAS patients showed significantly increased pSTAT1 levels compared to sHLH/MAS patients in remission and a trend to higher levels of pSTAT1 compared to active sJIA patients (**Figure 1A**). This was true for both sHLH and MAS patients.

TABLE 1 | Patient laboratory parameters.

	Other inflam.diseases (n=13)	Active sJIA patients (n=12)	Untreated sHLH/MAS (n=10)	Treated sHLH/MAS (n=14)	Remission sHLH/MAS (n=12)
White blood cells (cells/mL)	6500 (5815-7950)	9980 (6175-14408)	3880 (2060-6323)	6935 (2933-20798)	6145 (4093-8018)
Hemoglobin (gr/dL)	12.7 (11.65-13.2)	11 (9.6-11.3)	9.9 (9.2-11)	9.9 (8.4-10.6)	11.9 (10.2-12.8)
Platelets (x10^9/L)	277 (260-349.5)	284 (232-370)	124 (63.7-225.5)	133.5 (52.5-442.5)	244 (152.3-369.3)
Ferritin (ng/mL)	NA	327 (149-1457)	3718 (1270-10535)	2612 (1212-17682)	23.5 (15.7-136.4)
D-dimer (mg/mL)	NA	1.94 (1.2-3.4)	3.1 (2.0-6.1)	2.2 (0.82-6.1)	0.4 (0.3-1.2)
Fibrinogen (mg/dL)	NA	444.5 (361-626)	379.5 (191.8-493.3)	356 (228.3-552.3)	264 (232-381)
ALT (U/L)	23.5 (15.5-31.8)	15 (10.2-22)	59 (23-118.8)	129 (46-689.3)	27.5 (16.5-57.5)
AST (U/L)	29 (22.5-31.5)	32.5 (18.2-49.7)	80.5 (49.7-137.8)	67 (43.2-345.5)	31.5 (20.5-79.7)
LDH (U/L)	452.5 (396.5-522.8)	545 (345-684)	1066 (688.5-1848)	886.5 (609.8-1015)	499.5 (379.5-700.3)
GammaGT (U/L)	10 (7-19.2)	12.5 (9.25-19.3)	34.5 (14.2-123)	127.5 (53.5-313)	16 (9.2-52.2)
CRP (mg/dL)	0.57 (0.1-1.3)	4.7 (1.4-11.7)	6.9 (1.5-16.8)	3.2 (1.2-17.34)	0.2 (0.05-2.4)

Values are shown as median and interquartile range (IQR). NA, not available.

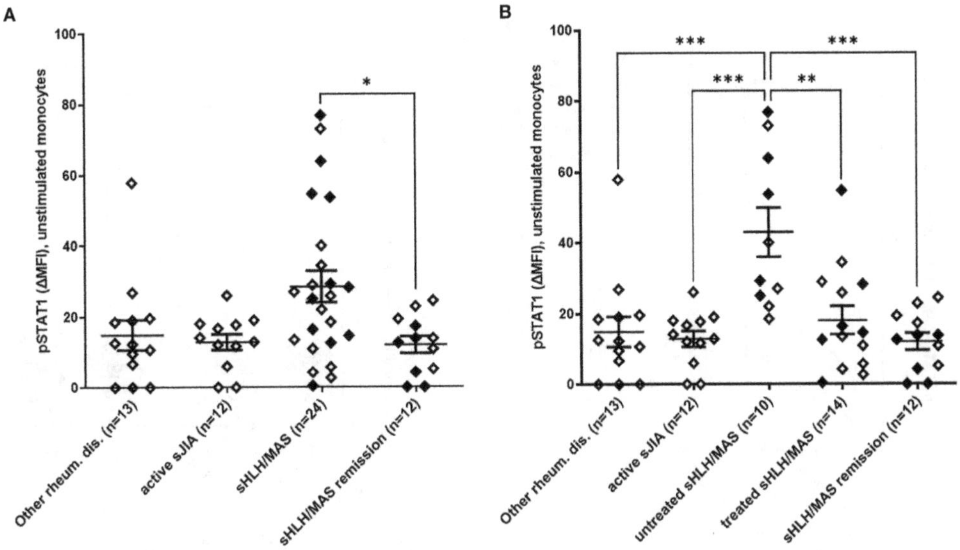

FIGURE 1 | Increased phosphorylated STAT1 (pSTAT1) levels in monocytes of untreated sHLH/MAS patients. **(A)** pSTAT1 levels were evaluated in unstimulated monocytes from sHLH/MAS patients and compared to levels observed in monocytes from patients with other rheumatic diseases, patients with active sJIA, patients with sHLH/MAS in a remission phase. **(B)** pSTAT1 levels were evaluated in sHLH/MAS patients not treated (untreated sHLH/MAS) and treated (treated sHLH/MAS) with glucocorticoids at sampling and compared with the other patient groups. Full diamonds indicate samples from MAS patients. **(A, B)** pSTAT1 levels were measured by flow cytometry and reported as Delta mean fluorescence intensity (ΔMFI, calculated by subtracting MFI values of isotype controls from sample MFI values). Differences between groups were analyzed using the one-way ANOVA test and the *post hoc* Bonferroni's for multiple comparisons test. The data shown represent mean (± SEM) values. $^{*}p \leq 0.05$, $^{**}p \leq 0.01$, $^{***}p \leq 0.001$.

Based on several data demonstrating that, *in vivo* and *ex vivo*, glucocorticoids inhibits IFNγ-mediated phosphorylation of STAT1 (9, 22), we divided sHLH/MAS patients into two groups: patients without any treatment at time of blood sampling (untreated patients, n=10) and patients who were already receiving glucocorticoids (treated patients, n=14). We found that untreated sHLH/MAS patients showed significantly higher basal pSTAT1 levels in monocytes compared to treated sHLH/MAS patients, as well as to all the other disease control groups (**Figure 1B**).

Monocytes From Untreated MAS/sHLH Patients Show Increased Responsiveness to IFNγ

To investigate potential perturbations in IFNγ signaling pathway activation in sHLH/MAS, we analyzed pSTAT1 levels in monocytes following *ex vivo* stimulation with increasing concentrations of IFNγ. As shown in **Figure 2**, we found that monocytes of untreated sHLH/MAS patients showed a significant increase in responsiveness to IFNγ stimulation (at 1 and 10 ng/ml of IFNγ), compared to all the other disease control groups. Notably, following IFNγ stimulation, monocytes from glucocorticoid-treated sHLH/MAS patients showed pSTAT1 levels superimposable to those of the other patient/control groups. In monocytes of untreated sHLH/MAS patients, levels of pSTAT1 following IFNγ stimulation were significantly correlated with basal pSTAT1 levels (IFNγ 10 ng/ml: p=0.01, r=0.77). This correlation was not observed in disease control groups. We also found a correlation of pSTAT1 levels in unstimulated (n=10, p=0.01, r=0,75) and IFNγ (10 ng/ml) stimulated monocytes (n=10, p=0.03, r=0.68) with *IFNG* mRNA expression in whole blood paired samples. Consistently, plasma levels of IFNγ were high in patients with sHLH/MAS (mean± SEM, 51 pg/ml ± 14.7, n=24) and were correlated with pSTAT1 levels in monocytes not stimulated (n=24, p=0.004, r=0.56) or stimulated with IFNγ (n=23, p<0.0001, r=0.72). These data suggest a relation between overexpression of IFNγ *in vivo* and enhanced pSTAT1 levels *ex vivo*. In contrast, in patients with active sJIA, circulating levels of IFNγ were undetectable and no statistically significant correlations between IFNG mRNA, circulating levels of IFNγ and pSTAT1 levels were observed.

We also measured by flow cytometry total STAT1 expression in unstimulated monocytes from a smaller number of patients. Due to the small number of samples analyzed, we found a trend for higher levels of STAT1 in untreated sHLH/MAS patients (**Supplementary Figure 1**). However, we found that total STAT1 levels significantly correlated with pSTAT1 levels in both unstimulated (p=0.04, r=0.5) (**Figure 3A**) and IFNγ-stimulated sHLH/MAS monocytes (p<0.0001, r=0.85) (**Figure 3B**). In contrast, no significant correlations were observed between total STAT1 levels and pSTAT1 levels in patients with active sJIA (**Figures 3C, D**).

Altogether, these results showed significantly higher levels of pSTAT1 both in unstimulated and *ex vivo* IFNγ-stimulated monocytes from patients with sHLH/MAS who were not receiving glucocorticoids. These levels correlated with mRNA expression and circulating levels of IFNγ. In addition,

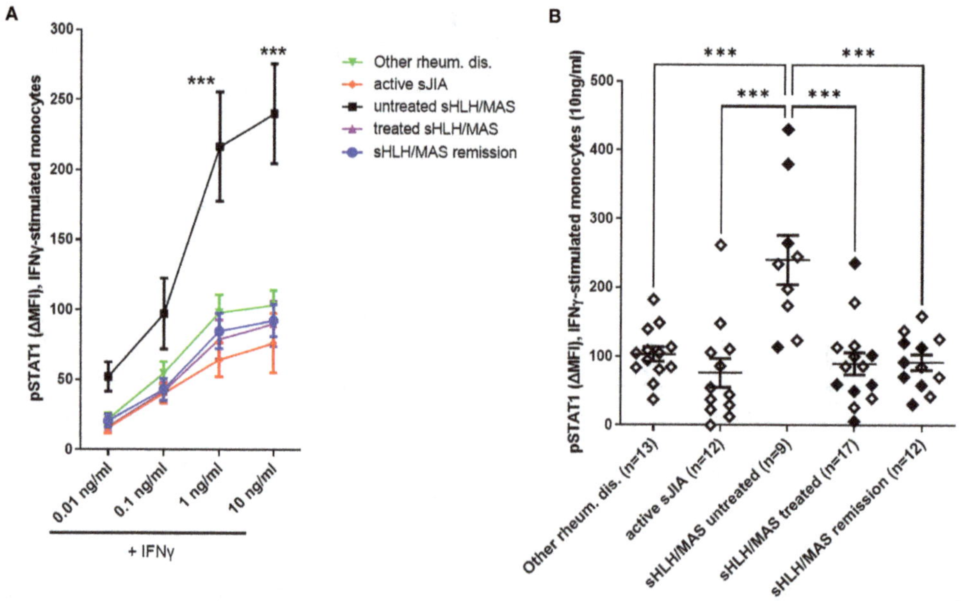

FIGURE 2 | Monocytes from untreated MAS/sHLH patients show increased responsiveness to IFNγ. **(A)** pSTAT1 levels were evaluated in monocytes from patients following *ex vivo* stimulation with increasing concentration of human recombinant IFNγ. Differences between groups were analyzed using the two-way ANOVA test and the *post hoc* Bonferroni's for multiple comparisons test. The data shown represent mean (± SEM) values; ****p* ≤ 0.001. In untreated sHLH/MAS patients, pSTAT1 levels following stimulation with 1 and 10 ng/ml of IFNγ were significantly higher than those observed in all the other patient groups ($p < 0.0001$). **(B)** pSTAT1 levels in monocytes stimulated with 10 ng/ml of IFNγ are reported in detail. Full diamonds indicate samples from MAS patients. **(A, B)** pSTAT1 levels were measured by flow cytometry and reported as Delta mean fluorescence intensity (ΔMFI, calculated by subtracting MFI values of isotype controls from sample MFI values). Untreated sHLH/MAS patients were 9 instead of 10, because for one patient there were not enough cells for IFNγ-stimulation experiments.

a correlation between total STAT1 levels and pSTAT1 levels in unstimulated and IFNγ–stimulated monocytes from sHLH/MAS not receiving glucocorticoids was also found. These results are consistent with the upregulation of IFNγ and the activation of IFNγ-mediated signaling pathway in patients with sHLH/MAS.

Clinical Relevance of pSTAT1 Levels in sHLH/MAS

In order to evaluate whether pSTAT1 levels could be used to identify HLH/MAS patients in a clinical setting, we performed receiver operating characteristic (ROC) curve analysis, by using as controls patients with active sJIA without MAS and patients with other rheumatic diseases. When untreated sHLH/MAS patients were analyzed, we found an area under the curve (AUC) of 0.93 [95% confidence interval (CI), 0.85-1.00, p<0.001] for pSTAT1 levels in unstimulated monocytes (**Figure 4A**) and an AUC of 0.92 (95% CI, 0.83-1.00, p<0.001) for pSTAT1 levels in monocytes stimulated with IFNγ (10 ng/ml) (**Figure 4B**). However, when all sHLH/MAS patients (untreated and treated with glucocorticoids at sampling) were analyzed, we found an AUC of 0.73 (95% CI, 0.58-0.87, p=0.006) for pSTAT1 levels in unstimulated monocytes (**Figure 4C**) and an AUC of 0.66 (95% CI, 0.50-0.81, p=0.06) for pSTAT1 levels in monocytes stimulated with IFNγ (10 ng/ml) (**Figure 4D**).

When we evaluated in untreated MAS/sHLH patients and in all MAS/sHLH patients (treated and untreated) the correlations of pSTAT1 and total STAT1 with clinical and laboratory parameters, including white blood cell count, platelet count, hemoglobin, ferritin, fibrinogen, we did not find any statistically significant correlation (data not shown).

DISCUSSION

A growing number of studies point to a pivotal role of IFNγ in the pathogenesis of primary and secondary HLH forms, including MAS (4, 7).

Consistently with the observations of high levels of IFNγ and IFNγ-inducible inflammatory mediators in blood of patients and in animal models with sHLH (5–7), we found that freshly isolated blood monocytes from patients with sHLH/MAS show increased levels of pSTAT1, further confirming the activation of the IFNγ signaling pathway in these patients. In particular, we found that blood monocytes of patients with sHLH/MAS not treated with glucocorticoids express significantly higher levels of pSTAT1 compared to patients with active sJIA, as well as compared to patients with sHLH/MAS treated with glucocorticoids or to sHLH/MAS patients during remission. In addition, we found a statistically significant correlation of total STAT1 levels with pSTAT1 levels in sHLH/MAS patients. These data are consistent with previous findings demonstrating that STAT1 and pSTAT1 levels are strongly increased in target tissues, such as liver and lung, of patients and animals with sHLH/MAS (5, 8, 9).

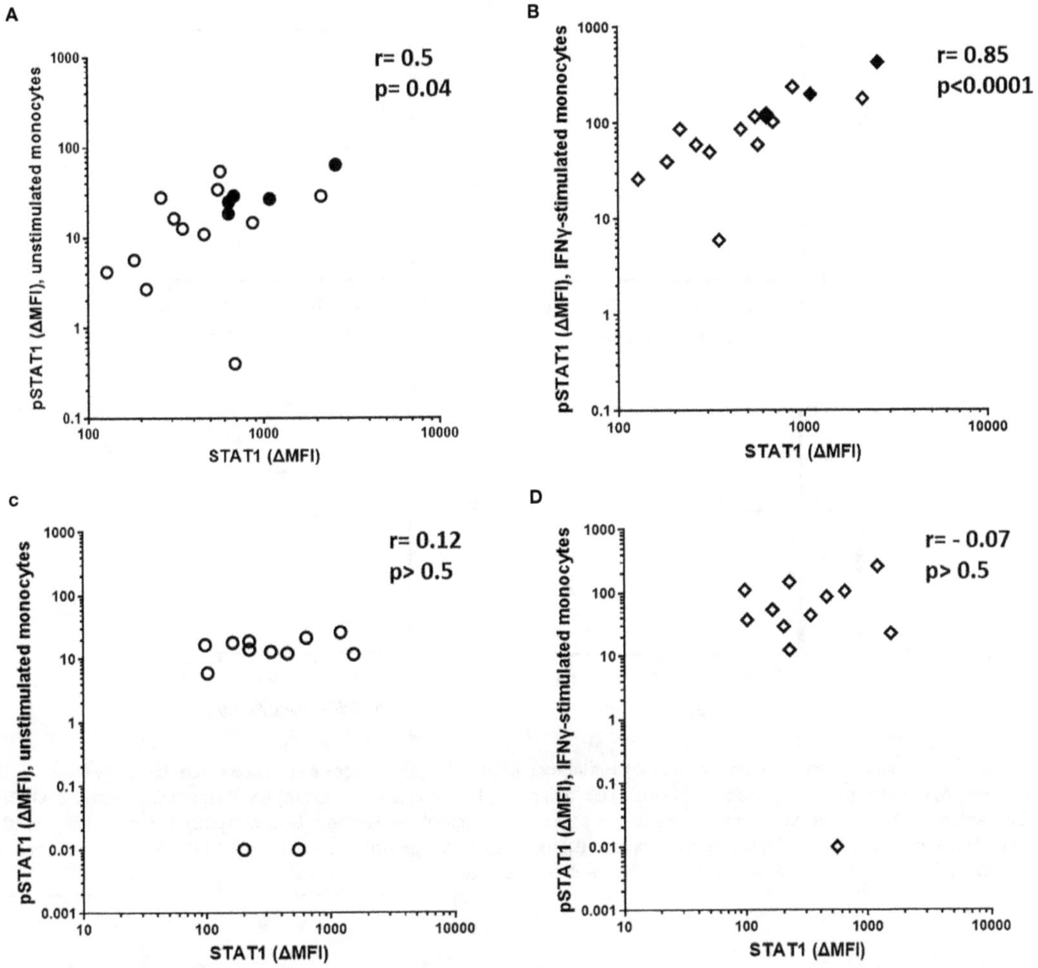

FIGURE 3 | Total STAT1 levels are significantly correlated with pSTAT1 levels in monocytes of sHLH/MAS patients, but not in those of active sJIA patients. **(A, B)** Total STAT1 levels were correlated with pSTAT1 levels in monocytes unstimulated (n=17) or stimulated (n=16) with IFNγ (10 ng/Mml) from sHLH/MAS patients. Full diamonds and circles indicate samples from untreated sHLH/MAS patients. **(C, D)** Total STAT1 levels were correlated with pSTAT1 levels in monocytes unstimulated (n=12) or stimulated (n=12) with IFNγ (10ng/ml) from active sJIA patients. Correlations were tested using Spearman's rank order test. A base-10 log scale is used for the y and x axes of graphs **(A–D)**.

Our data showing significant differences in pSTAT1 levels between untreated patients and glucocorticoid-treated patients are consistent with the known inhibitory effects, both *in vitro* and *in vivo*, of glucocorticoids on the IFNγ-mediated signaling pathway. Indeed, addition of dexamethasone to PBMC cultures has been demonstrated to result in the suppression of STAT1 expression and, therefore, in a dramatic inhibition of IFNγ signaling pathway activation, as revealed by suppression of IFNγ-inducible gene expression (22). Our observation also confirms our previous findings in PBMCs collected from one patient with sHLH: total STAT1 and pSTAT1 levels were significantly increased during the acute phase of the disease, but they underwent a marked decrease following initiation of treatment with glucocorticoids (9). Glucocorticoids are often used in the early phase of the disease to stabilize patients with rapidly progressive worsening disease. Indeed, we found that pSTAT1 levels in unstimulated and IFNγ-stimulated monocytes are sensitive and specific in discriminating sHLH/MAS patients not treated with glucocorticoids at sampling from patients with active sJIA and other rheumatic diseases. In contrast, they do not distinguish sHLH/MAS patients treated with glucocorticoids at sampling from disease controls. Altogether, these observations make it difficult to consider the measurement of pSTAT1 levels as a good biomarker for the identification of patients at early stages of sHLH/MAS in clinical practice.

To investigate potential perturbations in downstream IFNγ signaling pathway activation in monocytes of patients with sHLH/MAS, we also evaluated the activation of STAT1 following *ex vivo* stimulation of peripheral whole blood cells with increasing concentrations of recombinant IFNγ. We found that IFNγ stimulation was much more effective in inducing STAT1 phosphorylation in monocytes of sHLH/MAS patients not treated with glucocorticoids compared to all the other patient groups analyzed. These results are consistent with *in vitro*

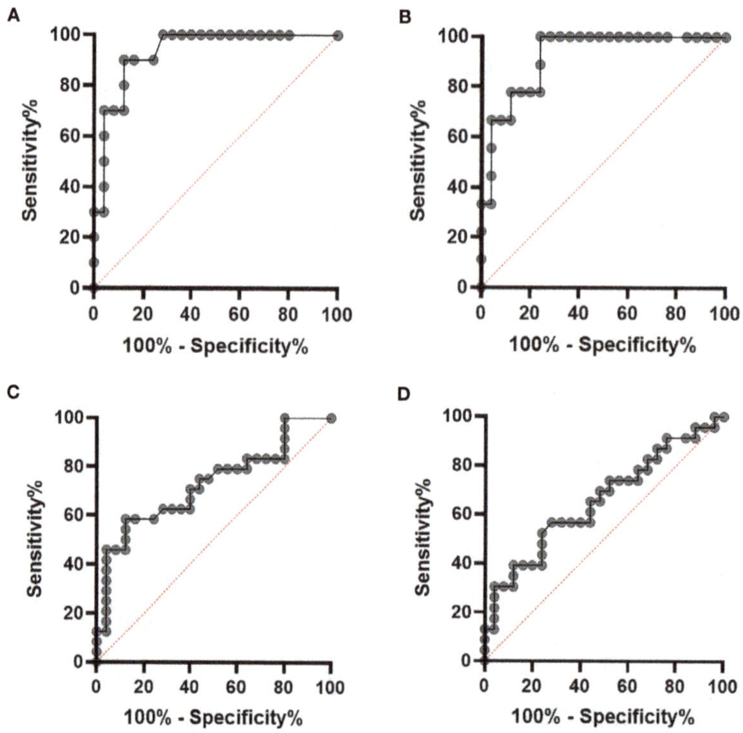

FIGURE 4 | pSTAT1 levels in monocytes distinguish patients with sHLH/MAS not treated with glucocorticoids at sampling from patients with active sJIA or with other rheumatic diseases. **(A, B)** receiver operating characteristic (ROC) curve of pSTAT1 levels in unstimulated **(A)** and IFNγ (10 ng/ml)–stimulated **(B)** monocytes distinguishing patients with sHLH/MAS not treated with glucocorticoids at sampling from patients with active sJIA or with other rheumatic diseases. **(C, D)** ROC curve of pSTAT1 levels in unstimulated **(C)** and IFNγ (10 ng/ml)–stimulated **(D)** monocytes distinguishing all patients with sHLH/MAS (not treated and treated with glucocorticoids at sampling) from patients with active sJIA or with other rheumatic diseases.

findings, demonstrating that in macrophages exposition to subthreshold concentrations of IFNγ increased their sensitivity to subsequent IFNγ stimulation, resulting in increased pSTAT1 and increased IFNγ–dependent gene expression (23). It is therefore conceivable that in patients with sHLH/MAS *in vivo* pre-exposure of monocytes to IFNγ (7) led to hyper-response to subsequent *ex vivo* IFNγ stimulation. Accordingly, we observed a correlation between *IFNG* mRNA expression levels in whole blood cells, circulating IFNγ levels and pSTAT1 levels in unstimulated and IFNγ-stimulated monocytes of sHLH/MAS patients. The exact mechanism involved in the hyper-responsiveness to IFNγ of monocytes from sHLH/MAS patients remains to be elucidated. Other cytokines or a particular inflammatory milieu may affect total STAT1 levels in patients with sHLH/MAS. For example, TNF has been demonstrated to induce sustained expression of STAT1 and IFN-response genes in monocytes and macrophages (24). Recently, a role for increased TRIM8 expression in enhancing macrophage responsiveness to IFNγ in patients with active sJIA and MAS has also been reported (25).

Our results demonstrating that the activation of the IFNγ–mediated signaling pathway in patients with active sJIA without MAS and in patients with sHLH/MAS in remission is comparable to that observed in patients with other rheumatologic diseases provide evidence of a normal response of monocytes to IFNγ in these conditions. These data are in agreement with previous results obtained by Sikora et al., demonstrating that monocytes of patients with active sJIA do not show a hyperresponsiveness to IFNγ stimulation (26). In this study, we showed that, during the active phase of sHLH/MAS, monocytes are more responsive to IFNγ stimulation. These results add new insights to the pathogenesis of sHLH, demonstrating that sHLH/MAS is not only characterized by increased production of IFNγ (7), but also by increased reactivity of monocytes to IFNγ stimulation.

The major limitation of this study is the small sample size, as the study was conducted at one hospital center only. This is mainly due to the need to use freshly isolated cells for the cytofluorimetric assay, as we found that cell cryopreservation affected pSTAT1 staining.

In summary, consistently with the activation of the IFNγ pathway, we report that pSTAT1 levels are increased in monocytes of patients with HLH/MAS. Given the major effect of glucocorticoid treatment, often required to stabilize patients, on *in vivo* pSTAT1 levels and the need for freshly isolated cells and the relatively sophisticated technique, pSTAT1 levels cannot be used in routine practice as a test to identify patients at early stages of HLH/MAS. The observed hyper-response to *ex vivo*

IFNγ stimulation suggests that both increased production of, and increased response to, IFNγ contribute to the amplification of hyperinflammation. Our results provide additional mechanistic support for the use of neutralizing IFNγ antibodies in the treatment of sHLH/MAS and, therefore, may have an impact on the justification of the dose of neutralizing antibody to be used.

ETHICS STATEMENT

The local Institutional Ethical Committee of Bambino Gesù Children's Hospital approved the study (number 1649/2018). Written informed consent to participate in this study was provided by the participants' legal guardian/next of kin.

AUTHOR CONTRIBUTIONS

GP, CB, and FDB conceived and designed the work. AP, IC, MNR, GMM, and VM performed the experiments. CB, AA, and MP enrolled patients and collected clinical data. GP and FDB wrote the manuscript. All authors contributed to the article and approved the submitted version.

REFERENCES

1. Risma KA, Marsh RA. Hemophagocytic Lymphohistiocytosis: Clinical Presentations and Diagnosis. *J Allergy Clin Immunol Practice* (2019) 7:824–32.
2. Griffin G, Shenoi S, Hughes GC. Hemophagocytic lymphohistiocytosis: An update on pathogenesis, diagnosis, and therapy. *Best Pract Res Clin Rheumatol* (2020) 34:101515.
3. Zoller EE, Lykens JE, Terrell CE, Aliberti J, Filipovich AH, Henson PM, et al. J Exp Med. *Hemophagocytosis Causes Consumptive Anemia Inflam* (2011) 208:1203–14.
4. Jordan MB, Hildeman D, Kappler J, Marrack P. An animal model of hemophagocytic lymphohistiocytosis (HLH): CD8+ T cells and interferon gamma are essential for the disorder. *Blood* (2004) 104:735–43.
5. Prencipe G, Caiello I, Pascarella A, Grom AA, Bracaglia C, Chatel L, et al. Neutralization of IFN-γ reverts clinical and laboratory features in a mouse model of macrophage activation syndrome. *J Allergy Clin Immunol* (2018) 141:1439–49.
6. Behrens EM, Canna SW, Slade K, Rao S, Kreiger PA, Paessler M, et al. Repeated TLR9 stimulation results in macrophage activation syndrome-like disease in mice. *J Clin Invest* (2011) 121:2264–77.
7. Bracaglia C, de Graaf K, Pires Marafon D, Guilhot F, Ferlin W, Prencipe G, et al. Elevated circulating levels of interferon-γ and interferon-γ-induced chemokines characterise patients with macrophage activation syndrome complicating systemic juvenile idiopathic arthritis. *Ann Rheum Dis* (2017) 76:166–72.
8. Schulert GS, Yasin S, Carey B, Chalk C, Do T, Schapiro AH, et al. Systemic juvenile idiopathic arthritis-associated lung disease: Characterization and risk factors. *Arthritis Rheumatol* (2019) 71:1943–54.
9. Prencipe G, Bracaglia C, Caiello I, Pascarella A, Francalanci P, Pardeo M, et al. The interferon-gamma pathway is selectively up-regulated in the liver of patients with secondary hemophagocytic lymphohistiocytosis. *PLoS One* (2019) 14:e0226043.
10. Takakura M, Shimizu M, Irabu H, Sakumura N, Inoue N, Mizuta M, et al. Comparison of serum biomarkers for the diagnosis of macrophage activation syndrome complicating systemic juvenile idiopathic arthritis. *Clin Immunol* (2019) 208:108252.
11. Locatelli F, Jordan MB, Allen C, Cesaro S, Rizzari C, Rao A, et al. Emapalumab in children with primary hemophagocytic lymphohistiocytosis. *N Engl J Med* (2020) 382:1811–22.
12. Gloude NJ, Dandoy CE, Davies SM, Myers KC, Jordan MB, Marsh RA, et al. Thinking Beyond HLH: Clinical Features of Patients with Concurrent Presentation of Hemophagocytic Lymphohistiocytosis and Thrombotic Microangiopathy. *J Clin Immunol* (2020) 40:699–707.
13. Gabr JB, Liu E, Mian S, Pillittere J, Bonilla E, Banki K, et al. Successful treatment of secondary macrophage activation syndrome with emapalumab in a patient with newly diagnosed adult-onset Still's disease: case report and review of the literature. *Ann Trans Med* (2020) 8:887.
14. Schoenborn JR, Wilson CB. Regulation of interferon-gamma during innate and adaptive immune responses. *Adv Immunol* (2007) 96:41–101.
15. Schroder K, Hertzog PJ, Ravasi T, Hume DA. Interferon-gamma: an overview of signals, mechanisms and functions. *J Leukoc Biol* (2004) 75:163–89.
16. Saha B, Jyothi Prasanna S, Chandrasekar B, Nandi D. Gene modulation and immunoregulatory roles of interferon gamma. *Cytokine* (2010) 50:1–14.
17. Petty RE, Southwood TR, Manners P, Baum J, Glass DN, Goldenberg J, et al. International League of Associations for Rheumatology classification of juvenile idiopathic arthritis: second revision, Edmonton, 2001. *J Rheumatol* (2004) 31:390–2.
18. Wallace CA, Ruperto N, Giannini E, Childhood A, Rheumatology Research APediatric Rheumatology International Trials O, et al. Preliminary criteria for clinical remission for select categories of juvenile idiopathic arthritis. *J Rheumatol* (2004) 31:2290–4.
19. Ravelli A, Minoia F, Davi S, Horne A, Bovis F, Pistorio A, et al. 2016 Classification Criteria for Macrophage Activation Syndrome Complicating Systemic Juvenile Idiopathic Arthritis: A European League Against Rheumatism/American College of Rheumatology/Paediatric Rheumatology International Trials Organisation Collaborative Initiative. *Ann Rheum Dis* (2016) 75:481–9. doi: 10.1136/annrheumdis-2015-208982
20. Henter JI, Horne A, Arico M, Egeler RM, Filipovich AH, Imashuku S, et al. HLH-2004: Diagnostic and therapeutic guidelines for hemophagocytic lymphohistiocytosis. *Pediatr Blood Cancer* (2007) 48:124–31.
21. De Benedetti F BP, Grom A, Quartier P, Schneider R, Antón J, Bracaglia C, et al. Interferon-gamma (IFN-γ) Neutralization with Emapalumab and Time to Response in Patients with Macrophage Activation Syndrome (MAS) Complicating Systemic Juvenile Idiopathic Arthritis (s-JIA) who failed High-Dose Glucocorticoids abstract. *Arthritis Rheumatol* (2019) 71(suppl 10):5229–30.
22. Hu X, Li WP, Meng C, Ivashkiv LB. Inhibition of IFN-gamma signaling by glucocorticoids. *J Immunol* (2003) 170:4833–9.
23. Hu X, Herrero C, Li WP, Antoniv TT, Falck-Pedersen E, Koch AE, et al. Sensitization of IFN-gamma Jak-STAT signaling during macrophage activation. *Nat Immunol* (2002) 3:859–66.
24. Yarilina A, Park-Min KH, Antoniv T, Hu X, Ivashkiv LB. TNF activates an IRF1-dependent autocrine loop leading to sustained expression of chemokines and STAT1-dependent type I interferon-response genes. *Nat Immunol* (2008) 9:378–87.
25. Schulert GS, Pickering AV, Do T, Dhakal S, Fall N, Schnell D, et al. Monocyte and bone marrow macrophage transcriptional phenotypes in systemic juvenile idiopathic arthritis reveal TRIM8 as a mediator of IFN-gamma hyper-responsiveness and risk for macrophage activation syndrome. *Ann Rheum Dis* (2020).
26. Sikora KA, Fall N, Thornton S, Grom AA. The limited role of interferon-gamma in systemic juvenile idiopathic arthritis cannot be explained by cellular hyporesponsiveness. *Arthritis Rheumatol* (2012) 64:3799–808.

Permissions

All chapters in this book were first published by Frontiers; hereby published with permission under the Creative Commons Attribution License or equivalent. Every chapter published in this book has been scrutinized by our experts. Their significance has been extensively debated. The topics covered herein carry significant findings which will fuel the growth of the discipline. They may even be implemented as practical applications or may be referred to as a beginning point for another development.

The contributors of this book come from diverse backgrounds, making this book a truly international effort. This book will bring forth new frontiers with its revolutionizing research information and detailed analysis of the nascent developments around the world.

We would like to thank all the contributing authors for lending their expertise to make the book truly unique. They have played a crucial role in the development of this book. Without their invaluable contributions this book wouldn't have been possible. They have made vital efforts to compile up to date information on the varied aspects of this subject to make this book a valuable addition to the collection of many professionals and students.

This book was conceptualized with the vision of imparting up-to-date information and advanced data in this field. To ensure the same, a matchless editorial board was set up. Every individual on the board went through rigorous rounds of assessment to prove their worth. After which they invested a large part of their time researching and compiling the most relevant data for our readers.

The editorial board has been involved in producing this book since its inception. They have spent rigorous hours researching and exploring the diverse topics which have resulted in the successful publishing of this book. They have passed on their knowledge of decades through this book. To expedite this challenging task, the publisher supported the team at every step. A small team of assistant editors was also appointed to further simplify the editing procedure and attain best results for the readers.

Apart from the editorial board, the designing team has also invested a significant amount of their time in understanding the subject and creating the most relevant covers. They scrutinized every image to scout for the most suitable representation of the subject and create an appropriate cover for the book.

The publishing team has been an ardent support to the editorial, designing and production team. Their endless efforts to recruit the best for this project, has resulted in the accomplishment of this book. They are a veteran in the field of academics and their pool of knowledge is as vast as their experience in printing. Their expertise and guidance has proved useful at every step. Their uncompromising quality standards have made this book an exceptional effort. Their encouragement from time to time has been an inspiration for everyone.

The publisher and the editorial board hope that this book will prove to be a valuable piece of knowledge for researchers, students, practitioners and scholars across the globe.

List of Contributors

Jose Manuel Sánchez-Maldonado, Antonio José Cabrera-Serrano, Ana Moñiz-Díez and Manuel Jurado
Genomic Oncology Area, Centre for Genomics and Oncological Research (GENYO), Parque tecnológico de la Salud (PTS) Granada, Granada, Spain
Hematology Depar.tment, Virgen de las Nieves University Hospital, Granada, Spain
Instituto de Investigación Biosanitaria (IBs) Granada, Granada, Spain

Rafael Cáliz
Genomic Oncology Area, Centre for Genomics and Oncological Research (GENYO), Parque tecnológico de la Salud (PTS) Granada, Granada, Spain
Instituto de Investigación Biosanitaria (IBs) Granada, Granada, Spain
Department of Rheumatology, Virgen de las Nieves University Hospital, Granada, Spain

Miguel Ángel López-Nevot
Instituto de Investigación Biosanitaria (IBs) Granada, Granada, Spain
Immunology Department, Virgen de las Nieves University Hospital, Granada, Spain

Helena Canhão
EpiDoC Unit, CEDOC, NOVA Medical School and National School of Public Health, Universidade Nova de Lisboa, Lisbon, Portugal
Comprehensive Health Research Center (CHRC), NOVA Medical School, Lisbon, Portugal

João E Fonseca
Rheumatology and Metabolic Bone Diseases Department, Hospital de Santa Maria, Centro Hospitalar Universitário Lisboa Norte (CHLN), Lisbon, Portugal
Rheumatology Research Unit, Instituto de Medicina Molecular, Faculty of Medicine, University of Lisbon, Lisbon Academic Medical Center, Lisbon, Portugal

Juan Sainz
Genomic Oncology Area, Centre for Genomics and Oncological Research (GENYO), Parque tecnológico de la Salud (PTS) Granada, Granada, Spain
Hematology Department, Virgen de las Nieves University Hospital, Granada, Spain
Instituto de Investigación Biosanitaria (IBs) Granada, Granada, Spain
Department of Biochemistry and Molecular Biology I, University of Granada, Granada, Spain

Rob Ter Horst
Department of Internal Medicine and Radboud Center for Infectious Diseases, Radboud University Nijmegen Medical Center, Nijmegen, Netherlands

Luca Quartuccio
Department of Medical Area, Clinic of Rheumatology, University of Udine, Udine, Italy

Signe B Sorensen
Molecular Diagnostic and Clinical Research Unit, IRSCenter Sonderjylland, University Hospital of Southern Jutland, Aabenraa, Denmark
Institute of Molecular Medicine, Faculty of Health Sciences, University of Southern Denmark, Odense, Denmark

Bente Glintborg and Merete L Hetland
The Danish Rheumatologic Biobank and Copenhagen Center for Arthritis Research (DANBIO) Registry The Danish Rheumatologic Biobank and Copenhagen Center for Arthritis Research (COPECARE), Center for Rheumatology and Spine Diseases, Centre of Head and Orthopaedics, Rigshospitalet, Glostrup, Denmark
Department of Clinical Medicine, Faculty of Health and Medical Sciences, University of Copenhagen, Copenhagen, Denmark

Ileana Filipescu
Rheumatology Department, University of Medicine and Pharmacy "Iuliu Hatieganu", Cluj-Napoca, Romania

Eva Pérez-Pampin
Rheumatology Unit, University Hospital of Santiago de Compostela, Santiago de Compostela, Spain

Pablo Conesa-Zamora
Clinical Analysis Department, Santa Lucía University Hospital, Cartagena, Spain

Jerzy Swierkot
Department of Rheumatology and Internal Medicine, Wroclaw Medical University, Wroclaw, Poland

Alfons A den Broeder
Radboud Institute for Health Sciences, Department of Rheumatology, Radboud University Medical Center, Nijmegen, Netherlands

Salvatore De Vita
Department of Medical Area, Clinic of Rheumatology, University of Udine, Udine, Italy

Eva Rabing Brix Petersen
Department of Biochemistry and Immunology, University Hospital of Southern Jutland, Aabenraa, Denmark

Yang Li
Department of Internal Medicine and Radboud Center for Infectious Diseases, Radboud University Nijmegen Medical Center, Nijmegen, Netherlands
Centre for Individualised Infection Medicine (CiiM) & Centre for Experimental and Clinical Infection Research (TWINCORE), Helmholtz-Centre for Infection Research (HZI) and The Hannover Medical School (MHH), Hannover, Germany

Miguel A Ferrer
Instituto de Investigación Biosanitaria (IBs) Granada, Granada, Spain

Alejandro Escudero and Eduardo Collantes
Rheumatology Department, Reina Sofía Hospital/ Instituto Maimónides de Investigación Biomédica de Córdoba (IMIBIC)/University of Córdoba, Córdoba, Spain

Mihai G Netea
Department of Internal Medicine and Radboud Center for Infectious Diseases, Radboud University Nijmegen Medical Center, Nijmegen, Netherlands
Department for Immunology & Metabolism, Life and Medical Sciences Institute (LIMES), University of Bonn, Bonn, Germany

Marieke J H Coenen
Radboud Institute for Health Sciences, Department of Human Genetics, Radboud University Medical Center, Nijmegen, Netherlands

Vibeke Andersen
Department of Medical Area, Clinic of Rheumatology, University of Udine, Udine, Italy
Molecular Diagnostic and Clinical Research Unit, IRSCenter Sonderjylland, University Hospital of Southern Jutland, Aabenraa, Denmark
Institute of Regional Research, Faculty of Health Sciences, University of Southern Denmark, Odense, Denmark

Katarzyna Bogunia-Kubik
Laboratory of Clinical Immunogenetics and Pharmacogenetics, Hirszfeld Institute of Immunology and Experimental Therapy, Polish Academy of Sciences, Wrocław, Poland

Yujie Cai, Renge Liang, Shibai Xiao, Qin Huang, Dingji Zhu, Qingqing Ouyang and Min Yang
Department of Rheumatology and Immunology, Nanfang Hospital, Southern Medical University, Guangzhou, China

Guo-Ping Shi
Department of Medicine, Brigham and Women's Hospital and Harvard Medical School, Boston, MA, United States

Hongjiang Liu
Department of Rheumatology and Immunology, Peking University People's Hospital & Beijing Key Laboratory for Rheumatism Mechanism and Immune Diagnosis (BZ0135), Beijing, China
Department of Rheumatology and Immunology, The People's Hospital of China Three Gorges University/ The First People's Hospital of Yichang, Yichang, China

Yundong Zou, Chen Chen, Yundi Tang and Jianping Guo
Department of Rheumatology and Immunology, Peking University People's Hospital & Beijing Key Laboratory for Rheumatism Mechanism and Immune Diagnosis (BZ0135), Beijing, China

Guillaume Larid and Pierre Lafforgue
Rhumatologie, Institut du Mouvement et de l'appareil Locomoteur (IML), Assistance Publique - Hôpitaux de Marseille (AP-HM), Marseille, France

Mikael Pancarte, Géraldine Offer, Cyril Clavel and Guy Serre
Université de Toulouse, INSERM, UMRs 1056, UDEAR, Hôpital Purpan, Toulouse, France

Marielle Martin and Isabelle Auger
Aix Marseille Université, INSERM UMRs 1097, Arthrites autoimmunes, Marseille, France

Vincent Pradel
CEIP de Marseille (PACA-Corse, Centre Associé), Laboratoire de Santé Publique, Faculté de Médecine, Marseille, France

Jean Roudier and Nathalie Balandraud
Rhumatologie, Institut du Mouvement et de l'appareil Locomoteur (IML), Assistance Publique - Hôpitaux de Marseille (AP-HM), Marseille, France
Aix Marseille Université, INSERM UMRs 1097, Arthrites autoimmunes, Marseille, France

Yunjuan Zhao
Department of Endocrinology, The Second Affiliated Hospital of Guangzhou Medical University, Guangzhou, China
Medical Inflammation Research, Department of Medical Biochemistry and Biophysics, Karolinska Institute, Stockholm, Sweden

Vilma Urbonaviciute, Bingze Xu, Weiwei Cai, Zeynep Sener, Changrong Ge and Rikard Holmdahl
Medical Inflammation Research, Department of Medical Biochemistry and Biophysics, Karolinska Institute, Stockholm, Sweden

Eric Toussirot
INSERM CIC-1431, Centre d'Investigation Clinique Biothérapie, Pôle Recherche, CHU de Besançon, Besançon, France
Fédération Hospitalo-Universitaire INCREASE, CHU de Besançon, Besançon, France
Rhumatologie, Pôle PACTE (Pathologies Aiguës Chroniques Transplantation Éducation), CHU de Besançon, Besançon, France
Département Universitaire de Thérapeutique, Université de Bourgogne Franche-Comté, Besançon, France
Univ. Bourgogne Franche-Comté, INSERM, EFS BFC, UMR1098, Interactions Hôte-Greffon-Tumeur/ Ingénierie Cellulaire et Génique, LabEx LipSTIC, Besançon, France

Francis Bonnefoy
Univ. Bourgogne Franche-Comté, INSERM, EFS BFC, UMR1098, Interactions Hôte-Greffon-Tumeur/ Ingénierie Cellulaire et Génique, LabEx LipSTIC, Besançon, France
MED'INN'Pharma, Besançon, France

Charline Vauchy
INSERM CIC-1431, Centre d'Investigation Clinique Biothérapie, Pôle Recherche, CHU de Besançon, Besançon, France
Univ. Bourgogne Franche-Comté, INSERM, EFS BFC, UMR1098, Interactions Hôte-Greffon-Tumeur/ Ingénierie Cellulaire et Génique, LabEx LipSTIC, Besançon, France

Sylvain Perruche
Fédération Hospitalo-Universitaire INCREASE, CHU de Besançon, Besançon, France
Univ. Bourgogne Franche-Comté, INSERM, EFS BFC, UMR1098, Interactions Hôte-Greffon-Tumeur/ Ingénierie Cellulaire et Génique, LabEx LipSTIC, Besançon, France
MED'INN'Pharma, Besançon, France

Philippe Saas
INSERM CIC-1431, Centre d'Investigation Clinique Biothérapie, Pôle Recherche, CHU de Besançon, Besançon, France
Fédération Hospitalo-Universitaire INCREASE, CHU de Besançon, Besançon, France
Univ. Bourgogne Franche-Comté, INSERM, EFS BFC, UMR1098, Interactions Hôte-Greffon-Tumeur/ Ingénierie Cellulaire et Génique, LabEx LipSTIC, Besançon, France

Iva Sorić Hosman
Department of Pediatrics, Zadar General Hospital, Zadar, Croatia

Ivanka Kos
Division of Nephrology, Dialysis and Transplantation, Department of Pediatrics, University Hospital Centre Zagreb, Zagreb, Croatia

Lovro Lamot
Division of Nephrology, Dialysis and Transplantation, Department of Pediatrics, University Hospital Centre Zagreb, Zagreb, Croatia
Department of Pediatrics, University of Zagreb School of Medicine, Zagreb, Croatia

Lan Yan, Mingge Liang, Tong Yang, Jinyu Ji and Goutham Sanker Jose Kumar Sreena
Medical College of China Three Gorges University, Yichang, China

Xiaoqiang Hou and Zhitao Feng
The Institute of Rheumatology, The First College of Clinical Medical Sciences, China Three Gorges University, Yichang, China

Meiqun Cao
Shenzhen Institute of Geriatrics, Shenzhen Second People's Hospital, The First Affiliated Hospital of Shenzhen University, Shenzhen, China

Milena Iwaszko, Joanna Wielińska and Monika Chaszczewska-Markowska
Laboratory of Clinical Immunogenetics and Pharmacogenetics, Hirszfeld Institute of Immunology and Experimental Therapy, Polish Academy of Sciences, Wrocław, Poland

Jerzy Świerkot, Renata Sokolik and Bartosz Bugaj
Department of Rheumatology and Internal Medicine, Wroclaw Medical University, Wrocław, Poland

Katarzyna Kolossa
Department of Rheumatology and Connective Tissue Diseases, Jan Biziel University Hospital No. 2, Bydgoszcz, Poland

Sławomir Jeka
Department of Rheumatology and Connective Tissue Diseases, Jan Biziel University Hospital No. 2, Bydgoszcz, Poland
Ludwik Rydygier Collegium Medicum in Bydgoszcz, Nicolaus Copernicus University, Toruń, Poland

Joel Jihwan Hwang
College of Public Health and Social Justice, Saint Louis University, St. Louis, MO, United States

Yoojun Nam
Catholic Induced Pluripotent Stem Cell Research Center, College of Medicine, The Catholic University of Korea, Seoul, South Korea

Jehan J. El-Jawhari and Yasser El-Sherbiny
Department of Biosciences, School of Science and Technology, Nottingham Trent University, Nottingham, United Kingdom
Department of Clinical Pathology, Faculty of Medicine, Mansoura University, Mansoura, Egypt

Dennis McGonagle and Elena Jones
Faculty of Medicine and Health, Leeds Institute of Rheumatic and Musculoskeletal Medicine, University of Leeds, Leeds, United Kingdom
The National Institute for Health Research Leeds Biomedical Research Centre, Chapel Allerton Hospital, Leeds, United Kingdom

Rei Nakano
Laboratory for Cellular Function Conversion Technology, RIKEN Center for Integrative Medical Sciences, Yokohama, Japan
Laboratory of Veterinary Radiology, Department of Veterinary Medicine, College of Bioresource Sciences, Nihon University, Fujisawa, Japan
Laboratory of Veterinary Biochemistry, Department of Veterinary Medicine, College of Bioresource Sciences, Nihon University, Fujisawa, Japan

Taku Kitanaka, Shinichi Namba, Nanako Kitanaka and Hiroshi Sugiya
Laboratory of Veterinary Radiology, Department of Veterinary Medicine, College of Bioresource Sciences, Nihon University, Fujisawa, Japan
Laboratory of Veterinary Biochemistry, Department of Veterinary Medicine, College of Bioresource Sciences, Nihon University, Fujisawa, Japan

Yoko Suwabe and Tomohiro Nakayama
Laboratory of Veterinary Radiology, Department of Veterinary Medicine, College of Bioresource Sciences, Nihon University, Fujisawa, Japan

Tadayoshi Konno
Laboratory of Veterinary Biochemistry, Department of Veterinary Medicine, College of Bioresource Sciences, Nihon University, Fujisawa, Japan

Jun Yamazaki
Laboratory of Veterinary Pharmacology, Department of Veterinary Medicine, College of Bioresource Sciences, Nihon University, Fujisawa, Japan

Matheus Braga, Fernanda Formaggi Lara-Armi and Janisleya Silva Ferreira Neves
Post Graduation Program in Biosciences and Physiopathology, Department of Clinical Analysis and Biomedicine, State University of Maringá, Paraná, Brazil

Marco Antônio Rocha-Loures
Rheumatology Division, Department of Medicine, State University of Maringá, Paraná, Brazil

Mariana de Souza Terron-Monich and Larissa Danielle Bahls-Pinto
Immunogenetics Laboratory, Department of Basic and Health Science, State University of Maringá, Paraná, Brazil

Quirino Alves de Lima Neto, Joana Maira Valentini Zacarias, Ana Maria Sell and Jeane Eliete Laguila Visentainer
Post Graduation Program in Biosciences and Physiopathology, Department of Clinical Analysis and Biomedicine, State University of Maringá, Paraná, Brazil
Immunogenetics Laboratory, Department of Basic and Health Science, State University of Maringá, Paraná, Brazil

Qi Huang and Wang-Dong Xu
Department of Evidence-Based Medicine, School of Public Health, Southwest Medical University, Luzhou, China

Lin-Chong Su
Department of Rheumatology and Immunology, Minda Hospital of Hubei Minzu University, Enshi, China

Xiao-Yan Liu
Department of Nutrition and Food Hygiene, School of Public Health, Southwest Medical University, Luzhou, China

An-Fang Huang
Department of Rheumatology and Immunology, Affiliated Hospital of Southwest Medical University, Luzhou, China

Myriam Martin, Rebecca Trattner and Anna M. Blom
Department of Translational Medicine, Section of Medical Protein Chemistry, Lund University, Malmö, Sweden
Region Skåne, Laboratory Medicine, Clinical Chemistry, Malmö, Sweden

Sara C. Nilsson
Department of Translational Medicine, Section of Medical Protein Chemistry, Lund University, Malmö, Sweden

Albin Björk
Department of Medicine, Division of Rheumatology, Karolinska Institutet, Stockholm, Sweden

Agneta Zickert and Iva Gunnarsson
Department of Medicine, Division of Rheumatology, Karolinska Institutet, Stockholm, Sweden
Rheumatology, Karolinska University Hospital, Stockholm, Sweden

Maria Luque-Tévar, Carlos Perez-Sanchez, Alejandra Ma Patiño-Trives, Nuria Barbarroja, Ivan Arias de la Rosa, Ma Carmen Abalos-Aguilera, Juan Antonio Marin-Sanz, Desiree Ruiz-Vilchez, Rafaela Ortega-Castro, Pilar Font, Clementina Lopez-Medina, Montserrat Romero-Gomez, M. Angeles Aguirre, Alejandro Escudero-Contreras, Eduardo Collantes-Estevez and Chary Lopez-Pedrera
Instituto Maimónides de Investigación Biomédica de Córdoba (IMIBIC), Hospital Reina Sofia, Universidad de Cordoba, Córdoba, Spain

Carlos Rodriguez-Escalera
Hospital Universitario de Jaen, Jaén, Spain

Jose Perez-Venegas, Ma Dolores Ruiz-Montesinos and Carmen Dominguez
Hospital Universitario Virgen Macarena, Sevilla, Spain

Carmen Romero-Barco
Hospital Clínico Universitario, Malaga, Spain

Antonio Fernandez-Nebro and Natalia Mena-Vazquez
Hospital Regional Universitario de Malaga, Malaga, Spain

Jose Luis Marenco and Julia Uceda-Montañez
Hospital Universitario Virgen de Valme, Sevilla, Spain

Mª Dolores Toledo-Coello
Hospital Universitario de Jerez de la Frontera, Cádiz, Spain

Guillaume Padern, Rosanna Ferreira, Said Assou, Christian Jorgensen and Yves-Marie Pers
IRMB, University of Montpellier, INSERM, CHU Montpellier, Montpellier, France

Claire Duflos and Maja Jurtela
Clinical Research and Epidemiology Unit, CHU Montpellier, Montpellier University, Montpellier, France

Philippe Guilpain and Alexandre Thibault Jacques Maria
IRMB, University of Montpellier, INSERM, CHU Montpellier, Montpellier, France
Internal Medicine and Multi-Organic Diseases Department, Hôpital Saint Éloi, CHU Montpellier, Montpellier, France

Radjiv Goulabchand
Internal Medicine Department, Caremeau University Hospital, Nîmes, France

Pascale Galea
BioRad Laboratory, Research and Development Department, Montpellier, France

Antonia Pascarella, Ivan Caiello, Gian Marco Moneta, Marianna Nicoletta Rossi, Valentina Matteo and Giusi Prencipe
Division of Rheumatology, IRCCS Ospedale Pediatrico Bambino Gesù, Rome, Italy

Claudia Bracaglia, Alessia Arduini, Manuela Pardeo and Fabrizio De Benedetti
Laboratory of Immuno-Rheumatology, IRCCS Ospedale Pediatrico Bambino Gesù, Rome, Italy

Index

www.ingramcontent.com/pod-product-compliance
Lightning Source LLC
LaVergne TN
LVHW082151200926
848484LV00008B/2141